Reading the Chest Radiograph
A Physiologic Approach

Reading the
Chest Radiograph

A Physiologic Approach

Eric N.C. Milne, MD, FRCR, FRCP (Ed)

Professor of Radiology and Medicine
Department of Radiologic Sciences
University of California, Irvine
Irvine, California

Massimo Pistolesi, MD

Associate Professor of Respiratory Pathophysiology
University of Pisa and
CNR Institute of Clinical Physiology
Pisa, Italy

*With **621** Illustrations and **2** Color Plates
with original illustrations by Eric N.C. Milne*

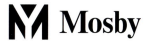

Mosby

St. Louis Baltimore Boston Chicago London Philadelphia Sydney Toronto

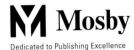
Mosby
Dedicated to Publishing Excellence

Publisher: George S. Stamathis
Editor: Anne S. Patterson
Developmental Editor: Maura K. Leib
Project Manager: Peggy Fagen
Book Designer: Susan Lane

Printed in the United States of America

Mosby–Year Book, Inc.
11830 Westline Industrial Drive
St. Louis, Missouri 63146

Library of Congress Cataloging in Publication Data

Milne, Eric N. C.
    Reading the chest radiograph : a physiologic approach / Eric N.C.
  Milne, Massimo Pistolesi.
        p.   cm.
    Includes bibliographical references and index.
    ISBN 0-8016-3303-6
    1. Chest—Radiography.   2. Chest—Pathophysiology.   I. Pistolesi,
  Massimo.   II. Title.
    [DNLM: 1. Lung Diseases—radiography.   WF 600 M659r]
  RC941.M55   1992
  617.5′407572—dc20
  DNLM/DLC   92-49492
    for Library of Congress   CIP

93 94 95 96 97 CL/MY 9 8 7 6 5 4 3 2 1

To those who taught us
> **Julius H. Comroe, Jr.**
> **Carlo Giuntini**
> **Leo G. Rigler**
> **Eric Samuel**
> **Morris Simon**
> **Robert E. Steiner**

and to the untamed and beautiful lands
which formed us
> **Scotland**
> *and*
> **Tuscany**

Preface

This book is the culmination of many years of radiologic, clinical, and physiologic observation that has led to the formulation and rigorous testing of several new hypotheses concerning radiologic/physiologic correlations. For anyone who needs to read chest films and would like to increase his or her ability to abstract functional data, this is a "how to do it" book. As such it should be of particular value to radiologists at all levels of training, from resident to chest expert. But this book does not simply contain information on how to abstract physiologic data from the chest radiograph; it also delves quite deeply into the physiologic and microanatomic changes underlying and causing the radiologic abnormalities from which the physiologic diagnoses can be made. Because of this, we believe the book will be of equal value to physiologists, pulmonologists, cardiologists, anesthesiologists, and critical care specialists. In fact, such readers may find that the unique ability of the chest radiograph to show chronologic changes in form occurring over hours, months, or years, in many thousands of live intact humans, permits the radiologic image to illuminate our knowledge of physiology even more than our physiologic knowledge illuminates our interpretation of the radiograph.

The book contains almost equal amounts of radiology and physiology, all of which is closely correlated. Some of the physiologic argumentation is painstaking and requires considerable concentration, but it is vital to establishing the validity of many of our radiologic/physiologic correlations and hypotheses. Where the argument might, by its complexity or length, interrupt the flow of logic—particularly for the reader primarily interested in the "how to do" rather than the "why it is so"—we have adapted the device of removing the more complex reasoning and analysis from the body of the chapter into an appendix at the end of that chapter. We hope the reader will find this an acceptable approach.

The book contains many new ideas and by design is often analytically critical of certain dogmas that we believe can be shown to be incorrect. In all cases where our views diverge from those presently accepted, we have tried to provide full documentation, argumentation, and often experimentation to support our views.

It is our hope that the reader—whether radiologist, physiologist, or clinician—will find this book of everyday practical value for interpreting the chest radiograph, but we also hope strongly that the book gives the reader a clearer understanding of some of the fundamental physiologic principles operating within the lung.

As with all attempts to codify old knowledge more accurately, to reclassify it more exactly, and to formulate new hypotheses and develop new knowledge, it is quite inevitable that time and new findings will show us to be wrong in some of our views. Unfortunately, we cannot foresee which ideas will stand and which will fall, but at least we can strongly encourage any reader who sees errors in our logic, or who has newer or more accurate information to offer, to write to us so that we can amend and incorporate this knowledge into our future thinking and writing.

Eric N.C. Milne
Massimo Pistolesi

Acknowledgments

We gratefully acknowledge the considerable assistance of Dr. Massimo Miniati, career investigator of the Italian National Research Council, in the clinical physiology laboratories at the University of Pisa, whose superb experimental and analytical skills contributed largely to the acquisition of the new physiologic data contained in this book.

The word processing and laying out of tables for this entire book has been carried out by Mrs. Elizabeth Trent, to whom we owe a deep debt of gratitude for the consistently superb quality of her work and for her unfailing dedication and support over many years.

Mr. James Ransome, our photographer, worked for many hours to expertly reproduce all of the detail we required in over 200 cases. He has been able to bring out better information in many intensive care unit radiographs than could be seen on the original. Our thanks go to Mr. Ransome for his consistently high standards and his willingness to persist with every case until the last possible detail has been reproduced.

Finally, we would like to thank Mrs. Kari Campbell Maloney for many years of loyal and cheerful assistance and, in particular, for her continued expertise in solving all of our logistic problems.

Contents

1 Reading the Chest Radiograph
The Value of Adding the Physiologic Approach

"Seeing" is based on the information content of the object, "perceiving" on the information content of the observer.

For generations the emphasis in radiologic training for the interpretation of chest films has been anatomic and pathologic, with relatively little regard for the physiologic alterations that either cause or stem from the change in anatomic form. The anatomic/pathologic approach (pattern recognition) remains the mainstay of radiologic interpretation, but it may fail to answer why a certain disease process should develop a particular pattern or may fail to provide information about the functional changes accompanying that pattern. The film reader with a knowledge of physiology is better able to determine why a particular pattern occurs and therefore to explain its functional significance. Physiologic knowledge may also permit the radiologist to deduce the meaning of variations from known patterns and even of patterns that have not been encountered before.

In the past much valid physiologic information provided by interpretation of the chest x-ray has gone unheeded because of a lack of belief in the radiologist's ability to derive such information. One of the reasons for this lack of confidence has been the widespread, simplistic view that it is not possible to abstract dynamic, quantitative data from a static radiograph. This incredulity barrier was first voiced to one of us many years ago by an eminent professor of physiology at a distinguished East Coast university. We were somewhat exercised in mind to find the best way to explain to him exactly how dynamic information *could* be derived from a static picture, until we hit upon the idea of showing him a picture of a large waterfall (Fig. 1-1) and asking him if the water was flowing. It was immediately obvious that the water *was* flowing and that there was no alternative answer—i.e., one was making a dynamic deduction from a static picture. Even if one suggested that the water was frozen, it clearly was not—from the evidence (also in the picture) of spray rebounding from the ground. There were, in addition, small human figures at the rim of the canyon that provided a scale from which the height, width, and (to a lesser extent) depth of the falls could be estimated. Since one knows the specific gravity of water, it would then become possible

to work out the amount of electricity that could be generated per hour. Clearly, dynamic quantitative information can be extracted from a static image, and the more knowledge we bring to our interpretation, the more information we can abstract from the image.

This relates to a second common criticism of the credibility of radiologic data—that radiographic interpretation is highly subjective. Phrases such as "guessing at shadows"[1] are not infrequently used to describe radiologic interpretation. However, we would argue that such statements demonstrate a considerable lack of understanding of the radiographic process. In the first place the film reader is observing, accumulating data, analyzing, and deducing (not "guessing"), and in the second place a radiograph is not a shadow. The word "shadow" implies that electromagnetic radiation has *not* been able to penetrate the object in question, whereas, for a radiologic image to be formed, radiation must pass through the object. The resultant image is not a "shadow" but is a complex, physically predictable summation of the passage of a polychromatic beam of x-rays through an object containing many areas of differing linear absorption coefficients, recorded on a film/screen combination with a nonlinear response to the intensity of light emitted from the surrounding intensifying screens by the nonabsorbed portion of the radiation. Although the nonlinearity of the system does preclude absolute densitometric measurements on plain films (a problem that has been largely overcome by computed tomography), this nonlinearity is well known and can be readily compensated for in interpretation.

If some error has occurred in the data-gathering process (e.g., under- or overexposure, partial rotation, inappropriate use of a grid, faulty development), it is immediately evident to a trained film reader. In such a case either an appropriate adjustment in interpretation is made or the film is retaken correctly (Fig. 1-2). This ability to recognize faulty data does not exist with any other type of medical data—i.e., the physician usually cannot know if the data being received, whether hemodynamic or biochemical, are true or have been affected by laboratory error (a frequent occurrence), such as a

1

Fig. 1-1   Human figures on the canyon rim *(arrow)* give an approximate scale, from which the height, width, and (less accurately) depth of the falls can be determined. From these data the quantity of electricity that could be generated per hour can be estimated.

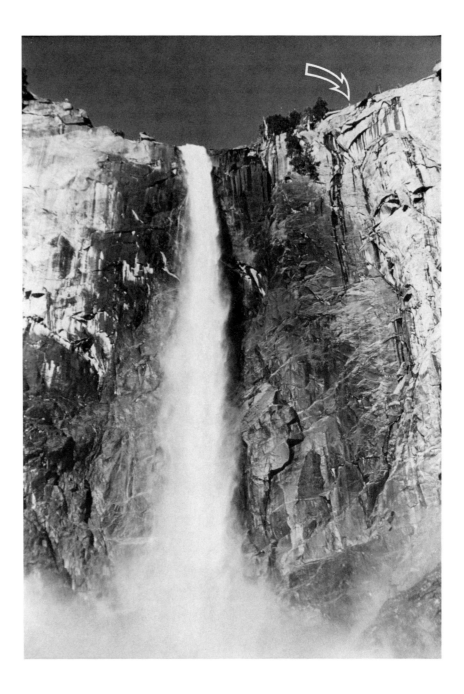

bubble or kink in a catheter, insensitivity of the recording system, or a drifting calibration. Many measurements, even when there is *no* technical fault, have such a wide range of accepted error that minor abnormalities are masked.[2] Without a priori knowledge of what numbers would be appropriate for that particular patient and disease, the clinician can only suspect that the data given are erroneous if they are at definite variance with an established preconception of what they should be. In contrast, every single radiograph provides the radiologist with an immediate check on the validity of the radiologic data, and in our view the information is therefore

"harder" than virtually any other type of medical data.

It is also still often stated that radiologic interpretation is an art rather than a science. While it is true that reading x-ray films does demand a perceptive ability that cannot always be taught, the same is true for the clinician's approach to numerical data. Some clinicians have an inherent ability to integrate and perceive the meaning of complex data—some do not and may not be able to acquire it. In the same way that radiologic visual data must be processed through the mind of the film-reader before a diagnosis or differential diagnosis can be made (i.e., making this a subjective process), so clin-

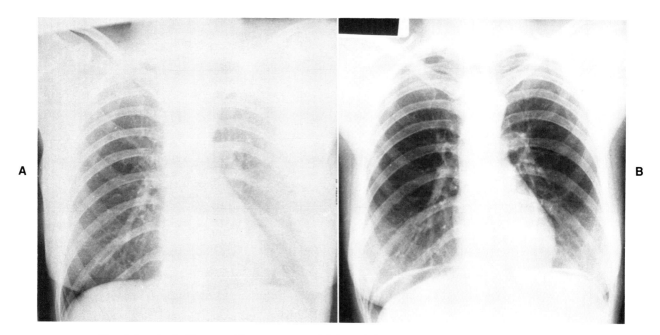

Fig. 1-2   A, A 45-year-old woman complaining of dyspnea and postoperative bilateral subscapular pain on inspiration. This supine AP film was initially interpreted as a probable pulmonary embolus. Blood gases (pH 7.44, Po_2 90, Pco_2 33) did not support this. NOTE: The right chest wall is much better penetrated than the left. The loss of rib visualization on the left clearly could not be caused by intrathoracic pathology, and yet there is no evidence of extrathoracic (chest wall) abnormality. (Bright-lighting showed that the right and left soft tissue thicknesses were the same.) The discrepancy in density is caused by faulty tube centering to the patient's right.   **B,** A repeat film 10 minutes later, made in the erect position and correctly centered, reveals the true cause of the patient's symptoms.

ical measurements must be processed through the mind of the clinician, making this process equally subjective. As discussed already, radiologic data are in themselves invariant or "hard"; the more the interpreter learns, the more "objective" the conclusions from these data will become. This ability with physiologic training to abstract increasing amounts of information from the same visual data is best illustrated by constructing a series of increasingly complex hypothetical diagnostic tasks and considering how well observers untrained in radiologic/physiologic correlation would do with exactly the same data compared first with a general radiologist and second with a radiologist specializing in chest radiology (Table 1-1).

A third reason for the belief that interpretation of chest radiographs is subjective is that the lung can react pathologically to an insult in only a few ways, so a wide spectrum of diseases may result in quite similar patterns. Such patterns (e.g., the honeycomb pattern of an end-stage lung or the pattern of fine interstitial nodulation) can fit the diagnosis of a score of different entities. Since these patterns are quite common and since different radiologists may give different sets of differential di-

agnoses for these patterns, it may appear that the reading must be very subjective. However, it would be more correct to say in these cases that the film simply does not contain enough information to make a diagnosis. It is note worthy that even direct lung biopsy in such cases has a low percentage of success in making a specific diagnosis, not because the histologic interpretation is "highly subjective" but because there are not sufficient data present.

In contrast to this difficulty in providing a specific diagnosis using pathologic/radiologic correlation, it is common in cases in which the problems are principally hemodynamic or physiologic to be able to provide a single diagnosis that is specific enough for the clinician to treat the patient without need for any further confirmatory investigation (Fig. 1-3). The more the film reader learns about the physiologic changes in these numerous cases, including cardiac failure, pulmonary hypertension, overhydration, renal failure, adult respiratory distress syndrome (ARDS), and chronic obstructive pulmonary disease (COPD), the more specific and accurate the diagnoses will become.

The physiologic approach to reading chest films that

Table 1-1 Predicted success in diagnostic interpretation of chest film by level of radiologic training

Diagnostic tasks (in increasing order of complexity)	Predicted success rate		
	Medical observer with no radiologic training (%)	Normally trained radiologist (%)	Trained chest radiologist (%)
To determine if there has been a total left pneumonectomy	100	100	100
To determine if there is right middle lobe consolidation	50	98	100
To determine if right middle lobe actelectasis is present	20	90	100
To detect moderately severe interstitial pulmonary edema	5	90	100
To detect moderate interstitial pulmonary edema	—	90	100
To detect minimal interstitial pulmonary edema	—	60	95
To detect moderate emphysema	—	60	95
To detect minimal emphysema	—	20	80

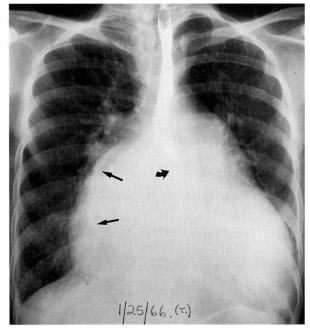

Fig. 1-3 A 40-year-old man with a massive left atrium manifested by a deviated barium column *(curved arrow),* calcification *(straight arrows),* and elevated left main bronchus. This, plus the very large main pulmonary artery, small aorta, inversion of flow, and biventricular enlargement, give the diagnosis of mitral regurgitation with pulmonary arterial and venous hypertension. Peribronchial cuffing, small effusion, and faint septal lines indicate that left-sided heart failure is present. At this stage no further investigation is necessary to institute medical treatment. (NOTE: The distinctive large lung volumes are very common in chronic mitral valve disease but much less so in chronic left-sided heart failure caused by coronary artery disease.)

we espouse is certainly not new, one of the most fundamental observations having been made in 1927 by Bjure and Laurell, who noted that in the erect position, blood, under the influence of gravity, occupied predominantly the lower zones of the lung and that the apices were devoid of blood, causing what they called "orthostatic apical anemia."[3] Bjure and Laurell also pointed out that in cows and horses it was the dorsum of the lungs that was anemic and in bats (hanging upside down) it was the bases of the lungs—and that these were precisely the areas in which these animals developed tuberculosis! It is salutary to remember that literally millions of chest films had been interpreted by a myriad of observers—many very skillful and thoughtful—prior to this observation and yet this obvious (once shown) gravitational distribution of blood flow had not been "perceived" before. Since that time many other equally "obvious" observations have been made, always prompting the query, "Now, why didn't I see that before?" and the comment, "Now that it has been pointed out to me, it seems quite obvious." It is certain, though it is always difficult to believe, that many more such fundamental observations remain to be made from the gold mine of the plain chest films that so many people seem to believe were worked out many years ago.

In 1959 Leo Rigler, revered as the greatest American chest radiologist, gave the Caldwell Lecture at the 59th Meeting of the American Roentgen Ray Society and entitled it "Functional Roentgen Diagnosis: Anatomical Image, Physiologic Interpretation."[4] At the end of this masterly paper he concluded: "For the younger generation there is here a challenge: The study of the Roentgenogram in terms of physiology, in terms of a living process. There is a great opportunity to use initiative, energy, and imagination to investigate the further possibilities, the still undiscovered potentialities in the interpretation of simple Roentgenograms."

Dr. Rigler's exhortation to his audience did not result in any stampede to the laboratory benches, partly because there has been little or no emphasis during radiologic training, or even in radiologic fellowships, on the importance of being able to recognize a research problem and to design and carry through appropriate experiments to solve the problem. However, over the years since Rigler gave this paper, one or two groups of investigators have been working steadily and consistently on the types of problems he described, and a new body of work concerning the correlation between radiologic cardiopulmonary changes and physiologic changes has been developed.

Unfortunately for the radiologic profession, much of this knowledge has been published in nonradiologic journals and presented at physiologic, cardiac, and critical care meetings. It has therefore been taken up not so much by radiologists but by cardiac, pulmonary, and critical care specialists. These nonradiologically trained physicians, presumably because of their training in physiology, presently appear better able than radiologists to weigh and appreciate the value of these new findings. In addition, with the advent of computed tomography (CT), nonradiologic physicians have become much more willing to accept the fact that accurate information about function can be derived from a radiologic image. Their familiarity with numerical data in their own specialties and the digital nature of CT make them more comfortable in accepting that valid quantitative data can be obtained from an image. This increasing willingness to use images to derive dynamic quantitative information has fortunately spilled over into a belated acceptance of the value of plain films for the same purpose.

The physiologic approach to interpretation has been taken back from meeting rooms to universities, hospitals, and practices and is creating increasing pressure on both radiologists and nonradiologists to acquire new interpretive skills. Unfortunately, this pressure is occurring at a time when trainee radiologists are being asked to spend more and more time on ever-expanding technical procedures such as CT, ultrasound, nuclear medicine, and magnetic resonance imaging (MRI) and are actually learning less about chest film interpretation than ever before. This is particularly regrettable since, although CT and MRI are invaluable problem-solvers, the problems they solve are almost invariably derived from prior interpretation of the plain chest film. Plain chest radiography remains the primary imaging technique for over 98% of chest diagnoses in the United States and for an even higher percentage in other countries, being of cardinal importance in critical care units and trauma centers.

Those diseases that cause the greatest morbidity and mortality—bronchitis, emphysema, cardiac decompensation, and combinations of all of these—are also the most common diseases for which chest x-rays are taken. A conservative estimate would suggest that over 35 million films per year are taken in the United States for this particular group of diseases, all of which require physiologic knowledge for their proper interpretation.

If the physiologic approach is so useful, why then is it not already in general use by the majority of radiologists? To understand this we must look back to the 1940s and early 1950s at which time a great deal of material was being published by radiologists and radiologic/clinical teams about the correlations between radiologic and hemodynamic/physiologic changes. At that time radiologists had developed a good deal of confidence in their ability to judge pulmonary vascular pressures and flows from chest radiographs.[5-11] Then some criticisms of the accuracy of the criteria on which these assessments were based began to be published. Unfortunately, since research methodology and experimental design have never been a part of radiologic training, the radiologic profession's response to the publication of these criticisms was not to try and find out why the anomalies existed (and therefore be able to factor them correctly into the diagnosis) but, regrettably, to lower their own confidence in their abilities to abstract hemodynamic data from radiographs. Even though they had produced some excellent work, most radiologists ceased publishing on these topics and even became somewhat apologetic for ever suggesting that the radiograph was a good source of hemodynamic data. One or two investigators did, however, continue to work consistently on the problems of pulmonary and cardiac radiologic/physiologic correlation. The results of their work, showing that good hemodynamic data could be abstracted (noninterventionally) from a plain chest film, began to intrigue several groups of investigative physiologists and experimental pathologists, and excellent hard physiologic/hemodynamic experimental data have now been developed that strongly support the fact that clinically valuable physiologic data can be derived from plain chest films.[2,12]

While all this step-by-step radiologic/physiologic correlation has been going on over the years, most of the radiologic community (certainly in the United States) has been looking the other way, at technologies that glittered a good deal more than the plain chest film (e.g., CT, ultrasound, and MRI). Radiologists in general have not yet turned their attention to the fact that they can now resume their former confidence in their physiologic diagnostic abilities. The pendulum has swung over to the realization that radiologic data are sound and that the nonradiologic test methods used initially to throw doubt on the radiologic conclusions were themselves often in error. A particularly good example of this inaccuracy of the "gold" standard involves the use of thermodilution techniques to determine whether pulmonary edema is present. The accuracy of plain film radiologic quantitation of pulmonary edema was questioned extensively, on the basis that the results did not correlate well with those of thermodilution studies made in the same patients,[13,14] the assumption being that it was the radiographic estimate that was in error. However, careful examination of these critical studies[15] revealed that it was the thermodilution method itself that was in error.[16,17] The thermodilution technique has now been shown to be inaccurate when abnormal pulmonary blood flow distribution exists,[12] and the chest radiograph is now becoming accepted as the gold standard for determining the presence and quantity of edema.[18]

A classic example of the way in which prior problems concerning the accuracy of radiologic/physiologic correlation have been solved is provided by the estimation of left atrial pressure (LAP) from the chest radiograph. All of the initial work on pressure estimation was carried out in patients with mitral valve disease, and all authors obtained very good results—correlations on the order of 0.85 being obtained between LAP estimations by x-ray and those by cardiac catheterization.[5,7,8,11] However, when cases of chronic left-sided heart failure were then analyzed using the same criteria (developed for mitral stenosis) for estimating pressure, the results became less accurate; when acute left-sided heart failure cases were also added, accuracy became unacceptably low. Despite the change in case material, there had been no change in the *criteria* used to estimate LAP. The use of the radiograph for estimating LAP thus fell into disrepute.

A number of years later critical care units and trauma centers began to assume great importance, and interest redeveloped in the possibility of deriving physiologic data from the chest radiograph "noninterventionally." However, when investigators tried to assess LAP in critical care unit patients using the previously published radiologic criteria, the level of accuracy was even lower than in prior papers. The reason for this is quite simple. If one includes a *mixture* of patients—some with edema from injury (capillary permeability) (in which the LAP is usually normal), some with renal failure and overhydration (in which case the LAP is usually only slightly elevated), and some with both acute and chronic cardiac failure (in which the LAP is usually high but distribution of blood flow varies depending upon whether organic or functional changes are present) and then applies to this heterogeneous mixture the radiologic criteria that were initially developed for estimating LAP in mitral stenosis, the result will of course be a very low level of accuracy. However, if the film reader learns to distinguish from the plain film what *type* of

edema is present (a skill to be taught later in this book), current newly developed criteria for each edema type can then be applied and the results of LAP estimation will again become accurate and of clinical value[11] (Figs. 1-2 and 1-4).

So many of the questions that previously raised doubts as to the accuracy of physiologic interpretation have now been answered that it is appropriate and indeed essential that film interpreters incorporate this knowledge into their daily reading of chest films.

The ability to think and talk in sophisticated physiologic terms is an essential way of improving that communication between the radiologist and the referring clinician so vital to the accuracy of diagnosis and to the rapid transfer of radiologic information for immediate incorporation into the treatment of patients. The information that the film reader derives from the radiograph *must* be iterated immediately with the data available from the referring physician, to allow its full value to be abstracted.[2]

Let us look at an example of the importance of this iteration. A clinician in the burn unit is having prob-

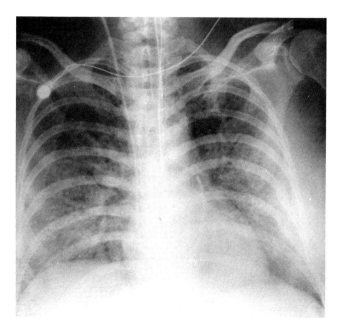

Fig. 1-4 A 30-year-old man in septic shock. The radiographic signs on the AP erect chest film are classic for injury edema—a normal vascular pedicle, normal pulmonary blood volume, air bronchograms, no effusions, and little evidence of peribronchial cuffing despite the severity of the edema. With this type of edema the left atrial pressure should be normal, but the Swan-Ganz catheter reading was 30 mm Hg and the patient was about to undergo diuresis for presumed cardiac failure. In view of the radiologic findings the catheterization data were checked and found to be erroneous (calibration error). As a result potentially fatal diuresis was not instituted.

lems resuscitating a patient with a 60% second- and third-degree surface area burn. He has taken a chest radiograph and is consulting with the radiologist. The radiologist points out that the patient's soft tissues are increasing in thickness while the systemic blood volume (manifested by a narrower vascular pedicle [see Chapter 4]) is actually less than on the previous day (Fig. 1-5). When this is integrated with the clinician's information that the patient is 8 L of fluid ahead but remains hypotensive, it becomes clear that the patient is "third-spacing" more rapidly into the burned tissues than the rate of fluid replacement and that the circulating blood volume is actually progressively *diminishing.*

The message is clear: the film reader must be able to speak and understand physiologic language very well to be able to deduce correctly from the radiograph what is happening to the patient and, in turn, to communicate these deductions to the person who is looking after the patient.

Physiologic knowledge also increases the radiologist's level of credibility and puts him or her in a much better position to argue the validity and importance of radiologic findings, particularly when these appear to be at variance with the clinical data.

Virtually all training departments of radiology have weekly or daily rounds wherein residents and fellows present radiology/pathology conferences, but it is quite

rare to have a radiology/*physiology* conference unless it is within the deparments of cardiology or pulmonary medicine. In many centers, almost certainly because of the radiologist's lack of specific training in physiology, cardiologists and pulmonologists prefer to interpret the films of their own patients. One would imagine that their extensive knowledge of cardiac or pulmonary physiology would result in a high level of diagnostic accuracy in their interpretations; unfortunately, the cardiologist has not usually been specifically trained in either radiodiagnosis or pulmonary physiology and may regard the lungs as more or less an impediment between the right and left sides of the heart, while the pulmonologist may similarly regard the heart as merely an impediment between the lungs. In both specialties extensive knowledge of the patient's *clinical* findings results in an almost irresistible tendency for physicians to read into the films what they think would fit their clinical understanding of the laboratory data—a dangerous approach! To eliminate this seductive and often misleading bias, it is our established practice to interpret films initially with no knowledge of the patient, apart from age and sex. Clinical information is brought into consideration only *after* we have analyzed the films and formulated a preliminary opinion. Similarly, when we consult on a problem case, we ask for the clinical information to be withheld initially (often to the distress

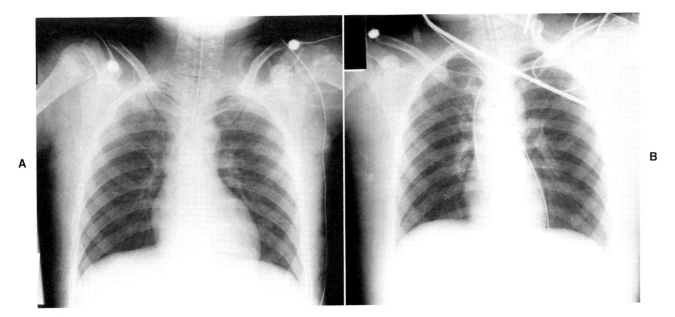

A   B

Fig. 1-5   A, A 30-year-old man with a severe burn of both chest walls (note the abnormal texture and the irregularity and thickness of chest wall tissues). The patient is hypotensive.   **B,** The following day the patient remains hypotensive despite being 8 L of fluid "ahead." The reduced vascular pedicle width and cardiac volume are incontrovertible evidence of actual *loss* of intravascular fluid since the previous day. The gross increase in thickness of the soft tissues of the chest wall shows that the patient is "third-spacing," explaining the persistent state of shock.

of the referring physician), until we have studied the films. Quite frequently a single diagnosis can be made from the films alone, but often several diagnoses fit the radiologic findings equally well and it is at this point that we request the clinical information and indeed may ask for further information concerning pressure measurements, state of hydration, etc. to narrow down the diagnosis. Without a balanced knowledge of pulmonary and cardiac physiology and specific training in diagnostic radiology—which has its own particular knowledge base, part technical, part anatomic, part perceptual—the chest film cannot be interpreted properly and without bias.

It is in no way the intent of this book to suggest that the physiologic approach to reading chest films should or could replace the traditional anatomic/pathologic approach. However, in a large number of cardiac and pulmonary cases the physiologic approach *will* be the primary one; and in *all* cases, since it is the physiologic effects of the anatomic alterations that produce symptomatology and dictate the severity of the disease, physiologic knowledge should be an integral part of the radiologic interpretation. We believe that physicians who learn to use the physiologic approach will find that they have made a major gain in their diagnostic capabilities, whether they are interpreting plain films, computed tomograms, or magnetic resonance images of the lungs. In fact, the advent of new imaging techniques (e.g., MRI flow studies) has made it increasingly necessary to understand the underlying physiology of the disease process being studied and to factor this into the diagnosis.

REFERENCES

1. Staub NC: Only the shadow knows (editorial), *AJR* 144:1086, 1985.
2. Milne ENC: A physiological approach to reading critical care unit films, *J Thorac Imag* 1(3):60, 1986.
3. Bjure A, Laurell H: Abnormal static circulatory phenomena and their symptoms; arterial orthostatic anemia as neglected clinical picture, *Ups Lakaref Forh* 33:1, 1927.
4. Rigler LG: Functional Roentgen diagnosis: anatomical image, physiologic interpretation. Caldwell Lecture, 59th Annual Meeting, American Roentgen Ray Society, *AJR* 82:1, 1959.
5. Davies G, Goodwin JF, Steiner RE, Van Leuven BD: Clinical and radiological assessment of pulmonary arterial pressure in mitral stenosis, *Br Heart J* 15:393, 1953.
6. Fleming PR, Simon M: The hemodynamic significance of intrapulmonary septal lymphatic lines (lines B of Kerley), *J Fac Radiologists* 9:33, 1958.
7. Kerley P: Lung changes in acquired heart disease, *AJR* 80:256, 1958.
8. Milne ENC: Physiological interpretation of the plain film in mitral stenosis including a review of criteria for the estimation of pulmonary arterial and venous pressures, *Br J Radiol* 36:902, 1963.
9. Simon M: The pulmonary veins in mitral stenosis, *J Fac Radiol* 9:25, 1958.
10. Steinbach HL, Keats TE, Sheline AE: The Roentgen appearance of the pulmonary veins in heart disease, *Radiology* 65:157, 1955.
11. Milne ENC, Carlssen E: Physiological interpretation of the plain radiograph following mitral valvotomy and prosthetic replacement, *Radiology* 92:1201, 1966.
12. Miniati M, Pistolesi M, Milne ENC, Giuntini C: Detection of lung edema, *Crit Care Med* 15(12):1146, 1987.
13. Baudendistel L, Shields JB, Kaminski DL: Comparison of double indicator thermodilution measurements of extravascular lung water (EVLW) with radiographic estimation of lung water in trauma patients, *J Trauma* 22:983:1982.
14. Sibbald WJ, Cunningham DR, Chin DN: Non-cardiac or cardiac pulmonary edema? A practical approach to clinical differentiation in critically ill patients, *Chest* 84:452, 1983.
15. Grover M, Slutsky RA, Higgins CB, Shabratai R: Extravascular lung water in patients with congestive heart failure, *Radiology* 147:659, 1983.
16. Carlile PV, Gray BA: Type of lung injury influences the thermal dye estimation of extravascular lung water, *J Appl Physiol* 51:680, 1984.
17. Oppenheimer L, Elings VB, Lewis FR: Thermal dye lung water measurements: effects of edema and embolisation, *J Surg Res* 26:504, 1979.
18. Staub NC: Clinical use of lung water measurements. Report of a workshop, *Chest* 90:588, 1986.

2 Radiologic Appearances of Pulmonary Edema
Anatomic and physiologic basis

It might appear at first that the ultrastructure of the lung as shown by electron microscopy, with its resolution measurable in angstroms, is far removed from our analyses of chest radiographs, with their crude resolution of 3 to 4 line pairs per millimeter (more than a million times larger than the structures seen with the electron microscope). But knowing how the ultrastructural architecture of the lung influences the amount and direction of water flow within the lung, and what happens to this flow when ultrastructure is deformed or destroyed, allows the film-reader to extrapolate backward, from the gross changes seen on chest radiographs to what is happening at the ultrastructural level, and thereby to assist the referring clinician materially in deciding upon the correct therapy.

APPLIED ANATOMY OF GAS EXCHANGE AND FLUID FORMATION

Atmospheric gases enter the lung via a single large cartilage-supported, thick-walled bronchus that termi-nates, after 23 divisions, into 300 million to 500 million exquisitely thin-walled air sacs approximately 250 μm in diameter, with a surface area for gas exchange (per lung) the size of a tennis court (75 m^2).[1] A single large pulmonary artery carrying hypoxic blood to each lung for reoxygenation accompanies the bronchus and divides approximately 28 times to terminate by forming a vast network of capillaries, some 8 to 10 μm in diameter, ramifying over the surfaces of the alveoli and containing a volume (per lung) of only 90 to 120 ml of blood, but again having a huge surface area (closely matching the inner alveolar surface area of approximately 70 m^2).

Alveolar/Capillary Interface

The basement membrane of the endothelial wall of a capillary facing the alveolus is actually fused with the basement membrane of the alveolar epithelium (Fig. 2-1). By contrast, the capillary wall facing away from the alveolar wall is separated from the neighboring alveolus (forming the opposite wall of the intraalveolar septum) by interstitial space (Fig. 2-2). Where the capillary wall is fused with the alveolus, no interstitial space exists and gas can pass very easily in either direction, between alveolus and capillary, across only two thin fused basement membranes. This structural arrangement of the alveolocapillary interface is called the "thin" side, in contrast to the opposite side of the capillary (facing the interstitial space), where capillary endothelium, interstitial space and its contents, and alveolar epithelium all intervene between the alveolar and capillary lumina and must be traversed by gas passing from alveolus to capillary. This is called the "thick" side of the alveolocapillary interface, and on this side fluid, both normal and abnormal, can accumulate (Figs. 2-1 and 2-2).

Because water cannot accumulate on the thin side, gas exchange continues efficiently even when interstitial edema is present.* To facilitate gas exchange still further, the capillaries fused to the alveolar wall actually bulge into the lumen of the alveolus, looking rather like air conditioning ducts hanging from a ceiling,

*See footnote on p.10.

Fig. 2-1 Normal human lung, septum between two alveoli *(A)*. The alveolus in the *lower* half of the diaphragm is separated from the capillary *(C)* by only the fused basement membranes *(double arrow)* of the alveolar epithelium *(Bep)* and the capillary endothelium *(Ben)*, the "thin" side of the alveolocapillary membrane. The alveolus in the upper half is separated from the capillary *(L)* by the (1) lining layer (remnant of surfactant) of the alveolus, (2) alveolar epithelium (cell nucleus and prolongation, *Ep 1)*, (3) interstitial space filled with fibroblasts *(F)*, fibrils *(f)*, and small pools of free liquid (*), and (4) capillary endothelium *(En)*, forming the "thick" side of the septum. Endothelial cell junctions *(J)* are frequent and "loose" in structure. Epithelial cell junctions *(Jep)* are less frequent and are "tight." (Reprinted from Bachofen H, Bachofen M, Weibel ER: *J Thorac Imaging* 3[3]:1, 1988.)

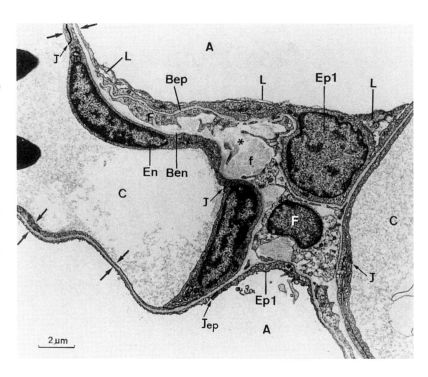

which further markedly increases the surface available for gas exchange, giving a huge surface area, which by its structure is protected from the development of interstitial edema.

To ensure the relative dryness of the alveoli, the epithelial cells that form the walls of the alveoli are fastened together at their periphery by junctions that are impermeable to water and solutes and are called "tight" junctions (Fig. 2-2). In contrast to this, the endothelial cells that form the walls of the capillaries have junctions that are much wider and are therefore more permeable to water and solutes, so-called "loose" junctions (Fig. 2-2). This arrangement means that water and solutes

passing out of the capillaries, largely via the loose endothelial cell junctions, under the effect of intra- and extraluminal hydrostatic and oncotic forces (Starling forces), will pass freely into the thick side of the interstitial space but will then be prevented from passing into the alveoli by the tight interepithelial cell junctions.*

Some authors have visualized this normal very slow movement of fluid from the capillary lumen into the interalveolar septa as "dripping" and have called the junctional portions of the interstitial space "drip channels."[4] (This term, while certainly evocative of a slow leaking of fluid, is not entirely satisfactory since drips can form only where fluid passes into either a gaseous medium or a vacuum.)

It is important to be aware that the intercellular junc-

---

*This is why patients with pure interstitial edema, even when severe, have relatively little disturbance in gas exchange. The difference in functional impairment between severe interstitial edema in a patient with renal failure or overhydration and that in a patient with cardiac failure is very great. But the difference has nothing to do with the quantity of edema—it has to do with the underlying causative disease. For example, in renal failure the heart is *not* usually abnormal; in fact, cardiac output is supernormal and can increase still further if the patient is put on a treadmill.[2] Although there may be a small reduction in oxygenation, there is still plenty of blood—due to the increased circulating volume and the large cardiac output—to carry oxygen to the tissues. Patients with renal failure and quite severe interstitial edema will often walk into the department without any evidence of dyspnea and have their films taken standing erect. This is so striking that, if one sees a chest film with severe interstitial edema made with the patient standing, it is virtually certain the diagnosis is going to be renal/overhydration, not cardiac. With the same amount of edema the cardiac patient would be in the critical care unit because of the low cardiac output, which would make it impossible to carry sufficient oxygen to the tissues.

*Although the presence of loose endothelial cell junctions certainly provides a reasonable explanation as to how water and solutes pass from the capillaries to the interstitial space and vice versa, under the influence of altered hydrostatic pressure it is doubtful that this is the only mechanism operating; i.e., the endothelial cytoplasm contains vast numbers of vesicles that do appear to play a role in water transport but whose function is not yet clearly explained. Similarly, clusters of water molecules appear to exchange freely across the capillary endothelium, unaffected by Starling factors,[3] with no change in the actual quantity of fluid on each side of the membrane. We would caution, therefore, that explanations of hydrostatic water flow based only on the presence of "holes" caused by the cell junctions may later have to be modified. Similarly, when endothelial cell junctions are opened so wide that proteins can pass through freely, the role of the oncotic factors in the Starling equation becomes difficult to assess and may be dependent upon the length and area of intact endothelium intervening between successive open cell junctions.

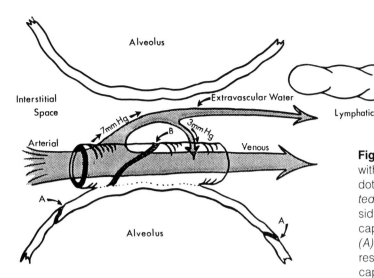

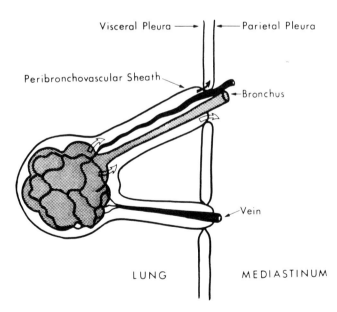

Fig. 2-2 Interstitial space between two alveoli (compare with Fig. 2-1). The basement membrane of the capillary endothelium is fused with that of the alveolar epithelium *(dotted line)* on one side only (the "thin" side). On the nonfused side much more tissue intervenes between alveolus and capillary (the "thick" side). Alveolar epithelial cell junctions *(A)* are tight and endothelial cell junctions *(B)* loose. The result of the various Starling forces operating on the capillaries is that fluid transudes out of the arterial end of the capillary (approximate transmural pressure +7.0 mm Hg) and is partially reabsorbed (transmural pressure −3 mm Hg) at the venous end of the capillary. The continual excess water formed flows toward the lymphatics where it is picked up and removed. (NOTE: In this diagram water is shown passing across the endothelium but, as discussed more fully in the text and appendix, water flow may take place primarily—or completely—at the cell *junctions.*) (See also Fig. 2-5.)

tions in the capillaries are closed by minute interdigitating projections, like a Velcro fastener, and can be pulled apart widely by increased intravascular pressure, only to come together again without apparent damage when the pressure drops. The cellular junctions at the venular end of the alveolar capillary are even looser than those at the arterial end.[5]

Anatomy of the Interstitial Space

As the bronchi and accompanying pulmonary artery enter the lung, they are enveloped by a sheath of tissue (the peribronchovascular sheath) that matches the bifurcations of the bronchi and vessels from the hilum out to the periphery of the lung until it merges with the interalveolar septal spaces, which in turn are continuous with the subpleural space. A continuous space therefore exists, extending from the inner visceral pleural surface to the hilum of the lung, forming a pathway along which liquid and solutes (provided they are not viscous) can move more or less freely, through the contents of this space from the outermost portions of the lung, to the hilum.

Centrally, where the hilar structures emerge from the lung into the mediastinum, the peribronchovascular sheath is sealed at the mediastinal pleural surface[6] (Fig. 2-3). It has been suggested by some authors[7] that the peribronchovascular sheaths, and therefore the interstitium of the lung, are open to the mediastinum and that clearance of liquid through this opening into the mediastinum could be an important route for removal of edema. This view is in contrast to several anatomic and clinical observations[6,8]:

First, when air is injected into the mediastinum, it does not dissect into the lungs to cause interstitial emphysema (as one would expect if the sheath were open) but causes pneumothoraces instead.[9]

Fig. 2-3 Bronchus and artery entering the lung, ramifying to form capillaries surrounding an alveolus and draining via the pulmonary vein through the mediastinal surface of the lung. The peribronchovascular sheath surrounding the bronchi and vessels is *fused* to the pleura at the mediastinal surface. Fluid (or air) entering the peribronchovascular sheath cannot pass into the pleura *(black arrow)* or into the mediastinum unless the sheath is ruptured *(open arrow).*

Second, when extensive high-pressure bleeding occurs into the mediastinum or an intravenous infusion infiltrates into the mediastinum this fluid does not pass into the interstitium of the lung.

Third, when interstitial emphysema develops in the lung as the result of positive pressure ventilation and barotrauma, it often confines itself to the lung and produces a pneumomediastinum in only in a small percentage of cases. When pneumomediastinum does occur, it is almost certainly because the sheath has ruptured from the high distending pressures.[8]

Fourth, on computed tomography, scans of patients with cardiac edema will show distended sheaths within the lungs, without evidence of extravascular liquid in the mediastinum.

Fifth, dissection studies of the human lung have shown fusion of the layers of peribronchovascular sheaths to the vessels and bronchi where they emerge from the lung.[6]

Reexamination of the animal and human cadaver studies[10-12] that originally contributed to the belief that peribronchovascular sheaths are open to the mediastinum reveals that the air and contrast media used in these studies were injected at very high pressures (far above physiological pressures) and it is virtually certain that this led to traumatic rupture of the sheaths.

As we have stated elsewhere,[8] we have no problem with the concept that some edema fluid can pass from the lungs into the mediastinal tissues. We have seen, at thoracotomy, hilar nodes "weeping" edema fluid in patients with cardiac decompensation, but this fluid comes from the lung interstitium via lymphatics to the lymph nodes, not from open peribronchovascular sheaths. It is conceivable that fluid could pass directly through the sheath wall into the mediastinum—as it does from the interstitium across the visceral pleura into the pleural space—but the area of sheath contiguous with the mediastinum is so small that it is difficult to believe it could be a significant mechanism for draining fluid from the lung.

Interstitial Space Contents

To support and strengthen what appears to be a very fragile structure of millions of minute thin-walled balloons and enable them to withstand the lifelong stresses of inspiration, expiration, Valsalva maneuvers, coughing, etc., the interstitial space contains an extensive fibrillar skeleton of connective tissue fibers that extend centrifugally from the hilum to the alveolar ducts along the branching path of pulmonary vessels and airways. A second group of fibers, originating from the visceral pleura, penetrates centripetally into the lung parenchyma within the interlobular septa, to meet a third group of fibers within the alveolar septa. This third group interdigitates with both the centrifugal and the

centripetal fibers to establish a fibrous tension skeleton that extends from the hilum to the visceral pleura and distributes mechanical forces of the respiratory cycle evenly throughout the lung[13] (Fig. 2-4).

The interalveolar interstitial space has a huge cross-sectional area. It is continuous peripherally with the subpleural and septal spaces and centrally with the peribronchovascular sheaths. These sheaths can hold a large volume of fluid and are sometimes referred to as a liquid "sump."

The alveolar septa are not inert but contain numerous fibroblasts with contractile properties.[14] These cells have cytoplasmic processes that, in addition to linking the basement membranes of alveolar epithelial cells with those of endothelial cells, extend across the alveolar septa to connect contiguous alveoli. It has been speculated[14] that these contractile fibroblasts may play an important role in the regulation of alveolar septal interstitial volume and compliance and fluid drainage. (They may also play a causative role in the pattern of "butterfly" or "batswing" edema.) The intraalveolar septa do not contain any lymphatic capillaries, but the nearby peribronchovascular sheaths do.[15] The ends of the lymphatic capillaries within the sheaths have a fenestrated endothelial layer and discontinuous basement membrane.

The interalveolar septal interstitial liquid compartment forms a waterway from which liquid and macromolecules flow centrally into the peribronchovascular sheaths and from there toward the hilum via two parallel channels: (1) within the sheaths, surrounding the fibrillar skeleton (an extralymphatic interstitial pathway), and (2) within the pulmonary lymphatic vessels.

The extralymphatic interstitial pathway within the peribronchovascular sheaths is not, as it might initially appear, a freely negotiable channel for liquid and solutes but is in fact a complex network of lymph vessels, many types of collagen and elastic fibers, and a dense matrix of proteoglycans and glycosaminoglycans.[16] Whereas these mucopolysaccharides may facilitate the transport of water and small ions through the labyrinth of inner spaces, they also partially exclude proteins.[17] (The structure and contents of the peribronchovascular space are discussed more fully in Appendix A of this chapter.)

The special anatomic features just described combine, under normal circumstances, to provide efficient drainage of the liquid that is continuously being filtered from the capillaries while, at the same time, permitting gas to interchange between capillaries and alveoli—both events occurring in the same anatomic structures.

PHYSIOLOGIC FACTORS DETERMINING LUNG FLUID FLOW

The physiologic factors determining the rate of liquid and solute exchange across a capillary wall are (1) intra-

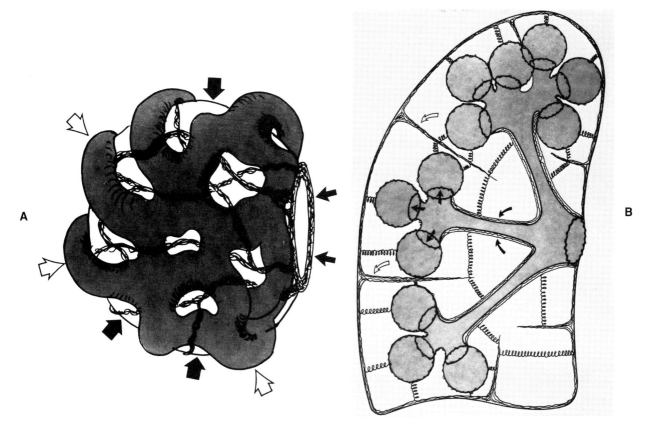

Fig. 2-4 A, Alveolus *(wide black arrows)* with surrounding capillary bed *(open arrows).* Fibrous strands arising from the alveolar duct *(narrow black arrows)* interlace between and around the capillaries. **B,** "Skeleton" of the lung. Starting from the hilum, fibrous strands extend through the peribronchovascular sheath *(curved arrows)* to become attached peripherally to rings of fibrous tissue around the alveolar ducts *(straight arrows).* Connective tissue passing into the lung via interlobular septa *(open arrows)* connects with the fibers emanating from the hilum *(coiled springs),* forming a complete fibrous skeleton from hilum to pleural surface. (Modified from Weibel ER. In Fishman AP, Macklem PT, Mead JS, editors: *Handbook of physiology. The respiratory system,* section 3, vol 3, part 1, Washington DC, 1986, American Physiological Society, p 89.)

vascular hydrostatic pressure (HPiv), (2) extravascular (interstitial) hydrostatic pressure (HPev), (3) intravascular oncotic pressure (OPiv), and (4) extravascular (interstitial) oncotic pressure (OPev).

These factors, in turn, have a certain dependency on the anatomic features of the capillary wall.

Capillary walls function as semipermeable membranes or (more correctly) as dialyzable membranes.[18] The differing physiologic behavior of brain, lung, and systemic and glomerular capillaries (which have differing numbers and tightness of endothelial cell junctions but the same endothelial structure) suggests that their physiologic functions (both oncotic and hydrostatic) may be mediated through the capillary wall endothelial cell junctions, and not across the endothelial wall.[18]

Since oncotic pressure acts in a direction opposite to hydrostatic pressure, then, if the effective combination of hydrostatic (HP) and oncotic (OP) *intra*vascular pressures (HPiv + OPiv) is higher than the effective combined *extra*vascular pressures (HPev + OPev) within the interstitium, fluid will flow out of the vessel. Conversely, if the total effective pressure is higher in the interstitium than within the capillary, fluid will flow into the capillary. However, the picture is not quite as simple as this. Oncotic flow is modified by the particular resistance of the given capillary wall to the passage of solutes (expressed in the Starling equation as the "oncotic reflection coefficient," σ), which, as indicated above, may be a function primarily of the width of the endothelial cell gaps. Small plasma components (e.g., electrolytes) pass freely across the microvascular barrier, and their concentration in the plasma is approximately equal to that in the perimicrovascular interstitium. As a consequence, these substances do not exert any osmotic activity across the capillary wall. By contrast, larger solutes (plasma proteins) are restricted (in proportion to their molecular radius)[19] and have a higher concentration in plasma than in the interstitium. The osmotic activity across the capillary wall is therefore essentially exerted by plasma proteins (σ close to 1), and σ appears to vary normally from the arterial to the venous end of the pulmonary capillaries (being approximately ten times greater at the venous end).[18] It may be altered pathophysiologically by high intravascular pressure (causing increased width of the junction) and pathologically by inflammation (injury lung edema).

Similarly, *hydrostatic* flow is modified by the "hydraulic conductivity" of the capillary wall (the resistance to the passage of water across the capillary junctions caused by a change in hydrostatic pressure), which appears to be a function of both the number and the size of "pores" in the endothelium. (The only "pores" physically detectable by present microscopic technique are the endothelial cell junctions.) It would appear, therefore, that endothelial cell junction morphology and morphometry may determine both the oncotic reflection coefficient (σ in the Starling equation) and the hydraulic conductivity. Hydraulic conductivity is not a separate term in the Starling equation but is one of several factors included in the multifactorial Kf term (usually called the "conductance" of the capillary wall).

Let us consider how endothelial cell junction numbers and size may affect the passage of water into or out of a capillary. If the *number* of endothelial cell junctions per unit area is increased but their gap size is kept unchanged (e.g., glomerular capillaries, which have many more "gaps" than pulmonary capillaries), hydraulic conductivity (and as a result Kf) will increase materially but the oncotic reflection coefficient (σ) should not be affected (since it appears to be a function of gap *size*). In contrast, if the number of junctions per unit area is kept unchanged but their *gap size* is increased (e.g., by marked elevation of intravascular hydrostatic pressure), hydraulic conductivity will again increase (causing Kf to increase) but oncotic pressure effects may progressively diminish (σ will become less) (Fig. 2-5). Carried to extremes, if the cell junctions are pushed so far apart that protein molecules can pass across freely (e.g., as in high altitude pulmonary edema and neurogenic edema) or are "allowed" to open under neurohormonal control, or if actual "holes" appear in the capillary wall, then all oncotic effects at this point may disappear (Fig. 2-5)—which can occur in injury lung edema.

If these deductions are correct, then there appear to be some fallacies in employing the Starling equation, as it is customarily used, to calculate the change in water flow that should occur as a result of change in hydrostatic pressure. For the interested reader the logic behind this critique is more fully explored, and examples given, in Appendix B of this chapter.

Leaving aside for the moment these possible objections to use of the Starling equation, and using it as it is presently employed, one can determine theoretically the amount of liquid that will be filtered per unit area per unit time (Qf)[20]:

$$Qf = Kf[(HPiv - HPev) - \sigma (OPiv - OPev)]$$

Or, since the total quantity filtered per unit time will depend upon the surface area of the capillaries involved, *net* flow per unit time (Qf net) may be derived by multiplying the total of the righthand terms in the Starling equation by the area involved:

$$Qf\ net = Area \times Kf[(HPiv-HPev)-\sigma(OPiv-OPev)]$$

Most of the variables in this equation cannot be measured directly, but some values have been derived by experimentation and some have been deduced. Although the numbers used by different authors have varied, it has been generally accepted[19,21-25] that in normal subjects the net filtration pressure in the lung exceeds the net absorption pressure by a few millimeters of mercury and, as a consequence, there is a small net outward movement of liquid from the microvessels into the interstitium (Fig. 2-2). This is in keeping with the observation that there is a continuous flow of lymph from the normal lung.

Under physiologic conditions the inflow of liquid into the pulmonary interstitium and the outflow from the lung are in a state of continuous equilibrium so that the interstitial volume remains essentially constant. Under these conditions lymph flow equals the Qf (net) of the Starling equation.[19] It has been deduced from animal studies[26] that in the normal human lung lymph flow should range from approximately 10 to 20 ml/hr.

If we accept that there are some 3,000,000 capillaries in the lung (with a surface area of 75 m^2), that 10 to 20 ml/hr of transudation occurs from the whole lung, and that approximately two thirds of the capillaries are recruited in the normal subject (50 m^2), then it can be deduced that the fluid flow from a single capillary will approximate 0.05 to 0.1 millionth of a milliliter every hour.

The exchange of liquid and solute in the lung is probably much more complicated than described by the Starling equation alone, and readers who are interested in a fuller analysis—including the mechanical factors involved—are referred to Appendixes A, B, and C of this chapter.

PATHOPHYSIOLOGY OF EDEMA FORMATION

With the proviso already stated against accepting Starling mechanisms as a complete explanation of fluid flow across capillaries, there are fundamentally only two ways in which flow of water out of the capillaries can be increased. These are (1) by increasing transmu-

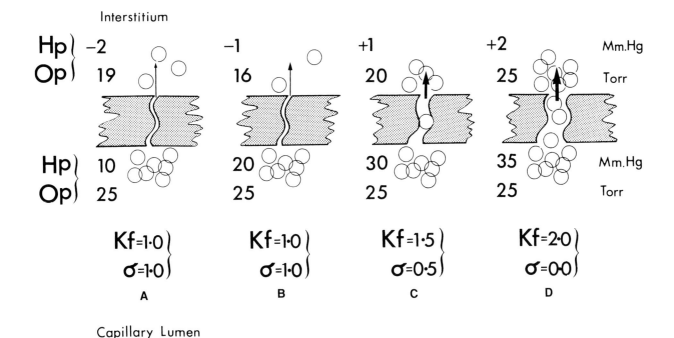

Interstitium

Capillary Lumen

Fig. 2-5 Hypothesis of the effects of increasing intracapillary hydrostatic pressure *(Kf)* on conductance of water and the oncotic reflection coefficient (σ). *Open circles* represent protein molecules, *screened areas* the capillary endothelium interrupted by endothelial cell junctions. *Arrows* show the direction of water flow, and arrow size the amount of flow.

Column A, Normal pulmonary capillary pressures (arterial end). Protein cannot pass through the narrow junctions; σ = 1, Kf = 1. The differences in extravascular and intravascular hydrostatic and oncotic pressures result in a very small efflux of water. Absorption at the venous end of the capillary along with lymph flow will keep interstitial fluid from accumulating and the extravascular protein will not be diluted (though its concentration may vary slightly from the arterial end to the venous end of the capillary).

Column B, Increasing hydrostatic pressure from 10 to 25 mm Hg results in increasing flow of water, but with no appreciable change in junction width and therefore no change in either Kf or σ. Some dilution of extravascular pro-

tein occurs because of the increased interstitial fluid volume, causing a drop in OPev (from 19 to, say, 16). There also will be a slight increase in HPev (from −2 to −1). Both factors help prevent further efflux.

Column C, Further increase in HPiv, to 30 mm Hg, may result in widening of the junctions to the point that some protein is able to pass through. The increased diameter of the junctions would cause a major change in Kf (because of Poiseuille's law—see Appendix B) and in σ. Note that there would now also be an *increase* in extravascular protein and further increase in HPev (from −2 to, say, +1).

Column D, With a very high HPiv (35 mm Hg +) the junctions may be pushed far enough apart to permit free passage of proteins (see also Fig. 2-6, column *4*) and there may no longer be any semipermeable membrane effect; σ would therefore disappear (= 0), but Kf would increase greatly. This is probably the situation in very high pressure (e.g., neurogenic) edema (see Fig. 2-6, column *4*, and Table 2-1).

ral pressure (hydrostatic and/or oncotic) and (2) by damaging the capillary walls and/or endothelial cell junctions. This damage may be reversible or non reversible. Combinations of both etiologies are common.

It has been suggested[7] that simply increasing the surface area of capillaries will cause edema; however, if more capillaries are recruited (e.g., by increasing circulating blood volume, though this will certainly cause normal physiological transudation to occur in the recruited area [which was formerly dry], giving an increased *total* extravascular lung water), the regional

quantity of water per milliliter of lung will remain normal and edema (defined as an excess of lung water) will not therefore occur.[8]

Elevated Pressure Edema

Elevated pressure gradients across the capillary walls may be either hydrostatic or oncotic, but it should be pointed out immediately that increasing the transudation of water from the capillaries into the interstitium will simultaneously alter the oncotic pressure of the extravascular space. Hydrostatic pressure changes are therefore always accompanied by a concomitant change in oncotic pressure.

Transmural increase in hydrostatic pressure can occur at either the venous end of the capillary (e.g., by elevation of left atrial pressure) or along the whole length of the capillary (by diminishing interstitial pressure, for example, secondary to very negative pleural pressures induced by the Müller maneuver or by inspiration against an edematous glottis [croup]). Much more rarely, transmural pressure can be increased primarily at the arterial end of the capillaries by elevation

of *arterial* pressure (e.g., high altitude edema or neurogenic edema) (Fig. 2-6 and Table 2-1).

There are many ways in which capillary transmural pressure may be elevated, but the commonest causes are certainly cardiac (i.e., left heart decompensation and mitral valve disease) (Fig. 2-6 and Table 2-1).

Low to Moderate Transmural Pressure Elevations (10 to 25 mm Hg) (Fig. 2-6, column 2).. Low to moderate elevations in capillary transmural pressure will cause the loose endothelial cell junctions to be pushed slightly apart, leading to an increased flow of water and low mo-

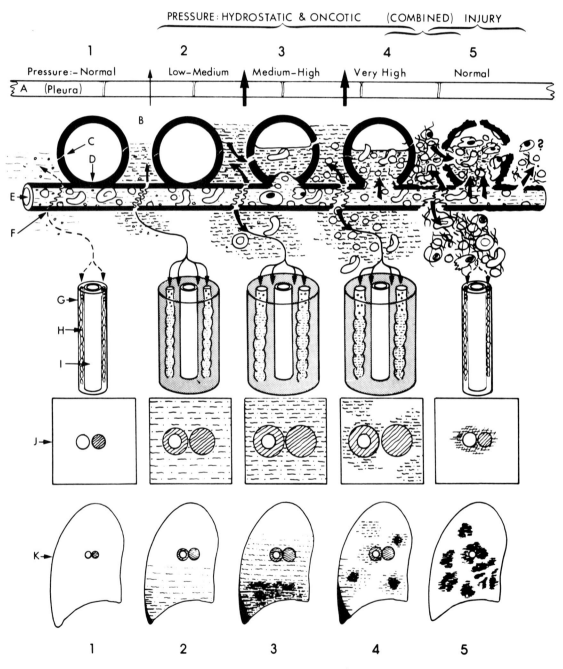

Fig. 2-6   For legend see opposite page.

lecular weight electrolytes into the interstitium and causing (initially) increased lymphatic flow and pure interstitial edema with minimal dilation of the peribronchovascular sheaths.

If fluid continues to transude from the capillaries, the increasing edema will recruit the peribronchovascular "sumps" and will occupy the subpleural interstitial space, eventually causing the passage of water from this space across the visceral pleura to form effusions.[7,27] (See Chapter 5.) At this stage the alveolar epithelial cell junctions (tight junctions) remain closed and no water, protein, or cells enter the alveolus (Fig. 2-6, column 2).

Moderate to High Transmural Pressure Elevations (25 to 40 mm Hg) (Fig. 2-6, column 3). Column 3 of Fig. 2-6 shows the effects of a further increase in transmural pressure. The peribronchovascular sumps become completely filled, at which point "interstitial tamponade" will develop, causing a sudden rise in pressure and forcing apart the tight junctions between alveolar epithelial cells, with the result that water will then pass into the alveoli.

It appears that the junctions may be opened enough in severe edema to permit some protein and red cells to enter both the interstitium and the alveoli.[28-30] Such a mechanism would certainly fit well with the clinical and pathologic findings of blood in the edema fluid of patients with severe cardiac failure. It has also been shown[4,30] that, with high intravascular pressures, the fused basement membranes (thin side) may be damaged and may bulge as a very thin membrane into the alveolar lumen (Fig. 2-6, column 3). This may be a further pathway for the passage of red cells and protein into the alveoli.*

Very High Transmural Pressure Elevations (more than 35 to 40 mm Hg). In neurogenic as well as high altitude edema the transmural pressures may be extremely high[31-33]; and it has been shown experimentally [34] that, with very high transmural pressures, particularly if the pressure elevation is abrupt, as indeed it is in neuro-

---

*The fact that protein can be found in the alveoli with pure elevated venous pressure would appear to make the usage of plasma protein/alveolar protein ratios of doubtful value in distinguishing between hydrostatic and injury lung edema. This should be taken into account when evaluating papers that have used these protein ratios as a "gold standard" to discount the value of the chest radiograph in making such a differentiation. (See Chapter 7.)

Fig. 2-6 Pathophysiologic (and resultant radiologic) changes in edema due to elevated transmural pressure (columns *2* to *4*) versus normal pressure ("injury") lung edema (column *5*). (NOTE: Very high pressure edema [column *4*] has combined elements of pressure and injury.) *A,* Pleura; *B,* interstitial space; *C,* "tight" epithelial cell junctions in the alveolar wall; *D,* fused basement membranes of an alveolus and capillary ("thin" side); *E,* capillary lumen; *F,* "loose" endothelial cell junctions; *G,* peribronchovascular sheaths; *H,* lymphatics within sheaths; *I,* lumen of a vessel (artery or vein); *J,* appearance of a bronchus and accompanying artery (end-on); *K,* appearance of the whole lung.

Column *1* (normal pressure), A small quantity of water is present in the interstitial space, but no protein or red cells. The alveoli are dry, with no pleural fluid. Normal peribronchial sheath and radiograph.

Column *2* (low to medium elevation of pressure), Endothelial junctions are slightly widened, increasing fluid in the interstitium (mild to moderate interstitial edema). There is beginning pleural effusion, and peribronchial cuffing (no protein or red cells in the interstitium, alveoli dry). The radiograph shows gravitationally distributed interstitial edema, peribronchial cuffing, and beginning pleural effusion.

Column *3* (medium to high elevation of pressure), Endothelial cell junctions are pushed apart (severe interstitial edema), causing elevated interstitial pressure, opening of the alveolar epithelial cell junctions, and alveolar edema. Occasional protein molecules and red cells are in the interstitium. The radiograph shows widely distended peribronchial sheaths, gravitationally distributed interstitial and alveolar edema, and pleural effusions. Advancing alveolar edema makes the lung progressively radiopaque and the outer walls of cuffs more difficult to see. Air bronchograms, however, are rare. (NOTE: Thinning and bulging of the *basement membrane* into the lumen of the alveolus may be a pathway for the development of alveolar edema and the presence of red cells.)

Column *4* (very high pressure), Extreme elevation is rare in humans and probably can only be caused by high altitude or neurogenic edema. Severe combined interstitial and alveolar edema with some protein and red cells in both the interstitium and the alveoli is probably due to wide separation of endothelial cell junctions *(curved arrow)* and rupture of fused basement membranes *(straight arrow)*. Pleural effusion is variable—peribronchial cuffing usually present and radiographically the distribution of edema is nongravitational and patchy. (NOTE: The presence of protein and red cells gives very high pressure edema some of the characteristics, including drop in lung compliance, of injury lung edema. Columns *4* and *5* are therefore linked under the heading "combined.")

Column *5* (normal pressure: capillary injury), The alveolar and, to a lesser extent, capillary endothelium shows extensive damage—with passage of fibrin, desquamated cells, protein, and red cells into the interstitium *(curved arrows)* and alveoli *(double arrows)* via ruptured fused basement membranes. Only a small amount of this viscid material can flow, and peribronchovascular cuffing is usually absent. Pleural effusions are also absent or minimal. The radiograph shows nongravitational random alveolar edema with air bronchograms (little or no evidence of cuffing or effusions).

Table 2-1   New, simplified classification of pulmonary edema

| Elevated pressure (hydrostatic/oncotic) | | | Normal pressure | |
Low to medium (10 to 25 mm Hg)	Medium to high (25 to 40 mm Hg)	Very high (40 mm +)	Allergic (potentially reversible)	Injury (irreversible)
Left heart failure (mild to moderate) Renal failure[1] Overhydration[1] Near-drowning[2] Decreased interstitial pressure (croup, re-expansion)[3] Lymphatic blockage Pulmonary venous thrombosis	Left heart failure (severe to acute) Left heart failure [4] (severe-chronic) Mitral valve disease[4] Left atrial myxoma Hyperperfusion (post-pneumonectomy, single-lung transplant) Postembolic	Neurogenic[6] High altitude[6] (?) Extreme effort	Drugs (hypersensitivity) Hormonal (peripartum) Transfusion reaction Leukoagglutinin reaction Organic allergens	Sepsis Hypotension ("Vietnam lung," "DaNang lung," "shock lung") O_2 toxicity Aspiration Noxious inhalation (includes cocaine) Embolism (air, fat, amniotic) Pancreatitis Disseminated intravascular coagulation "Pump" lung Virulent pneumonias Drugs (cytotoxic and noncytotoxic)

1. The combination of mildly elevated left atrial pressure and a drop in intravascular oncotic pressure, causes edema
2. A form of oncotic edema that may be complicated by *injury* edema if the aspirated water is contaminated, plus an element of low *interstitial* pressure because of inspiration against a closed glottis
3. A combination of increased transmural pressure (low negative interstitial pressure because of the negative pleural pressures used to induce reinflation) and an element of capillary injury; may lead to regional ARDS
4. Chronic LHF and mitral valve disease share lung lymphatic hypertrophy, permitting patients to survive long-term high elevation of LAP without overt edema
5. Postembolic edema, which appears to have both pressure (hyperperfusion of the *non*embolized lung) and chemical (released from the clot) factors operating
6. All these edemas are proteinaceous but usually reversible; they can all, however, progress to ARDS and may be classified as spanning both categories.

genic and high altitude edema, there is (in addition to widening of the endothelial cell junctions, allowing protein and red cells to spill into the interstitium) an actual disruption of the thin side. The resultant passage of proteins and red cells directly into the alveoli is analogous to the alveolar hemorrhage that occurs with great frequency in race horses at the end of a race[34] (Fig. 2-6, column 4). It is not clear in these circumstances whether there is also any disruption of the alveolar tight junctions.

Injury Lung Edema

It would seem clear, from the progressive increase in width of the loose interendothelial cell junctions occurring with elevated transmural capillary pressure, that pure *mechanical* stress can change the "permeability" of the capillaries (Fig. 2-6, columns 3 and 4) but that such changes are frequently reversible (i.e., as previously suggested, the Velcro fastener construction of the loose junctions permits them to return to normal when the intravascular pressure drops[4]). When the junctions are wide open, however, the functioning of capillaries as a semipermeable membrane is clearly affected. So long as the junctions are narrow enough to prevent plasma protein from passing through, this change will affect hydraulic permeability only and the capillary wall should still function as a semipermeable membrane (i.e., only the Kf term in the Starling equation will be affected). However, as mentioned, if the cell junctions are pushed far enough apart for proteins to pass out into the interstitium—in these areas certainly, there will no longer be a semipermeable membrane effect and the σ factor in the Starling equation will also be affected (Fig. 2-5).

The evidence indicates that it is possible for all these changes in "permeability" to occur on a purely mechanical basis; and since protein and red cells can appear in the interstitium and alveoli with simple hydrostatic edema, the use of the term "capillary permeability" to distinguish between hydrostatic edema and edema due to capillary injury does not appear to be well founded. We believe that the terms "high pressure" (or hydrostatic) and "normal pressure" edema would be more accurate and would not convey the probably erroneous impression that there are "holes" in the vessel walls in one variety of edema but not in the other.

The classification "normal pressure edema" should in turn be subdivided for clarity into "normal pressure noninjury" and "normal pressure injury" types (Table 2-1 and Fig. 2-6).

Normal Pressure Noninjury Edema. The principal cause of this category of edema appears to be hypersensitivity, mainly from drugs but also from organic allergens and from transfusion and leukoagglutinin reactions (Table 2-1). A type of edema that occurs in the peripartum period might also be included in this normal pressure/noninjury category since it can occur in the absence of any pressure elevation and without any history of drug administration. The causation does not appear to be allergic and may be hormonal. It should be pointed out that, though they can usually be reversed (e.g., through the use of intravenous antihistamines or steroids), the allergic edemas may also become irreversible, leading to *injury* edema and the development of ARDS.

Normal Pressure Injury Edema. This is the group presently referred to by most authors and clinicians as "capillary permeability edema" and for which we prefer, as stated, the term "injury" edema.

The causes of injury lung edema are numerous (Table 2-1), but the commonest in our experience are hypotension and/or sepsis ("shock lung"). The mechanisms that intervene between the insult to the lung and the development of injury to the capillaries and alveolar epithelium remain the subject of extensive research, but the one unifying factor that emerges from many studies and theories[35-38] appears to be inflammatory damage. Again, despite the virtually universal use of the term "capillary permeability" edema, it has been clearly shown[4,39] that the principal damage is not to the capillaries but to the alveolar epithelium. Fig. 2-6, column 5, illustrates diagrammatically the changes that occur.

There is extensive damage to the *alveolar epithelium*, with changes ranging from cytoplasmic swelling to actual fragmentation. There are also endothelial wall defects, which often are plugged with aggregations of platelets and fibrin strands or microthrombi.[4,39]

The alveoli become filled with proteins, cells, erythrocytes, leukocytes, macrophages, cell debris, and sheets of hyaline membrane. The same admixture of cells, debris, and proteins is found in the perialveolar interstitium contiguous with the areas of injury (Fig. 2-6, column 5). These changes occur in a very patchy fashion throughout the lung, often with apparently normal areas intervening. There is only minor evidence of migration of this exudate into the peribronchovascular sheaths.[4,25,40,41] The exudative material appears too viscid to migrate through the cell and gel phases and fibrillar content of the interstitial spaces[18,25,42] and, unlike hydrostatic edema, it does not therefore usually form septal lines or peribronchial cuffs, nor does it have a gravitational distribution[25,43,44] (Fig. 2-6). These differences are clearly manifested on the chest radiograph

and assist in the differentiation between high pressure and normal pressure injury edema.[21,25,43] (See Chapter 7.)

Because in injury lung edema the alveolar epithelium and vascular endothelium are simultaneously damaged, there is an *almost simultaneous* flooding of the perialveolar and intraalveolar spaces.[4] The sequence of development of normal pressure injury edema is therefore quite different from that of elevated pressure hydrostatic edema [21,25,43-45]; and since this is an important factor in the radiologic distinction between the two, it will be discussed more fully in the ensuing pages.

Sequence of Development of High Pressure Versus Normal Pressure Injury Lung Edema. Although it is now well known that lung edema due to pressure and that due to injury are two very different entities, the sequence of events leading to lung liquid and solute accumulation is still widely reported to be the same[46] (i.e., excess water from the microvessels "recruits" the juxtaalveolar interstitium, leaving at this stage the width of the alveolar septum unaltered) (Fig. 2-7). Part of this filtered liquid can exit the lung via the lymphatics, but excess liquid that cannot be cleared by the lymphatics then moves into the connective tissue sheaths surrounding successively larger vessels and bronchi. The interlobular septa may also be engorged at this stage, together with the subpleural interstitium and the pleural space (Fig. 2-8, *A* and *B*). As edema increases further, pleural fluid formation increases, as does lymph flow; and, with increasing pressure in the sheaths and juxtaalveolar interstitium, fluid then begins to distend the alveolar septa (perimicrovascular interstitium) (Fig. 2-8, *C*). Finally, when the interstitium can hold no more and pressure rises abruptly (interstitial tamponade), liquid breaks through into the alveoli[22,47] (Fig. 2-8, *D*).

In complete contrast to this sequence (which actually occurs only in pressure forms of edema), in injury lung edema there is *simultaneous* appearance of alveolar and interstitial edema, with much greater emphasis on the filling of alveoli than filling of the interstitium (Figs. 2-6, column 5, and 2-9).

The belief that the same sequence is followed in both pressure edema and injury edema came originally not from human observations but from a paper published in 1967 by Staub, Nagano, and Pearce[46] in which the same sequence of events was reported to occur in dogs with hydrostatic and injury lung edema. The authors concluded that lung water accumulates in the same fashion, irrespective of the etiologic mechanisms causing the edema. This is quite contrary to what can be seen happening in human patients, and we and others[4,39] believe that, in the paper by Staub et al.,[46] the authors came to incorrect conclusions. (Readers interested in a fuller critique of the errors in this often-

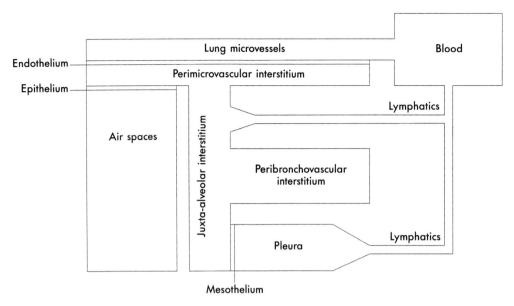

Fig. 2-7 Compartmentalization of extravascular lung water spaces. Liquid and solute are filtered from the lung microvessels into perimicrovascular interstitial spaces. Connections (in series) exist between the perimicrovascular interstitium and both the juxtaalveolar interstitium and the air spaces. The air spaces are sealed by tight interepithelial junctions (see Fig. 2-1) whereas the juxtaalveolar interstitium forms a waterway leading to lymphatics, loose connective peribronchovascular interstitium (cuffs), and in its more peripheral extension the pleural space. Lymphatics return liquid and solute recovered from the interstitial spaces and pleura to the systemic circulation. (The size of the compartments is not intended to be proportional to the true anatomic size.)

quoted experiment are referred to Appendix C of this chapter.)

FACTORS RESTRICTING DEVELOPMENT OF EDEMA

As fluid accumulates within the interstitial space, two pressure changes occur—one hydrostatic and the other oncotic. Because of rising hydrostatic pressure within the interstitial space as edema accumulates, there is a progressive drop in the hydrostatic pressure gradient across the capillary wall[48-50] (Figs. 2-5 and 2-10). As the interstitial pressure rises, transudation tends to diminish. Concomitantly, because of dilution of the proteins within the interstitial space, oncotic pressure drops, increasing still further the pressure gradient from the capillary lumen to the interstitium and opposing filtration of fluid from the microvessels (Fig. 2-10). It has been estimated[22] that 50% of the lung tissue's ability to counteract edema formation is due to the increased colloid/osmotic gradient and the remaining 50% is divided equally between increased interstitial tissue pressure and increased lymph flow.

These mechanisms restricting edema formation are effective only in pressure forms of edema and do not take place in injury edema, wherein the protein concentration of the edema liquid is close to that of plasma[22] and in which the viscous edema fluid cannot fill the peribronchovascular sheaths but recruits instead the high capacitance, low resistance compartment formed by the air spaces.

As a result the interstitial pressure does not rise as much as it does in pressure edema. Indeed, because of the drop in lung compliance caused by injury lung edema and the resultant increase in respiratory effort, the interstitial pressure may become more negative than usual, which would tend to increase the outflow of water from the capillaries.[35]

MECHANISMS OF CLEARANCE OF LUNG EDEMA
Pressure Edema (Interstitium)

As has already been described, the interstitial space forms an anatomic continuum from the visceral subpleural space, through the interalveolar septa and juxtaalveolar interstitium, into the peribronchovascular sheaths (Figs. 2-6 to 2-9) (also see Fig. 5-2). Drainage of liquid from the interstitial space can occur via several mechanisms (Fig. 2-1)—the lymphatics, the reversal of pressure gradients (hydrostatic and oncotic) between capillary lumen and interstitium, the passage of fluid

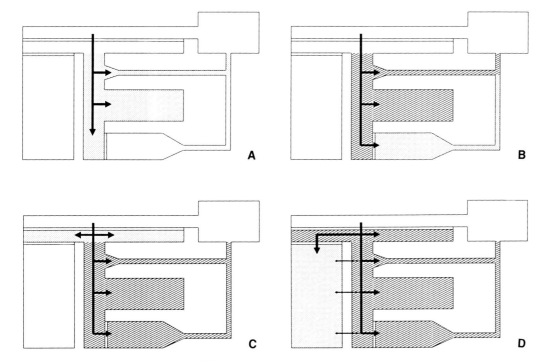

Fig. 2-8   Possible sequence of filling of lung liquid compartments in the course of "pure" hydrostatic (pressure) lung edema. (For the denomination of compartments, see Fig. 2-7.) Arrows indicate the direction of flow of extravascular liquid. Light and dark shaded areas denote the sequential invasion of compartments by extravascular liquid. **A,** Some of the liquid filtered in excess bypasses lung lymphatics (which absorb only a portion of it) and begins to fill the juxtaalveolar interstitium and peribronchovascular sheaths. **B,** Continued liquid filtration causes further filling of the peribronchovascular sheaths and transudation into the pleural space. **C,** As more liquid filters, the alveolar septal interstitium begins to swell. **D,** When all interstitial tissues are filled, flooding of the air spaces takes place through interepithelial alveolar junctions or, possibly, by retrograde filling from the terminal airway epithelium *(thin arrows).*

across the visceral pleura into the pleural space, and the passage of fluid into the alveoli (Fig. 2-10).

Lymph drainage occurs from the peribronchovascular sheaths via the lymphatics to mediastinal lymph nodes and trunks (the jugulomediastinal trunk on the right and the thoracic duct on the left) that enter the venous system at the junction of the right and left jugular subclavian veins respectively, terminating in the right atrium. It must be pointed out, however, that the major function of the lung lymphatics, rather than absorbing liquid, is to return protein and interstitial material unabsorbable by blood vessels into the systemic circulation.[51] Despite the fact that the lung has an extensive

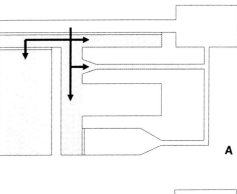

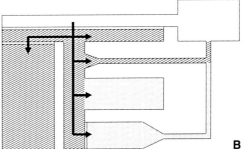

Fig. 2-9   Possible sequence of filling of extravascular lung liquid compartments in the course of "pure" injury lung edema. **A,** Liquid filtered through the injured microvessels causes increased lymph flow and fills the alveolar septum and juxtaalveolar interstitium. Alveolar flooding occurs early by concomitant injury of the alveolar epithelial cells. **B,** Persistence of injury causes greater air space flooding, with relative sparing of the peribronchovascular interstitium and pleural space. (Same notations as Fig. 2-7.)

Fig. 2-10 Starling factors affecting fluid re-absorption. *Hp,* Hydrostatic pressure; *Op,* oncotic pressure. **A,** Normal pressures resulting in a transudation force at the arterial end and a reabsorptive force at the venous end. Minimal lymphatic flow. **B,** Capillary pressure elevated by 20 mm Hg. Transudation force at the arterial end 27, at the venous end 17. Marked increase in lymph flow. If lymph flow cannot keep up with transudation, fluid accumulates in the interstitium, Hp rises (to approximately +5), and Op falls (to approximately 9) (see **C**). **C,** If capillary pressure then drops to normal, there is no transudation but there is now resorptive force of 11 at the arterial end and 18 at the venous end of the capillary.

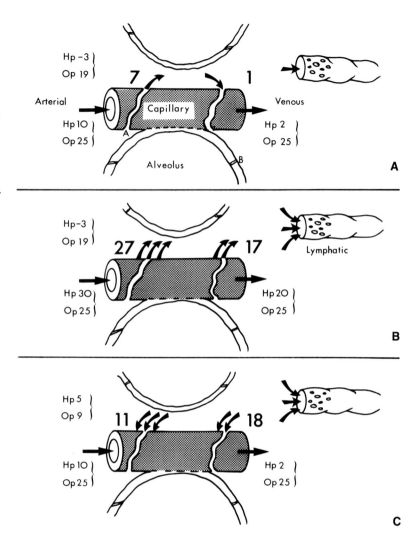

network of lymphatics, lymph flow is usually dynamically inadequate to keep pace, in terms of removal, with abnormal increases in liquid filtration. In acute edema only a small fraction of the liquid and solute that leave the microvessels is removed in the form of lymph.[51]

Increasing the volume of liquid in the pulmonary interstitium increases the driving pressure for liquid to pass into the terminal lymphatics.[52-56] Lymph pressure must increase, from subatmospheric in the terminal lymph capillaries within the juxtaalveolar connective tissue to positive in the collecting ducts draining out of the lungs into systemic veins.[48] Lymph propulsion takes place both passively (by respiratory motion) and actively (by intrinsic muscular contraction of lymphatic walls).[22] Although lymph flow under acute conditions increases severalfold, the response is slow and insufficient to keep up with the increased rate of fluid accumulation[55-58]; and where alveolar flooding develops, there is usually no further increase in lymph flow since most of the extravasating fluid is now accommodated in

the low-resistance, high-capacitance compartment of the air spaces and bronchi.[22,24,56]

If, however, there is *chronic* elevation of capillary transmural pressure (e.g., in chronic left-sided heart failure or mitral stenosis), compensatory morphologic changes occur, such as lymphatic dilation, thickening of the alveolar capillary basement membranes, and interstitial fibroblastic proliferation.[4,59-61] These changes can be regarded as additional protective mechanisms, (1) restricting the development of pulmonary edema and (2) markedly increasing lymph flow from the lung. They explain why a long-standing increase in microvascular filtration pressure (even at the 30 mm Hg level, as in mitral stenosis) is often associated with either dry lungs (radiologically) or a predominantly interstitial edema whereas an *acute* left heart failure, for comparable levels of increased left atrial pressure, will present with severe edema, often alveolar[62] (Fig. 2-11).

The greater lymphatic safety factor that develops in chronic, compared to acute, left heart failure (LHF) has been clearly demonstrated by animal studies. Uhley et

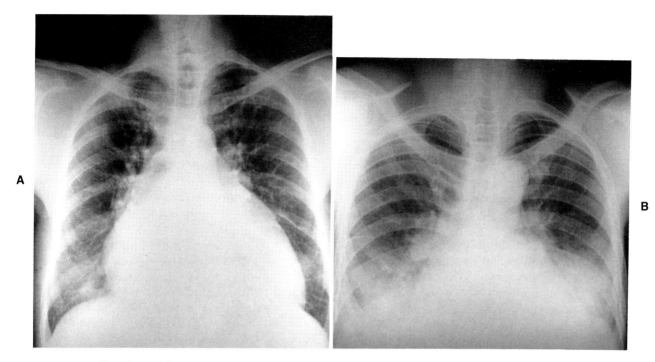

Fig. 2-11   A, A 30-year-old man with long-standing rheumatic mitral stenosis and incompetence as well as tricuspid incompetence. Left atrial pressure is 30 mm Hg. Septal lines are present, but there is no alveolar edema. **B,** A 50-year-old man with myocardial infarction and acute left heart failure. Left atrial pressure 30 mm Hg (as in **A**) but florid alveolar edema is present.

al.[58,63] showed that in dogs with acute pulmonary venous hypertension, raising the level of left atrial pressure caused the lymph flow from the right lymph duct to be only minimally increased above the baseline value of 4 ml/hr whereas in dogs in which congestive heart failure was *chronically* induced the flow was above 100 ml/hr.[58,63]

Hydrostatic Pressure. Because of the enormous surface area of the capillary bed, removal of edema fluid can be very rapid as transmural filtration pressures are restored to normal. Recall that when intravascular and interstitial pressures are normal there is usually a gradient of pressure at the venous end of the capillary and this favors *absorption* of fluid into the capillaries (Fig. 2-10). When left atrial pressure drops (e.g., with successful treatment of left heart failure), not only will this normal reabsorption take place but it will be greater than under normal circumstances because the interstitial pressure will remain elevated (increasing the driving force into the capillaries) until the quantity of fluid in the interstitial space begins to drop (Fig. 2-10).

Oncotic Pressure. Under normal circumstances the oncotic pressure gradient across the capillary wall junctions, which favors absorption of fluid into the capillaries, overcomes the hydrostatic pressure at the venous end of the capillary and resultant absorption takes place

(Fig. 2-10). At the arterial end of the capillary, however, oncotic pressure is normally overcome by the hydrostatic pressure and transudation takes place (Fig. 2-10). With the drop in oncotic interstitial pressure caused by interstitial edema, the oncotic gradient favoring absorption increases and, when intracapillary hydrostatic pressure drops back to normal, absorption may take place not only at the venous end of the capillary but also at the arterial end (Fig. 2-10). This mechanism is analogous to the transition from fetal to newborn life, when pulmonary vascular hydrostatic pressure drops abruptly and, because of the oncotic pressure difference, the extravascular water is rapidly absorbed into the bloodstream.[7] Note that when pulmonary edema is caused (or contributed to) by low oncotic pressure (common in overhydration and renal failure) the oncotic pressure is low not only in the pulmonary capillaries and subpleural visceral capillaries but also in the *parietal* pleural capillaries, causing increased formation of pleural fluid concomitant with the development of pulmonary edema (i.e., there may be no [or only a reduced] "lag period") (see Chapter 5). Similarly, when the oncotic pressure is raised by treatment it rises simultaneously in the pulmonary and systemic capillaries (including the parietal pleural capillaries), facilitating reabsorption of pleural fluid, and there may be no "lag period" between the resolution of pulmonary edema and the reabsorption of pleural effusions.

Pleural Fluid. As shown in Chapter 5, pleural fluid is normally formed by the parietal pleura; but when pulmonary edema develops, interstitial lung water can pass across the visceral pleura into the pleural space, draining via the parietal stomata into the lymphatics, back to the right atrium (see Fig. 5-12, *A*). This provides an additional clearance mechanism for pulmonary edema, but it would appear that as the intrapulmonary mechanisms for clearing edema go into effect and interstitial edema begins to clear there is a cessation of fluid flow into the pleural space. Certainly, hydrostatic edema clears much more rapidly than the effusions (i.e., there is a "lag" period between the two), suggesting that the clearance of pulmonary edema via the pleura is of much less importance than clearance via the lung capillaries.

Alveolar Fluid. Apart from liquid that is coughed up or removed by ciliary action, the major pathway for alveolar liquid clearance is through the interstitium.[64,65] Water and electrolytes are cleared more quickly than proteins so that the clearance rate of alveolar edema liquid is inversely related to its initial protein content.[66,67] The more rapid clearance of water compared with protein causes a process of relative protein concentration in the alveoli with subsequent slowing of clearance.[68]* There is also some evidence that active metabolic processes (demonstrated by selective enhancement or inhibition by pharmacologic agents) may play an important role in continuing the reabsorption of liquid against the colloid osmotic gradient.[67,68]

Protein leaves the alveoli by an exceedingly slow process (1% per hour), whose main mechanisms are not completely understood.[68] It has been hypothesized that protein may be removed from the alveoli primarily by epithelial cell vesicular transport or, secondarily, by engulfment in macrophages.

Injury Edema

The mechanisms in pressure edema just described, which lead to the flow of edema fluid from the alveolar septa into the peribronchovascular sheaths, do not operate in injury edema. One reason for this is the early damage to alveolar walls and filling of the alveoli—opening up low-resistance pathways to the flow of edema. Because of this, and due to the loss of surfactant, the normal liquid dynamics of the alveolar interstitium is lost and liquid in the septa does not flow toward the extraalveolar sumps. The loose interstitial spaces—with their sol, gel, and fibrillar content—appear to form a barrier to the highly proteinaceous, cell-

and debris-containing capillary exudate. Even the diffusion of water molecules along the extravascular tissue space is hampered by the high oncotic activity of the extravasated plasma proteins. Using NMR relaxation times to differentiate between pressure and injury lung edema, preliminary studies have shown that free water is increased more in the pulmonary lymph of animals with pressure edema compared to injury edema, in which the water bound to macromolecules predominates.[69-71] Thus further evidence has been provided that in injury edema a considerable fraction of the edema fluid cannot diffuse freely into the peribronchovascular sheaths, interlobular septa, subpleural space, or pleura.[72]

In injury edema, since the most important of the safety factors against edema formation (i.e., the increased plasma-to-interstitium colloid osmotic gradient and increased interstitial pressure) are lost, liquid and protein clearance is largely dependent upon the function of the lymphatic system.[51] Lymphatic vessels, however, have been shown to respond slowly to an increase in the net filtration rate[55] and, furthermore, their function may be impaired in the course of lung injury.[73] As long as injury persists, therefore, the lymphatic system cannot satisfactorily remove excess liquid and solute.

In pressure edema it has been shown[73] that perivascular protein exchanges very slowly with other liquid compartments in the interstitial space—which may result in a lower protein content in the interstitium (diluted with edema fluid) than around the larger vessels, thereby establishing a colloid/osmotic gradient along which water molecules could diffuse centrally from the periphery of the lung. It would also provide, together with the interstitial liquid hydrostatic gradient, an extra propulsive mechanism to move edema fluid away from the alveolar area, possibly explaining the central distribution of edema that is frequently seen radiologically.[43-45,74] This mechanism is lost in injury edema.

For all these reasons the clearance of injury edema is very slow, taking usually as many days as pressure edema takes hours (an important radiologic feature).

PATHOPHYSIOLOGIC/RADIOLOGIC CORRELATIONS

The relationships between each stage in the development of pressure edema and of normal pressure noninjury, and injury, lung edema are demonstrated diagrammatically in Figs. 2-6 to 2-9. It is clear that the very different pathophysiologic mechanisms in pressure and injury edema cause profoundly different clinical and radiologic presentations.* These differences are more fully described in Chapter 8.

---

*A further argument for the lack of specificity in using alveolar/plasma protein ratios to distinguish between pressure and nonpressure (injury) edema.

*References 21, 25, 43-45, 72, 74-78.

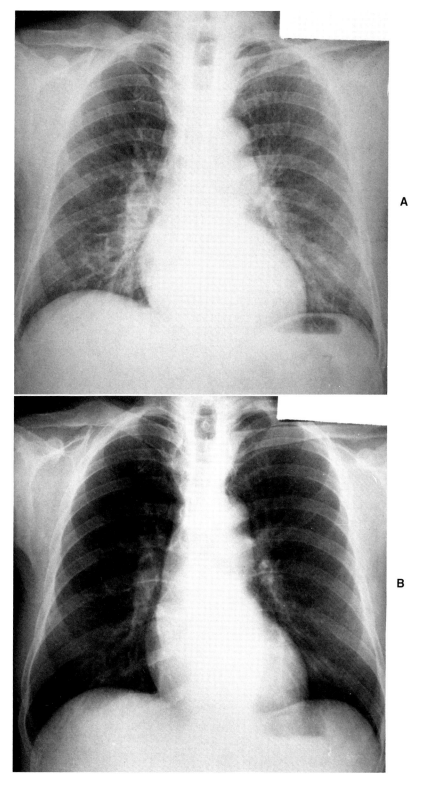

Fig. 2-12   Change of radiographic lung density in the chest radiographs of a patient with acute myocardial infarction, from the acute phase **A,** to recovery, **B.** The hilar blurring disappears after recovery. (NOTE: Some of the initial density is due to scattering from edema of the chest wall.)

Pressure Edema

In left heart failure, renal failure, overhydration, and low oncotic pressure edema the sequence of development of edema is virtually identical, modified only by the severity of the underlying pathology and how abruptly the edema develops (Figs. 2-6 to 2-8).

Although the interstitium of the lung normally contains a small amount of liquid, its presence is not usually radiologically recognizable; however, in patients who are dehydrated, and in emphysema patients, the abnormal dryness of the lung is manifested by unusual sharpness of the vessel margins both en face and in profile. The very slight unsharpness of vessel walls that we see in *normal* subjects may therefore be due not simply

to the poor resolution of the radiographic system but possibly to the *normal* extravascular water content.

As transmural pressure is increased and fluid begins to transude into the loose interstitial tissues (Fig. 2-6, column *2*), there is early loss of definition of vessel margins and a slight diminution in the blackness of the lung, without recognizable (to the eye) development of peribronchial cuffing. At this stage the slight loss of lucency of the lung surrounding the bronchi may make the end-on air-filled lumen stand out somewhat more than normal. The changes may be confined to the bases but are also often generally distributed throughout the lung, without apparent gravitational effect (Figs. 2-12 to 2-14). (The radiologic appearances in Figs. 2-12 and

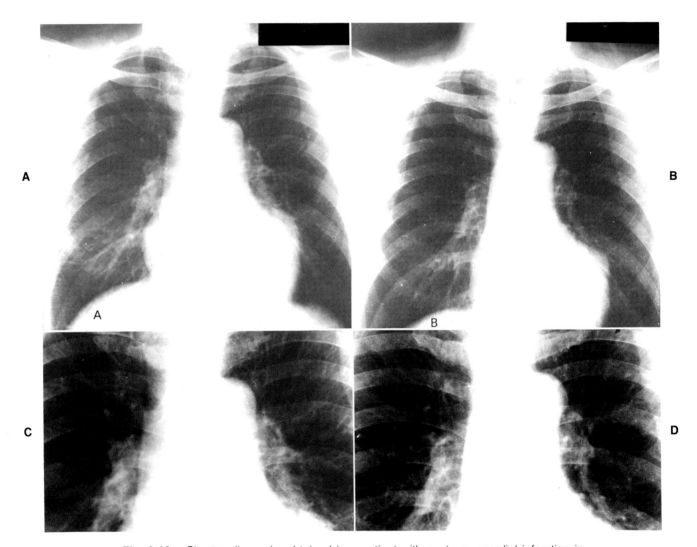

Fig. 2-13   Chest radiographs obtained in a patient with acute myocardial infarction in the acute phase, **A,** and after recovery, **B.** Note in **A** the radiographic signs of interstitial edema, including blurring of the hilar vessels and Kerley B lines at the right lung base, when the patient had no clinical signs compatible with lung edema. In **B,** 5 days later, the hilar vessels are no longer blurred and the Kerley B lines have disappeared. **C** and **D** are closeup views of the hilar regions showing changes in the blurring.

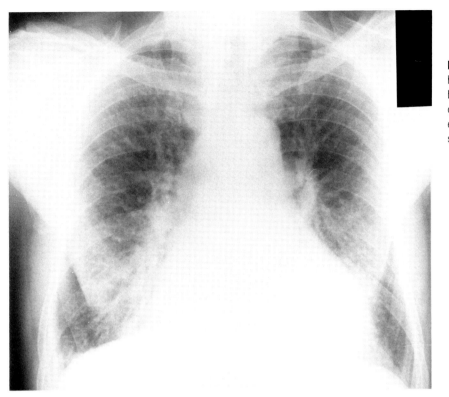

Fig. 2-14 Patient with recurrent left heart failure showing blurring of the hilar vessels, a diffuse increase in density, and moderately large pleural effusion on the right with lamellar effusion on the left.

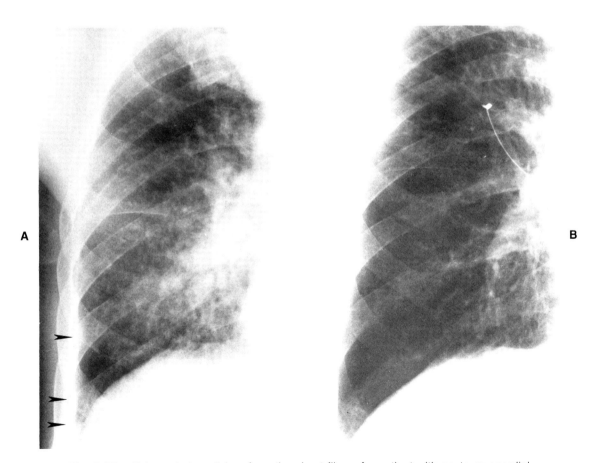

Fig. 2-15 Enlarged views taken from the chest films of a patient with acute myocardial infarction in the acute phase, **A,** showing an extensive perihilar haze, widening of the horizontal fissure, and pleural effusion *(arrowheads),* with obscuration of the small background vessels. After recovery, **B,** the hilar blurring has disappeared and the background vasculature is once again visible.

2-13 would correspond to an extravascular lung water of 50 to 60 ml/L of lung, i.e., "borderline interstitial edema.") (See Table 3-3.)

If edema continues to develop, central migration of edema fluid within the interstitium will cause progressive blurring of the larger vessels within the hilum, and a further loss of lung lucency. The small vessel pattern in the background, between large conducting vessels, becomes progressively more difficult to see (Fig. 2-15). (These radiologic findings would correspond to an extravascular lung water of 60 to 70 ml H$_2$O, i.e., "mild interstitial edema;" see Table 3-3.) At this stage definite bronchial cuffing is not seen.

As increasing amounts of interstitial edema develop and the peribronchovascular sheaths fill, definite bronchial cuffs can be identified[79-84] (Figs. 2-6, column 2, 2-16, and 2-17).* The presence of cuffs around medium-sized vessels seen end-on gives a "micronodular" appearance[79,81,83] (Fig. 2-18). Pleural effusion will not

---

*It has been hypothesized that cuffing is caused by transudation of fluid from the bronchial vessels supplying the walls and mucosa of the bronchi rather than by migration of fluid from the pulmonary capillaries into the cuffs.[84] However, the bronchial circulation supplying the perihilar area (where the larger bronchi are seen end-on) drains to the *right* side of the heart and would not be expected to be affected by elevation of left heart pressure. Also, when right heart pressure increases (e.g., after LHF), instead of bronchial mucosal edema (the cause of cardiac asthma) becoming worse (as one would anticipate if the bronchial circulation were implicated in cuffing), it actually becomes better, making it unlikely that the bronchial circulation is in fact the cause of bronchial wall thickening.

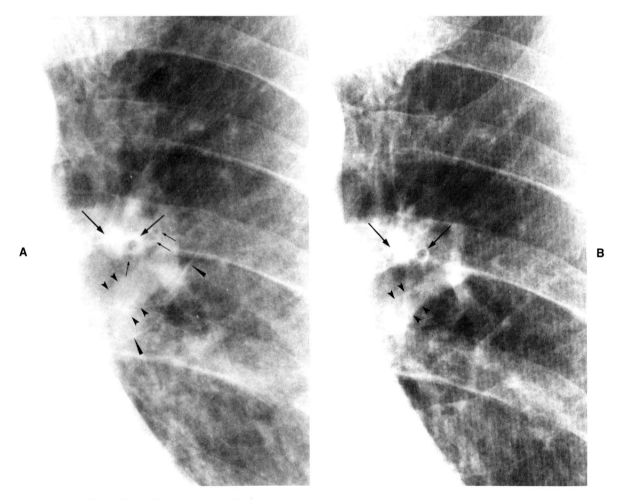

Fig. 2-16 Closeup views of the left perihilar region obtained from the chest films of a patient with chronic left heart decompensation while in failure, **A,** and after cardiotonic and diuretic treatment, **B.** Peribronchial and perivascular cuffs *(long arrows)* change markedly after treatment, together with an overall reduction of lung density and the disappearance of Kerley A septal lines *(long arrowheads)*. Note the marked reduction in width of the superior veins *(small arrowheads)* and the disappearance of small bronchi, seen end-on only during failure *(small arrows)*.

usually develop until interstitial edema is already present (i.e., pleural fluid formation lags, typically 24 hours or so, behind the development of edema) (Figs. 2-14 and 2-15). These radiologic appearances correspond to 70 to 80 ml H$_2$O, that is, "moderate interstitial edema" (Table 3-3).

Filling of the subpleural interstitium by edema can result in apparent thickening of pleural fissures and the impression that a small pleural effusion is present, particularly in the horizontal fissure. There is some controversy in the literature as to whether thickened fissures are due to subpleural interstitial edema[76,83-86] or to true intrapleural effusions.[79,87] It is difficult to distinguish between these two conditions, which in most cases coexist radiologically, since pleural effusion is a direct

consequence of subpleural edema. (See Chapter 5.) We believe that the presence of subpleural effusion may be identified by the loss of definition of the fissure margins (Fig. 2-19), in contrast to a fissure widened by a small pleural effusion, which is sharply defined[79] (Fig. 2-20). The presence of a thickened fissure does not necessarily mean that there must be interstitial edema in the subpleural interstitium directly bordering the fissure itself—excess pleural liquid may migrate into pleural fissures from remote pleural regions, following gradients of intrapleural liquid pressure.[27,88-91] Intrapleural collection of liquid may also cause accessory fissures to stand out where they could not be seen previously[79,92] (Fig. 2-20). The relationship between lung edema and pleural space involvement is described in Chapter 5.

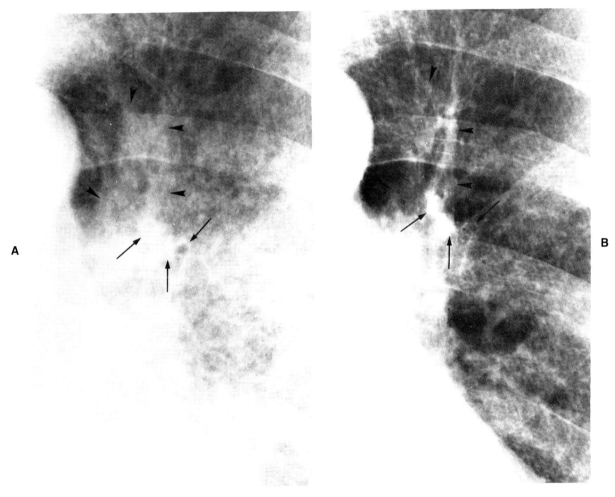

Fig. 2-17   Closeup views of the left perihilar region in a patient with acute myocardial infarction, **A,** while there were clinical and radiographic signs of alveolar edema and, **B,** after recovery. In **A** confluent areas of alveolar edema are associated with peribronchovascular cuffing *(arrows)* and blurring of vascular shadows *(arrowheads).* In **B** note the marked change in perivascular density and the sharp margins of the upper lobe vessels. These vessels were obscured by edema in **A** and became visible only when the patient recovered *(arrowheads).*

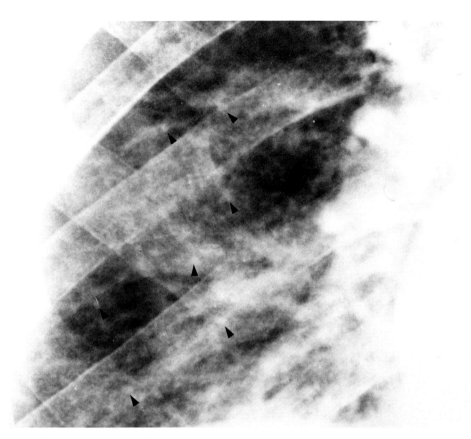

Fig. 2-18 Micronodulation of the right lung base in the chest film of a patient with acute myocardial infarction. Micronoduli (some of them indicated by arrowheads) are consistently observed along the vascular shadows of medium-sized vessels.

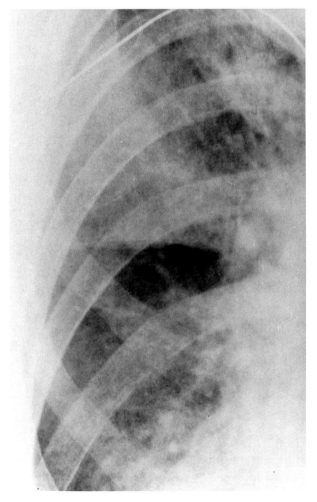

Fig. 2-19 Subpleural effusion in the chest film of a patient with acute myocardial infarction. Peripheral extension of the edema liquid recruits the interstitial space continuous with the pleural layer forming the horizontal fissure. Note the difference between this appearance and that of actual fluid (effusion) within the fissure, as shown in Figs. 2-15 and 2-20, A.

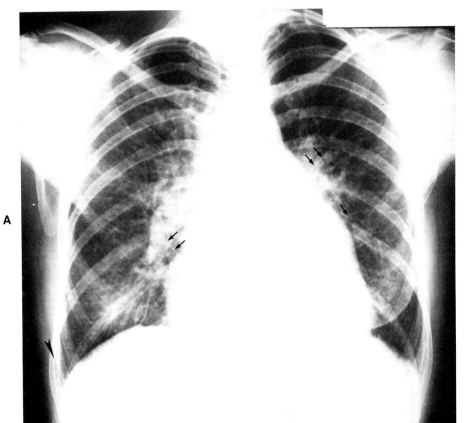

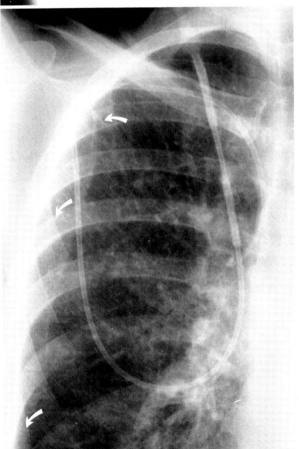

Fig. 2-20   A, The chest film of a woman with acute detachment of a mitral valve prosthesis shows bilateral blurring of the hilar vessels, Kerley A *(small arrows)* and B lines, and widening of the fissures. The widening of the horizontal and median basal accessory fissures (in the right cardiophrenic angle, *open arrow*) is associated with a small pleural effusion *(arrowhead)*. Note that the fissure margins are sharp. **B,** Septal lines in a 20-year-old man with subacute bacterial endocarditis. Note that the septal lines extend up to the clavicle and, as they near the apex, become progressively more vertical *(curved arrows)*.

Kerley's Septal Lines. In addition to subpleural fluid collections and pleural effusions, extension of interstitial edema to the periphery of the lung may cause Kerley's septal lines (Figs. 2-14, 2-15, 2-20, and 2-21). These findings often occur simultaneously since they represent different radiographic aspects of the same event (i.e., collection of edema liquid in the submesothelial pleural interstitium with passage through the visceral pleura into the pleural space).

Kerley's septal lines are the radiographic expression of liquid accumulation within the interlobular septa, which dip into the lung parenchyma from the visceral pleura.[93,94] Kerley described A, B, and C lines. The commonest seen are the *B lines*, very short, thin, unusually dense, and sharply defined (as if drawn with a pen and white ink). These lines occur usually at the base of the lungs, at right angles to the pleural surface, and almost invariably are accompanied by a lamellar effusion. They are only horizontally positioned when they occur just above the diaphragms because the interlobular septa happen to be horizontal at this point. In some cases, where edema is florid, septal lines may extend as high as the apices, at which point they are *vertical* (Fig. 2-20). *A lines* occur in the medial third of the lungs and are frequently seen perpendicular to or crossing the left

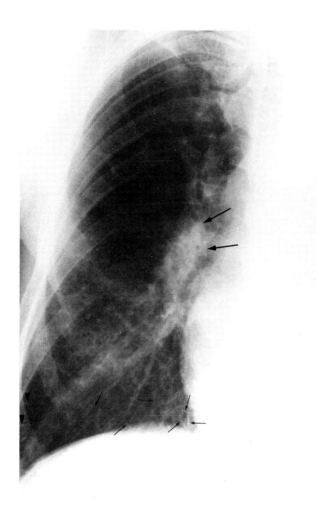

Fig. 2-21   Enlarged view of the right lung taken from the chest film of a patient with recurrent myocardial infarction during decompensation, showing blurring of the hilar vessels and Kerley A *(large arrows)*, B *(arrowheads)*, and C *(small arrows)* septal lines.

heart border diagonally. They are often said to radiate from the hilum, but in fact they usually do not (Figs. 2-20 and 2-21). (The statement that they "radiate from the hilum" probably arose from the old and now disproven[95] belief that Kerley lines were caused by distended lymphatics.) A lines are usually longer and more randomly distributed than B lines because the interlobular septa become sparser and much larger and more irregular as the center of the lung is approached. They share with B lines the unusually sharp margins (in a lung in which all other sharp edges are effaced by edema) and the surprising density (Fig. 2-20). As we have shown, this apparent density is not a physical function of their front-to-back depth but an optical illusion (Mach effect).[95]

C lines are simply the same interlobular septa seen

end-on, encircling the lobule and therefore forming a coarse network pattern (Fig. 2-21). In our experience C lines are rarely sharply defined because of their sloping orientation to the x-ray beam, are much rarer than A or B lines, and are best seen on lateral views.

Septal lines tend to occur when venous pressure rises abruptly, less often when it rises gradually. A lines, in particular, are seen to occur with abrupt changes in venous pressure[79,87,96-98] (e.g., ruptured valve, torn papillary muscle) and may occur without B lines' being seen. It used to be popular to say that B lines in chronic left heart failure could be caused by the presence of fibrous tissue in the interlobular septa[83,93] rather than edema. These lines were said to remain even in mitral valve cases following "successful" surgery. However, in a series of cases that we have analyzed[99] septal lines persisted only in patients in whom the operation was *unsuccessful* (as defined by catheterization), usually following closed finger-fracture of the valve, an operation that was frequently unsuccessful hemodynamically; if the patient had a prosthetic valve inserted, the alleged fibrotic lines abruptly disappeared.

When the interstitial space is completely filled, alveolar edema develops, often quite abruptly (Fig. 2-6, column *4*). The vessels in areas of alveolar edema can no longer be seen because of loss of the air that usually surrounds them (Fig. 2-22) and, for the same reason, the outer borders of peribronchial cuffs and the hilum may become impossible to see (Fig. 2-17). These appearances would accord with an extravascular lung water of 100 to 120 ml H_2O, that is, mild alveolar edema (Table 3-3).

Bats-wing Edema. In contrast to the sequence of edema accumulation just described, in which there is a relatively gradual elevation of pressure, if cardiac (or renal) decompensation is *abrupt* and massive there may be no detectable interstitial phase. It is probable that the interstitium does flood first, even with abrupt decompensation, but this may occur so rapidly as not to be captured radiographically; instead, the initial radiograph may show extensive alveolar flooding. Curiously, when such abrupt decompensation occurs, approximately 10% of cases will show a central distribution of edema (Fig. 2-23) and in a smaller percentage there will be the striking "bats-wing" distribution (Chapter 3), with sharply demarcated outer borders and a lung periphery largely devoid of edema (Fig. 2-24). This distribution is most common in abrupt severe cardiac decompensation (e.g., from a ruptured valve leaflet or massive myocardial infarct, or in severe renal failure).

A curious and partly unexplained finding we have observed in some cases of "bats-wing" edema is that, despite the presence of florid alveolar edema, there is relatively little peribronchovascular cuffing in the area of edema, suggesting that at least some of the initial filling

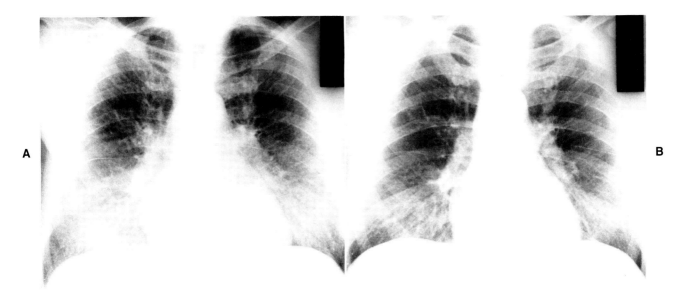

Fig. 2-22 Chest films of a patient with recurrent left heart failure obtained while in failure, **A,** and after partial recovery, **B.** In **A** the diffuse increase of radiographic density in the lower regions of both lungs is associated with confluent areas of alveolar edema obscuring the vessels. Note that from **A** to **B** the blurring of hilar vessels and peribronchovascular cuffs disappears and the vessels "reappear."

phase has been bypassed. An explanation for this could lie in the structure and content of the peribronchovascular sheaths—that is, increasing interstitial tissue edema usually increases liquid conductance, for the following reasons: Within the interstitium (including the peribronchovascular sheaths) water and small ions may percolate through tiny, freely negotiable paths surrounding connective tissue fibers, which, at all lung volumes, are under tension. The ground substance, filling the spaces between the fibers, is formed by a gel of mucopolysaccharides that acts like a molecular sieve. It exerts substantial resistance to liquid and solute flux under conditions of normal hydration but, when tissue hydration increases (i.e., as edema develops), allows water to pass more freely through the interstitium; in other words, its hydraulic conductivity increases. It may be that attempts to increase the peribronchovascular volume *abruptly* will not permit this usual increase in hydraulic conductivity to occur, with the result that interstitial pressure rises abruptly before the sheath space is fully recruited (i.e., before cuffs are fully developed) and fluid passes immediately into the alveoli, without a fully developed preceding interstitial phase.

Several theoretical explanations have been offered for the striking appearance of bats-wing edema,[100,101] of which the most tenable appear to be those of Herrnheiser and Hinson[102] and Fleischner,[103] who suggested that the better pumping action of the periphery of the lung on inspiration and expiration forces fluid centrally.

This mechanism certainly occurs and can be seen quite dramatically in the intensive care unit when a patient with generalized pulmonary edema is put onto high levels of positive-pressure ventilation (Fig. 2-25). The periphery of the lung immediately appears much clearer than the center; however, the characteristic sharp edge of true butterfly edema is not seen under these circumstances and the characteristic lucency along the upper and lower borders of the horizontal fissure is also missing. Thus, although the appearances are somewhat similar, increased ventilation of the periphery of the lung does not appear to offer a complete explanation for true bats-wing edema.

It is tempting to speculate that the *contractility of the alveolar septa,* apparently *designed* to keep them from filling with fluid, may play a role in development of the butterfly pattern by expelling fluid from the peripheral interstitium toward the center of the lung; this would explain why the periphery of all the lung lobes is clear of edema. Incidentally, bats-wing edema has no gravitational component. On lateral films and CT scans the dorsum (or dependent portion) of the lungs is also quite clear in its periphery (Fig. 2-26). Normally, any form of pressure edema would gravitate freely through the interstitial space of the lungs to the bases in the erect position and to the dorsum in the supine position. The fact that this does not occur in bats-wing edema strongly suggests that the peripheral interstitium of the lung may in fact be "closed-off" (by alveolar septal con-

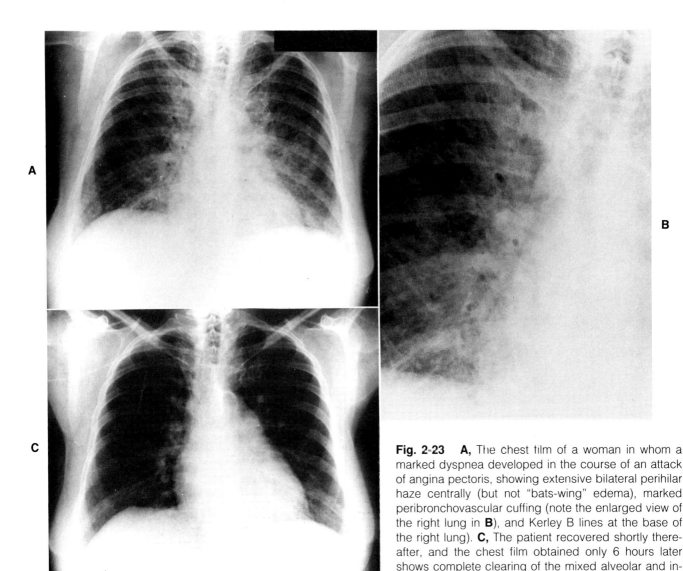

Fig. 2-23 **A,** The chest film of a woman in whom a marked dyspnea developed in the course of an attack of angina pectoris, showing extensive bilateral perihilar haze centrally (but not "bats-wing" edema), marked peribronchovascular cuffing (note the enlarged view of the right lung in **B**), and Kerley B lines at the base of the right lung). **C,** The patient recovered shortly thereafter, and the chest film obtained only 6 hours later shows complete clearing of the mixed alveolar and interstitial edema.

traction?). This explanation would also fit with *our* observation that in bats-wing edema the sharply defined margin of the edema (outlined by the clear edema-free peripheral [cortical] zone) is, in the left lung, unbroken from apex to just above the diaphragm, where it turns medially to leave a clear zone above the diaphragm, but on the right side is broken at the horizontal fissure, where it turns medially (paralleling the horizontal fissure) to leave clear cortical zones along the inferior aspect of the anterior upper lobe and the superior aspect of the middle lobe.

Because of the structural complexity and contents of the lung interstitium, the sequence of development of pulmonary edema is not quite as simple at the microscopic level as would appear from the foregoing descriptions. The reader interested in greater detail on the behavior of fluid within the interstitium is referred to Appendix A of this chapter.

Fig. 2-24 Chest radiographs obtained within a 24-hour period in a patient with acute myocardial infarction. An initial "butterfly" pattern of increased lung density is associated with the radiographic findings of alveolar edema. From **B** to **F** there is progressive clearing of the lung fields and perihilar density with therapy. (Note that peribronchial cuffing is "concealed" in **A** by the surrounding alveolar edema and is best seen in **D** as the alveolar edema is clearing.)

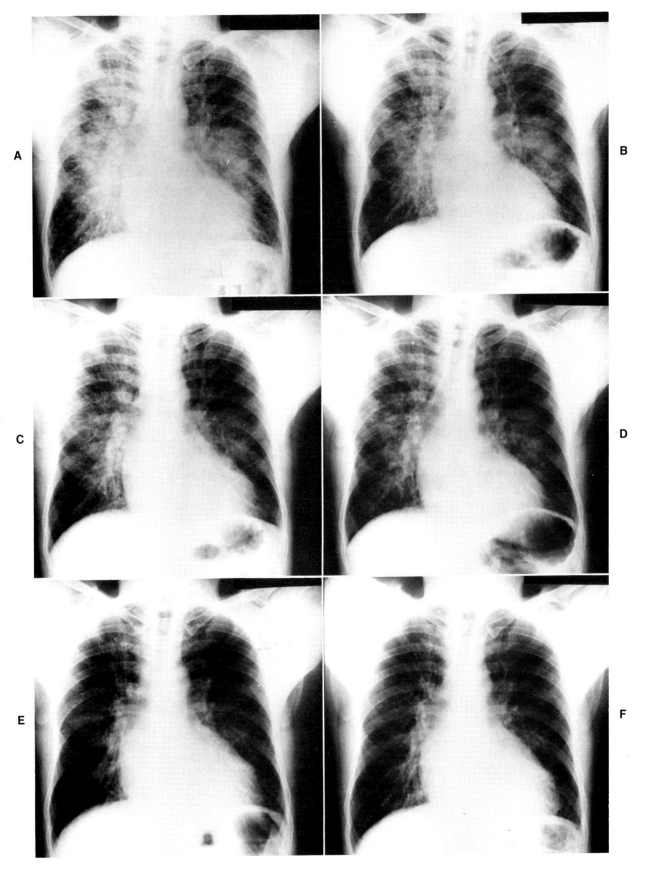

Fig. 2-24   For legend see opposite page.

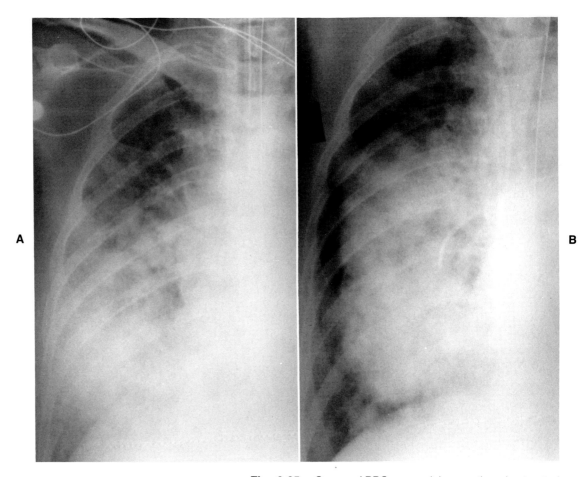

Fig. 2-25 Severe ARDS caused by septicemia, treated with positive-pressure ventilation. **A,** Peak pressure 40, PEEP 15. Edema extends to the periphery of the lung. **B,** Peak pressure increased to 96, PEEP 25. The periphery of the lung seems to clear, giving a "pseudo-bats-wing" appearance.

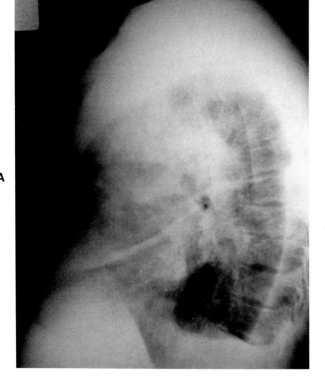

Fig. 2-26 **A,** Lateral view of a patient with renal failure and batswing edema showing the edema to be central and not affected by gravity. **B,** One year later extensive pulmonary ossification has developed that exactly duplicates the distribution of the bats-wing edema. **C** to **E,** Successive CT cuts from the apices to just above the carina show that the ossification, following the bats-wing pattern, completely spares the periphery. (Note the beautiful demonstration of lung lobulation in **C.**)

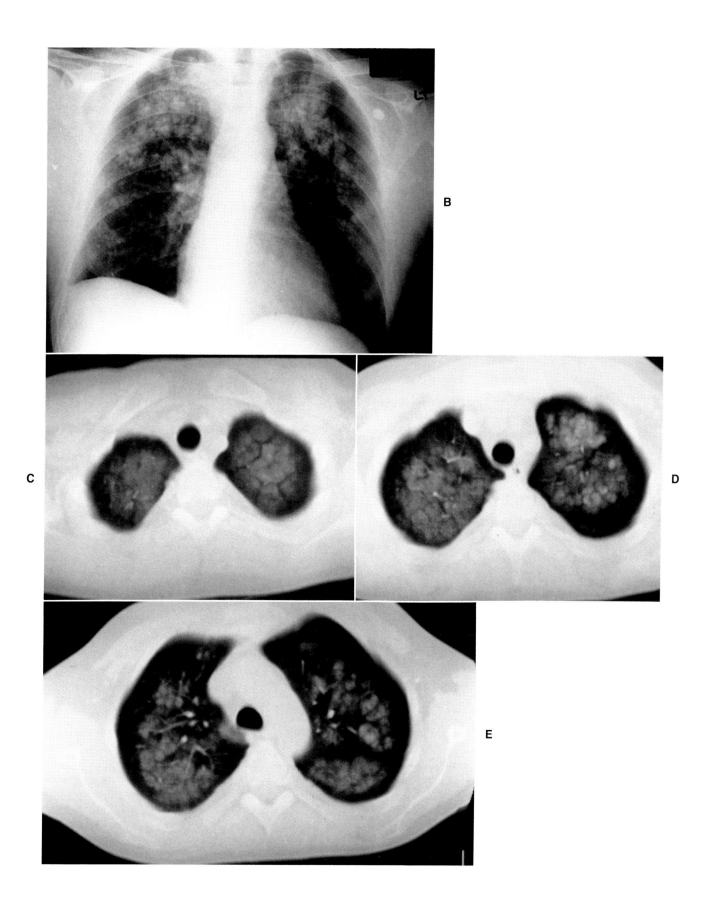

Injury Edema

In injury edema, as previously discussed, the chest radiographic pattern does not follow the characteristic sequence observed in progressive edema (i.e., beginning as an interstitial process and later becoming alveolar).

The first stages of injury edema, when ultrastructural damage is occurring to the epithelium and endothelium, seem to precede the radiologic development of edema. Certainly, the pathophysiologic changes of hypoxemia and diminishing lung compliance and the clinical symptoms of dyspnea occur some 12 to 24 hours before there is radiologic evidence of edema, although occasionally a faint increase in interstitial markings may take place. When the edema does manifest itself, it usually appears quite abruptly in a mixed alveolar and interstitial form,[104] causing a patchy randomly distributed pattern (tending toward a peripheral localization), with little or no evidence of cuffing and no septal lines or evidence of gravitational distribution. The costophrenic angles are often completely spared

(Fig. 2-27). Pleural effusions are rare and when present are usually small (Figs. 2-27 and 2-28). (See Chapters 3 and 8.)

Filling of the air spaces by proteinaceous liquid (Fig. 2-6, column 5) causes air bronchograms to be present in 80% of cases (Fig. 2-28). By contrast, air bronchograms are quite rare in pressure edema, even when alveolar edema is extensive.[21,25,43]* The development of injury edema is usually complete within a 24- to 36-hour period. It is then very characteristic for this pattern, no matter how random or bizarre, to stay quite unchanged for days. In fact, any abrupt change in the pattern strongly suggests the superimposition of some other pathology (aspiration, overhydration, pneumonia, or bleeding) whereas abrupt clearing makes it evident that

---

*We hypothesize that in injury edema the viscid alveolar fluid cannot flow centrally into the bronchi, which therefore remain filled with air, whereas in hydrostatic edema the alveolar fluid can flow into the bronchi, rendering them radiopaque.

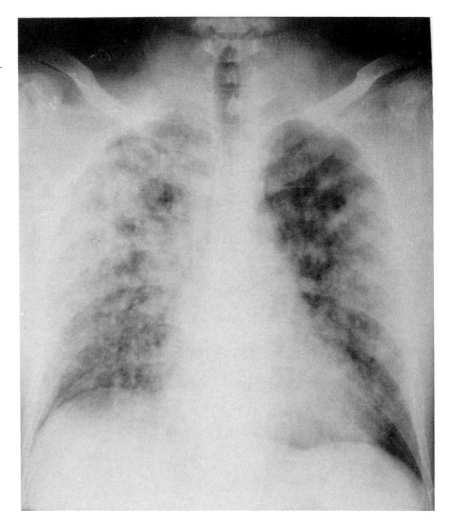

Fig. 2-27   Patient with ARDS after trauma. Note the confluent areas of alveolar edema, more prominent in the periphery of the lungs The costophrenic angles are spared.

the initial diagnosis of injury lung edema was erroneous.

The distribution of the alveolar changes is somewhat dependent upon the etiology. For example, if there has been inhalation of *noxious fumes*, the edema may be largely basal; if there has been *gastric acid aspiration* (often resulting in a gasping inspiration), the edema may be spread from apex to base, though its most frequent distribution, particularly following septicemia or hypovolemic shock, is patchy, random, and nongravitational, with a tendency to spare the costophrenic angles; with *normal pressure injury* lung edema, septal lines (in our experience) are never seen and cuffs are relatively rare (Figs. 2-27 to 2-29). Septal lines may, however, be seen sometimes in association with a viral pneumonia, later leading to injury lung edema (Fig. 2-30) or in normal pressure noninjury (allergic) edema (Fig. 2-31).

Although it is tempting to visualize the presence of open "holes" in the walls of the capillaries in injury lung edema, the holes in fact appear to be blocked very rapidly by fibrin and cells after the initial damage. [4] Electron microscopic evidence for this fits well with the radiologic observation that peribronchovascular cuffing is absent or rare in injury lung edema.[25]

The absence of cuffing in injury lung edema persists unless hydrostatic pressure edema develops on top of the injury edema, as it frequently does, because of fluid administration (extremely common), renal failure, low oncotic pressure, or heart failure. (See Chapter 8.) Under these circumstances endothelial cell junctions that have *not* been injured are free to respond to the increased pressure by opening, recruiting the interstitial space, and causing peribronchovascular cuffing with septal lines. This ties in well with the radiologic observation that *unaffected* areas of lung, interspersed

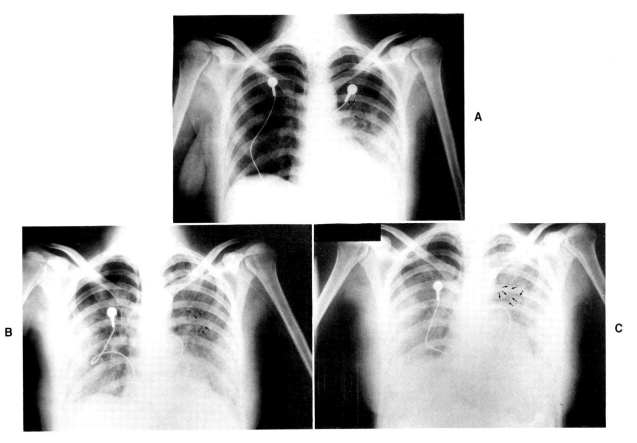

Fig. 2-28   Chest films of a woman obtained, **A,** 1, **B,** 3, and **C,** 4 days after brain hemorrhage following a car accident. The development of patchy increased density in the lower regions of the left lung **(A)** is followed by further ipsilateral and contralateral extension **(B)** until, shortly before the patient's death, an extensive white density develops in both lungs **(C)**. Air bronchograms are prominent throughout the evolution *(arrows)*. In **C** the lumen of the upper lobe bronchus stands out in the consolidated lung. The narrow vascular pedicle and, in the final radiograph, thin soft tissues of the chest wall indicate that no overhydration is present.

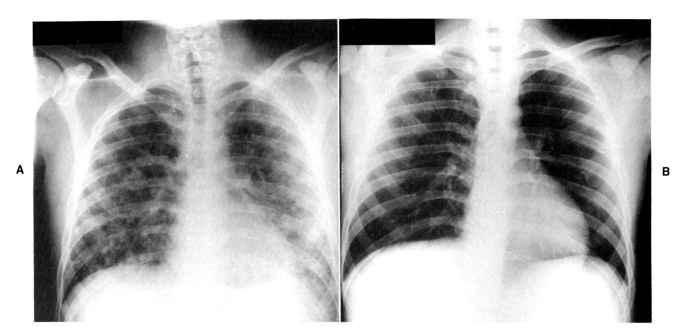

Fig. 2-29   Chest films of a patient with ARDS obtained, **A,** 24 hours after massive trauma to the lower limbs and, **B,** 1 month later, after recovery. In **A** patchy confluent areas of increased lung density involve both lungs, mostly the outer portions. Note the absence of typical radiographic findings of interstitial edema. In **B** the clear right costophrenic angle shows no gravitational distribution of edema.

among the random areas of damage in injury lung edema, become edematous when hydration edema develops. Stated another way, the water is not (as is commonly but, we believe, erroneously suggested) pouring out of "open" holes into the damaged areas.

If resolution occurs (as it does in approximately 35% of the cases of ARDS), it is manifested by a gradual (over several days) sharpening of the borders of each area or patch of consolidation, with slowly progressive (days to weeks) disappearance of the areas of consolidation, leaving some parenchymal scarring; the picture often appears mild compared to the previous full-blown picture of injury edema in that patient (Fig. 2-29).

In hydrostatic edema the much more rapid resolution of alveolar edema is paralleled by the rapid recovery of gas exchange whereas in injury edema the deterioration of respiratory function persists long after visible resolution of the alveolar edema, indicating that repair processes (still ongoing) continue to impair the diffusion of gases through the endothelial/epithelial barrier[105,106] (Fig. 2-32).

APPENDIX A: MECHANICS OF THE INTERSTITIAL SPACE

To explain the dynamic processes involved in the movement of liquid through the interstitium, it is essential to consider the effects of the mechanical forces exerted on the delicate lung structures involved in liquid and solute exchange. Almost all transvascular filtration in the lung takes place from alveolar capillaries and small extraalveolar vessels because they have thin walls, devoid of media and adventitia, and a huge surface area.[24,107] There are three mechanical forces that normally exert pressure on these vessels[108]—tissue tension, capillary distending pressure, and surface tension.

Tissue tension results from the traction exerted during the respiratory cycle on fibers within the alveolar wall. These fibers are anchored at the mouths of the alveoli (the alveolar ducts) to connective tissue fibers that radiate centrifugally from the hilum (Fig. 2-4). They also are connected peripherally at the level of the interlobular septa to fibers that pass centripetally into the lung from the visceral pleura (Figs. 2-4 and 2-33). As the lung expands, the fibers within the alveolar septa are unfolded and stretched along the midplane of the septum (Fig. 2-34). Since these fibers are interwoven with the capillaries (Fig. 2-4, *A*), the tension exerted on them produces a pressure on the capillaries that is normal to the fiber axis and proportional to the degree of lung inflation. The net result of this septal fiber straightening is displacement of the capillaries (whose basement membranes are fused to the alveoli) to one side or the other of the septum while the true intersti-

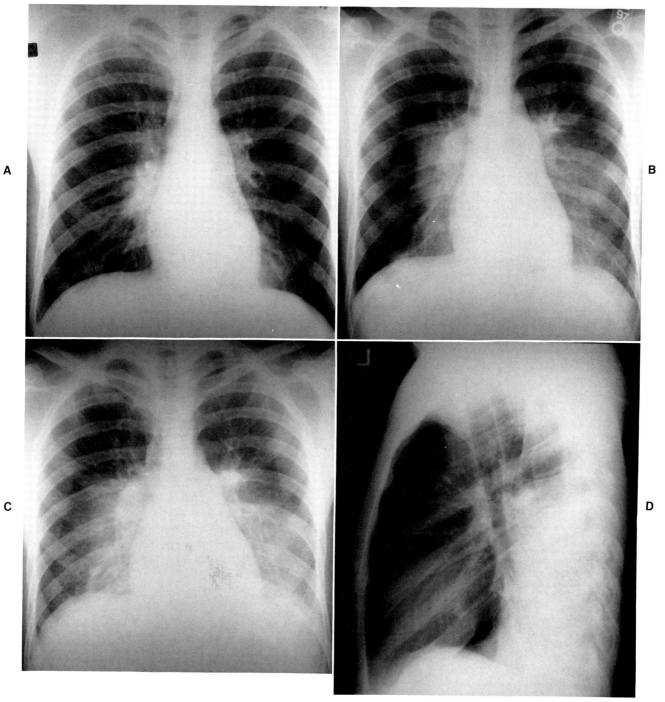

Fig. 2-30 A 24-year-old man with ARDS. **A,** Supine film. Rapidly developing right lymphadenopathy and obscuration of the hilar structure suggest underlying consolidation on the right plus beginning consolidation at the left base. **B,** Twelve hours later another supine film shows rapid development of consolidation, very sharply marginated on the right, giving a pseudo-bats-wing appearance. Note that the heart borders are sharply defined, indicating that the consolidation is posterior. Note also the rapid further enlargement of the right hilar nodes. **C,** Eighteen hours later a third supine film shows peribronchial cuffing and faint septal lines. These are rare in pure ARDS but can be seen with a fulminating pneumonia. In this patient the cause was *Hemophilus influenzae*. **D,** A lateral view shows that the entire process of consolidation is posterior. We believe that fulminating *Hemophilus* pneumonia in the lower lobe caused extremely rapid and massive exudation that, in the supine position, filled the paravertebral gutters gravitationally, giving the sharply defined outer edge, seen in **B.**

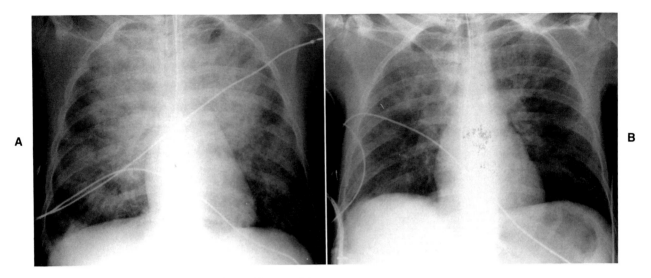

Fig. 2-31   **A,** Leukoagglutinin reaction in a 30-year-old man. Septal lines are present at the right base. **B,** Edema clearing rapidly after intravenous corticosteroids.

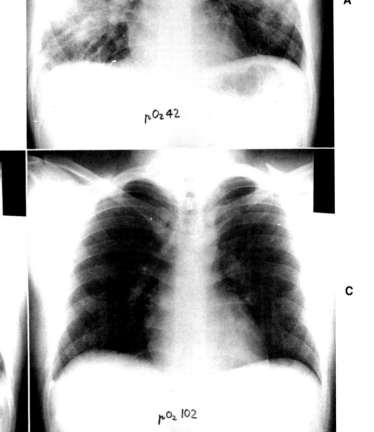

Fig. 2-32   Chest film of a patient with ARDS due to viral pneumonia. In the acute phase, **A,** confluent areas of patchy increased density (with predominantly nongravitational and peripheral distribution) involve both lungs. Arterial oxygen tension while breathing room air is 42 mm Hg. Two days later, **B,** although the lung fields have almost completely cleared, arterial oxygen tension is still remarkably low (64 mm Hg). Four more days, **C,** are needed for arterial oxygen tension to return to normal (102 mm Hg). In **A,** despite the marked increase in size and density (compare with **C**), the hilar vessels are not blurred. See also the hilar vessels in cases of hydrostatic lung edema in previous figures.

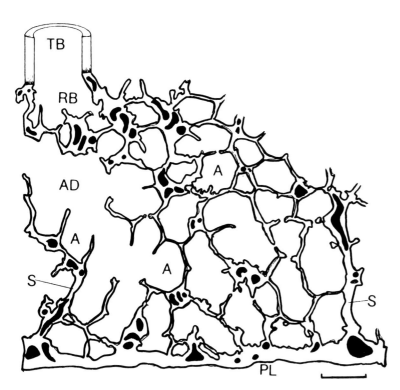

Fig. 2-33 Connective tissue spaces of the distal airways. The septal walls of alveoli *(A)* are contiguous with connective tissue emanating from the hilum and reaching the alveolar ducts *(AD)* around terminal *(TB)* and respiratory *(RB)* bronchioles. Connective tissue dipping into the lung from the visceral pleura *(PL)* is represented by two interlobular septa *(S)*. The black structures are arterioles, venules, and lymphatics in juxtaalveolar connective tissue spaces. (Scale 200 μm.) (Modified from Weibel ER. In Fishman AP, Macklem PT, Mead JS, editors: *Handbook of physiology. The respiratory system,* Section 3, vol 3, part 1. Bethesda, MD, 1986, American Physiological Society, p 89.)

tial space, through which water can flow, remains in the septal midplane[108] (Fig. 2-34).

Capillary distending pressure, generated by the intravascular hydrostatic pressure, has the effect of increasing the bulging of septal capillaries into the alveolar lumen (Fig. 2-34).

Surface tension is produced at the air/liquid interface of the alveolar surfactant lining layer by local deformation forces that tend to keep alveolar surface area to a minimum. The surface force is proportional to the level of alveolar inflation and is directed inward over convex portions of the alveolar surface where capillaries bulge, and outward in the concave depressions between capillaries (Fig. 2-34). Alveoli would tend to collapse if these surface forces were not counteracted by surfactant. Alveolar surfactant reduces the surface tension by pooling in pits between the protruding capillaries. This produces a rather smooth air/liquid interface whose surface area is significantly smaller than that covered by the epithelial cells. Furthermore, as alveoli become progressively smaller under the effect of surface tension forces, the compression exerted on the phospholipid layer of the alveolar surfactant generates an opposing reduction in surface tension.

• • •

The combined effect of tissue tension, capillary distending pressure, and surface tension on liquid dynamics in the alveolar septum is to produce a gradient of interstitial hydrostatic pressure from the compressed pericapillary space toward the intercapillary "pits," where the true interstitial space is located (Fig. 2-34). Because of this gradient, liquid filtered from capillaries is forced along the collagen support fibers in the midplane of the septa and into the alveolar corners, where three septa meet (triple junctions) (Fig. 2-34). The curvature radius at triple junctions is greater than that in the flat portion of the septum, causing a greater surface tension and consequently a lower interstitial hydrostatic pressure in these regions.[22,108] The migration of liquid from the pericapillary space to the intercapillary pits and from there along the fiber system toward triple junction lines, along a gradient of progressively more negative interstitial pressure, is similar to that of ink deposited on the flat surface of soap froth. The ink is sucked into triple junctions and moves along these lines, bypassing flat surfaces.[22,24]

Migrating liquid next enters the juxtaalveolar connective tissue spaces in the interlobular septa and alveolar duct regions, and the sheaths around distal bronchioles, which serve as liquid sumps and contain terminal lymphatics. This movement of liquid from the site of filtration to tissue spaces relatively remote from the alveolar septa is facilitated by cyclic lung inflation. Increased transpulmonary pressure and lung inflation enhance surface tension forces at triple junctions and produce traction on the juxtaalveolar connective tissue sumps, to which alveolar walls are firmly attached. The interstitial hydrostatic pressure becomes thus more and more negative, proceeding from the pericapillary space

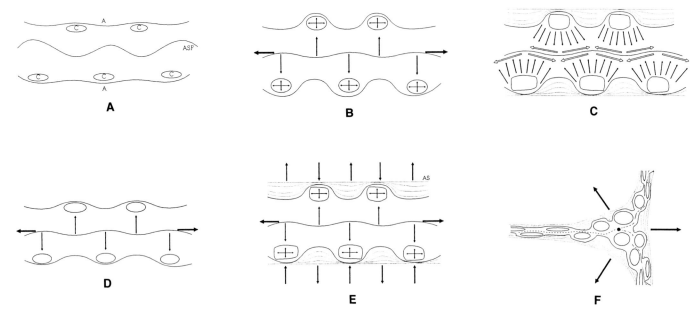

Fig. 2-34 Effects of mechanical forces on alveolar geometry and septal liquid movement. **A,** Main anatomic structures of the alveolar septum on which or by which mechanical forces are exerted. Each septum with its extensive network of capillaries (C) has two epithelial surfaces in contact with air in the alveoli (A). Collagen alveolar septal fibers (ASF) are located in the septal midplane. **B,** *Tissue tension.* Alveolar septal fibers are straightened and unfolded by lung inflation. Capillaries bulge into the alveolar lumina. **C,** *Capillary distending pressure.* Intraluminal hydrostatic capillary pressure enhances the bulging of capillaries into the alveolar lumina. **D,** *Surface tension.* At the air-liquid interface, pressure is exerted, alternately, toward the alveolus over concave surfaces (*between* bulging capillaries) and toward the septum over convex surfaces (*over* bulging capillaries). Alveolar surfactant (AS) deposited in thin layers over the capillaries and lying in small pools between the capillaries reduces the effects of surface tension forces on alveolar geometry. **E,** *Composite effect of tissue tension, capillary distending pressure, and surface tension.* Hydrostatic pressure is lower in the intercapillary pits and the septal midplane with respect to the pericapillary space. Liquid filtered from the capillaries is moved along the pressure gradient from the pericapillary interstitium toward the septal midplane (*thin arrows*), where it can spread along septal connective fibers and associated interstitial liquid spaces (*open arrows*). **F,** Interstitial pressure at triple junctions of alveolar walls. Because of greater curvature at the alveolar corners, surface tension forces are higher (*thick arrows*) and interstitial pressure is lower in the regions where three septa meet than on flat portions of the septa. Liquid is moved along this pressure gradient (*dashed lines*) toward the triple junctions. Note that the alveolar "corner" vessels are more widely opened than the capillaries along the flat surface of the septum.

in the alveolar septa to the juxtaalveolar connective tissue.

Lung vessels may be subdivided into *extraalveolar* and *alveolar* according to their behavior as the lung is inflated (Fig. 2-35). Small (extraalveolar) arterioles and venules located in juxtaalveolar connective tissue sheaths actually expand when the lung is inflated, in contrast to the alveolar vessels (in the flat portion of the septum), which may close on inflation. Because of the local increase in surface tension forces, vessels located in the corners of triple junctions (*corner* vessels) do not close even at high intraalveolar pressures.[109] The behavior of corner vessels is, in this respect, intermediate between the behaviors of extraalveolar and alveolar vessels, since at high transpulmonary pressures they do not expand as extraalveolar vessels do, but they do not collapse either, as alveolar vessels do (Fig. 2-35).

These mechanical forces operating on the lung microvessels may affect not only their resistance to flow but also their liquid and solute exchange properties. The walls of extraalveolar vessels and, to a lesser extent, of corner vessels are under greater tension than the walls of vessels in the flat portion of the septum. This may lead to a greater degree of stretching of the endothelial intercellular junctions in the extraalveolar vessels, and as a consequence plasma protein may leak more easily through these vessel walls in the junctional tissue than through septal capillaries.[48] This could be of

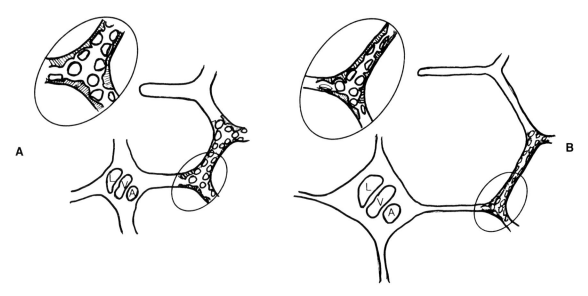

Fig. 2-35   Effects of lung expansion on alveolar and extraalveolar vessels. During lung inflation (from low, **A,** to high, **B,** intraalveolar pressure) the microvessels behave differently (according to their location, which affects the pressures "seen" by the vessels). Capillaries (alveolar vessels) of the flat surface of the septum are flattened and may be closed. The septal "corner" vessels remain open while arterioles *(A)*, venules *(V)*, and (juxtaalveolar) lymphatics *(L)* within the juxtaalveolar connective tissue actually dilate.

importance in the turnover of lung interstitial protein, since a substantial fraction of the overall protein leakage may take place in the same anatomic locations in which the terminal lymphatics are located.

The gradient of interstitial hydrostatic pressure from the alveolar septa to the juxtaalveolar regions continues along successively larger bronchi and vessels toward the perihilar connective tissue spaces,[49,50,110] whose compliance has been estimated to be up to 10 times the normal interstitial compliance for the whole lung.[22] These perihilar spaces can therefore be considered to be sumps with a high capacity for liquid collection. Under normal conditions the highly compliant peribronchovascular space is empty because the lymphatics can return all sorts of liquid and protein to the systemic circulation.

In conclusion, it is clear that an interlinked series of anatomic and physiologic features keeps the lung at work as both a gas and a liquid and solute exchanger. The most relevant pathophysiologic and clinical consequence of interference with these two functions is the presence of excess liquid in the gas exchange apparatus (i.e., the development of pulmonary edema).

APPENDIX B: SOME CONCERNS ABOUT THE APPLICATION OF THE STARLING EQUATION

When the Starling equation is used to assess how much change in water flow across a capillary wall will occur in response to a given change in intra- or extravascular pressure, the fact that the change in pressure may cause simultaneous changes in Kf and σ (particularly at high pressure levels) is not usually factored into the calculation. Fig. 2-5 illustrates that as intravascular pressure rises the endothelial cell junctions may begin to open (probably in the 25+ mm Hg range) and at this point Kf and, to a lesser extent, σ will begin to change. Fig. 2-5 should be compared with Fig. 2-6. If changes in Kf and σ are not factored into the Starling calculations, there may be a progressive underestimation of the amount of water flow with progressive elevation of hydrostatic pressure, as shown by the examples below. (Note, however, that if the change occurs only in *oncotic* pressure and not in hydrostatic pressure, since there will then be no change in Kf or σ, the standard Starling calculation should give a more correct assessment of the change in flow.)

Starling equation

$$Qf = Kf([HPiv - OPiv] - \sigma [HPev - OPev])$$

Example I. Static situation—normal pressures

Where HPiv = 10 mm Hg, OPiv = 25 mm Hg, HPev = −3 mm Hg, and OPev = 19 mm Hg.

Kf is taken to be 1, and for simplicity σ is also 1 (often quoted from experimental data as 0.96).

$$Qf= 1 ([10-(-3)] - 1 [25-19])$$
$$= 7 \text{ ml } H_2O/min/mm \text{ Hg/unit area}$$

Example II. If HPiv is now raised to 30 mm Hg and the effects of this elevation on Kf and σ are *ignored (as they usually are).*

$$Qf = 1 ([30-(-3)] - 1 [25-19])$$
$$= 27 \text{ ml } H_2O/\text{min/mm Hg/unit area}$$

Example III. If Kf and σ change as a result of the widened endothelial cell junctions, suppose that Kf now = 2 and σ = 0.5 (arbitrary numbers).

$$Qf = 2 ([30-(-3)]) - 0.5 [25-19])$$
$$= 60 \text{ ml } H_2O/\text{min/mm Hg/unit area}$$

For simplicity, the effects of the changing oncotic pressures in the interstitium (caused by dilution) and shown in Fig. 2-5 are not included in this calculation.

There are other factors that make the problems of understanding the Starling equation and applying it rationally even more difficult:

1. The meaning of Kf appears to vary from author to author. Kf is clearly not a constant but is more a "fudge factor" and appears to include several components (including, it has been suggested, pore size, pore length, pore area, and viscosity), all of which dictate hydraulic conductivity and may also affect the oncotic reflection coefficient.[18] Indeed, some authors[18] appear to include σ within the Kf rather than use it as a separate factor in the Starling equation.

2. If the hypothesis is correct that water exchange occurs at the endothelial cell junctions only (or largely), then, since by Poiseuille's law resistance to flow through a channel is proportional to the fourth power of its radius, very small changes in junction diameter will have quite major effects on flow whereas much larger changes may be required to produce a change in σ (the oncotic reflection coefficient). This is reflected in Fig. 2-5.

3. There is evidence that Kf may vary considerably anatomically from the arterial to the venous end of a capillary and that there is a neurohormonal mechanism controlling the width of the capillary venular endothelial cell junctions (and thus Kf and σ).[18]

As we have already indicated, these objections refer only to the way in which the Starling equation may be used and do not cast doubt on the principles of capillary filtration enunciated by Starling.[20]

APPENDIX C: SEQUENCE OF ACCUMULATION IN PRESSURE VERSUS INJURY LUNG EDEMA

A paper by Staub et al[46] is often cited as evidence that the sequence of edema formation in pressure and injury edema is the same. It must be stressed, however, that in this paper the microscopic specimens used for demonstrating the sequence of lung liquid accumulation were all obtained at the *end* of the experiment and cannot therefore be directly related to either (1) the physiologic variables measured in the dog from which the tissue samples were obtained or (2) the different phases of the experimental procedure chosen to induce lung edema. In both pressure edema and injury edema, tissue samples showing mild edema (interstitial) were used to describe the "earliest" stages of lung liquid accumulation whereas tissue samples showing severe edema (alveolar) were used to describe the later stages of such accumulation.

It is clear from this experimental design that inferring a temporal sequence from an observation made at one time (the end of the experiment) is somewhat artificial. To illustrate the sequence of extravascular compartment filling by edema, the paper needed to show temporally matched anatomic and physiologic data in different animals with differing grades of edema. It would be more correct to conclude that this work simply indicated that microscopic specimens with mild or moderate edema (resulting from either pressure or injury) showed no flooding of the alveolar compartment. This appearance could equally well have reflected the early phases of pressure edema or mild injury edema (i.e., in dogs in which alloxan did not cause any catastrophic injury of the endothelial/epithelial barrier). The dogs injected with alloxan received doses ranging from 50 to 150 mg/kg, but there was no reported correlation between the amount of alloxan injected and the severity of the edema.[46] It has been suggested that alloxan may induce, soon after injection, pulmonary venous constriction[111,112] and that this may, at least in the early stage of lung edema induction, cause excess liquid filtration by a *hydrostatic* mechanism. In the series of dogs injected with alloxan, there was indeed an initial transient rise of mean pulmonary arterial pressure. The authors denied that there could have been any hydrostatic component of edema, however, because the dogs had low left ventricular end-diastolic pressures throughout the experiment and, at least in the early phases, normal values of extravascular lung water. However, normal left ventricular filling pressures do not exclude hemodynamic alterations caused by regional pulmonary venous constriction (or by increasing negative interstitial pressure). Also the "normal" values of extravascular lung water calculated soon after injection of alloxan were obtained in only 3 of the 12 dogs—using the standard isotopic double-indicator dilution method, which has been shown to be quite insensitive, particularly in the earlier phases of edema formation (Chapter 3).

The authors' conclusion that the sequence of filling of extravascular lung compartments is the same in hydrostatic and injury edema is further weakened by the very different degree of involvement of the gas exchange apparatus in the two types of edema. In both the early and the late stages of edema induction, using the physiologic data reported in their own paper,[46] it can be seen that the carbon monoxide diffusing capacity and alveolar/arterial oxygen gradients were much more impaired in the dogs with injury edema than in those with pressure edema.

In the same year that the paper by Staub et al. was published, Cottrell et al.[40] showed by electron microscopy that, for comparable amounts of edema (confirmed gravimetrically) in dogs with pressure edema, the liquid accumulation was confined to the interstitial portion of the septum and the epithelial/endothelial layers were intact. By contrast, the dogs with injury edema, in which liquid was found in all portions of the septum and in the alveoli, had severe damage to both endothelium and epithelium. These authors concluded[40] that "the hemodynamic type of pulmonary edema appears to result from an accentuation of the normal process of fluid exchange within the lung. Alloxan-induced edema (i.e., injury edema), on the other hand, is a pathologic process."

These experimental observations are in keeping with the clinical findings that patients with injury lung edema have a greater and earlier impairment of respiratory function than patients with hydrostatic pulmonary edema, in whom gas exchange is not severely affected until alveolar edema develops. The work indicates, furthermore, that the sequence of edema formation under discussion (i.e., filling of peribronchovascular fluid sumps followed by thickening of the alveolar septum and eventually by flooding of alveoli) occurs only in hydrostatic forms of lung edema whereas in injury lung edema there appears to be earlier and more severe invasion of the air spaces, possibly before the interstitial fluid sumps are recruited.

Recently, in keeping with this interpretation, it has been shown by electron microscopy[4,39,41] that in both experimental and clinical conditions of injury edema, early and severe damage to the *epithelial* barrier is the primary factor, explaining the remarkably different pathophysiologic and clinical alterations seen in injury compared to pressure lung edema. The paper of Montaner et al.[41] shows that with the same amount of fluid accumulation, abnormalities of gas exchange were worse in the dogs with injury lung edema than in those with pressure edema. In the dogs injected with oleic acid to produce injury, light microscopy showed that 5% of the specimens examined had no edema, 14% had interstitial edema, and *81%* had alveolar edema. By contrast, in the dogs with pressure edema the same figures were 33%, 35%, and 30%. The peribronchovascular cuffs in the dogs with pressure edema were of much larger area than in those with injury edema. These results indicate that with comparable amounts of edema there is a far greater degree of alveolar flooding in injury edema than in hydrostatic edema (in which, by

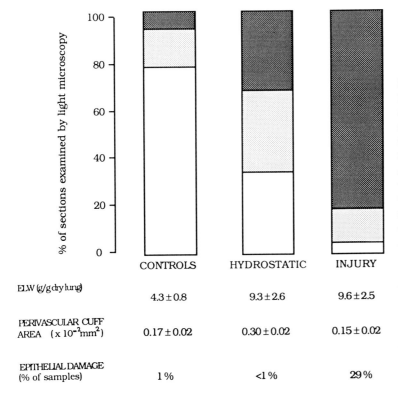

□ no edema
□ interstitial edema
▓ alveolar edema

Fig. 2-36 Relative distribution of extravascular lung liquid between interstitial and alveolar compartments in dogs with hydrostatic edema (n = 6) (induced either by increasing left ventricle filling pressure or by overhydration) (n = 6) and injury edema (induced by injection of oleic acid) (n = 6). In both conditions extravascular lung water *(ELW)* is increased to the same amount compared to controls (n = 6). As assessed by light microscopy, dogs with injury lung edema show a much greater degree of alveolar flooding and dogs with hydrostatic lung edema greater distention of the interstitial space. Perivascular cuff area is twice as large in hydrostatic edema. The injury cases show electron microscopic evidence of extensive alveolar epithelial damage. [Modified from Montaner JSG, Tsang J, Evans KG, et al: *J Clin Invest* 77:1786, 1986.]

	CONTROLS	HYDROSTATIC	INJURY
ELW (g/g dry lung)	4.3 ± 0.8	9.3 ± 2.6	9.6 ± 2.5
PERIVASCULAR CUFF AREA (x 10⁻²mm²)	0.17 ± 0.02	0.30 ± 0.02	0.15 ± 0.02
EPITHELIAL DAMAGE (% of samples)	1%	<1%	29%

contrast, there is much more distention of the interstitial space) (Fig. 2-36).

It is clear that, although the interstitial space of the lung has a large capacity to accumulate edema, in *injury* lung edema it is the air spaces that are flooded even when the interstitial liquid sumps contain little fluid. Damage to the epithelial barrier (Fig. 2-36), allowing liquid and solute to flood the alveoli, is the critical factor distinguishing the sequence of events of liquid accumulation in injury as compared to pressure edema.

REFERENCES

1. Dunnill MS: Morphology of the human lung in health and disease. In Hunt C (ed): *Form and function in the human lung*, Baltimore, 1968, Williams & Wilkins, p 19.
2. Guz A, Noble MIM, Trenchard D: The significance of a raised central venous pressure during sodium and water retention, *Clin Sci* 30:295, 1966.
3. Chinard FP, Enns T, Nolan MR: Indicator-dilution studies with "diffusible" indicators, *Circ Res* 10:473, 1962.
4. Bachofen H, Bachofen M, Weibel ER. Ultrastructural aspects of pulmonary edema, *J Thorac Imaging* 3(3):1, 1988.
5. Schneeberger EE: Structure of intercellular junctions in different segments of the intrapulmonary vasculature, *Ann NY Acad Sci* 384:54, 1982.
6. Cyrlak D, Milne ENC: Pneumomediastinum: a diagnostic problem, *CRC Crit Rev Diagn Imag* 23:75, 1984.
7. Staub NC: New concepts about the pathophysiology of pulmonary edema, *J Thorac Imaging* 3(3):8, 1988.
8. Milne ENC: Editorial, *J Thorac Imaging* 3(3):6, 1988.
9. Goldberg JD, Mitchell N: Mediastinal emphysema and pneumothorax following tracheotomy for croup, *Am J Surg* 106:448, 1942.
10. Macklin CC: Pneumothorax with massive collapse from experimental local overinflation of the lung substance, *Can Med Assoc J* 36:414, 1937.
11. Macklin CC: Transport of air along sheaths of pulmonic blood vessels from alveoli to mediastium: clinical implications, *Arch Intern Med* 64:913, 1939.
12. Marchand P: The anatomy and applied anatomy of the mediastinal fascia, *Thorax* 6:359, 1951.
13. Weibel ER, Bachofen H: Structural design of the alveolar septum and fluid exchange. In Fishman AP, Renkin EM (eds): *Pulmonary edema*, Bethesda, 1979, American Physiological Society, p 1.
14. Kapanci Y, Assimacopoulos A, Zwahlen A, et al: "Contractile interstitial cells" in pulmonary alveolar septa, *J Cell Biol* 60:375, 1974.
15. Lauweryns JM: The juxta-alveolar lymphatics in human adult lung, *Am Rev Respir Dis* 102:877, 1970.
16. Gil J: Lung interstitium, vascular and alveolar membranes. In Staub NC (ed): *Lung water and solute exchange*, New York, 1978, Marcel Dekker, p 49.
17. Vreim CE, Snashall PD, Staub NC: Protein composition of lung fluids in anesthetized dogs with acute cardiogenic edema, *Am J Physiol* 231:1466, 1976.
18. Honig CR: *Modern cardiovascular physiology*, ed 2, Boston, 1988, Little, Brown.
19. Taylor AE, Parker JC, Kvietys PR, Perry MA: The pulmonary interstitium in capillary exchange, *Ann NY Acad Sci* 384:146, 1982.
20. Starling EH: On the absorption of fluid from the connective tissue spaces, *J Physiol* 19:312, 1896.
21. Milne ENC, Pistolesi M: Pulmonary edema—cardiac and noncardiac. In Putman CE (ed): *Diagnostic imaging of the lung*, New York, 1990, Marcel Dekker, p 253.
22. Taylor AE, Parker JC: Pulmonary interstitial spaces and lymphatics. In Fishman AP, Fisher AB (eds): *Handbook of physiology. The respiratory system I*, Bethesda, 1985, American Physiological Society, p 167.
23. Flick MR: Pulmonary edema and acute lung injury. In Murray JF, Nadel JA (eds): *Textbook of respiratory medicine*, Philadelphia, 1988, WB Saunders, p 1359.
24. Staub NC: Pulmonary edema, *Physiol Rev* 54:678, 1974.
25. Milne ENC, Pistolesi M, Miniati M, Giuntini C: The radiologic distinction of cardiogenic and non-cardiogenic edema, *AJR* 144:879, 1985.
26. Staub NC: Pulmonary edema: physiologic approaches to management, *Chest* 74:559, 1978.
27. Pistolesi M, Miniati M, Giuntini C: State of the art: pleural liquid and solute exchange, *Am Rev Respir Dis* 140:825, 1989.
28. Bachofen M, Bachofen H, Weibel ER: Lung edema in the adult respiratory distress syndrome. In Fishman AP, Renkin EM (eds): *Pulmonary edema*, Bethesda, 1979, American Physiological Society, p. 241.
29. Bachofen M, Weibel ER: Structural alterations of lung parenchyma in the adult respiratory distress syndrome, *Clin Chest Med* 3:35, 1982.
30. Bachofen M: Personal communication.
31. Whayne TF, Severinghaus JW: Experimental hypoxic pulmonary edema in the rat, *J Appl Physiol* 25(6):729, 1968.
32. Schoene RB: Pulmonary edema at high altitude. Review, pathophysiology, and update, *Clin Chest Med* 6:491, 1985.
33. Colice GL: Neurogenic pulmonary edema, *Clin Chest Med* 6:473, 1985.
34. West JB, Tsukimoto K, Mathieu-Costello O, Prediletto R: Stress failure in pulmonary capillaries, *J Appl Physiol* 70:1731, 1991.
35. Iannuzzi M, Petty TL: The diagnosis, pathogenesis and treatment of adult respiratory distress syndrome, *J Thorac Imaging* 1(3):1, 1986.
36. Fowler AA, Hamman RF, Good JT, et al: Adult respiratory distress syndrome: risk with common predisposition, *Ann Intern Med* 98:593, 1983.
37. Matthay MA: Pathophysiology of pulmonary edema, *Clin Chest Med* 6:301, 1985.
38. Andreadis N, Petty TL: Adult respiratory distress syndrome: problems and progress, *Am Rev Respir Dis* 132:1344, 1985.
39. Bachofen M, Weibel ER: Alterations of the gas exchange apparatus in adult respiratory insufficiency associated with septicemia, *Am Rev Respir Dis* 116:589, 1977.
40. Cottrel TS, Levine OR, Senior RM, et al: Electron microscopic alterations at the alveolar level in pulmonary edema, *Circ Res* 21:783, 1967.
41. Montaner JSG, Tsang J, Evans KG, et al: Alveolar epithelial damage. A critical difference between high pressure and oleic acid–induced low pressure pulmonary edema, *J Clin Invest* 77:1786, 1986.
42. Comper WD, Laurent TC: Physiological function of connective tissue polysaccharides, *Physiol Rev* 58:255, 1978.
43. Miniati M, Pistolesi M, Paoletti P, et al: Objective radiographic criteria to differentiate cardiac, renal and injury lung edema, *Invest Radiol* 23:433, 1988.
44. Pistolesi M, Miniati M, Milne ENC, Giuntini C: Pulmonary edema. In Sperber M (ed): *Radiologic diagnosis of chest disease*, New York, 1990, Springer-Verlag, p 355.
45. Milne ENC: A physiologic approach to reading critical care unit films, *J Thorac Imaging* 1(3):60, 1986.
46. Staub NC, Nagano H, Pearce ML: Pulmonary edema in dogs,

especially the sequence of fluid accumulation in lungs, *J Appl Physiol* 22:227, 1967.

47. Ingram RH, Braunwald E: Pulmonary edema: cardiogenic and non-cardiogenic. In Braunwald E (ed): *Heart disease. A textbook of cardiovascular medicine*, ed 3, Philadelphia, 1988, WB Saunders p 544.

48. Guyton AC, Parker JC, Taylor AE, et al: Forces governing water movement in the lung. In Fishman AP, Renkin EM (eds): *Pulmonary edema*, Bethesda, 1979, American Physiological Society, p 65.

49. Inoue H, Inoue C, Hildebrandt J: Vascular and airway pressures and interstitial edema affect peribronchial fluid pressure, *J Appl Physiol* 48:177, 1980.

50. Lai-Fook SJ, Toporoff B: Pressure-volume behavior of perivascular interstitium measured in isolated dog lung, *J Appl Physiol* 48:939, 1980.

51. Drinker CD: *Pulmonary edema and inflammation*, Cambridge Mass, 1947, Harvard University Press.

52. Parker JC, Crain M, Grimbert F, et al: Total lung lymph flow and fluid compartmentation in edematous dog lungs, *J Appl Physiol* 51:1268, 1981.

53. Gee MH, Donovan KA: The flow and composition of pulmonary lymph in dogs with edema, *Lymphology* 12:125, 1979.

54. Nicoll PA, Taylor AE: Lymph formation and flow, *Ann Rev Physiol* 39:73, 1977.

55. Gee MH, Spath JA Jr: The dynamics of the lung fluid filtration system in dogs with edema, *Circ Res* 46:796, 1980.

56. Nakahara K, Nanjo S, Maeda M, Kawashima Y: Dynamic insufficiency of lung lymph flow from the right lymph duct in dogs with acute filtration edema, *Am Rev Respir Dis* 127:67, 1983.

57. Rabin ER, Meyer EC: Cardiopulmonary effects of pulmonary venous hypertension with special reference to pulmonary lymphatic flow, *Circ Res* 8:324, 1960.

58. Uhley H, Leeds SE, Sampson JJ, Friedman M: Some observations on the role of the lymphatics in experimental acute pulmonary edema, *Circ Res* 9:688, 1961.

59. Coalson JJ, Jacques WE, Campbell GS: Ultrastructure of the alveolar-capillary membrane in congenital and acquired heart disease, *Arch Pathol* 83:377, 1967.

60. Harris P, Heath D: *The human pulmonary circulation*, Edinburgh, 1977, Churchill-Livingstone, p 332.

61. Spencer H: *Pathology of the lung*, New York, 1977, Pergamon Press, p 116.

62. Giuntini C, Pistolesi M, Miniati M: Pulmonary venous hypertension. Mechanisms and consequences. In Wagenvoort CA, Denolin M (eds): *Pulmonary circulation*, Amsterdam, 1989, Elsevier, p 131.

63. Uhley MN, Leeds SE, Sampson JJ, Friedman M: Role of pulmonary lymphatics in chronic pulmonary edema, *Circ Res* 11:966:1962.

64. Gee MH, Staub NC: Role of bulk fluid flow in protein permeability of the dog lung alveolar membrane, *J Appl Physiol* 42:144, 1977.

65. Havill AM, Gee MH: Role of interstitium in clearance of alveolar fluid in normal and injured lungs, *J Appl Physiol* 57:1, 1984.

66. Matthay MA, Landolt CC, Staub NC: Differential liquid and protein clearance from the alveoli of anesthetized sheep, *J Appl Physiol* 53:96, 1982.

67. Matthay MA, Berthiaume Y, Staub NC: Long-term clearance of liquid and protein from the lungs of unanesthetized sheep, *J Appl Physiol* 59:928, 1985.

68. Matthay MA: Resolution of pulmonary edema. Mechanisms of liquid, protein, and cellular clearance from the lung, *Clin Chest Med* 6:521, 1985.

69. Cutillo AG, Morris AH, Ailion DC, et al: Quantitative assessment of pulmonary edema by nuclear magnetic resonance methods, *J Thorac Imaging* 3(3):51, 1988.

70. Morris AH, Cutillo AG, Ailion DC, et al: Pulmonary nuclear magnetic resonance: potential applications in ARDS. In Zapol WM, Lemaire F (eds): *Adult respiratory distress syndrome*, New York, 1991, Marcel Dekker, p 411.

71. Podgorski GT, Carrol FE, Parker RE: MR evaluation of pulmonary interstitial and intravascular fluids, *Invest Radiol* 21:478, 1986.

72. Pistolesi M, Miniati M, Ravelli V, Giuntini C: Injury versus hydrostatic lung edema: detection by chest x-ray, *Ann NY Acad Sci* 384:364, 1982.

73. Gee MH, Havill AM: The relationship between pulmonary perivascular cuff fluid and lung lymph in dogs with edema, *Microvasc Res* 19:209, 1980.

74. Pistolesi M, Miniati M, Milne ENC, Giuntini C: The chest roentgenogram in pulmonary edema, *Clin Chest Med* 6:315, 1985.

75. Smith RC, Mann H, Greenspan RH, et al: Radiographic differentiation between different etiologies of pulmonary edema, *Invest Radiol* 22:859, 1987.

76. Fraser RG, Paré JAP, Paré PD, et al: *Diagnosis of disease of the chest*, ed 3, vol 3, Philadelphia, 1990, WB Saunders, p 1823.

77. Murray JF: Disorders of the pulmonary circulation. General principles and diagnostic approach. In Murray JF, Nadel JA (eds): *Textbook of respiratory medicine*, Philadelphia, 1988, WB Saunders, p 1271.

78. Fishman AP: Pulmonary edema. In Fishman AP (ed): *Pulmonary diseases and disorders*, ed 2, vol 2, New York, 1988, McGraw-Hill, p 919.

79. Pistolesi M, Giuntini C: Assessment of extravascular lung water, *Radiol Clin North Am* 16:551, 1978.

80. Gleason DC, Steiner RE: The lateral roentgenogram in pulmonary edema, *AJR* 98:279, 1966.

81. Chait A: Interstitial pulmonary edema, *Circulation* 45:1323, 1972.

82. Basta LL, Lerona PT, January LE: Physical and radiologic examination of the lung in the evaluation of cardiac disease, *Am Heart J* 90:255, 1975.

83. Harrison MO, Conte PJ, Heitzman ER: Radiological detection of clinically occult cardiac failure following myocardial infarction, *Br J Radiol* 44:265, 1971.

84. Don C, Johnson R: The nature and significance of peribronchial cuffing in pulmonary edema, *Radiology* 125:577, 1977.

85. Logue RB, Rogers JV Jr, Gay BB Jr: Subtle roentgenographic signs of left heart failure, *Am Heart J* 65:464, 1963.

86. Heitzman ER, Ziter FM Jr: Acute interstitial pulmonary edema, *AJR* 98:281, 1966.

87. Meszaros WT: Lung changes in left heart failure, *Circulation* 47:859, 1973.

88. Courtice FC, Simmonds WJ: Absorption of fluids from the pleural cavities of rabbits and cats, *J Physiol* 109:17, 1949.

89. Cooray GH: Defensive mechanisms in the mediastinum, with special reference to the mechanisms of pleural absorption, *J Pathol Bacteriol* 61:551, 1949.

90. Miserocchi G, Nakamura T, Mariani E, Negrini D: Pleural liquid pressure over the interlobar, mediastinal and diaphragmatic surfaces of the lung, *Respir Physiol* 46:61, 1981.

91. Miserocchi G, Pistolesi M, Miniati M, et al: Pleural liquid pressure gradients and intrapleural distribution of injected bolus, *J Appl Physiol* 56:526, 1984.

92. Trapnell DH: The differential diagnosis of linear shadows in chest radiographs, *Radiol Clin North Am* 11:77, 1973.

93. Kerley P: Radiology in heart disease, *Br Med J* 2:594, 1933.

94. Kerley P: Lung changes in acquired heart disease, *AJR* 80:256, 1958.

95. Favre E, Milne ENC, Roeck WW: The anatomy of "A" lines, *Invest Radiol* 11(5):1, 1976.

96. Heitzman ER, Ziter FM Jr, Markanian B, et al: Kerley's interlobular septal lines: roentgen-pathologic correlation, *AJR* 100:578, 1967.

97. Fleischner FG, Reiner L: Linear x-ray shadows in acquired pulmonary hemosiderosis and congestion, *N Engl J Med* 250:900, 1954.

98. Jordan SC, Hicken P, Watson DA, et al: Pathology of the lung in mitral stenosis in relation to respiratory function and pulmonary hemodynamics, *Br Heart J* 28:101, 1966.

99. Milne ENC, Carlsson E: Physiological interpretation of the plain radiograph in mitral valve disease following valvotomy, valvuloplasty or valve replacement by prosthesis, *Radiology* 92:1201, 1969.

100. Hodson CJ: Pulmonary edema and "batswing" shadows, *J Fac Radiol* 1:176, 1950.

101. Nessa CB, Rigler LG: Roentgenological manifestations of pulmonary edema, *Radiology* 37:35, 1941.

102. Herrnheiser G, Hinson KFW: An anatomical explanation of the formation of butterfly shadows, *Thorax* 9:198, 1954.

103. Fleischner FG: The butterfly pattern of acute pulmonary edema. *Am J Cardiol* 20:39, 1967.

104. Joffe N: The adult respiratory distress syndrome, *AJR* 122:719, 1974.

105. Weibel ER: How does lung structure affect gas exchange, *Chest* 83:657, 1983.

106. Greene R: Adult respiratory distress syndrome: acute alveolar damage, *Radiology* 163:57, 1987.

107. Staub NC: The pathogenesis of pulmonary edema, *Progr Cardiovasc Dis* 23:53, 1980.

108. Weibel ER: Functional morphology of lung parenchyma. In Fishman AP, Macklem PT, Mead JS (eds), *Handbook of physiology. The respiratory system*, Section 3, vol 3, part 1, Bethesda, MD 1986, American Physiological Society, p 89.

109. Gil J: Alveolar wall relations, *NY Acad Sci* 384:31, 1982.

110. Bhattacharya J, Gropper MA, Staub NC: Interstitial fluid pressure gradient measured by micropuncture in excised dog lung, *J Appl Physiol* 56:271, 1984.

111. Aviado DM, Schmidt CF: Pathogenesis of pulmonary edema by alloxan, *Circ Res* 5:180, 1957.

112. Aviado DM: *The lung circulation*, New York, 1965 Pergamon Press, p 878.

3 Detection and Quantification of Pulmonary Edema

Although there has been a considerable increase in our knowledge of the etiology and pathogenesis of pulmonary edema in recent years, the detection, and particularly the quantification, of edema for clinical purposes remains the subject of great controversy. Is there in fact a real clinical *need* to detect and quantify lung edema in patients? The answer to this question differs, depending on whether one is considering patients with pressure edema (cardiac, renal, overhydration, neurogenic, or high altitude) or patients with injury lung edema.

Radiologic detection is of particular value in patients with pressure edema because it can detect the edema at a very early stage, whereas the clinician (using signs and symptoms) cannot diagnose edema until it is at an advanced stage (e.g., until it enters the alveoli). Furthermore, the chronology of development and clearing of edema, along with its regional distribution and quantity, correlate well with the underlying pathophysiology and severity of the illness and are of great value in determining, first, the etiology of the edema and, second, the efficacy of treatment.

By contrast, in normal pressure (injury) lung edema the accumulation of lung water is usually *preceded* by clinical signs and symptoms and its radiologic detection is therefore of less value for very early diagnosis. The quantity of edema and the chronology of its development do not correlate as well with the severity of disease in ARDS as they do in pressure edemas, but they are quite characteristic of lung injury edema and can therefore greatly aid in the frequent and clinically difficult problem of deciding whether a patient has injury edema, pressure edema, or a combination of the two.

CRITERIA FOR ACCURATELY DETECTING AND QUANTIFYING PULMONARY EDEMA

A recent workshop on the clinical use of lung water measurements[1] recommended that any method of quantitating pulmonary edema should, ideally, have the following characteristics: First, it should give accurate measurements of the actual amount of water present. Second, it should be sensitive enough to detect even small increases in lung water (i.e., making it possible to detect the early stages of fluid accumulation) when the edema is confined to the interstitium. (Air space edema can easily be diagnosed by auscultation.) Third, it should be noninvasive, reproducible, preferably inexpensive, and practical (i.e., easy to perform and capable of giving immediate results). Pulmonary edema is a dynamic process, and patients may require serial evaluations day by day, even hour by hour.

At the present time no method exists that completely fulfills all these criteria, and one of the most popular cardiology textbooks[2] states that "attempts to quantify pulmonary edema in its various stages of development are not yet sufficiently successful in terms of accuracy, sensitivity and reproducibility." However, the workshop on pulmonary edema referred to above concluded somewhat differently, that "the chest x-ray remains the reference standard against which other lung water content methods are compared. Its advantages include moderate accuracy, fair sensitivity, good reproducibility, noninvasiveness, practicality, availability, reliability, portability, ease of use in the emergency situation, and relatively low cost. It also provides excellent information about edema distribution." As we show later in this chapter, the accuracy and sensitivity of the radiologic methods can be greatly improved if an objective reading table is used.

In the last 10 years a large amount of evidence[3-11] has accumulated proving the superiority of the chest film for clinical assessment of lung edema, and several studies[12-17] have confirmed an earlier clinical belief that the chest x-ray becomes abnormal in cardiac failure well before clinical signs of pulmonary edema develop. It has also been shown[9,15,16] that the chest radiograph becomes positive for the presence of pulmonary edema while sophisticated indicator dilution techniques remain negative. (This will be discussed more fully later in the chapter.) There remains, however, a general reluctance to believe that the simple chest radiograph is the method of choice for quantifying lung water; and despite its universal availability, it is still considered by many referring physicians to be only semiquantitative, nonspecific, and too subjective to serve as the basis for clinical treatment. This idea is quite erroneous but has become deeply rooted. As a result the medical literature is now replete with articles attempting to prove the advantages of much more complicated techniques over the chest film. Because of this, many referring physicians, regrettably, will not accept that the chest film does contain valuable quantitative information about pulmonary edema. This, in turn, discourages film readers from developing the quite simple interpretive skills necessary to provide such quantitative information in the radiologic report. Since pulmonary edema is one of the commonest and most important pathophysiologic changes seen in hospital patients, it is of great importance clinically and logistically to break down this communications barrier. To do this, the person charged with reading the chest films must not only understand clearly the value of the chest radiograph in assessing lung water but also be able in discussions to substantiate this belief and marshal in argument the flaws that exist in alternative, more complex, techniques that the referring physicians might presently espouse. In this chapter we will therefore evaluate the sensitivity and accuracy of the chest radiograph for assessing lung water and will analyze and compare briefly the strengths and weaknesses of the more commonly used alternative techniques, with particular emphasis on indicator dilution measurements. These comparisons will be limited to *sensitivity* and *accuracy* since no other technique can be compared even tentatively with the chest radiograph in terms of availability, reproducibility, noninvasiveness, practicality, and cost.

METHODS FOR QUANTIFYING PULMONARY EDEMA

Table 3-1 lists techniques that have been applied or proposed for the detection and quantification of pulmonary edema in patients. Destructive methods, such as the gravimetric assessment of extravascular lung water[18,19] or histologic/morphometric evaluations,[20,21] have no clinical applications but are mentioned because they do provide reference standards for in vivo methods and help explain the different pathogenetic events in hydrostatic and injury lung edema.

Table 3-1 Methods of quantifying pulmonary edema

Physical changes	Tracer equilibration
Nonimaging techniques	
Transthoracic electrical impedance	Inhalation of soluble inert gas
Microwave radiation	Double-indicator dilution
Compton-scatter densitometry	Low molecular weight radioaerosol clearance
Transthoracic gamma ray attenuation	Protein external radioflux detection
Imaging techniques	
Chest radiography	
Positron emission tomography	
Computed tomography	
Nuclear magnetic resonance	

Physical Changes in the Lung (Nonimaging)

Transthoracic impedance to the passage of an electrical signal,[22,23] pulmonary transmission of microwaves,[24] and scattering and attenuation of gamma rays[25-27] all suffer from the fundamental disadvantage of not being able to differentiate changes in *intravascular* water (increasing or decreasing pulmonary blood volume) from changes in *extravascular* water (edema) (Fig. 3-1). They are also dependent on the degree of lung inflation and are subject to motion artifact and the positioning of signal detectors. They are not sufficiently sensitive, accurate, or reproducible to be of value in clinical practice.

Tracer Methods

Inhalation of Soluble Inert Gas. Acetylene is a highly soluble and inert gas that, when inhaled, equilibrates rapidly with the pulmonary tissues. Since most of the lung tissue is water, any increase in lung water should be reflected by the initial disappearance of the soluble gas.[28-30] Again, however, the technique does not distinguish between intra- and extravascular water. An increase in pulmonary blood volume will be erroneously read as an increase in extravascular lung water (EVLW), even when no edema is present (Fig. 3-1). Furthermore, in patients with alveolar edema the gas will not be convected into the alveoli and underestimation of water will result (Fig. 3-2). With the acetylene technique a wide range of EVLW values is found, even in normal subjects, which makes the technique insensitive to picking up the early changes of pulmonary edema. Its practical application is also lessened by the necessity for patient cooperation and by the intricacy of

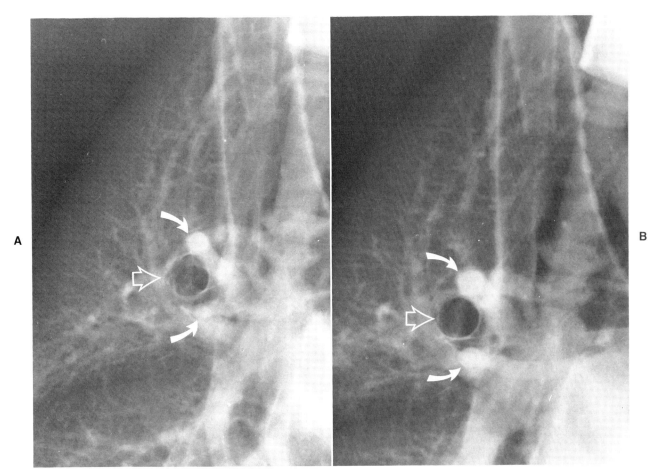

Fig. 3-1   A, Spot view of an inflated isolated lung with normal pulmonary blood volume. Note the size of the end-on vessels *(curved arrows)* above and below the bronchus *(open arrow).* There is no evidence of edema, and specifically no peribronchial cuffing. **B,** The intravascular blood volume has now been doubled. Note the increased size of all vessels; but there is still no pulmonary edema (normal bronchial wall). Most methods of estimating "lung water" cannot differentiate between *intra-* and *extravascular* water and would therefore indicate erroneously that this lung showed pulmonary edema. Peribronchial cuffing is not seen in this isolated lung preparation partly because the peribronchovascular sheath, during removal of the lung, has been ruptured and the fluid spilled out. In a patient with an intact lung, cuffing is easier to detect.

the computations, which does not allow an immediate reading to be given.

Double-Indicator Dilution. Apart from the chest film, indicator dilution techniques are now the most commonly used methods for quantifying lung edema. Two tracers are injected intravenously simultaneously. One is diffusible and equilibrates rapidly with both intra- and extravascular water. The other is nondiffusible and confines itself to the intravascular space (Fig. 3-3). The two, in their passage through the lungs, will therefore be diluted to a different extent—the more the EVLW, the greater the dilution of the diffusible tracer. Samples are then taken from a systemic artery and the different dilution volumes of the two tracers are calculated.[31,32] The approach, however, has been shown to be weak[33,34] and to provide an estimated EVLW that is considerably less than the amount measured from the same lungs by accurate in vitro gravimetric techniques.[18,35] Also it may fail to detect an increase in EVLW even in patients with obvious clinical signs of pulmonary edema.[36] An improvement in the methodology has been made by including *recirculating* tracer in the computation of the mean residence time of the tracer through the lungs.[15,34] Although this is a much more accurate method (providing there are no marked alterations in lung perfusion) and gives very similar results to those obtained gravimetrically,[15,16,34] the technique is invasive and the computerized mathematical analysis so complex that it cannot be used clinically. It is, nevertheless, valuable as a reference standard for

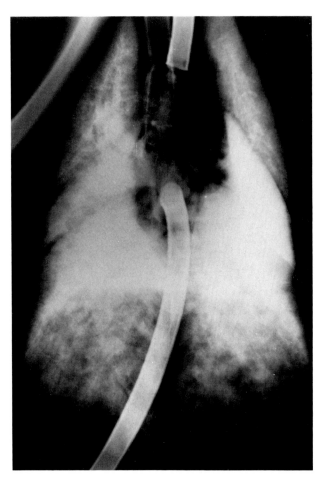

Fig. 3-2 Inflated isolated lung showing gross alveolar edema (high-pressure type). The alveoli are filled with fluid, and any technique using gas to measure lung water will be unsuccessful since the gas cannot be convected into the alveoli.

evaluating the sensitivity and accuracy of other techniques such as the chest film.

Another attempt to improve the accuracy of indicator dilution techniques has been made by using *heat* as the diffusible indicator. This diffuses through water 50 times faster than tritiated water.[33,37] The data derived can be microprocessor computed to provide on-line results.[38,39] The extravascular lung water estimates with this technique are similar to gravimetric determinations, but again the technique depends on the presence of perfusion within the edematous area.[33,34] This can be a particularly great disadvantage in patients with ARDS, in whom large amounts of EVLW may be present where there are pulmonary vascular occlusions.[40-43] Measurements are also affected by positive pressure ventilation, cardiac output, and pulmonary artery pressure.[44-46] It is therefore not appropriate to base critical therapeutic interventions on the "num-

bers" resulting from this technique of measurement. Nor, and we must emphasize this point strongly, is it appropriate to use this technique as the gold standard with which to assess the accuracy of the chest roentgenographic technique. We will discuss this in more detail later in the chapter.

In patients with ARDS, it may be that measurements of changes in the capillary endothelial barrier would be more useful clinically than measurements of edema alone.

Low Molecular Weight Radioaerosol Clearance (Injury Edema). Loss of integrity of the epithelial alveolar barrier in injury lung edema can be detected by assessing the rate of disappearance from the lungs of an aerosolized low molecular weight radiotracer. Technetium 99m diethylenetriamine pentaacetic acid (^{99m}Tc-DTPA) is deposited in the lungs as a submicronic aerosol, and its clearance measured with a gamma camera or a portable gamma ray probe.[47,48] Alveolar epithelial damage is a characteristic feature of ARDS,[20,21] and ^{99m}Tc-DTPA clearance is markedly increased in patients with established ARDS.[48-50] The technique is noninvasive, can be performed by portable apparatus, and will detect early alveolar damage[48,51]; unfortunately, it is not specific for ARDS, however, since the clearance rate is also markedly increased in smokers and in a variety of acute and chronic lung disorders[48,52]—to the extent that their distinction from patients with ARDS becomes obscure. Also positive end-expiratory pressure ventilation accelerates the clearance of ^{99m}Tc-DTPA,[53] and this fact, together with the intrinsic lack of specificity, greatly affects the interpretation of results in critically ill patients and consequently reduces the clinical value of the technique. Cardiogenic pulmonary edema alone does not increase the lung clearance rate of ^{99m}Tc-DTPA, but a considerable overlap of clearance rates has been observed[49,50] between ARDS and cardiac patients.

Protein External Radioflux Detection (Injury Edema). Increased lung microvascular permeability, resulting in increased plasma protein extravasation, is a specific hallmark of ARDS. Various experimental approaches[54-56] have been employed to study the rate of movement of plasma protein from the blood into the extravascular space of the lung. In general, a radiolabeled protein (albumin or transferrin) injected intravenously is monitored over the lung and corrected for the regional blood volume activity using a reference intravascular tracer such as radiolabeled red blood cells. The detecting system may be a gamma camera or a portable gamma ray probe. Protein external radioflux detection is potentially a very sensitive technique that may allow detection of abnormal lung solute transport. The technique can specifically detect increased permeability before definite edema has developed,[57,58] but results of

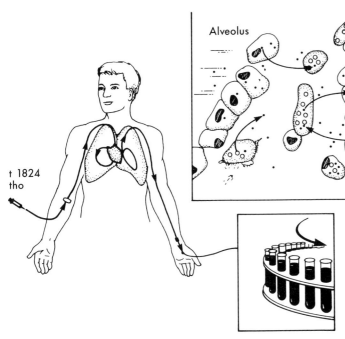

Fig. 3-3 Mixed nondiffusible indicator (blue dye *T 1824)* and diffusible (tritiated water, *THO, black dots*) are injected into the right atrium, and samples are collected from the radial artery on a rotating drum at 1 sec intervals. (The inset shows large T 1824 particles confined to the intravascular space while tiny THO molecules diffuse freely through intra- and extravascular water.) Dilution of the THO will result in a delayed transit time and therefore a different dilution curve from the reference T 1824. (Modified from Van de Water JM, Min-Sheh J, O'Connor E, et al: *J Trauma* 10:440-449, 1970.)

preliminary clinical applications are not encouraging. Although the technique has been shown to differentiate patients with established ARDS from normals or patients with left ventricular failure,[59] it has not been possible to draw conclusions as to its sensitivity in the *early* detection of lung injury since all patients studied have had radiographic evidence of late *(alveolar)* edema.[52,60,61] Large-scale clinical trials to assess the sensitivity of the technique in detecting early changes in patients with preclinical ARDS are beset by the complexity of the apparatus, the time required to make the measurement (more than an hour), and the unavailability of on-line results.

Imaging Techniques

Positron Emission Tomography (Pressure and Injury Edema). By combining positron emission tomography (PET) scanning of injected or inhaled positron-emitting isotopes with transmission scanning, it is possible to derive sensitive and accurate quantitative regional measurements of water, blood flow, hematocrit, extravascular density, and vascular permeability in the lung.[62-67] PET can depict the different regional distributions of extravascular lung density in various conditions of cardiogenic lung edema[68-70] (Fig. 3-4).

Compared to CT scanning, which depicts the regional distribution of whole lung density (and is unable to separate out the intra- and extravascular components), PET has the advantage that by subtraction techniques it *can* display intra- and extravascular lung density separately. PET is at present the most promising technique for the experimental pathophysiologic study of pulmonary edema, and in highly selected cases it

might be of use for clinical purposes; however, its cumbersome and costly apparatus and nonportability will, even in the future, seriously limit its clinical applicability.

Computed Tomography. CT can demonstrate very accurately the changes in lung density, lung weight, and distribution of pathology that occur in both pressure edema and injury edema[71-73]; and an excellent correlation has been shown[74] between dependent lung density and left ventricular end-diastolic pressure (LVEDP) in patients with cardiac failure (a relationship ,however, that one would expect to be much poorer during both the developing and the clearing phases of cardiac edema because of the lag that occurs between the drop in LVEDP and the reabsorption of edema). However, CT's inability to separate increased intravascular volume from extravascular volume, plus its nonportability, dollar expense, and radiation dosage, tends to relegate it (at least presently and as far as pressure edema is concerned) to the role of an animal research tool.[75-77] By contrast, it may be of some clinical value in injury lung edema.

The CT scan, when combined with a measurement of lung gas volume, is very useful to assess lung *weight* in vivo in patients with severe ARDS.[78] Since the weights obtained in vivo correlate well with those obtained at autopsy,[78] the CT scan may be of value for accurately assessing the severity and distribution of ARDS damage and assisting in treatment planning. In some cases the

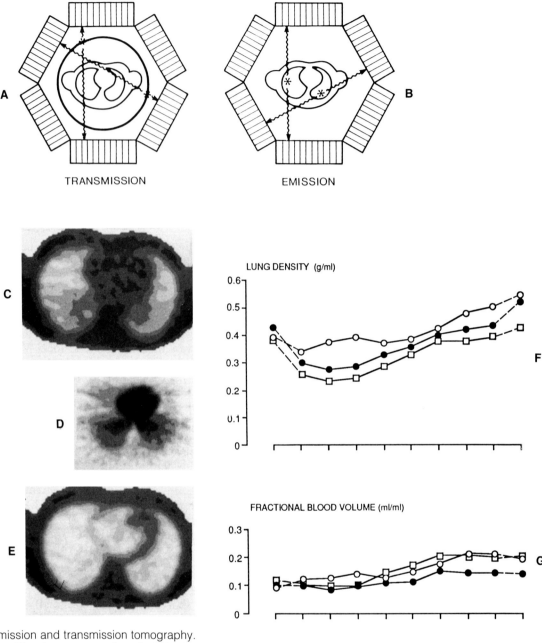

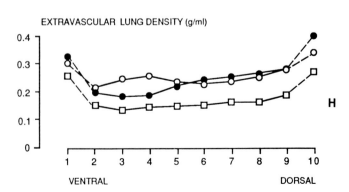

Fig. 3-4 Positron emission and transmission tomography. **A,** Transmission mode. The ring source, placed within the hexagonal array of detectors, contains ^{68}Ga and surrounds the thorax. Gamma ray emission, detected by the same counter pair, makes an identical journey through the thorax as in the emission sequence and corrects for attenuation; it is therefore directly proportional to the physical density in its path. **B,** Emission mode. A radionuclide within the lung gives off two 511 keV gamma rays in coincidence, detected by opposing counters. **C,** Density from the transmission scan. **D,** Red cell volume from the emission scan (after ^{11}CO inhalation). **E,** *Extravascular* density (water and tissue): Subtract **D** from **C. F** to **H,** Lung density, fractional blood volume, and extravascular lung density derived from tomographic slices (ventral-to-dorsal) of the supine lung. (Modified from Wollmer P, Rhodes CG: *J Thorac Imaging* 3[3]:44, 1988.)

value of this information might be felt to outweigh the dollar and radiation costs and the considerable logistic difficulties of transporting a very sick patient on positive pressure ventilation to the CT scanner.

Magnetic Resonance Imaging. Various MRI approaches to the in vivo measurement of lung water in animals and humans[79,80] have indicated a possible future role for this technique in the study of pulmonary edema. MRI has the potential advantage of giving no radiation exposure to the patient; however, MRI lung water determinations are presently susceptible to error from cardiac and respiratory motion and, again, from the inability to discriminate between intra- and extravascular hydrogen nuclei. Nonportability, long examination times, and high costs are other important limitations in the clinical application of MRI to the study of pulmonary edema.

CHEST RADIOGRAPHY

There is still a general reluctance (particularly among nonradiologists) to accept the chest film as a gold standard because of its alleged subjectivity and the possibility of iatrogenic variations introduced by changes in radiographic technique. In practice, changes in technique are not so great a problem as the nonradiologist might imagine. It is quite easy to recognize the usual variations in technique (overexposure, underexposure, expiratory film) from the radiograph itself and either to factor these into one's estimations or, if they are too great, to simply repeat the film using a correct technique. The matter of subjectivity is also probably overemphasized. The better the observer's training, the more objective the interpretation becomes; and we have shown in multiple observer studies that there is little variation between trained observers in quantitating pulmonary edema from the chest radiograph when a standardized reading table is used (e.g., Tables 3-2 and 3-3), as it should be to maintain consistency and objectivity. The training of a film reader is not a lengthy or difficult process. Most medical students will become competent at detecting and quantitating EVLW after a day or so of training, and a radiologist already trained in general chest interpretation can master the technique in 1 or 2 hours.

It is often stated that EVLW must increase by 35% before it can be detected on the chest radiograph,[81,82] but we believe this statement is based on a misinterpretation of a single experimental study in dogs.[83] Careful examination of the radiographs published in this animal study demonstrates that they *did* in fact show evi-

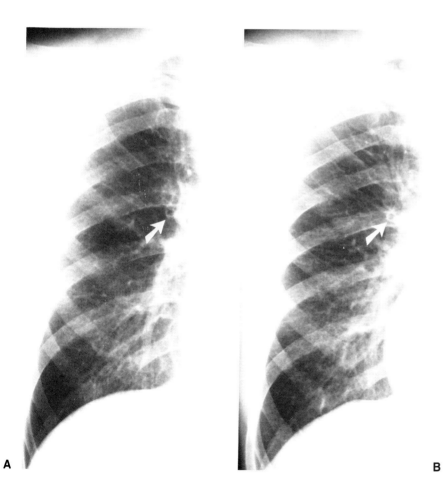

Fig. 3-5 **A,** Young man with renal disease. Hilum and large vessels—normal definition. Cuffing—definitely none *(arrow).* Lung lucency—normal. Background subsegmental vessels, —well seen. (From Table 3-3: no edema. EVLW, 40 to 50.) **B,** Same patient with worsening renal failure. Hilum and large vessels—definite mild blurring. Cuffing—definitely present *(arrow).* Lung lucency—questionable loss of blackness. Subsegmental vessels—definite early loss of visibility. (From Table 3-3: mild to moderate interstitial edema. EVLW, 65 to 75.)

A

B

dence of pulmonary edema with EVLW less than 35% and the authors themselves confirmed that. We have found[16] that an increase of 10% in EVLW is detectible and an increase of 35% (EVLW approximately 70 ml/L of lung at TLC) would be interpreted by our criteria as definite interstitial edema (Fig. 3-5). A more detailed analysis of the reasons for our belief that the oft-quoted study by Snashall has been misinterpreted, and that this misinterpretation has subsequently been handed down without reexamination from author to author, is offered in the appendix to this chapter.

The radiographic appearances of pressure and injury edema differ in many respects (Chapter 8), and the criteria for quantitating pressure edema must also therefore differ from those for injury edema.[84,85] The first task in quantitating pulmonary edema radiologically must then be to determine which *type* of edema is present. To do this, we use the radiologic method described in Chapter 8,[16,84-87] integrating it wherever possible with evidence from the patient's history and with clinical and instrumental findings—keeping in mind, however, that mixtures of types of edema are common. Even these mixtures can be handled successfully, provided one has a thorough knowledge of the appearance and behavior of each type of edema in its pure unadulterated form. (See Chapters 8 and 10.)

Quantification of Hydrostatic (Pressure) Edema

The radiographic features that we used initially to detect and quantify hydrostatic pulmonary edema include hilar size, density, and sharpness, blurring of vessel margins, thickening of fissures, peribronchial cuffing, septal lines, subpleural effusions, and "micronoduli" (probably caused by small-vessel perivascular cuffs seen end-on) (Table 3-2). These radiologic findings (discussed in Chapters 2 and 8) were derived initially from an extensive survey of the literature and from our own

Table 3-2 Criteria for grading pressure edema

Chest roentgenogram	Score
Hila	
Enlarged	1, 2, 3
Increased density	2, 4, 6
Blurred	3, 6, 9
Kerley lines	
A	4, 8
B	4, 8
C	4, 8
Micronoduli	4, 8
Widening of fissures	4, 8
Peribronchial and perivascular cuffs	4, 8, 12
Extensive perihilar haze	4, 8, 12
Subpleural effusion	5, 10
Diffuse increase of density	5, 10, 15

For each radiologic feature the lowest number indicates mild, the middle number moderate, and the highest number severe degrees of change.

analyses of the chest radiographs of a large series of cardiac patients.[15]

Our initial method of grading pressure pulmonary edema utilized eight of these factors and attached a weighted "score" to each sign, the level of the score depending upon the observer's estimate of the severity of that sign (Table 3-2). The scores were added to give a total numerical "index" (but not an actual quantification) of the severity of the edema. The total scores had previously been correlated with carefully determined indicator dilution measurements of lung water in the same patients, and if the film interpreter has this graph (Fig. 3-6) available, it is possible from the total score to derive the actual *quantity* of lung water present.

This rigorous approach is of particular value in both human and animal physiologic/radiologic correlation experiments but is time-consuming. Consequently, we have developed a quicker approach for use in daily clin-

Table 3-3 Rapid quantification of pressure edema

EVLW (ml H₂O/L of lung, at TLC)	Less than normal lung water (20 to 40 ml)	Normal lung water (40 to 50 ml)	Borderline interstitial edema (50 to 60 ml)	Mild interstitial edema (60 to 70 ml)	Moderate interstitial edema (70 to 80 ml)
Hilum and large vessels	Very sharp	Normal definition	Questionable blurring	Definite blurring (mild degree)	Definite blurring (mild degree)
Cuffing	Definitely none	Definitely none	Definitely none	Questionable	Definitely present
Lung lucency	Very black	Normal black	Questionable loss of blackness	Definite minimal graying	Changed from black to dark gray
Small (subsegmental) vessels	Very well-seen but sparse	Well-seen normal	Well-seen	Questionable loss of visibility	Definite early loss of visibility

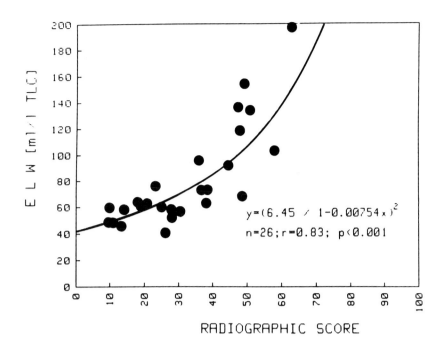

Fig. 3-6 Correlation between edema graded by x-ray and quantified by modified indicator dilution technique. (From Pistolesi M, Giuntini C: *Radiol Clin North Am* 16:551, 1978.)

ical practice embodying only four factors and allowing us to "read" the quantity of edema directly from our reading table (Table 3-3).

1. Clarity of vessel margins
2. Peribronchial cuffing
3. Change in lung lucency
4. Visibility of subsegmental vessels

Using both of these techniques—the first with eight factors and numerical weighting and the second with only four radiologic features—we quantified edema on 210 chest films in 77 cardiac patients with either ischemic or valvular disease. The correlation between the two methodologies was 0.91, p < 0.001 (Fig. 3-7). This confirmed that the simplified rapid assessment technique, using only four readily visualized and easily quantifiable radiologic features, is quite accurate for clinical purposes.

The table we use clinically for detecting and quantifying pressure edema (Table 3-3) provides a series of descriptions (covering 11 grades of edema severity) for each of the four features, and the film reader responds simply by choosing the description that matches the appearance of each of the features on the radiograph. From specific changes in these four features the quantity of edema in the lungs can then be read directly from the table (Figs. 3-5, 3-8, and 3-9). For example, if the film reader decides that the appearances on the radiograph match the table as follows

Feature	Description
Hilum and large vessels	Definite blurring (mild degree)
Cuffing	Definitely present
Lung lucency	Change from black to dark gray
Small subsegmental vessels	Definite loss of visibility

Severe interstitial edema (80 to 90 ml)	Questionable alveolar edema (90 to 100 ml)	Mild alveolar edema (100 to 120 ml)	Moderately severe alveolar edema (120 to 140 ml)	Severe alveolar edema (140 to 180 ml)	Fulminating alveolar edema (180 ml plus)
Definite blurring (moderate degree)	Definite blurring (moderate to severe)	Definite blurring (severe)	Becoming obscured by alveolar filling	Only larger vessels and hilum seen	Hilum and large vessels obscured ("white-out")
Definite	Definite	Becoming obscured by alveolar filling	Becoming obscured by alveolar filling	Obscured: questionable air bronchograms	"White-out"
Gray	Gray/white	Gray/white	White (regional)	White (extensive)	"White-out"
Vessels difficult to make out	Vessels very difficult to make out	Vessels obscured at bases	Vessels obscured at bases	Vessels obscured throughout lung	"White-out"

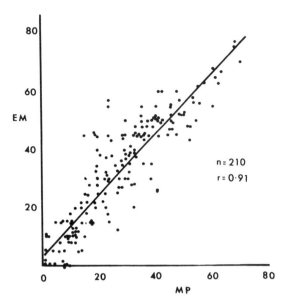

Fig. 3-7   Correlation between the method of "scoring" pulmonary edema listed in Table 3-2 and the method of quantifying pulmonary edema listed in Table 3-3. (NOTE: For the purposes of this correlative study both methods are listed in units of severity [from 0 to 80] and not in milliliters of water per liter of lung. On this scale 0 units would correspond to 20 ml EVLW 80 units to 140 to 180 ml EVLW.) *EM* = Eric Milne; *MP* = Massimo Pistolesi.

then the patient has "moderate interstitial edema" (70 to 80 ml EVLW/L of lung [at TLC]) (Figs. 3-5, *B*, and 3-8, *B*).

By contrast, if the appearances match

Hilum and large vessels	Becoming obscured by alveolar filling
Cuffing	Becoming obscured by alveolar filling
Lung lucence	White (regionally)
Small vessels	Obscured at bases

then the patient has moderately severe alveolar edema (120 to 140 ml EVLW/L of lung [at TLC]) (Figs. 3-8, *C*, and 3-9, *G* and *H*).

It is important to point out that when a radiologist uses the word "questionable" this is usually taken to signify an inability to make a decision; but, in fact, selecting the category "questionable" means that a decision *has* been made. For example, in choosing the category "questionable" to describe peribronchial cuffing, the radiologist has already made two decisions: that cuffing (1) is *not* definitely absent and (2) is *not* definitely present and has chosen the specific grading of "questionable" as lying between the two possibilities.

It might be thought that people untrained in recognizing the factors that characterize pulmonary edema, and using the table for the first time, would rely heavily on the "questionable" boxes, but in fact they do not.

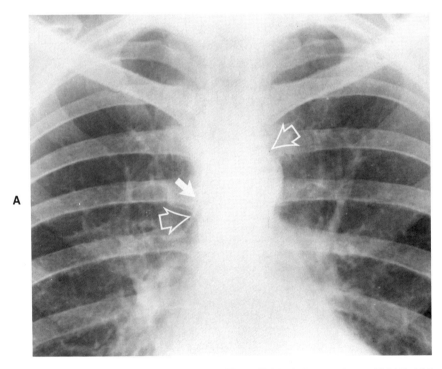

Fig. 3-8   A, Young man with renal failure. (From Table 3-3: no edema. EVLW, 40 to 50.) Compare the vena azygos *(solid arrow)* and vascular pedicle width *(open arrows)* with those in **C.**

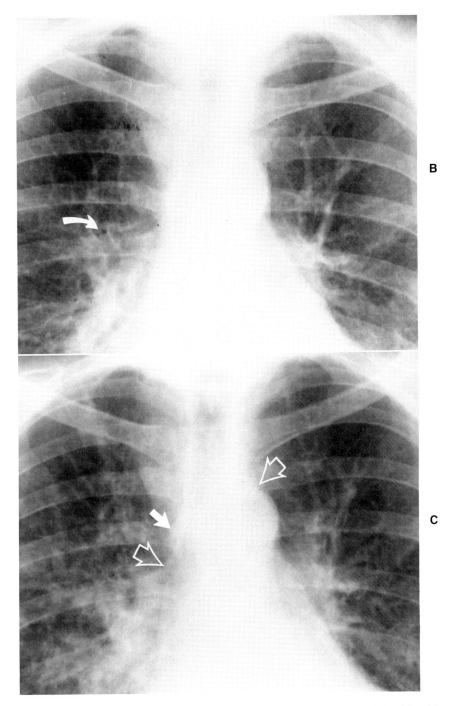

Fig. 3-8, cont'd   As renal failure worsens, **B,** the radiograph shows definite hilar blurring, questionable cuffing *(arrow),* and slight loss of lung lucency. There is also early loss of visibility of the subsegmental vessels. (From Table 3-3: mild, verging on moderate, interstitial edema. EVLW, 65 to 75.) Further worsening, **C** *(prior to dialysis).* Note the moderate to severe blurring of the hilum and larger vessels. Cuffing is present *(arrow).* The lung lucency has changed from black to dark gray. Subsegmental vessels are very difficult to make out. (From Table 3-3: questionable to mild alveolar edema. EVLW, 95 to 110.)   Note the progressive enlargement of the vascular pedicle from **A** to **C** *(open arrows)* and of the vena azygos *(solid arrow).* This patient shows both a progressively increased circulating blood volume (intravascular water) and an increase in lung water (extravascular).

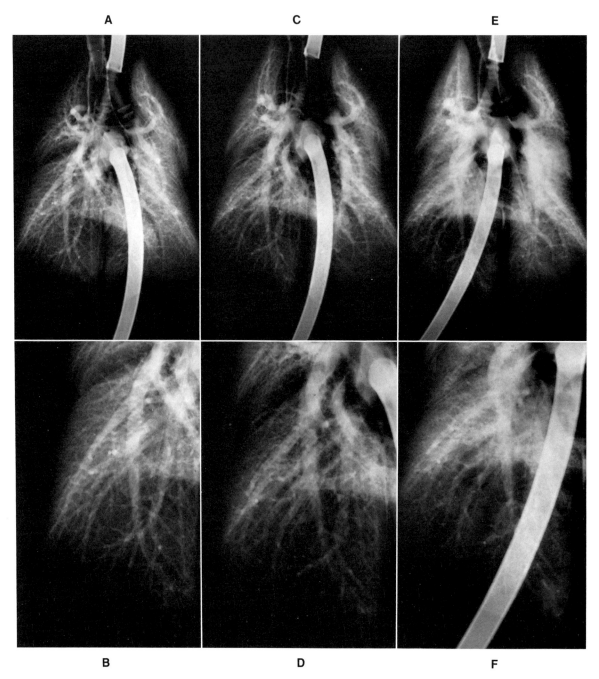

Fig. 3-9 **A** and **B,** Isolated lung preparation. Normal vascular pressures. Normal hilum, no cuffing. Lung lucency, normal. Subsegmental vessels, easily seen. (From Table 3-3: EVLW, 40 to 50 [normal].) **C** and **D,** Venous pressure has been elevated 10 to 15 mm Hg. Normal hilum, questionable blurring of large vessels; subsegmental vessels, still well seen. (From Table 3-3: EVLW, 50 to 60 [borderline interstitial edema].) **E** and **F,** Venous pressure elevated 10 to 15 mm Hg. Hilum and large vessels, definitely blurred. Lung lucency, some loss (graying). Subsegmental vessels, early loss of visibility. (From Table 3-3: EVLW, 70 to 80 [moderate interstitial edema].)

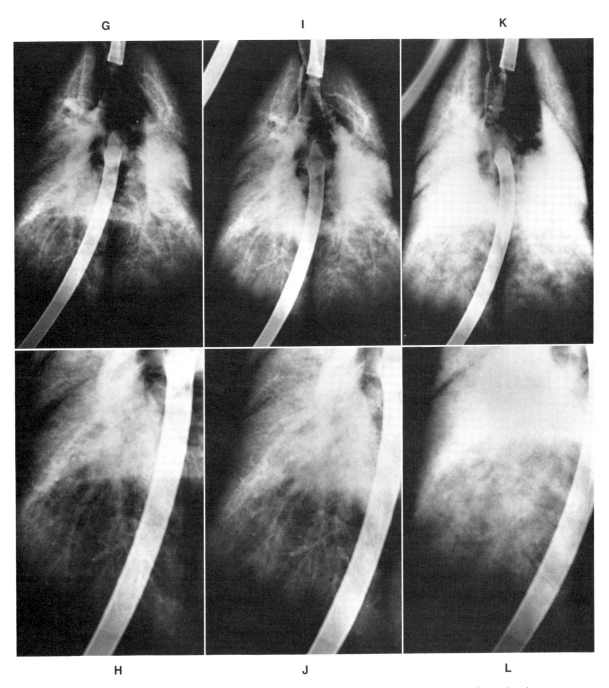

Fig. 3-9, cont'd **G** and **H,** Pulmonary arterial and venous pressures moderately elevated. Hilum and large vessels, becoming obscured by alveolar filling. Lung lucency, gray/white. Subsegmental vessels, becoming difficult to make out. (From Table 3-3: moderately severe alveolar edema. EVLW, 120.) **I** and **J,** Very high venous and arterial pressures (LAP 35, PAP 80 mm Hg). Hilum and large vessels, only larger vessels seen. Lung lucency, white (regional). Subsegmental vessels, obscured at bases. (From Table 3-3: severe alveolar edema. EVLW, 130 to 150.) **K** and **L,** LAP 35 PAP 110, mm Hg. Hilum and large vessels, obscured ("white-out"). Lung lucency ("white-out."). Subsegmental vessels, obscured by white-out. (From Table 3-3: fulminating alveolar edema. EVLW, 180+.)

Once the questions have been posed, e.g., are the hila and large vessels

Excessively sharp?

Of normal definition?

Questionably blurred?

Definitely blurred (mild)?

Definitely blurred (moderate)?

Definitely blurred (moderate to severe)?

Definitely blurred (severe)?

Becoming obscured by alveolar filling?

Partly seen (only the large ones)?

Totally obscured ("white-out")?

it becomes quite easy, even without previous experience, to pick the appropriate description. The reader is unlikely to classify "excessively sharp" or "definitely blurred (moderate)" as "questionable," because these degrees of change are easy to see; but, with inexperience, they might well not be able to distinguish between "normal definition," "questionable," and "definitely blurred (mild)." The reader is choosing here between a range of only ±10 ml EVLW/L of lung (a very small difference) and the initial lack of expertise would result in merely a slight underestimation of "mild interstitial edema" as "borderline" or a slight overestimation of "normal" as "borderline interstitial edema."

If a group of medical students with little or no experience reading chest films is asked to respond individually to the questions on the table, comparing them with the radiograph and each person's estimate is recorded secretly, when the results are compared there will rarely be more than a 10 ml EVLW variation between individual estimates of lung water and the correct figure. In other words, the use of this very specific reading table confers a high level of objectivity to the quantification of lung water and removes the need for a large radiologic experience in estimating lung water correctly.[*]

Although we have been able for the last 20 years to provide actual *numerical* quantification of pressure edema directly from the radiograph (quoted as "milliliters of EVLW/L of lung, at TLC for that patient"), these numbers appear presently to be of limited value to the referring clinician. Clinicians rarely seem to use actual numbers to determine how much extravascular lung water is present; rather, they still prefer to have the radiologist's estimate couched in descriptive terms of the type we have used in Table 3-3, e.g., "mild interstitial edema confined to the bases, slightly improved since the day before." This is why Table 3-3 contains, in addition to the numerical data, appropriate descriptions of the anatomic location (interstitial, alveolar, or mixed) and severity of edema.

By using this approach one can assess the severity of the underlying disease process causing the pulmonary edema (e.g., cardiac failure, renal failure, neurogenic damage) from the chest radiograph and use the information objectively to monitor and evaluate the effects of any therapeutic intervention.

In evaluating the chest films of patients with cardiac disease it is important that two points be kept in mind. First, pulmonary edema can in some cases persist ("lag") for a certain time after left atrial pressure (LAP) has been restored to normal by treatment. The length of time it persists in the face of a normal LAP varies greatly (from an hour or so to a day or more) depending upon the efficiency of the patient's lymphatic system, the vigor of respiratory motion, and the oncotic pressure of the plasma. Second, patients with chronic left heart failure (and long-standing pulmonary venous hypertension) may have a hypertrophied pulmonary lymphatic system and produce only interstitial edema even with large rises in LAP whereas patients with *acute* left heart failure and the same degree of LAP elevation but a normal nonhypertrophied lymphatic system may go into severe alveolar edema. These points are discussed more fully in Chapters 6 and 7.

Quantification of Capillary Permeability (Injury) Edema

The different criteria and weighting that we have developed for grading the severity of injury edema are listed in Table 3-4. It is important to realize that the scores from this table cannot be related directly to absolute quantities of extravascular lung water for the following reasons: First, as we have already discussed, no satisfactory nonradiologic method presently exists for the accurate in vivo quantification of injury edema that would calibrate with the radiographic estimate. Second, in ARDS the radiographic changes are caused not only by injury edema but also by areas of atelectasis, vascu-

Table 3-4 Criteria for grading injury edema

Chest roentgenographic findings	Score
Right-sided cardiac enlargement with bulging of main pulmonary artery	2, 4
Hilar abnormalities (size and density)	1, 2
Air bronchogram	2, 4
Lung density increase	
Hazy	
Central	1, 2
Peripheral	2, 4
Central and peripheral	3, 6
Patchy	
Central	2, 4
Peripheral	5, 10
Central and peripheral	7, 14
Extensive white density	20

Each lung is scored separately. (See footnote for Table 3-2.)

*Many of our radiologic clinicians carry a miniaturized version of the table with them.

lar occlusion, hemorrhage, and (at a later stage) hyaline membranes and fibrosis. Third, in ARDS the increase in lung water does not develop gradually as it does in pressure edema, beginning with a clear interstitial phase and progressing in recognizable quantifiable stages to alveolar edema (which may again progress to a final "white-out") but instead tends to appear quite abruptly. It usually has no identifiable separate interstitial phase but appears from its onset to be a mixture of interstitial and alveolar edema and (usually) to assume its final degree of severity almost immediately, staying apparently unchanged thereafter in both quantity and distribution for many days or weeks. In the small percentage of cases that survive, gradual organization is manifested by (1) increasing sharpness of margins of both the pulmonary vessels and the areas of consolidation and (2) a slow resolution manifested by gradual diminution in the quantity and density of the involved areas over a period of weeks to months.

For these reasons any method, whether radiologic or not, aimed at assessing simply the *quantity* of pulmonary edema in ARDS is unlikely to be of much value in either the early detection or the later follow-up of the syndrome. Also, in the early stage of lung injury, the turnover of fluid and solutes through the interstitial/lymphatic system may be increased substantially before any increase in extravascular lung water can be detected.[88] In ARDS the increase in lung water alone does not correlate well with the deterioration of gas exchange and does not predict the outcome of the disease process.[89] If some other radiologic features are added, however, as discussed below, x-ray assessment of the severity of ARDS becomes more useful.

The radiographic scores in Table 3-4 (ARDS) are based on the presence, qualitative features, regional distribution, extent, and intensity of a number of radiographic findings (more extensively described in Chapter 2). These features have been derived by us from an analysis of the chest radiographs of a large series of patients with ARDS[84-87] and include right-sided cardiac enlargement and bulging of the main pulmonary artery, changes in the size and density of the hila, the presence of air bronchograms, and changes in lung density and the regional distribution of these density changes. Some of these features (e.g., right-sided cardiac enlargement, enlarged main pulmonary artery) may actually precede the onset of radiologically detectable edema.[16,87] Each of the radiologic features in the table

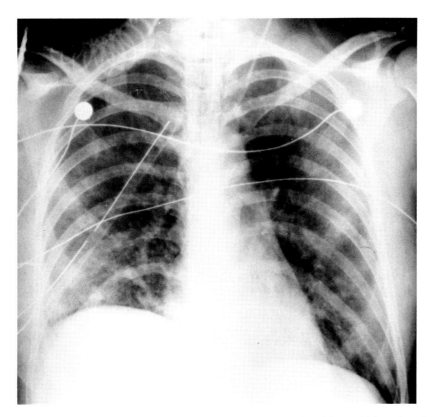

Fig. 3-10 Young man with ARDS following hypotension. Mixed interstitial and early alveolar edema still permit vascular structures to be seen (stage 1 severity).

carries a set of weighting numbers, according to its severity, and the sum of all these numbers gives an index to the severity of the injury edema. The cardiac changes reflect hemodynamic alterations (increased pulmonary vascular resistance and elevated pulmonary arterial pressure), which are consistent clinical features of ARDS[90-92]; but, because they cannot be considered specific for injury edema, they have been assigned a lower weighting in the scoring table (Table 3-4).

The terms used in Table 3-4 to describe *qualitatively* the patterns of radiographic increase in lung density match with three degrees of lung involvement:

1. Mixed interstitial and alveolar edema ("hazy", i.e., ill-defined, partially radiopaque densities that still allow the underlying vascular structures to be seen) (Fig. 3-10)
2. Alveolar edema ("patchy," i.e., scattered radiopaque densities that completely obscure the underlying vascular structures locally) (Figs. 3-11 and 3-12)
3. Extensive lung consolidation (referred to in the table as "extensive white density" (Fig. 3-13)

A peripheral distribution of increased lung density (as in Fig. 3-12) is given a higher score than a central distribution (Fig. 3-14) because it represents a more severe degree of involvement of the gas exchange sites.[16,84] In the scoring procedure each lung must be considered *separately* since lung injury edema is often asymmetric (Fig. 3-15) or even unilateral (Fig. 3-16).*

To assess the ability of the chest radiograph to determine the severity of ARDS, instead of comparing the radiographic score with the amount of extravascular lung water determined by indicator dilution studies (which, as we have shown, are not accurate), it would seem more realistic to compare it with other parameters (e.g., blood gas, compliance) that reflect the severity of ARDS with greater accuracy.

---

*On supine CT scans ARDS often appears to be gravitational (i.e., located in the dorsal paravertebral regions); but if the patient is turned into the *prone* position, the CT will reveal an *instant* shift of the dorsal densities to the ventral surface, showing that the densities were due to severe atelectasis from the weight of the ARDS lung, *not* to injury edema (which cannot move throughout the lung).

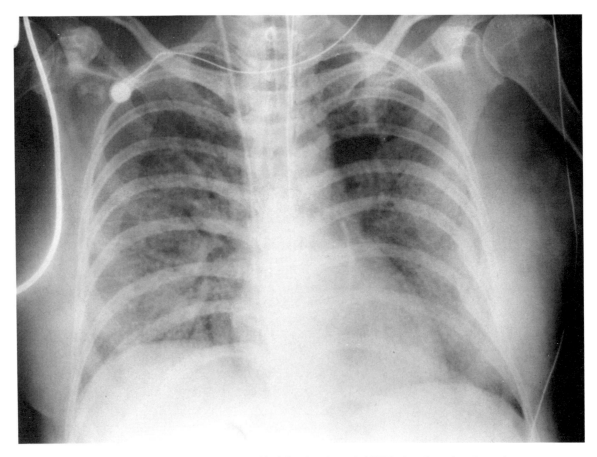

Fig. 3-11 A 36-year-old woman with fully developed ARDS showing alveolar edema, somewhat patchy but completely obscuring the vascular structure in areas (stage 3 severity). (Compare with Fig. 3-19, showing the same patient 2 days earlier.)

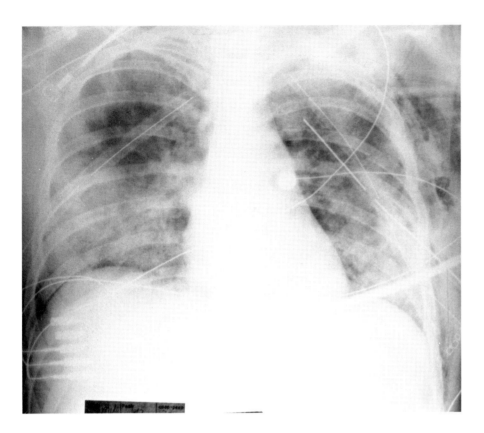

Fig. 3-12 A 34-year-old man with ARDS following septicemic shock. The patchiness and random distribution of the capillary permeability edema are typical but have been further modified by high positive ventilatory pressures (peak 70 cm, PEEP 25 cm H_2O), causing expansion of the *normal* areas of lung. Barotrauma was present with bilateral pneumothorax (stage 2 severity).

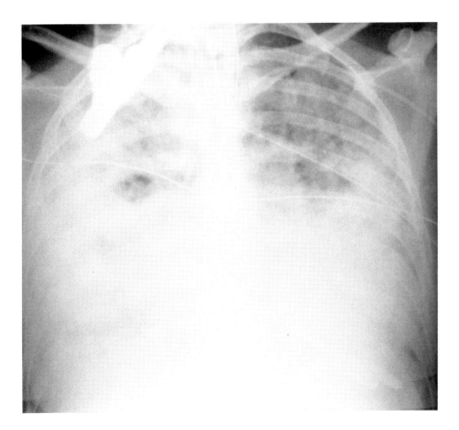

Fig. 3-13 A 28-year-old man with severe ARDS following septicemia, showing the appearances referred to as "extensive white density" (stage 3 severity).

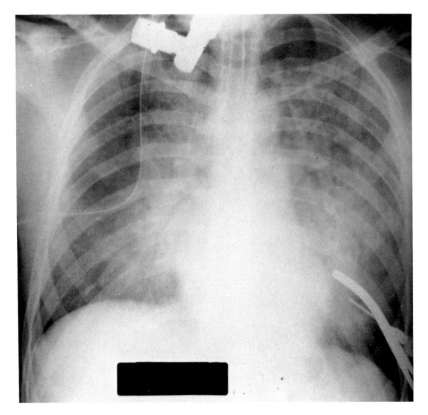

Fig. 3-14   A 20-year-old man resuscitated following profuse bleeding from a stab wound and severe hypotension. Note the *central* distribution of capillary permeability edema and the slightly increased convexity of the main pulmonary artery (indicating elevated pulmonary artery pressure).

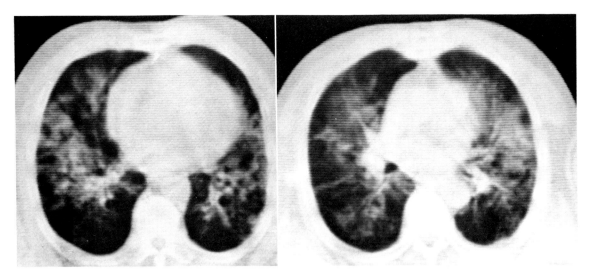

Fig. 3-15   Two CT cuts through the lungs of a patient with moderately severe ARDS showing the characteristic nongravitional patchy distribution with intervening areas of spared lung. The distribution in this case appears more peripheral just above the diaphragm and more central at a higher level.

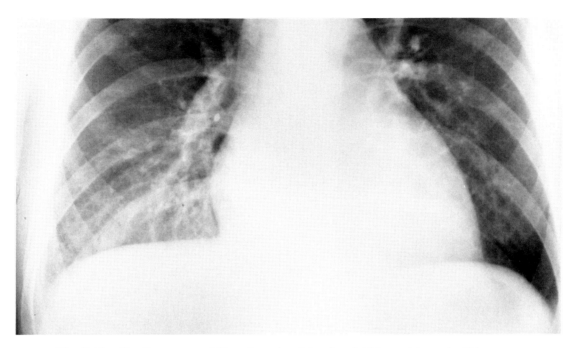

Fig. 3-16 Capillary permeability edema involving the right lower lobe only. This young man self-injected minced marijuana suspended in milk intravenously while lying curled on the floor on his right side.

Radiographic Grading of Severity Correlated with Hypoxemia in ARDS. Arterial blood samples were taken at the time the chest x-ray was obtained. Most of the patients were not intubated while the blood gas measurements were being made since the determinations were performed at the time of the patient's admission to the intensive care unit or following recovery from the acute phase of ARDS. In patients receiving positive pressure ventilation the PEEP was stopped prior to blood sampling. In any case, arterial oxygen tension values were expressed as "standard arterial oxygen tension" (correcting the measured values by using the Mays diagram[93]). Standard arterial oxygen tension quantitates gas exchange impairment at any level of alveolar ventilation better than measured arterial oxygen tension does.[93] A highly significant correlation was found between the radiographic score and standard arterial oxygen tension (Fig. 3-17). The curvilinear shape of this correlation indicates that, in some instances, standard arterial oxygen tension may be significantly reduced even in the presence of relatively moderate radiographic abnormalities. This could occur either in the very early stages of ARDS, when extravascular lung water is not appreciably increased or in the recovery phase of the syndrome, when alveolar flooding has been replaced by tissue repair[94] (Fig. 3-18). At both stages the lung fields may appear relatively clear on the chest radiograph and yet marked

hypoxemia can be found. This finding further confirms that in ARDS, factors other than lung water accumulation are responsible for the derangement of gas exchange and that in the clinical evaluation of patients it is important to combine the information derived from the chest x-ray and the blood gas data. It is worth noting, however, that in no instance was the chest x-ray scored as normal when significant hypoxemia was present.

Cardiac and pulmonary vascular abnormalities (e.g., a bulging main pulmonary artery, enlarged right side of the heart) in association with clear lung fields are often the only radiographic findings in the early stage of ARDS (Figs. 3-11 and 3-19). Once the diagnosis of pulmonary embolism has been ruled out, the occurrence of such a radiographic pattern in patients with predisposing risk factors should give rise to a suspicion of impending ARDS.[95,96] Pulmonary embolism is the only condition likely to present with a similar combination of clinical, blood gas, and radiographic data.[9,16,95-97] Thus even a chest radiograph with minimal or no evidence of edema can still be useful in the early detection of ARDS if cardiac or pulmonary vascular changes are present.

Chest X-ray and Impairment of Lung Perfusion. Injury to the pulmonary vessels is believed to be of major importance in the development of ARDS. The central role of the pulmonary circulation is demonstrated by bi-

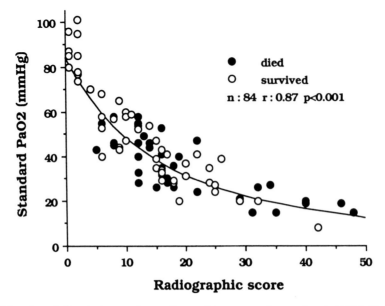

Fig. 3-17   Correlation between the radiographic score of severity of ARDS (Table 3-4) and standard Po$_2$.

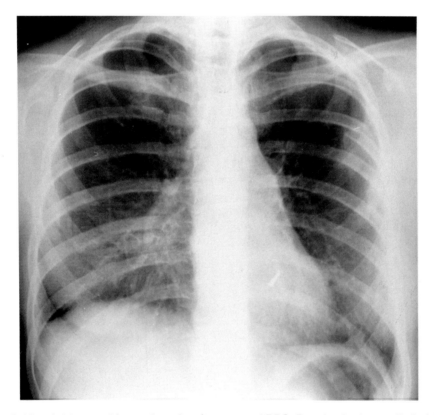

Fig. 3-18   A 34-year-old man 4 weeks after severe ARDS. Despite the "normality" of the lung fields, standard O$_2$ tension was significantly reduced.

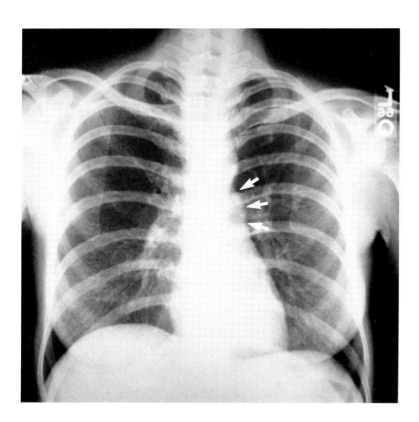

Fig. 3-19 A 36-year-old woman following severe bleeding from a duodenal ulcer. Note the increased convexity of the main pulmonary artery *(arrows)*. At this stage her Po$_2$ had dropped abruptly. The lungs show no radiologic abnormality. (Compare with Fig. 3-11, same patient 3 days later in full ARDS.)

opsies and postmortem studies performed in patients with ARDS[41,98,99]—which show acute endothelial injury, intimal fibrosis, thromboembolization of capillary and precapillary vessels, increased arterial wall thickness, and extension of smooth muscle into normally nonmuscular pulmonary arterioles. These pathologic findings may explain the common clinical occurrence of pulmonary hypertension at elevated pulmonary vascular resistance in patients with ARDS.[90-92] Furthermore, pulmonary vascular occlusive disease has been demonstrated by bedside pulmonary angiography in the early stages of ARDS[40-42] (Fig. 3-20). The presence of angiographic filling defects correlates with the severity of respiratory failure, mortality, the presence of intravascular coagulation, and increased pulmonary vascular resistance.[40] Such alterations are more easily detected by lung perfusion examinations than by the plain chest film.

In a series of patients with ARDS we showed[43] that scintigraphic perfusion abnormalities are the rule throughout the evolving syndrome (Fig. 3-21). These abnormalities include focal nonsegmental defects, mostly peripheral and dorsal, with perfusion redistribution away from the dependent lung zones. Perfusion abnormalities correlate with the severity of ARDS as expressed by gas exchange impairment, increased pulmonary artery pressure, and vascular resistance.[43] Even though perfusion defects do not necessarily correspond to increased radiographic densities, their extent on the

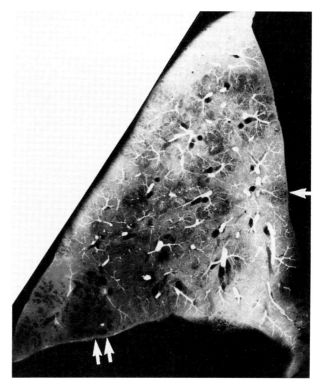

Fig. 3-20 Barium sulfate injected postmortem into the lungs of a patient who died of severe ARDS following pneumonia reveals several subpleural areas of oligemia *(single arrow)* and a large area of ischemic necrosis *(twin arrows)*. (From Greene R: *J Thorac Imaging* 1[3]:31, 1986.)

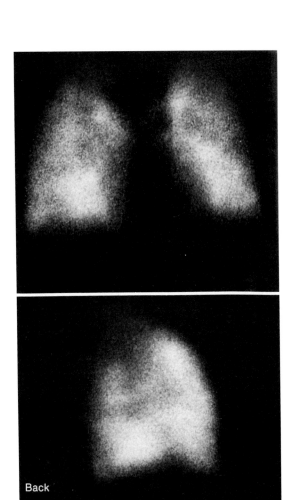

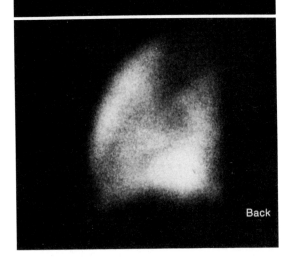

Fig. 3-21 Perfusion lung scans of a young man with severe ARDS following septicemic shock. Note the bilateral large nonsegmental perfusion defects in apical, central, and dorsal regions of the lungs. From Pistolesi M, Miniati M, DiRicco G, et al: *J Thorac Imaging* 1[3]:11, 1986.)

lung scan shows a positive linear correlation with the radiographic score of ARDS[43]—further recommending the chest x-ray for assessment of lung dysfunction in patients with ARDS (in whom pulmonary angiography or lung perfusion scans cannot be routinely performed).

Chest X-ray, Lung Compliance, and Increased Lung Density. Another demonstration of the chest x-ray's ability to reflect the severity of ARDS comes from preliminary work in which it has been demonstrated that the radiographic score increases with reduction in static compliance[100] and with increases in the overall lung density determined by CT[101] in patients with ARDS.

Since the x-ray scoring method is strongly correlated with the indices of ARDS severity such as impairment of gas exchange, lung perfusion abnormalities, reduction in lung compliance, and increase in the specific gravity of the lung, the plain chest radiograph can now be accepted not only as the gold standard for detecting and quantifying *hydrostatic* edema but also as the simplest and most objective method of monitoring the clinical progress of patients with ARDS.

Relative Accuracy of Chest Radiography and Indicator Dilution Measurements for Quantifying Pressure Edema

Many papers, most of which have been published since the advent of thermodilution techniques, declare that the chest x-ray is not a reliable method for evaluating pulmonary edema because x-ray assessments do not correlate with the amount of pulmonary edema measured by indicator dilution methods. It is important to point out that (1) most of these comparisons have been obtained using poorly standardized radiographic methods for assessing pulmonary edema and (2) the measurement of extravascular lung water by indicator dilution techniques has in most reports been considered (inappropriately) the "gold standard" by which the radiographic appearances must be critically appraised. These two problems affect the correctness of the conclusions of the majority of these papers since, as we have already shown,[34] the measurement of extravascular lung water by indicator dilution is less accurate than usually believed. The standard isotopic indicator dilution method underestimates EVLW by approximately 50% in basal conditions and even more when edema is present.[15,16,18]

Standardization of the chest reading technique, using the same film reading table for every film and every observer (e.g., Table 3-3), is essential to introduce objectivity, consistency, and accuracy into the interpretation. When authors use very simplistic inadequate x-ray analytic techniques to assess extravascular lung water and then compare these findings with an indicator dilution technique that is not in itself sufficiently sensitive to detect early edema at the lower end of the scale, and becomes progressively less and less accurate in detecting edema at the upper end of the scale (as alveolar edema develops),[102] it is not surprising that so many erroneous conclusions have been drawn about the accuracy of the radiographic assessment technique. For example, in one report alleging that the indicator dilution method had a higher sensitivity than the x-ray approach,[103] the only radiologic criterion used for detecting and quantitating edema was the presence of Kerley lines, which, as we have shown,[15,84,104] occur in only 30% of patients with cardiac edema.

Once the film reader has become completely familiar with the many radiologic signs of pulmonary edema, accuracy in reading is affected surprisingly little by variations in radiologic technique or patient positioning. One observation that does have a profound effect on the accuracy of edema measurements is inadequate inspiration; but, as we have detailed elsewhere in this book, inadvertent expiratory films are much less common than usually supposed and can be quite readily recognized in a chronologic series of films—not by the level of the diaphragm but by the reduction in *width* of the thorax that occurs in expiration. Nevertheless, careful standardization of the way the radiograph is taken can add to the accuracy of interpretation.

It goes without saying that maximum power and minimum exposure times should be employed and that, once a satisfactory set of exposure factors has been achieved (kV, mA, time), these should be recorded and used for all sequential films. In addition, however, the film reader must know whether the patient was erect or supine, how far the film was from the x-ray tube, and whether the patient was receiving positive pressure ventilation and, if so, the levels of peak pressure and PEEP (remembering that the film reader sees [hopefully] a fully inspiratory film, at which point peak—or more correctly "plateau" pressure—is in effect, not PEEP). All these data must be recorded directly on the film so they can be factored into the radiologic analysis. (The type of label we have developed for this purpose has been described elsewhere[86] and will be discussed more fully in Chapter 10.)

Probably more important than any of these factors is proper technologist training—such as the holding of regular educational (in-service) sessions with the technologists to ensure that they are aware of *their* importance in helping the patient recover. Human nature being what it is, "refresher" in-service talks are necessary rather frequently to keep the technologists' level of participatory enthusiasm high! (See Chapter 10.)

With the combination of standardized radiographic and reading techniques, achieved by use of the same reading table for all readers (Table 3-3), the "subjectivity" so often referred to as one of the major problems in using the chest radiograph to detect and quantitate edema can be markedly reduced (and, for experienced trained observers, virtually eliminated.)[84]

The low sensitivity of the older indicator dilution methods is clearly revealed in a report[103] in which the authors found that the indicator dilution values increased above normal only when the patients had developed gross clinical pulmonary edema. More recently, with the thermal indicator dilution technique,[82] which is more accurate than the older unmodified isotopic technique, better correlations have been obtained between x-ray measurements and thermal dilution methods. However, since reduction in the indicator dilution measurements of extravascular lung water after therapy was matched by simultaneous radiographic clearing of edema, it is evident that the thermal dilution measurement does not offer any advantage over the x-ray in follow-up of patients with cardiac edema. It is also important to note that, in the publications quoted,[82] a normal chest radiograph was always associated with normal indicator dilution values. Therefore, in cardiac patients, if the chest x-ray shows no evidence of edema, there is no indication to use thermal dilution techniques.

Our initial study[17] (the first ever made of the accuracy of chest radiographs in quantitating pulmonary edema) was carried out using the older unmodified, less accurate, double indicator dilution technique; but even with this limitation, by using a standardized scoring technique, rigorously applied, we found a good correlation between x-ray and indicator dilution assessments in a mixture of patients with cardiac, overhydration, and injury lung edema (Fig. 3-22).

We later repeated this study in a group of cardiac patients using more refined radiologic criteria and a more accurate indicator dilution method modified by ourselves,[15,16] and again there was excellent correlation between our radiographic scoring technique and the modified indicator dilution technique (Fig. 3-6). It is important to point out that the correlation we obtained is not linear. At first, the x-ray score of edema increases while the indicator dilution measurements remain normal; then the indicator values rise sharply and there is an approximately linear correlation with the x-ray score (Fig. 3-6). The initial rise in the x-ray score, while the indicator dilution studies remained unchanged, reveals the extraordinary ability of the chest radiograph to disclose subtle signs of early interstitial edema that are undetectable by the less sensitive isotope techniques (even though the complex modified isotope technique we used in this study was much more accurate than the standard technique employed clinically).

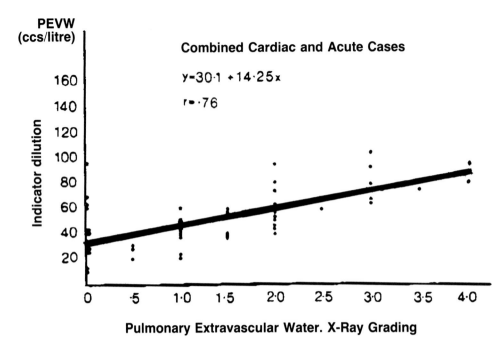

Fig. 3-22 Correlation between edema (EVLW) graded by x-ray and by indicator dilution technique. (Modified from Milne ENC: *Radiol Clin North Am* 11:17, 1973.)

Relative Accuracy of Chest Radiography and Indicator Dilution Measurements for Quantifying Injury Edema (ARDS)

As we have discussed previously, indicator dilution techniques are strongly dependent upon perfusion. When heat is used as the indicator, this dependence appears to diminish but is still present. The effect of perfusion on the accuracy of indicator dilution estimates of extravascular lung water is of particular importance in patients with ARDS, in whom perfusion defects are much commoner than in patients with hydrostatic edema. Several papers have been published[83,105-115] comparing the measurement of extravascular lung water by indicator dilution techniques with the chest radiographic appearances in ARDS. In most of these reports heat was used as the diffusible indicator. With few exceptions,[109,110,112] the amount of extravascular lung water measured by dilution techniques increased in parallel with increasing severity of the radiographic findings.* However, cases showing definite radiographic edema (even alveolar edema) with *normal* extravascular thermal values are common in many of these reports.† Failure to appreciate that in these patients extravascular lung water may be greatly underestimated, because of either inherent inaccuracies in the thermal dilution technique[33,34,44,116] or the presence of

unperfused lung regions,[10-43] has led to the erroneous conclusion that if the chest x-ray shows definite signs of lung edema, and the thermal dilution value is normal, the chest x-ray is falsely positive.* Since it is most unlikely that the specific radiographic findings of pulmonary edema can occur without edema being present, the absence of any detectable increase in thermal dilution estimates of lung water in such cases[9,33,34,44] suggests that it is the accuracy of the thermal dilution method (not the radiographic method) that requires a rigorous and critical reappraisal, particularly when applied to the monitoring of pulmonary edema in patients with ARDS.

It could be correctly argued that the appearance of increased lung densities in intensive care unit patients with ARDS is caused by processes such as atelectasis or fibrosis, in which extravascular lung water may not be elevated. However, the chest radiograph (and in particular sequential radiographs) will often permit the correct etiology of the lung densities to be diagnosed and the radiologist can then exclude these findings from the evaluation of edema.

It is important also to point out that figures for lung water derived from dilution studies represent a *mean* value of all the perfused regions of the lung, some of which may be grossly edematous and others quite free of edema. This regional variation in intensity of edema

---

*References 82, 105-108, 113-115.
†References 82, 107, 108, 113-115.

*References 105, 107, 109, 112, 113.

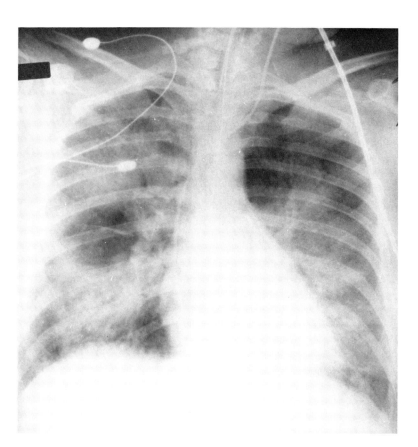

Fig. 3-23   Characteristic distribution of injury edema in a case or ARDS. The regional distribution of the edema is clearly visible.

is readily recognized on the chest film (Fig. 3-23) but is impossible to abstract from the indicator dilution numbers—another distinct clinical advantage for the chest film.

It has been reported[82] that patients with injury edema have greater amounts of extravascular lung water than patients with the same radiologic grade of pressure edema. This belief is probably related to the incorrect application of criteria developed specifically for *hydrostatic* (pressure) edema to score injury edema, for which (as we have shown[16,84,85]) quite different radiographic criteria must be used. Furthermore, in these studies no attempt was made to standardize the actual *taking* of the chest radiograph, the authors simply declaring* that standardization was deliberately not carried out so that the "real life" setting would be duplicated. This is like rejecting a priori the valuable information that can be obtained from the chest x-ray simply to avoid having to make a few technical adjustments, which are incomparably simpler than those necessary for the acquisition of most data in the complex environment of the intensive care unit. However, even with *poorly* standardized chest radiographs, an important common result of these papers (as with the cardiac edema papers) was that in the presence of a chest x-ray

with no detectable signs of edema (score = 0) the mean thermal dilution value of extravascular lung water was also consistently normal.* This means that when the chest x-ray is normal it is quite improbable that extravascular lung water is increased to a level that can be detected by any indicator dilution method. It appears, therefore, that using the invasive, expensive, and complex thermal dilution method to measure extravascular lung water in ARDS when the chest x-ray has proved normal is valueless. Similarly, the indicator dilution method does not offer any advantage over the chest x-ray for early detection of edema in patients at risk of ARDS.

The comparisons between indicator dilution values of extravascular lung water and chest x-ray evaluations, in both pressure edema and injury edema, clearly confirm that the chest x-ray must now be considered the "gold standard" for detecting and monitoring pulmonary edema. The amount of information that can be derived from it in patients with pulmonary edema is much greater than presently generally appreciated. As the experience and skill of film readers increase, it can be expected that yet more clinical information will be extracted from the plain chest film.

---

*References 105, 107, 112, 115.

*References 82, 105, 106, 111, 113, 114.

APPENDIX: EXAMINATION OF THE WIDELY HELD BELIEF THAT AN INCREASE IN LUNG WATER OF OVER 35% IS REQUIRED BEFORE EDEMA CAN BE RECOGNIZED ON THE CHEST RADIOGRAPH

This belief is based on an experimental study in dogs[83] in which pulmonary edema was induced by fluid overload or alloxan injection and a chest radiograph was obtained before and after the development of edema. The radiograph obtained shortly before death was used for comparison with a gravimetric assessment of extravascular lung water. As stated by the authors of this study,

In all cases where the extravascular water/dry lung weight ratio was increased more than 35%, definite oedema was diagnosed.

Since the publication of this paper, "35%" has become a magic number in the literature and, without being further confirmed or even discussed, has been handed down from author to author as the radiographic threshold for early detection of lung edema.* This was not the message of the original paper, however, since the authors only accepted that "definite edema" was present if the films showed "shadowing that caused blurring and obscuring of vessel, cardiac, and diaphragmatic outlines." However they also described the early phase of lung water accumulation as "abnormal shadowing but *insufficient* to blur or obscure vessel shadows" and *this* radiographic appearance was present and recognized by the authors in *every dog* subjected to an edematogenic procedure, even when the increase in extravascular lung water was less than 35% by gravimetric methods or too small to be detected gravimetrically. Therefore this paper, instead of implying (as is usually stated) that lung water must be increased by 35% to be detectible radiologically, in fact confirmed that the chest radiograph has a much higher sensitivity than this for the detection of pulmonary edema.

An increase in extravascular lung water of 35% would, in the human, approximate to 70 ml H_2O per liter of TLC. This would rank (Table 3-3) as "moderate" interstitial edema, which should be very easily recognized.

It is known that a fluid gain of 35% can be accommodated in the peribronchovascular interstitium prior to the development of alveolar flooding.[123] If one were to accept that there must be a 35% gain in EVLW before pulmonary edema can be diagnosed radiologically, this would imply that only *alveolar* edema can be reliably detected by the chest radiograph—a conclusion at complete variance with clinical and experimental data.[12-17]

Extrapolation of the results of animal studies to humans is always hazardous, but in this case it appears safe to conclude that the sensitivity obtained in human patients will be even greater than that in dogs since the narrow transverse and deep anteroposterior diameters of the canine thorax, the large area obscured by the canine heart, and the absence of canine interlobular septa (obviating the development of septal lines) all make it more difficult to see edema in dogs than in humans.

From these considerations it appears that in humans (1) the radiographic threshold for the detection of pulmonary edema is considerably lower than in dogs and (2) the approximate value of a 10% increase in lung water (derived from comparison of radiologic estimates with indicator dilution values) may be closer to reality than the more oft-quoted 35%.[16]

REFERENCES

1. Staub NC: Clinical use of lung water measurements. Report of a workshop, *Chest* 90:589, 1986.
2. Ingram RH, Braunwald E. Pulmonary edema: cardiogenic and noncardiogenic. In Braunwald E (ed): *Heart disease. A textbook of cardiovascular medicine*, ed 3, Philadelphia, 1988, WB Saunders, p 1870.
3. Casaburi R, Wasserman K, Effros RM: Detection and measurement of pulmonary edema. In Staub NC (ed): *Lung water and solute exchange*, New York, 1978, Marcel Dekker, p 323.
4. Snashall PD, Hughes JMB: Lung water balance, *Rev Physiol Biochem Pharmacol* 89:5, 1981.
5. Prichard JS: Diagnostic methods and clinical measurement of pulmonary edema. In Prichard JS,: *Edema of the lung*, Springfield Ill, 1982, Charles C Thomas, p 227.
6. Hogg JC: The assessment of pulmonary microvascular permeability and edema. In Said SI (ed): *The pulmonary circulation and acute lung injury*, Mount Kisco NY, 1985, Futura Publishing, p 209.
7. Murray JF: The lungs and heart failure, *Hosp Pract* 4:55, 1985.
8. Cutillo AG: The clinical assessment of lung water, *Chest* 92:319, 1987.
9. Miniati M, Pistolesi M, Milne ENC, Giuntini C: Detection of lung edema, *Crit Care Med* 15:1146, 1987.
10. Fishman AP: Pulmonary edema. In Fishman AP (ed): *Pulmonary diseases and disorders*, ed 2, vol 2, New York, 1988, McGraw-Hill, p 919.
11. Flick MR: Pulmonary edema and acute lung injury. In Murray JF, Nadel JA (eds): *Textbook of respiratory medicine*, Philadelphia, 1988, WB Saunders, p 1359.
12. Logue RB, Rogers JV Jr, Gray BB Jr: Subtle roentgenographic findings of left heart failure, *Am Heart J* 65:464, 1963.
13. Harrison MO, Conte PJ, Heitzman ER: Radiological detection of clinically occult cardiac failure following myocardial infarction, *Br J Radiol* 44:265, 1971.
14. Chait A, Cohen ME, Meltzer LE, Van Durme JP: The bedside chest radiograph in the evaluation of incipient left heart failure, *Radiology* 105:563, 1972.
15. Pistolesi M, Giuntini C: Assessment of extravascular lung water, *Radiol Clin North Am* 16:551, 1978.
16. Pistolesi M, Miniati M, Milne ENC, Giuntini C: The chest roentgenogram in pulmonary edema, *Clin Chest Med* 6:315, 1985.
17. Milne ENC: Correlation of physiologic findings with chest roentgenology, *Radiol Clin North Am* 11:17, 1973.
18. Staub NC: Pulmonary edema, *Physiol Rev* 54:678, 1974.
19. Gump FE: Lung fluid and solute compartments. In Staub NC

*References 1, 11, 44, 82, 105-108, 117-122.

(ed): *Lung water and solute exchange*, New York, 1978, Marcel Dekker, p 75.

20. Montaner JSG, Tsang J, Evans KJ, et al: Alveolar epithelial damage. A critical difference between high pressure and oleic acid-induced low pressure pulmonary edema, *J Clin Invest* 77:1786, 1986.

21. Bachofen H, Bachofen M, Weibel ER: Ultrastructural aspects of pulmonary edema, *J Thorac Imaging* 3(3):1, 1988.

22. Severinghaus JW, Catron C, Noble W: A focusing electrode bridge for unilateral lung resistance, *J Appl Physiol* 32:526, 1972.

23. Fein A, Grossman RF, Jones JG, et al: Evaluation of transthoracic electrical impedance in the diagnosis of pulmonary edema, *Circulation* 60:156, 1979.

24. Iskander MF, Durney CH: Microwave methods of measuring changes in lung water, *J Microwave Power* 18:265, 1983.

25. Gamsu G, Kauffman L, Swann SJ, Brito AC: Absolute lung density in experimental canine lung edema, *Invest Radiol* 14:261, 1979.

26. Webber LE, Coates G: A clinical system for the in vivo measurement of lung density, *Med Phys* 9:473, 1982.

27. Simon DS, Murray JF, Staub NC: Measurement of pulmonary edema in intact dogs by transthoracic gamma ray attenuation, *J Appl Physiol* 47:1228, 1979.

28. Cander L, Forster RE: Determination of pulmonary parenchymal tissue volume and pulmonary capillary blood flow in men, *J Appl Physiol* 14:541, 1959.

29. Overland ES, Gupta RN, Huchon GJ, Murray JF: Measurement of pulmonary volume and blood flow in persons with normal and edematous lungs, *J Appl Physiol* 51:1375, 1981.

30. Kallay MC, Hyde RW, Fahey PJ, et al: Effect of the rebreathing pattern on pulmonary tissue volume and capillary blood flow, *J Appl Physiol* 58:188, 1985.

31. Chinard FP, Enns T: Transcapillary pulmonary exchange of water in the dog, *Am J Physiol* 178:197, 1954.

32. Zierler KL: Theoretical bases of indicator dilution methods of measuring flow and volume, *Circ Res* 10:393, 1962.

33. Effros RM: Lung water measurements with the mean transit time approach, *J Appl Physiol* 59:673, 1985.

34. Giuntini C, Pistolesi M, Miniati M, Fazio F: Theoretical and practical considerations of measuring extravascular lung water, *J Thorac Imaging* 3(3):36, 1988.

35. Pearce ML, Yamashita J, Beazell J: Measurement of pulmonary edema, *Circ Res* 16:482, 1965.

36. Kirk BW, Zylak C, Bristow GK: Gas exchange and extravascular water in acute myocardial infarction. In Giuntini C (ed): *Central hemodynamics and gas exchange*, Torino, 1971, Minerva Medica, p 333.

37. Lewis FR, Elings VB, Hill SL, Christensen JM: The measurement of extravascular lung water by thermal-green dye indicator dilution, *Ann NY Acad Sci* 384:394, 1982.

38. Noble WM, Severinghaus JW: Thermal and conductivity dilution curves for rapid quantitation of pulmonary edema, *J Appl Physiol* 32:770, 1972.

39. Lewis FR, Elings VB: Microprocessor determination of lung water using thermal-green dye double indicator dilution, *Surg Forum* 29:182, 1978.

40. Greene R, Zapol WM, Snider M, et al: Early bedside detection of pulmonary vascular occlusion during acute respiratory failure, *Am Rev Respir Dis* 124:593, 1981.

41. Tomashewski JF Jr, Davies P, Boggis C, et al: The pulmonary vascular lesions of the adult respiratory distress syndrome, *Am J Pathol* 112:112, 1983.

42. Greene R: Pulmonary vascular obstruction in the adult respiratory distress syndrome, *J Thorac Imaging* 1(3):31, 1986.

43. Pistolesi M, Miniati M, DiRicco G, et al: Perfusion lung imaging in the adult respiratory distress syndrome, *J Thorac Imaging* 1(3):11, 1986.

44. Allison RC, Carlile VP, Gray BA: Thermodilution measurement of lung water, *Clin Chest Med* 6:439, 1985.

45. Noble WH, Kay JC: Effects of emboli, positive-pressure ventilation, and airway water on lung water measurements, *J Appl Physiol* 65:156, 1988.

46. Carlile PV, Hagan SF, Gray BA: Perfusion distribution and lung thermal volume in canine hydrochloric acid aspiration, *J Appl Physiol* 65:750, 1988.

47. Effros RM, Mason GR: Measurements of pulmonary epithelial permeability in vivo, *Am Rev Respir Dis* 127(suppl):59, 1983.

48. Coates G, O'Brodovich H, Dolovich M: Lung clearance of ^{99m}Tc-DTPA in patients with acute lung injury and pulmonary edema, *J Thorac Imaging* 3(3):21, 1988.

49. Jones JC, Minty BD, Royston D: The physiology of leaky lungs, *Br J Anaesth* 1982;54:705.

50. Mason GR, Effros RM, Unsler JM, Mena I: Small solute clearance from the lungs of patients with cardiogenic and noncardiogenic pulmonary edema, *Chest* 88:327, 1985.

51. Tennenberg SD, Jacobs MP, Solomkin JS, et al: Increased pulmonary alveolar-capillary permeability in patients at risk for adult respiratory distress syndrome, *Crit Care Med* 15:289, 1987.

52. Braude S, Nolop KB, Hughes JMB, et al: Comparison of lung vascular and epithelial permeability indices in the adult respiratory distress syndrome, *Am Rev Respir Dis* 132:1002, 1986.

53. Marks JD, Luce JM, Lazar NM, et al: Effect of increases in lung volume on clearance of aerosolized solute from human lungs, *J Appl Physiol* 59:1242, 1985.

54. Gorin AB, Weidner WJ, Demling RM, Staub NC: Noninvasive measurement of pulmonary transvascular protein flux in sheep, *J Appl Physiol* 45:225, 1978.

55. Prichard JS, Lee G de J: Measurement of water distribution and transcapillary solute flux in dog lung by external counting, *Clin Sci* 57:145, 1979.

56. Gorin AB, Kohler J, DeNardo G: Noninvasive measurement of pulmonary transvascular protein flux in normal man, *J Clin Invest* 66:869, 1980.

57. Sugerman HJ, Strash AM, Hirsch JT, et al: Sensitivity of scintigraphy for detection of pulmonary capillary albumin leak in canine oleic acid ARDS, *J Trauma* 21:520, 1981.

58. Dauber IM, Pluss WT, VanGrondelle A, et al: Specificity and sensitivity of noninvasive measurement of pulmonary vascular protein leak, *J Appl Physiol* 59:674, 1985.

59. Basran GS, Hardy JG: Monitoring pulmonary vascular permeability using radiolabelled transferrin, *J Thorac Imaging* 3(3):28, 1988.

60. Tatum JL, Burke TS, Sugerman HJ, et al: Computerized scintigraphic technique for evaluation of adult respiratory distress syndrome: initial clinical trials, *Radiology* 143:237, 1982.

61. Sugerman HJ, Tatum JL, Burke TS, et al: Gamma scintigraphic analysis of albumin flux in patients with acute respiratory distress, *Surgery* 95:674, 1984.

62. Rhodes CG, Wollmer P, Fazio F, Jones T: Quantitative measurement of regional extravascular lung density using positron emission and transmission tomography, *J Comput Assist Tomogr* 5:783, 1981.

63. Schuster DP, Mintun MA, Green MA, Ter-Pogossian MM: Regional lung water and hematocrit determined by positron emission tomography. *J Appl Physiol* 1985;59:860.

64. Mintun MA, Ter-Pogossian MM, Green MA, et al: Quantitative measurement of regional pulmonary blood flow with positron emission tomography, *J Appl Physiol* 60:317, 1986.

65. Schuster DP, Marklin GF, Mintun MA: Regional changes in extravascular lung water detected by positron emission tomography, *J Appl Physiol* 60:1170, 1986.

66. Mintun MA, Dennis DR, Welch MJ, et al: Measurements of pulmonary vascular permeability with PET and Gallium-68 transferrin, *J Nucl Med* 28:1704, 1987.

67. Calandrino FS, Anderson DJ, Mintun MA, Schuster DP: Pulmonary vascular permeability during the adult respiratory distress syndrome: a positron emission tomographic study, *Am Rev Respir Dis* 138:421, 1988.

68. Wollmer P, Rhodes CG: Positron emission tomography in pulmonary edema, *J Thorac Imaging* 3(3):44, 1988.

69. Wollmer P, Rhodes CG, Deanfield J, et al: Regional extravascular lung density of the lung in patients with acute pulmonary edema, *J Appl Physiol* 63:1890, 1987.

70. Wollmer P, Rhodes CG, Allan RM, et al: Regional extravascular lung density and fractional blood volume in patients with chronic pulmonary venous hypertension, *Clin Physiol* 3:241, 1983.

71. Wegener OH, Koeppe P, Oeser M: Measurement of lung density by computed tomography, *J Comput Assist Tomogr* 2:263, 1978.

72. Rosenblum LJ, Mauceri RA, Wellenstein DE, et al: Density patterns in the normal lung as determined by computed tomography, *Radiology* 137:406, 1980.

73. Hedlund LW, Jones DP, Effmann EL, et al: A computed tomographic study of the dog lung during hemorrhagic shock and after resuscitation, *Invest Radiol* 16:446, 1981.

74. Slutski RA, Peck WW, Higgins CB, Mancini GBJ: Pulmonary density distribution in experimental and clinical cardiogenic pulmonary edema evaluated by computed transmission tomography, *Am Heart J* 108:401, 1984.

75. Hedlund LW, Vock P, Effmann EL: Computed tomography of the lung. Densitometric studies, *Radiol Clin North Am* 21:775, 1983.

76. Hedlund LW, Vock P, Effmann EL, et al: Hydrostatic pulmonary edema: an analysis of lung density changes by computed tomography, *Invest Radiol* 19:254, 1984.

77. Hedlund LW, Vock P, Effmann EL, Putman CE: Morphology of oleic acid-induced lung injury, *Invest Radiol* 20:2, 1985.

78. Gattinoni L, Pesenti A, Baglioni S, et al: Inflammatory pulmonary edema and positive end-expiratory pressure: correlations between imaging and physiologic studies, *J Thorac Imaging* 3(3):59, 1988.

79. Cutillo AG, Morris AM, Ailion DC, et al: Determination of lung water content and distribution by nuclear magnetic resonance imaging, *J Thorac Imaging* 1(3):39, 1986.

80. Cutillo AG, Morris AM, Ailion DC, et al: Quantitative assessment of pulmonary edema by nuclear magnetic resonance methods. *J Thorac Imaging* 3(3):51, 1988.

81. Staub NC, Hogg JC: Clinical measurement of lung water content, *Chest* 79:3, 1981.

82. Sibbald WJ, Warshawski FJ, Short AK, et al: Clinical studies of measuring extravascular lung water by the thermal dye technique in critically ill patients, *Chest* 83:725, 1983.

83. Snashall PD, Keyes SJ, Morgan BM, et al: The radiographic detection of acute pulmonary oedema. A comparison of radiographic appearances, densitometry and lung water in dogs, *Br J Radiol* 54:277, 1981.

84. Milne ENC, Pistolesi M, Miniati M, Giuntini C: The radiologic distinction of cardiogenic and noncardiogenic edema, *AJR* 144:879, 1985.

85. Miniati M, Pistolesi M, Paoletti P, et al: Objective radiographic criteria to differentiate cardiac, renal, and injury lung edema, *Invest Radiol* 23:433, 1988.

86. Milne ENC: A physiologic approach to reading critical care unit films, *J Thorac Imaging* 1(3):60, 1986.

87. Pistolesi M, Miniati M, Ravelli V, Giuntini C: Injury versus hydrostatic edema: detection by chest x-ray, *Ann NY Acad Sci* 384:364, 1982.

88. Brigham KL, Woolverton WC, Bland LM, Staub NC: Increased sheep lung vascular permeability caused by pseudomonas bacteremia, *J Clin Invest* 54:792, 1974.

89. Brigham KL, Kariman K, Harris TR, et al: Correlation of oxygenation with vascular permeability-surface area but not with lung water in humans with acute respiratory failure and pulmonary edema, *J Clin Invest* 72:339, 1983.

90. Zapol WM, Snider MT: Pulmonary hypertension in severe acute respiratory failure, *N Engl J Med* 296:476, 1977.

91. Shoemaker WC, Appel P, Czer LSC, et al: Pathogenesis of respiratory failure (ARDS) after hemorrhage and trauma. I. Cardiorespiratory patterns preceding the development of ARDS, *Crit Care Med* 8:504, 1980.

92. Zimmerman GA, Morris AM, Gengiz M: Cardiovascular alterations in the adult respiratory distress syndrome, *Am J Med* 73:25, 1980.

93. Mays EE: An arterial blood gas diagram for clinical use, *Chest* 63:793, 1973.

94. Greene R: Adult respiratory distress syndrome: acute alveolar damage, *Radiology* 163:57, 1987.

95. Fowler AA, Hamman RF, Good JT, et al: Adult respiratory distress syndrome: risk with common predisposition, *Ann Intern Med* 98:593, 1983.

96. Iannuzzi M, Petty TL: The diagnosis, pathogenesis, and treatment of adult respiratory distress syndrome, *J Thorac Imaging* 1(3):1, 1986.

97. Joffe N: The adult respiratory distress syndrome, *AJR* 122:719, 1974.

98. Eeles GH, Sevitt S: Microthrombosis in injured and burned patients. *J Pathol Bacteriol* 93:275, 1967.

99. Reid LM: Pathology of adult respiratory distress syndrome and experimental injury, with emphasis on vascular changes. In Andreadis NA, Petty TL (eds): *New basic and clinical science in adult respiratory distress syndrome.* Seminars in respiratory medicine, New York, 1986, Thieme Medical Publishers, p. 29.

100. Bernasconi M, Miniati M, Brandolese R, et al: Noninvasive quantification of edema in ARDS: respiratory mechanics versus portable chest x-ray, *Am Rev Respir Dis* 137(suppl):47A, 1988.

101. Bombino M, Gattinoni L, Pesenti A, et al: The value of portable chest roentgenography in adult respiratory distress syndrome: comparison with computed tomography, *Chest* 100:762, 1991.

102. Crosbie Wa, Snowden S, Parsons V: Change in lung capillary permeability in renal failure, *Br Med J* 4:388, 1972.

103. McCredie RM: The measurement of pulmonary edema in vascular heart disease, *Circulation* 36:381, 1967.

104. Jordan SC, Hicken P, Watson DA, et al: Pathology of the lungs in mitral stenosis in relation to respiratory function and pulmonary hemodynamics, *Br Heart J* 28:101, 1966.

105. Baudendistel L, Shields JB, Kaminski DL: Comparison of double indicator thermodilution measurements of extravascular lung water (EVLW) with radiographic estimation of lung water in trauma patients, *J Trauma* 22:983, 1982.

106. Laggner A, Kleinberger G, Haller J, et al: Bedside estimation of extravascular lung water in critically ill patients: comparison of the chest radiograph and the thermal dye technique, *Intens Care Med* 10:309, 1984.

107. Halperin BD, Feeley TW, Mihm FG, et al: Evaluation of the portable chest roentgenogram for quantitating extravascular lung water in critically ill adults, *Chest* 88:649, 1985.

108. Heinrichs W, Kraft B, Schild M, Halmagyi M: Beurteilung des Flussigkeitsgehaltes der Lunge anhand des Thorax-Roentgenbildes, *Deutsch Med Wochenschr* 113:1583, 1988.

109. Liebman PR, Philips E, Weisel R, et al: Diagnostic value of the portable chest x-ray technique in pulmonary edema, *Am J Surg* 135:604, 1978.

110. Meignan M, George C, Lemaire F: Eau pulmonaire extravascu-

laire au cours du syndrome de détresse respiratoire aigue de l'adulte, *Bull Europ Physiopath Resp* 14:617, 1978.

111. Lewis FR, Elings V, Sturm JA: Bedside measurement of lung water, *J Surg Res* 27:250, 1979.

112. Sivak ED, Richmond BJ, O'Donovan PB, Borkowski GP: Value of extravascular lung water measurement vs. portable chest x-ray in the management of pulmonary edema, *Crit Care Med* 11:498, 1983.

113. Haller VJ, Czembirek M, Salomonowitz E, et al: Die Thorax-bettaufnahme und extravaskulare Lungenwasserbestimmung bei Intensivpatienten, *Fortschr Roentgenstr* 142:68, 1985.

114. Zadrobilek E, Schindler I, Jantsch H, et al: Die Bewertung der thermalen Messtechnik zur quantitativen Bestimmung des extravaskularen Lungenvassers, *Anaesthesist* 34:582, 1985.

115. Eisenberg PR, Hansbrough JR, Anderson D, Schuster DP: A prospective study of lung water measurements during patient management in intensive care unit, *Am Rev Respir Dis* 136:66, 1987.

116. Milne ENC: Chest radiology in surgical patients, *Surg Clin North Am* 60:1503, 1980.

117. Staub NC, Hogg JC: Conference report of a workshop on the measurement of lung water, *Crit Care Med* 8:752, 1980.

118. Staub NC, Hogg JC: Clinical measurement of lung water content, *Chest* 79:3, 1981.

119. Staub NC: The measurement of lung water content, *J Microwave Power* 18:259, 1983.

120. Schuster DP, Anderson DJ: Lung water measurement in intensive care units, *Am Rev Respir Dis* 137:747, 1988.

121. Sibbald WJ, Short AK, Warshawski FJ, et al: Thermal dye measurement of extravascular lung water in critically ill patients, *Chest* 87:585, 1985.

122. Loyd E, Newman JH, Brigham KL: Permeability pulmonary edema. Diagnosis and treatment, *Arch Intern Med* 144:143, 1984.

123. Taylor AE, Parker JC: Pulmonary interstitial spaces and lymphatics. In Fishman AP, Fisher AB (eds): *Handbook of physiology. The respiratory system*, vol 1, Bethesda, 1985, American Physiological Society, p 167.

4 Assessing Systemic Intra- and Extravascular Water

In addition to the information that can be obtained from the plain chest film regarding pulmonary intravascular and extravascular volume (pulmonary edema), valuable information can be derived about *systemic* intravascular and extravascular volume (systemic edema).

Our anatomic source for the derivation of data on systemic *intra*vascular volume is the vascular pedicle, and for systemic *extra*vascular water volume the soft tissues of the chest wall. We will consider, first, how systemic intravascular volume can be quantitated using the vascular pedicle and, second, how the soft tissues of the chest wall can be utilized to give a measure of systemic extravascular volume.

VASCULAR PEDICLE

We introduced the term "vascular pedicle"[1] in the 1970s to describe the leash of large systemic vessels extending from the thoracic inlet to the heart and forming virtually the entire mediastinal density on a frontal view. The term "vascular pedicle" was preferred to "mediastinum," because it conveys better the idea that the mediastinum is made up largely of vessels and that these are not simply static anatomic structures but react to alterations in circulating blood volume and pressure by becoming distended or dilated. The vascular pedicle therefore displays dynamic (physiologic) changes—from which the radiologist can abstract useful physiologic data—and should be regarded as a dynamic physiologic structure rather than a purely static anatomic one.

Our first study of the value of the vascular pedicle in diagnosis was carried out to test the (seemingly self-evident) postulate that increasing the circulating blood volume—for example, by infusing fluids intravenously—would cause an increase in the width of the vascular pedicle and that measurement of this increase on the chest film should give an estimate of the increase in circulating blood volume. Before the results of this study are discussed, it is necessary to consider the anatomy of the pedicle and to show how it relates to the radiologic changes observed.

Anatomy

The vascular pedicle is made up of the largest systemic arteries and veins in the body. The upper half of its right-hand border is formed by the right brachiocephalic vein, which is joined just above the vena azygos by the left brachiocephalic vein to form the superior vena cava, which then constitutes the lower half of the right-hand border of the pedicle (Fig. 4-1, *A*). The right-hand border is therefore entirely venous.

The left-hand border is formed in its lower portion by the arch of the aorta and in its upper portion by the left subclavian artery, curving upward and outward toward the apex of the lung. Although the left subclavian vein actually extends further laterally into the left hemithorax than the artery, it is not usually seen on the

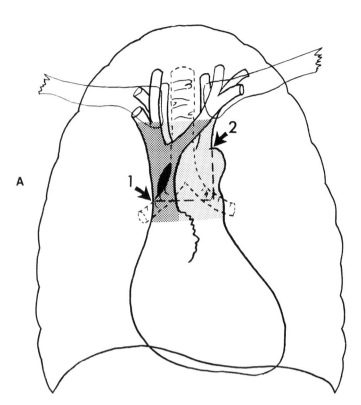

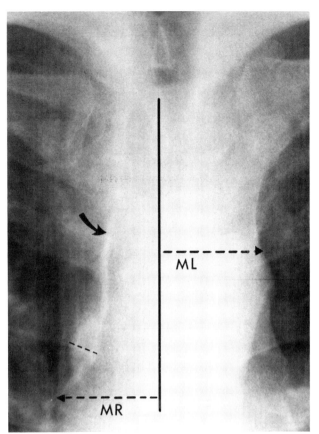

Fig. 4-1 **A,** The right-hand border of the pedicle *(dark stippling)* is formed by the right brachiocephalic vein above and the superior vena cava below. Since it is entirely venous and therefore thin-walled, it is very compliant. The left-hand border *(light stippling)* is formed by the aorta below and the left subclavian artery above. It is therefore entirely arterial and is thick-walled and much less compliant. The left subclavian vein does not usually contribute to the left-hand border. The azygos vein *(black ovoid)* arches over the top of the right main bronchus and is seen end-on as it enters the back of the superior vena cava. Arrows *1* and *2* indicate the points at which the vascular pedicle is measured. **B,** Radiograph of the vascular pedicle in an erect patient. Note that the distances from the midline to the left measuring point *(ML)* and to the right measuring point *(MR)* are approximately equal. The *short dotted line* illustrates how the azygos vein width is measured, across its maximum diameter. The *curved arrow* points to the paratracheal stripe.

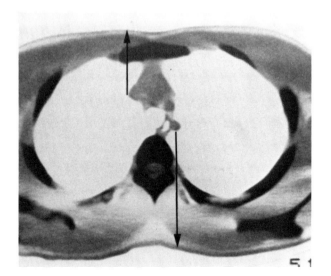

Fig. 4-2 CT scan of the thorax above the aortic arch. The right-hand boundary of the pedicle is formed by the outer edge of the superior vena cava, and the left-hand boundary by the left subclavian artery. Note that the right-hand border lies quite far anterior to the left border, at a shorter distance from the anterior chest wall *(short arrow)*. The left-hand border lies somewhat further away from the posterior chest wall *(long arrow)*.

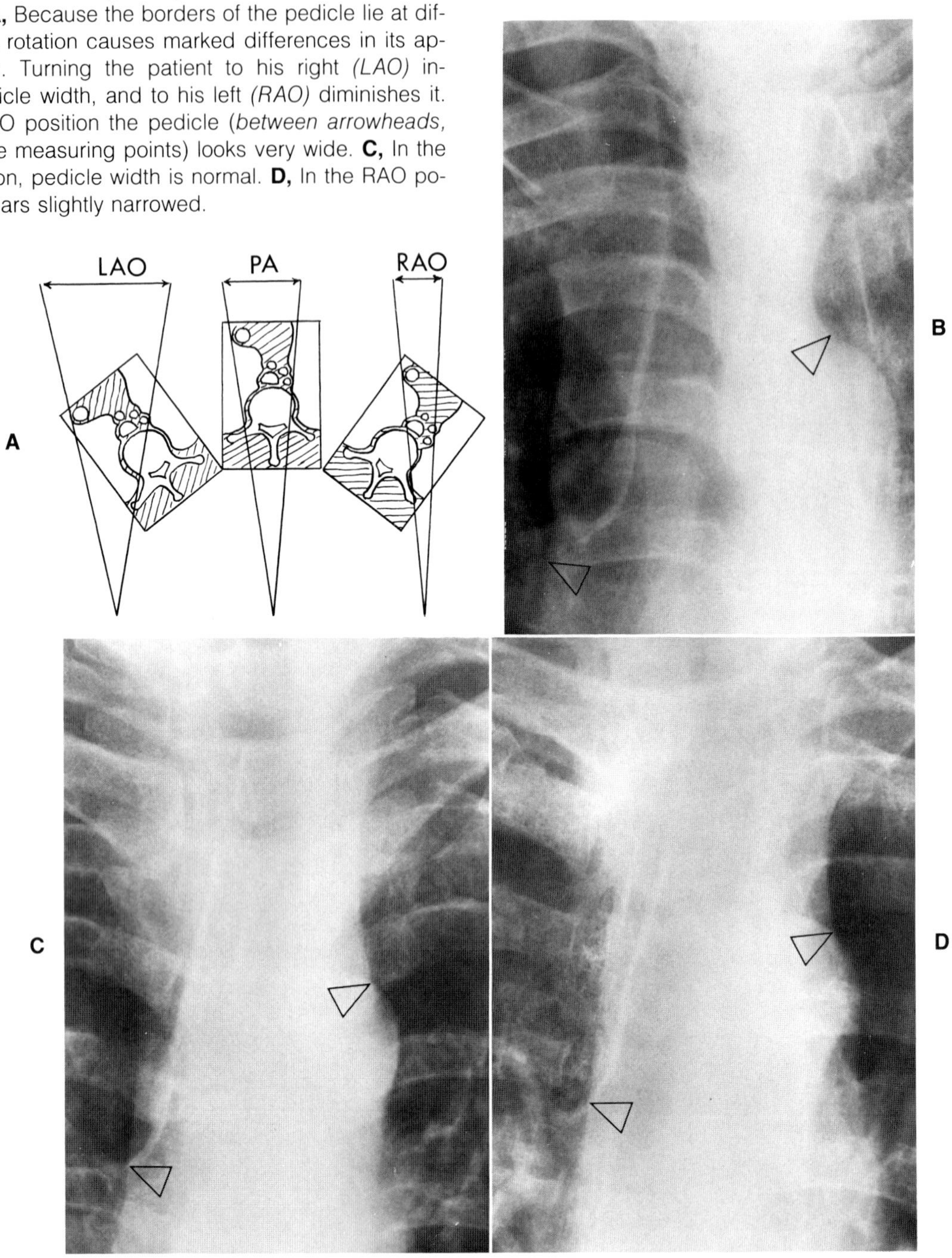

Fig. 4-3 Section through the pedicle at the same level as Figure 4-2. **A,** Because the borders of the pedicle lie at different levels, rotation causes marked differences in its apparent width. Turning the patient to his right (LAO) increases pedicle width, and to his left (RAO) diminishes it. **B,** In the LAO position the pedicle (between arrowheads, indicating the measuring points) looks very wide. **C,** In the frontal position, pedicle width is normal. **D,** In the RAO position it appears slightly narrowed.

plain film because it lies on top of and does not indent the lung whereas the left subclavian artery does indent the lung and can be visualized by virtue of the surrounding air.

Because the right-hand border of the pedicle is entirely venous, it is thin-walled and highly compliant and will respond much more readily to changes in volume and pressure than the left left-hand border, which is entirely arterial and less compliant. This point has very important implications for diagnosis.

Other diagnostically significant anatomic features within the pedicle include the azygos vein, which is seen end-on as it enters the back of the superior vena cava, and the paratracheal stripe (Fig. 4-1, *B*), which is formed by the right wall of the trachea, outlined medially by a column of air within the trachea and laterally by aerated lung in the right upper lobe. Thus the stripe is formed by tracheal wall, its surrounding fascia, and two layers of pleura (visceral and parietal), all of which together constitute a thin white band (usually 2 to 3

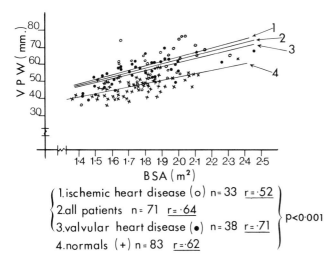

1. ischemic heart disease (o) n= 33 r=·52
2. all patients n= 71 r=·64   } p<0·001
3. valvular heart disease (●) n= 38 r=·71
4. normals (+) n= 83 r=·62

Fig. 4-4   Vascular pedicle width correlated with body surface area. In 38 patients with valvular heart disease the correlation is 0.71, in 33 patients with ischemic heart disease 0.52, and in 83 normal subjects 0.62 (p < 0.001).

Table 4-1   Linear correlation analysis of vascular pedicle width (VPW) and morphometric parameters in 83 normal subjects (44 men, 39 women)*

	Regression equations	r	p
VPW vs body weight (kg)	y = 0.29x + 27.72	0.64	<0.001
VPW vs body height (cm)	y = 0.26x + 3.69	0.45	<0.01
VPW vs body surface area (m^2)	y = 18.39x + 15.37	0.62	<0.001

*Determined from chest radiographs.
r, Correlation coefficient; p, level of significance using the z transform of r.

mm wide[2,3]) between tracheal and pulmonary air. The region appears to widen in its lower portion to "enclose" the end-on density of the vena azygos (Fig. 4-1, B). A *left* paratracheal stripe is not usually seen, since the great vessels from the left side of the aortic arch intervene between the trachea and the apex of the left lung. If the lung is markedly hyperexpanded, it will very occasionally extend between and behind these vessels to contact the tracheal wall; and under these circumstances a left paratracheal stripe may be seen.

A CT scan of the vascular pedicle (Fig. 4-2) reveals that its right-hand border lies much further anterior than its left-hand border. This has important implications for the effects of patient rotation on the apparent width of the pedicle. Turning the patient to the right (LAO) will artifactually widen the pedicle, and to the left (RAO) artifactually narrow it (Fig. 4-3). The effects of rotation must be known so they can be factored into assessments and comparisons of vascular pedicle width.

To be able to determine whether the vascular pedicle is abnormal in width, it is obviously necessary to be familiar with its normal behavior and, in particular, what constitutes "normal" width and what the effects are of the supine position, inspiration, expiration, and positive-pressure ventilation.

Normal Pedicle

We have measured vascular pedicle width (VPW) in 83 normal subjects and 71 patients with cardiac disease[4] and correlated these measurements with circulating blood volume determinations (in 105 of the subjects). The normal width of the vascular pedicle is 4.8 cm ± 5 mm and correlates fairly well with body weight and surface area but poorly with height (Fig. 4-4 and Table

4-1). Combining these two statements and expressing them in imaging terms, we can say (somewhat simplistically, but nevertheless correctly) that "large fat patients will have large wide pedicles, and small skinny patients small narrow pedicles"[4] (Fig. 4-5).

This is a fortunate relationship, since radiologists already carry in their visual memories the appearance of normal pedicles in a very large number of patients of all sizes and can usually recognize readily the inappropriateness (abnormality) of a wide vascular pedicle in a small thin patient, or a narrow pedicle in a large obese patient, without the tedious routine of applying a ruler to all chest films.

Measurement of Pedicle Width

We have determined by extensive experimentation[4] that the least interobserver variation (±2%) in determining pedicle width is obtained if the two measuring points shown in Fig. 4-6 are used. The measuring point on the right-hand border is located where the upper border of the right main bronchus crosses the superior vena cava (usually detectable even on underpenetrated films). This point occurs on the vertical noncurving portion of the pedicle border, which allows for greater objectivity in measurement. On the left side the measuring point is where the left subclavian artery leaves the aorta (Figs. 4-1, A, and 4-6). In some cases, particularly with obese patients and underexposed films, this point is impossible to see and in such cases the most medial point of concavity of the curve of the left subclavian artery is used. From the left-hand measuring point, a perpendicular is dropped to meet a horizontal line from the right-hand point. The distance from the right-hand border to this intercept is the width of the pedicle. Note that this measurement does not include the aorta. Since the aortic size is often markedly increased by atheroma, which bears no relationship to the circulating blood volume, excluding it greatly increases measurement accuracy.

Although for our initial study, done to confirm the

Fig. 4-5 The mean value for VPW is 48 ± 5 mm. Ninety-five percent of all people will fall within two standard deviations of this mean (i.e., from *38* to *58* mm). For a small thin patient a VPW of 38 mm is normal, and for a tall obese patient a VPW of 58 mm is normal. The patient's build, assessed by the radiologist from the chest film, is therefore of great importance in deciding whether the vascular pedicle width is within normal limits.

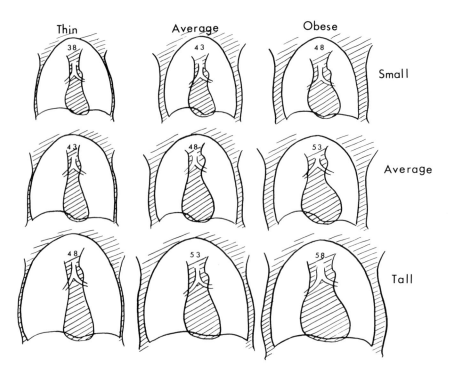

relationship between vascular pedicle width and circulating blood volume, we were required to mark these points and draw the various lines (a somewhat time-consuming procedure). In clinical practice we no longer do this. We simply mark the two measuring points, put the edge of a sheet of paper (usually the patient's requisition form) against the right-hand border marker, slide the paper up until its top edge touches the left-hand marker, and mark off this point on the edge of the paper (Fig. 4-6). It is then quite simple, using the same paper, to repeat this on any film for comparison. The difference, if any, between two or more vascular pedicle widths is rapidly and easily distinguished.

Effects of the Supine Position. In the erect position, with the patient nonrotated, the distance from the (midline) spinous processes to the left-hand border of the pedicle (ML) will be roughly equal to the distance from the midline to the right-hand border (MR) (Fig. 4-7). This is an important diagnostic observation, which should be emphasized. When the patient is placed in the *supine* position, there is an increased venous return from the legs and, because the vessels on the right are so much more compliant than those on the left, the pedicle enlarges more to the right (47% ± 37%) than to the left (7% ± 48%)[4] (Fig. 4-7). We will show later that this observation of the normal behavior of the pedicle is important in distinguishing between increased width of the vascular pedicle from *intra*vascular fluid and increased width from *extra*vascular fluid (e.g., bleeding into the mediastinum) (see Chapter 10).

There is considerable variability in the amount by

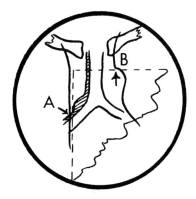

Fig. 4-6 Instead of drawing lines on films and dropping a perpendicular, we simply place the edge of a sheet of paper (usually the patient's requisition) against point *A* (where the right main bronchus crosses the superior vena cava) and move it up until its upper edge is at the level of point *B* (where the left subclavian artery leaves the aorta). This point is marked on the edge of the paper, and the distance can then be measured from the left-hand border to the marked point. However, it is more common to have two films to compare; and if this maneuver is merely repeated on the second film, using the same piece of paper, it becomes quite simple to see how much change has taken place in pedicle width and from this to derive the change in circulating blood volume (*1 cm of difference in vascular pedicle width approximates a 2 L difference in circulating blood volume*).

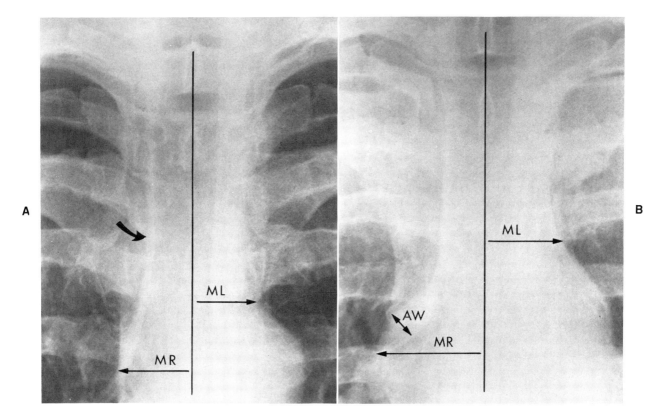

Fig. 4-7 **A,** Normal vascular pedicle, patient erect. *MR* and *ML* are equal. The paratracheal stripe is clearly identified running into a small azygos vein. **B,** Minutes later, supine position. The total width of the vascular pedicle has increased from 52 to 67 mm (29%), but *MR* (reflecting the compliant venous side of the pedicle) has increased 73% and *ML* (reflecting the less compliant arterial side) only 12%. Azygos width *(AW)* has increased from 5 to 11 mm (120%).

Table 4-2 Change in vascular pedicle width (VPW) and azygos width (AW) at various angles from erect to supine

Patient		[1]90° to 80° (erect) (% change)	80° to 60° (% change)	60° to 30° (% change)	30° to 0° (supine) (% change)	Total change from erect to supine (%)
1	VPW	↓5	7	0	13	2
	AW	↓29	70	41	↓17	71
2	VPW	2	16	2	3	12
	AW	NS	NS	NS	0	NS
3	VPW	15	11	12	4	19
	AW	↓28	60	0	25	15
4	VPW	↓6	18	↓2	↓5	16
	AW	NS	NS	37	18	NS
5	VPW	↓7	12	15	↓8	21
	AW	↓11	75	↓21	25	44
6	VPW	7	2	8	0	0
	AW	NS	0	13	14	NS
7	VPW	2	2	9	2	13
	AW	20	0	11	20	33
8	VPW	7	0	9	↓4	17
	AW	6	47	12	↓26	75
9	VPW	14	12	3	↓3	31
	AW	40	57	↓18	0	80
10	VPW	11	8	7	↓14	28
	AW	80	0	11	↓10	100

[1]Percent increase in VPW or AW. *NS,* Not seen. ↓ = decrease.

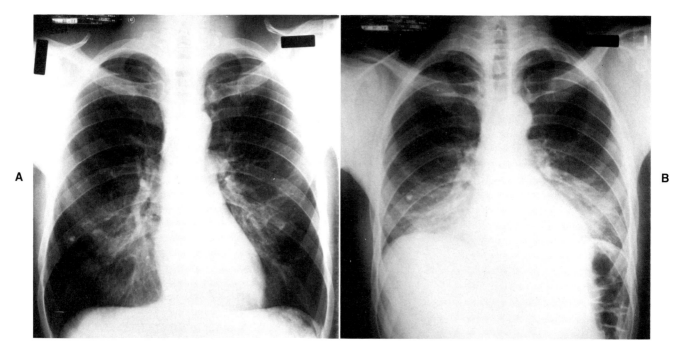

Fig. 4-8   A, Inspiratory view. Note the width of the pedicle. **B,** Same patient, forced expiratory view. Despite the great change in lung volume, there is no measurable change in vascular pedicle width.

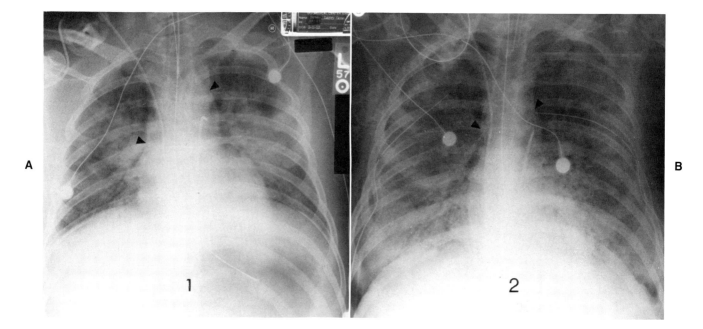

Fig. 4-9   A, Young man with ARDS on assist-control ventilation. Positive end-expiratory pressure (PEEP) is 5 cm H_2O. **B,** Same patient 24 hours later. PEEP is now 20 cm H_2O. Note the marked reduction in VPW despite the fact that there has been no change in the patient's circulating blood volume between the two radiographs. The narrowing of the vascular pedicle in this instance is related to increased intrathoracic pressure.

which the pedicle increases in the supine position.[4] When we first observed this, we presumed it was due to individual variations in vascular compliance, which were more likely caused by variations in vasomotor tone than by variations in histologic structure. We confirmed this[5] by taking AP radiographs and measuring the width of the pedicles at differing degrees (80, 60, 30, 10 degrees) as subjects (a group of 10 volunteers) were tilted back from vertical to horizontal (Table 4-2). One might have anticipated that as the thorax inclined backward from the vertical toward the horizontal the VPW would increase progressively. In some patients it did exactly this, but in others it began to widen until the patient was about 60 degrees from the horizontal and then it narrowed again, strongly suggesting that increasing intraluminal vascular pressure and volume, caused by the return of blood from the lower limbs, had triggered an increase in vasomotor tone. This may be part of the reason why there is so much variation from patient to patient in the percentage increase in VPWs obtained in the supine position. Note, however, that in all the subjects examined, even with what appeared to be episodes of vasoconstriction at certain degrees of angulation, the *supine* pedicle was never smaller (and in 9 of 10 cases was actually larger) than in the erect position (Table 4-2).

Effects of Respiration. Most experienced radiologists when questioned express the belief that the mediastinum (vascular pedicle) widens on expiratory films, and certainly this is the standard textbook statement. However, when we performed actual measurements of vascular pedicle width on inspiratory and expiratory films, we found that there was usually little or no difference in width of the pedicle on expiration—sometimes a small increase, sometimes a small decrease (Fig. 4-8). We believe the expiratory film gives an *impression* that the mediastinum has widened because the eye automatically relates and compares the width of the mediastinum to the width of the thorax, which of course is narrowed on the expiratory film. In fact, on inspiration, though the pedicle may tend to be narrowed by the downward pull of the diaphagm, this is overcome by the increased filling of the vessels caused by the negative inspiratory pressure in the thorax, sucking blood into the large vessels of the pedicle. On expiration, although the vascular pedicle is compacted from below and therefore tends to widen, this is counteracted by blood being pumped *out* of the intrathoracic vessels by the raised intrathoracic pressure of expiration.

This behavior pattern is important to recognize, particularly in the large numbers of ICU patients who are placed on positive-pressure ventilation. As ventilatory pressure is increased, the vascular pedicle width progressively diminishes. It is therefore *essential* when reading intensive care unit films to know precisely what

the ventilating pressure was at the moment the film was taken (peak pressure) and what the pressure was on expiration (PEEP)[6] (Fig. 4-9) (see Chapter 10). Without this knowledge, misdiagnoses can be made. Similar narrowing of the pedicle by increased intrathoracic pressure is seen in patients performing a Valsalva maneuver (deliberately or otherwise) and in some patients in status asthmaticus.

The same mechanism may be responsible for the fact that the vascular pedicle is narrower than normal in patients with pure emphysema[7] (Table 4-3), in whom air trapping occurs and intraalveolar pressure is elevated (particularly on expiration) (Fig. 4-10) and the usual negative interstitial pressure, which assists in keeping vessels and bronchi open, is lost. This narrowing is *not* seen in patients with pure chronic bronchitis, in whom the pedicle is often slightly wider than normal.[7] We believe this slight widening in those with chronic bronchitis is caused *not* by lessened intrathoracic pressure but by the frequent concomitant presence of left heart decompensation[8] and hypoperfusion of the kidneys, with resultant increase in circulating blood volume (i.e., a widened pedicle is another radiologic feature of the chronic bronchitic "blue bloater") —and possibly by secondary polycythemia.

It should be noted that, although the normal size of the vascular pedicle was initially determined in an Italian population,[4] a repeat study in non-Italian subjects (in San Francisco)[7] produced virtually the same figures for normal vascular pedicle width as our original study.

Effects of Distance and Anteroposterior Versus Posteroanterior Radiographic Projection

PA Versus AP Position. As previously mentioned, the right-hand border of the pedicle lies quite far anteriorly and the left-hand border posteriorly; as a result there is only a minor variation in the distance of the pedicle margins from the film, whether the film is taken AP or PA, and there is thus little appreciable change in width of the pedicle between the two positions (Fig. 4-2). However, since the azygos vein enters the back of the superior vena cava somewhat closer to the front chest wall than to the back chest wall, changing from the PA

Table 4-3 Differences in vascular pedicle width between patients with emphysema and patients with chronic bronchitis

Population	VPW (mm)
Normal (n = 93)	48.8 ± 4.9
Emphysema (n = 40)	44.5 ± 5.3
Chronic bronchitis (n = 26)	52.0 ± 7.7

The differences between normals and patients, and between the two groups of patients, are statistically significant, with a p < 0.001 (Student's t test for unpaired data).

to the AP position will cause a small geometric enlargement in the azygos width.

Tube-to-Film Distance. When 72-inch films are compared with 40-inch films, a small difference is seen amounting to a geometric increase of approximately 5% in both vascular pedicle width and azygos width on the 40-inch films.

Relationship Between Vascular Pedicle Width and Circulating Blood Volume. We measured the vascular pedicle width and circulating blood volume (CBV) in two groups of patients,[4,9] the first with ischemic heart disease and the second with rheumatic valvular disease. An excellent correlation was found in both groups (Fig. 4-11), but the relationship was stronger (r = 0.90) in patients with valvular disease than in those with ischemic heart disease (r = 0.67). We believe the reason for this lies in the age differences between the two groups. The ischemic heart disease group was, on average, 20 years older than the valvular disease group and suffered (partially by preselection, since we chose to examine patients with ischemic heart disease) from atherosclerosis affecting the great vessels arising from the aorta and passing up into the neck. This caused increased tortuosity and artifactually increased the width of the pedicle in the absence of any increase in circulating blood volume (Fig. 4-12).

There was also a statistically significant correlation between the vascular pedicle width and mean right atrial pressure (Fig. 4-13), but this was not as strong as the relationship between vascular pedicle width and circulating blood volume.

Although the correlation between vascular pedicle width and CBV is statistically good and clinically useful, it is much less strong statistically and much less important diagnostically than the relationship between *change* in width of the vascular pedicle and change in the CBV.[9] This change in circulating blood volume is a major part of the information one needs to determine whether a patient in cardiac failure is improving, whether fluid therapy in hypovolemic and septic shock and in burn patients has succeeded in restoring normal CBV, and whether diuresis has removed fluid predominantly from the intravascular or extravascular compartment or equally from both.[6]

Fig. 4-10   A, A 60-year-old man with moderately severe emphysema. Note the marked narrowing of the pedicle *(between arrows)* and the barely visible, very small vena azygos *(right-hand arrow).* **B,** A 58-year-old man with chronic bronchitis. Note the wide vascular pedicle *(straight arrows)* and the large vena azygos *(curved arrow).*

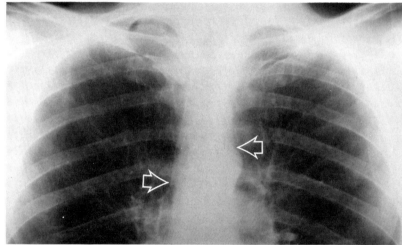

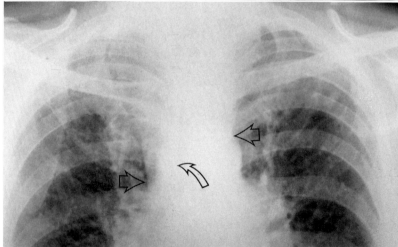

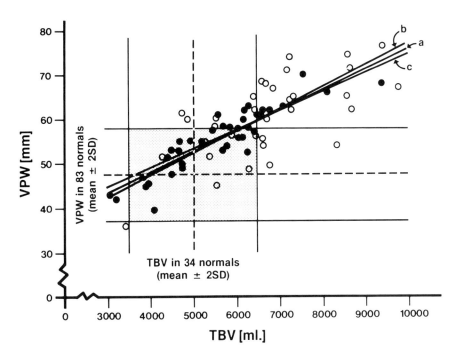

Fig. 4-11 Correlation between total blood volume (TBV) and vascular pedicle width (VPW) in 71 radiographs (linear regression line a, *open plus solid circles*). Thirty-eight of the radiographs are of patients with valvular disease (linear regression line b, *solid circles*) and 33 of patients with ischemic heart disease (linear regression line c, *open circles*). Normal values of VPW 47.6 ± 5.2 mm; normal values of TBV 4986 ± 740 ml. The shaded area is made by the crossing of the mean ±2 SD of normal values of VPW and TBV. In a population with gaussian distribution the mean ±2 SD sets confidence levels of 95.45%.

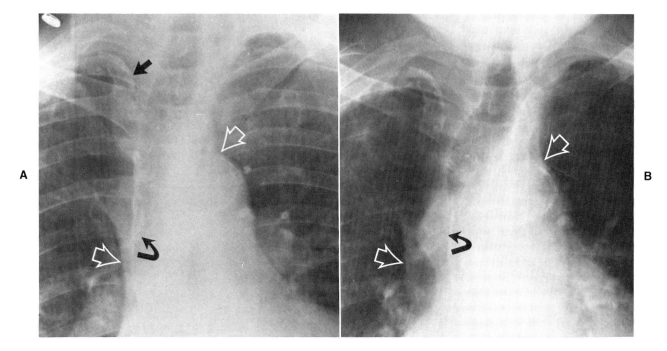

Fig. 4-12 **A,** A 60-year-old man with extensive vascular calcification. Note the right subclavian *(straight black arrow),* arising from a tortuous innominate artery, and the calcified aorta. No evidence of cardiac failure. VPW is indicated by the white arrows, and the azygos vein by the curved black arrow. **B,** One and a half years later the patient is now in cardiac failure. Note the considerable increase in VPW *(white arrows),* particularly to the *right,* and the increase in azygos vein size *(curved black arrow).* The presence of atherosclerosis does not affect the ability of the vascular pedicle to enlarge in response to increased circulating blood volume.

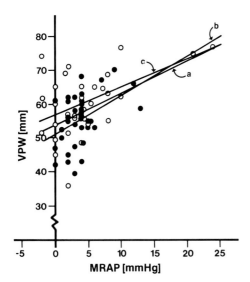

Fig. 4-13 Correlation between vascular pedicle width *(VPW)* and mean right atrial pressure *(MRAP)* in 67 cardiac patients (linear regression line *a, open plus solid circles*), of whom 36 had valvular disease (linear regression line *b, solid circles*) and 31 had ischemic heart disease (linear regression line *c, open circles*).

Relationship Between Change in Vascular Pedicle Width and Change in CBV. By measuring VPW and CBV sequentially in patients recovering from cardiac failure as well as changes in CBV following dialysis in renal patients and in normal persons giving blood or receiving intravenous fluids (experimentally), we have shown a remarkably close correlation between the change in volume of the circulating blood and the altered width of the vascular pedicle (Fig. 4-14). Although derived initially from only a small number of cases, these correlations (r = 0.93, p < 0.001) appeared quite remarkable for in vivo biologic data. Since then, extensive clinical experience[9] has shown that the measurement of changes in width of the vascular pedicle is one of the most objective (and certainly the simplest) ways of determining changes in circulating blood volume.

We began by correlating changes in vascular pedicle width with changes in the *total* circulating blood volume (i.e., systemic plus pulmonary volume) but on reflection realized that it was quite possible for the pulmonary and systemic blood volumes to behave differently—to change in different directions. For example, with left-to-right intracardiac shunts (e.g., an ASD) the

Fig. 4-14   A, This graph compares changes in vascular pedicle width *(VPW)* with changes in total blood volume *(TBV)* in 10 cardiac patients (9 ischemic and 1 valvular *[solid circles]*) and 3 normal individuals *(x)*. (Two of these patients had been given 2 L of saline, and one had had 450 ml of blood removed.) Equation *a* represents the linear correlation for the ten cardiac patients *(solid line)*. By simply extending this line *(dotted portion)* it is evident that it also closely fits the three normals. If the regression is recalculated (equation *b*) to include the three normals, the line remains virtually unchanged and the r value becomes 0.97. **B,** Linear regression in 8 of the 10 cardiac patients in whom PBV was also measured. The change in VPW is now correlated with the systemic blood volume (i.e., *TBV-PBV*). (The normal individual from whom 450 ml of blood was removed is shown in Fig. 4-16.)

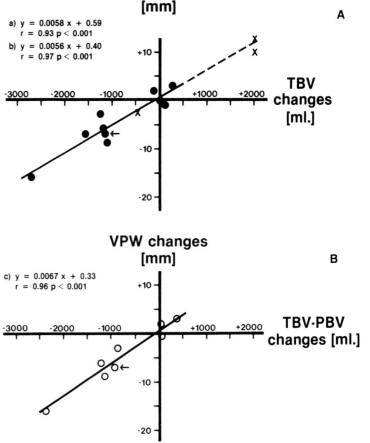

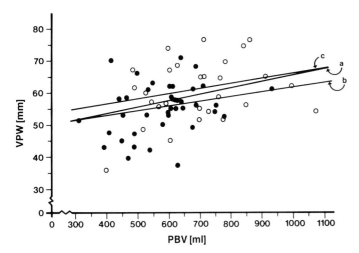

Fig. 4-15 Correlation between pulmonary blood volume and the width of the vascular pedicle in 69 radiographs. Linear regression line *a* refers to all cases *(solid plus open circles)*. There are 38 radiographs of patients with valvular disease (linear regression line *b, solid circles*) and 31 of patients with ischemic heart disease (linear regression line *c, open circles*). No significant correlation between *VPW* and *PBV*.

pulmonary blood volume enlarges (reflecting the large right heart output) but the systemic blood volume remains small (reflecting a small left ventricular output); and the vascular pedicle is therefore also small (reflecting the *systemic* blood volume only, not the total CBV). A decoupling of systemic blood volume and pulmonary

blood volume in the opposite direction can be caused, for example, by pericardial tamponade, in which the pulmonary blood volume becomes smaller and the systemic blood volume larger (reflected by enlargement of the vascular pedicle). We have shown [9] that the width of the vascular pedicle does *not*, in fact, correlate with pulmonary blood volume (Fig. 4-15). We therefore measured the pulmonary blood volume, as well as the total circulating blood volume, in several patients and subtracted this figure from their total blood volume to give their systemic blood volume. We then correlated the change in *systemic* blood volume with the change in vascular pedicle width, which resulted in a further improvement of the already strong correlation (r = 0.96, p < .001) (Fig. 4-14, *B*).

Fig. 4-14 shows a simple relationship, which is easy to memorize and of daily diagnostic value—*a change in width of the vascular pedicle of 1 cm approximates a change in systemic blood volume of 2 L* (Figs. 4-16 and 4-17).

Consideration of Fig. 4-14 shows that the line of identity passes almost exactly through the zero axis—which, translated into usable radiologic terms, means that if there has been no change in width of the vascular pedicle between one film and the next there can have been no change in systemic blood volume. This *lack* of change in VPW can be of great diagnostic value. For example, Fig. 4-18, *A*, shows a woman who had been stabbed, was bleeding profusely, and had a narrow pedicle, reflecting her low systemic volume. The next morning (Fig. 4-18, *B*) she was 9 L ahead on fluids

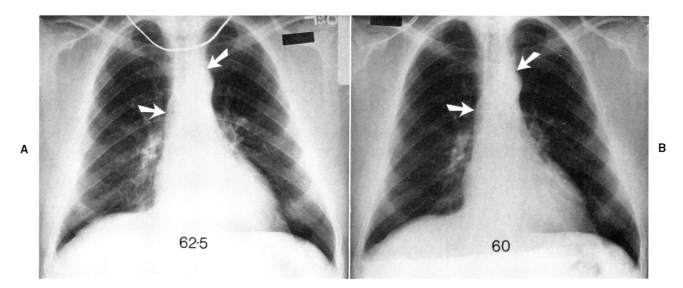

Fig. 4-16 A 50-year-old healthy athletic man, erect PA film. **A,** Prior to donating blood, the VPW is 62.5 mm. **B,** Following donation of 450 ml of blood, the VPW has decreased to 60 mm. Exposure factors are identical for **A** and **B,** and the films were processed simultaneously. As shown in Fig. 4-5, a change of 1 cm in the VPW corresponds to a change of 2.0L in circulating blood volume.

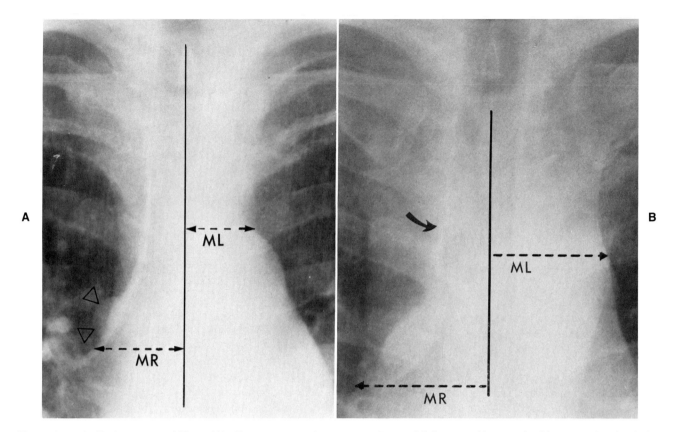

Fig. 4-17   A, Patient erect, *MR = ML*. The azygos vein should not extend beyond the confines of the SVC. The bulge marked by the arrowheads is actually a transverse process, not the azygos. **B,** Same patient, still erect but now in renal failure—with a marked increase in circulating blood volume. The VPW is considerably enlarged, more to the right than to the left. Note the increased size of the azygos vein (180%).

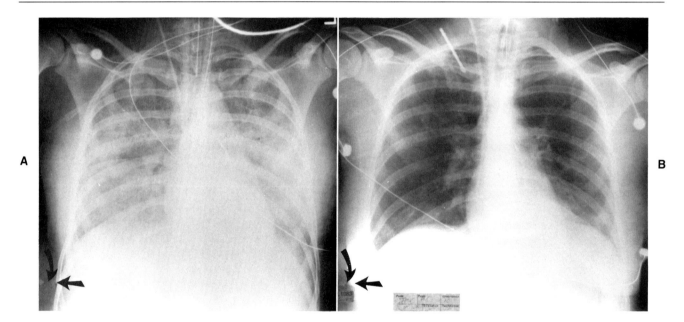

Fig. 4-18   A, Admission film of a young woman stabbed several times with a slender blade (like an icepick). This supine film was obtained after resuscitation with several liters of low–molecular weight fluids. Despite the hydration, her pedicle is narrow, indicating reduced circulating blood volume. The soft tissues of the right flank *(arrows)* are very thin. **B,** Twenty-four hours later, supine film. The patient is 9 L "ahead" on fluids, but clearly the fluids are not in the circulating blood volume (because the pedicle is even narrower than on the day before) and are not in the soft tissues of the chest wall (compare with **A**). At operation an unsuspected liver puncture was found, with 9 L of blood in the abdomen. The edema previously present because of very low oncotic pressure cleared following therapy with packed cells and restoration of normal oncotic pressure.

but the VPW had *not* increased, indicating that the 9 L of fluid were located somewhere *extra*vascular. The soft tissues had not increased, so it was deduced that the 9 L must be in the abdomen. At operation an unsuspected liver puncture was found and there were 9 L of blood in the abdominal cavity.

VENA AZYGOS
Anatomy

The vena azygos arises in the abdomen at the level of the first or second lumbar vertebra. Formed by branches of the right lumbar veins and sometimes by branches from the right renal vein or the inferior vena cava, it passes up into the thorax along the right antero-

lateral aspect of the vertebral column and through the aortic opening (Fig. 4-19, *A*). Around the level of the fourth or fifth dorsal vertebra (close to the carina) it arches forward (looking from the lateral view, somewhat like the curved handle of a walking stick) and over the top of the right main bronchus into the back of the superior vena cava before this passes into the pericardium. Since there is air in the lung on its superolateral aspect, air in the trachea on its medial aspect, and air in the right main bronchus on its inferomedial aspect, the vena azygos is easily seen in a high percentage of chest radiographs (approximately 85%).[10,11] There is often a single valve where the azygos vein passes into the superior vena cava. This valve does not usually appear to be

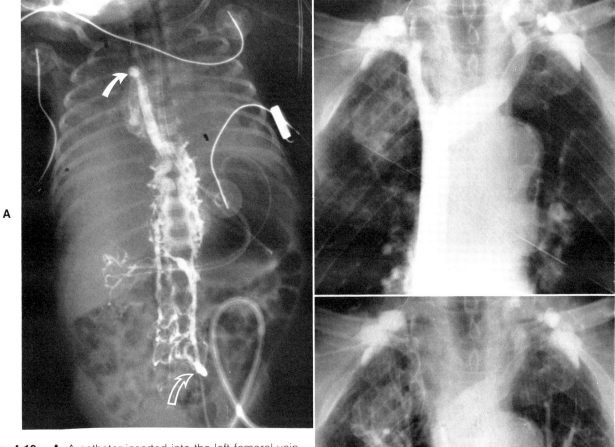

Fig. 4-19   A, A catheter inserted into the left femoral vein of a newborn infant has entered an ascending lumbar vein *(open arrow)*. Injection of contrast to determine its position provides an excellent serendipitous display of the anatomy of the vena azygos *(solid arrow)*. **B** and **C,** A 49-year-old man with superior vena caval syndrome. In **B** the intravenous contrast shows a tumor compressing the SVC. In **C** (a late film) some reflux of contrast into the vena azygos can be seen. The contrast is trapped behind leaves of the azygos valve, giving the characteristic coffee-bean (or lobster claw) appearance *(arrow)*.

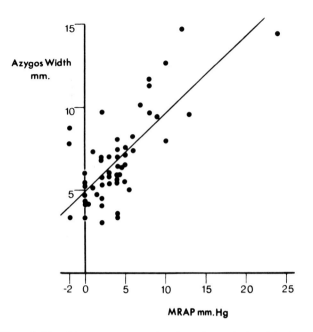

Fig. 4-20 Measurements showing the relationship between azygos vein width and mean right atrial pressure *(MRAP)*. Each azygos width measurement is the mean of two independent observations. (For the linear regression n = 57, r = 0.74, p < 0.001. y = 0.46x + 4.97.)

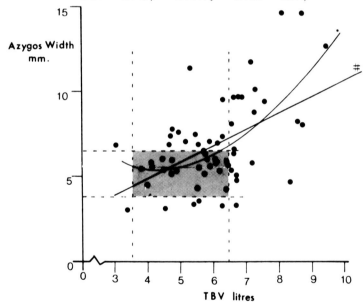

Fig. 4-21 Correlation of azygos vein width and total blood volume in the same group of patients as in Fig. 4-20. Each azygos width measurement is the mean of two independent observations. The cross-hatched area indicates the mean values ±2 SD of TBV in 34 normals and azygos vein width in another group of 82 normals. (For the linear regression [n = 57, r = 0.50, p < 0.01. y = 0.00960x + 1.03].) The parabolic relationship (*) shows a slightly better correlation (r = 0.55, p < 0.01).

$$y = 0.0000024x^2 - 0.002025x + 9.79$$

Where TBV increases, the azygos vein generally also increases but the correlation is still poor.

competent, but its presence should be known to the radiologist, since it can give a peculiar "lobster claw" or "coffee bean" appearance when it traps contrast beneath the valve cusps at angiography[12] (Fig. 4-19, *B* and *C*).

Relationship of Vena Azygos Width to Systemic Blood Volume and Right Atrial Pressure

The behavior of the azygos vein provides a valuable cross-check on the behavior of the vascular pedicle, but it differs slightly from behavior of the pedicle in that the width of the azygos vein is somewhat better related to mean right atrial pressure (Fig. 4-20) than it is to systemic blood volume (Fig. 4-21). This is the reverse of vascular pedicle width relationships and can be stated approximately as follows:

The width of the vascular pedicle reflects circulating blood volume better than it reflects right atrial pressure, and the width of the azygos vein reflects right atrial pressure slightly better than circulating blood volume.

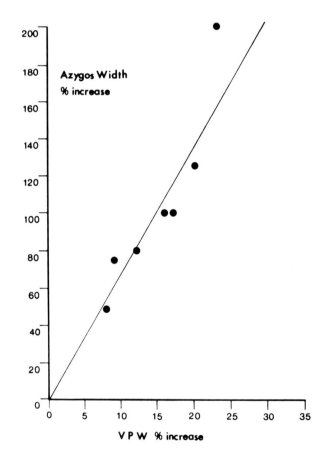

Fig. 4-22 The percent increase in width of the vena azygos is closely related to the percent increase in width of the vascular pedicle (i.e., the width of the pedicle and that of the azygos normally change together and in the same direction). Any discrepancy in this behavior should be investigated. (See Fig. 4-23.)

However, a *change* in width of the azygos usually exactly parallels a change in width of the pedicle (Fig. 4-22). The slope of this relationship shows that the azygos vein increases (in percentage) seven times more than the pedicle. In other words, if the pedicle increases 20% the azygos width increases 140%. There are rare causes of dissociation between the behavior of the the vena azygos and that of the vascular pedicle— e.g., in the presence of inferior vena caval block or compression, the vena azygos can form an anastomotic connection between vessels proximal to the blocked IVC and the right atrium. In such cases the azygos can enlarge enormously *without* reflecting any change in either CBV or right atrial pressure (Fig. 4-23). There would then be a discrepancy between the very large azygos vein and the normal pedicle width, which should suggest the diagnosis.

At this point we must mention that the azygos is not

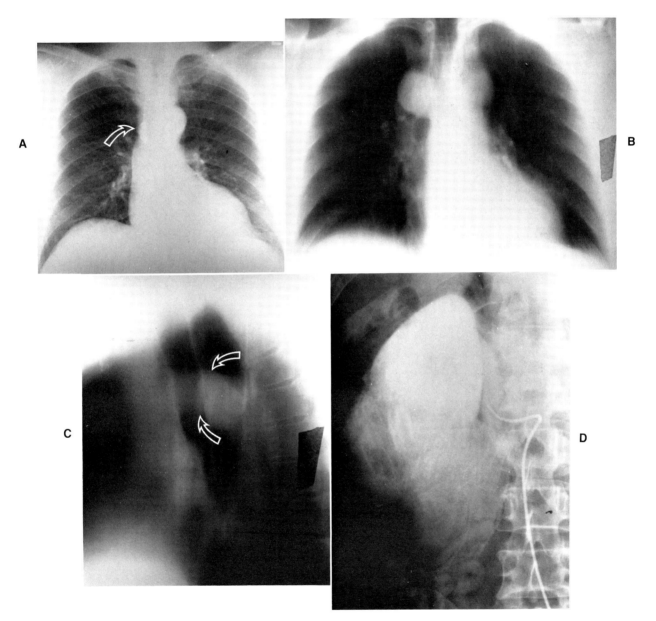

Fig. 4-23 A 40-year-old man with renal cell carcinoma. **A,** Erect PA chest film. Note the unusual shape of the azygos vein *(arrow)*. **B,** On the same day, in the supine position, the azygos enlarges enormously but the pedicle does not (linear tomogram). **C,** On a lateral (decubitus) tomogram the azygos is so large *(between arrows)* that it could readily be mistaken for the aorta. **D,** Renal angiogram showing a massive tumor with extensive collateral vein formation. The IVC was completely blocked by tumor, causing anastomotic flow through the vena azygos.

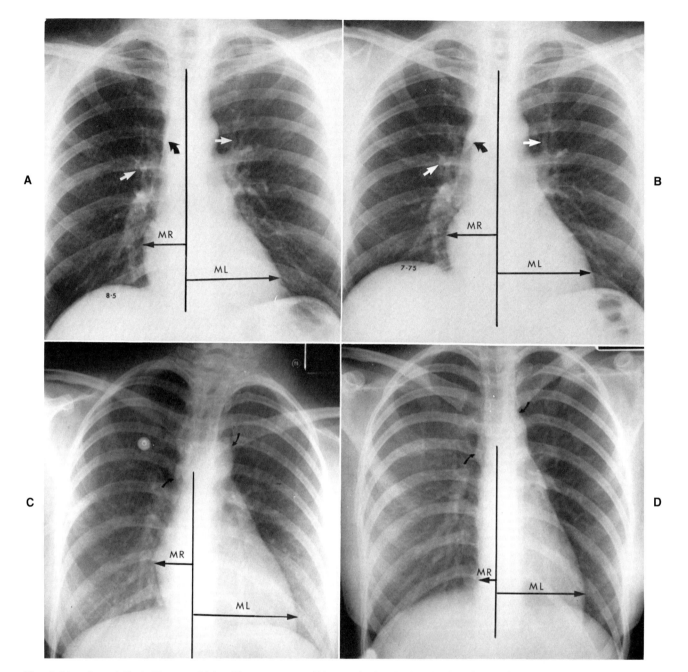

Fig. 4-24 **A** and **B,** A 38-year-old healthy man, erect PA radiographs. Note in **A** the distances from midline to the right *(MR)* and left *(ML)* heart borders. The black arrow indicates a small azygos vein. MR and ML of the pedicle are equal. The white arrows point to small upper lobe vessels. In **B,** made 20 minutes later, after intravenous infusion of 2 L of saline, the left side of the heart has not changed but the right has enlarged, matching the increase in width of the pedicle to the right and the increased size of the azygos vein *(black arrow).* Note that the upper lobe vessels have enlarged *(white arrows)* and a : (balanced) flow distri- bution is developing due to the general increase in circulat- ing blood volume. **C** and **D,** A 19-year-old female marathon runner who had a seizure following a long run in hot sun- shine. The chest film on admission, **C,** is normal. Twelve hours following deliberate dehydration to reduce intracra- nial pressure, **D,** note the only minor reduction in *ML* but the major reduction in *MR.* These alterations would be even more graphic except for some rotation, which diminishes the cardiac changes and decreases the width of the pedi- cle *(curved arrows).*

the only means of cross-checking the behavior of the vascular pedicle. In the same way that increasing systemic blood volume will cause a preferential increase in the right side of the pedicle, it will cause an increase in size of the right side of the heart (Fig. 4-24), and for exactly the same reasons (i.e., the right heart is thin-walled and very compliant compared to the left, which is thick-walled and much less compliant). A strong cor-

relation in patients undergoing dialysis for renal failure has been shown[13] between changes in circulating blood volume and changes in the transverse diameter of the heart. This relationship is much stronger if enlargement of only the *right* side of the heart is considered (i.e., from the midline of the thorax to the outermost convexity of the right heart border) rather than of the total cardiac diameter (Figs. 4-25 and 4-26), and it may help in deciding whether hydrostatic edema seen on a chest film is of cardiac or renal (overhydration) origin. Whereas the classic cardiac configuration in pure left heart failure does not usually show much in the way of right heart enlargement, the classic configuration in overhydration and renal failure shows enlargement of the heart more to the right than to the left (Figs. 4-24 and 4-27).

Pulmonary blood volume and flow distribution provide a further cross-check on estimations of circulating blood volume. An increase in CBV will cause *all* of the following:

1. Enlargement of the vascular pedicle predominantly to the right
2. Enlargement of the azygos vein
3. Increase in cardiac diameter, more to the right than to the left
4. Increase in pulmonary blood volume, with development of a one-to-one or "balanced" flow distribution, due to progressive recruitment of the upper lobe vessels by the increasing blood volume (Fig. 4-27)

To make full use of vascular pedicle observations, one must integrate them with clinical data concerning the patient's input and output of fluids and with radiologic observations of change (or absence of change) in the soft tissues of the chest wall. These soft tissues are often well-visualized on a chest film and contain valuable diagnostic information. In our experience they are rarely commented on by radiologists and may often change dramatically without exciting any radiologic comment, despite the fact that change in the soft tissues is virtually the only source of radiologic information about the behavior of extravascular water outside the lung (i.e., soft tissue edema as opposed to pulmonary edema).

SOFT TISSUE THICKNESS AND WATER BALANCE

The radiologic changes that characterize an increase in pulmonary extravascular water have been fully described,[14-19] but to our knowledge little has been written about determining radiologic changes in *systemic* extravascular water. Yet without this knowledge of what is happening to the systemic extravascular water, it is impossible to understand clearly what is happening to a patient's total fluid balance (i.e., to determine whether

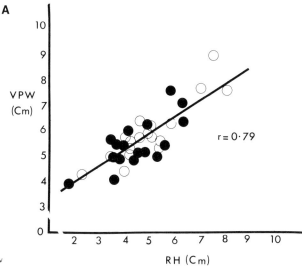

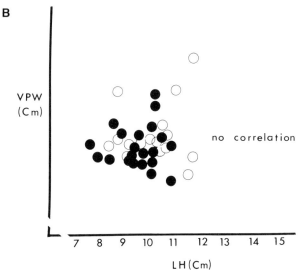

Fig. 4-25 Analysis of 63 x-rays in 21 renal patients. Open circles indicate predialysis films, solid circles postdialysis films. **A,** *VPW* versus *RH* (an index of right heart size) measured as in Fig. 4-24 from the midline to the outermost convexity of the right heart border). Good correlation (r = 0.79, p < 0.001)—the thin-walled right side of the heart behaves analogously to the thin-walled right side of the pedicle (as a reservoir, not a pump) and serves as a useful radiologic cross-check to the vascular pedicle on changes in circulating blood volume. **B,** *VPW* versus *LH* (midline to left border of the heart) shows *no* correlation.

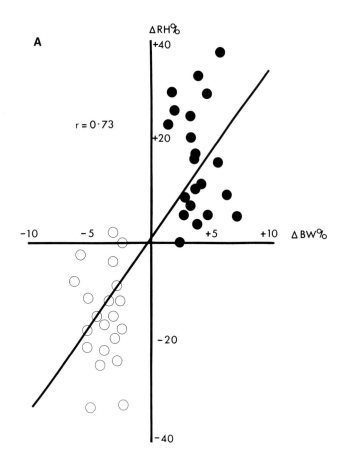

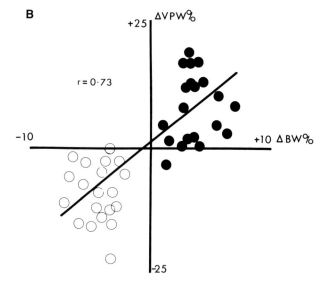

Fig. 4-26 Analysis of 21 patients predialysis *(solid circles)* and postdialysis *(open circles)*. **A,** Percentage change in size of the right side of the heart *(RH)* versus change in body weight. Good correlation (r = 0.73, p < 0.001). **B,** Percentage change in *VPW* versus change in body weight. Identical correlation.

the intravascular or extravascular components are increasing, whether one is increasing relative to the other, and whether there is matching pulmonary and systemic edema or *only* systemic or pulmonary edema). Even if we know a patient's fluid input and output, it is impossible to characterize the distribution of fluid within the patient by purely clinical means. It may be possible to do this by using radioisotopes, but such techniques are interventional, lengthy, expensive, and not repeatable and are therefore almost never used clinically. It *is*, however, quite easy to characterize the distribution of fluids (an essential piece of knowledge, particularly in ICU patients) by considering simultaneously on a plain chest radiograph the vascular pedicle, the azygos vein, the pulmonary blood volume and distribution, the pulmonary extravascular water, *and* the soft tissue thickness.

One might object that the soft tissues are so variable and deformable, particularly in the supine position, that they cannot be measured with any degree of accuracy; but, in fact, when one begins to do such measurements one finds this is not the case. Except for overlying and easily distinguishable breast shadows, and extremely obese patients, the soft tissues change very little in

their thickness from the erect to the supine position. A brief survey of CT scans will confirm that the thickness of the soft tissues is much the same anteriorly and along the lateral chest walls. On plain films the outer border of the soft tissues often requires "bright-lighting" but is usually sharply defined (Fig. 4-28, *A* and *B*). To maintain constancy of measurement from one film to another, we usually make our first measurement from the greatest outermost convexity of the thoracic cage to the skin surface and note which rib forms the greatest convexity (Fig. 4-28, *C*). On subsequent films (Fig. 4-28, *D*) we measure from the outermost margin of this same rib to the skin surface.

A study of patients in renal failure undergoing dialysis showed fairly good correlation (Fig. 4-29) between loss of body weight and decrease in soft tissue thickness. It is clear, however, that, since we did not try in this particular study to determine how much of the fluid was lost from the *intravascular* volume (i.e., by using change in vascular pedicle width) versus that lost from the *extravascular* volume, the correlation obtained could not be much better. For example, if the patient had been dialyzed to lose 2 kg in weight (2 L of

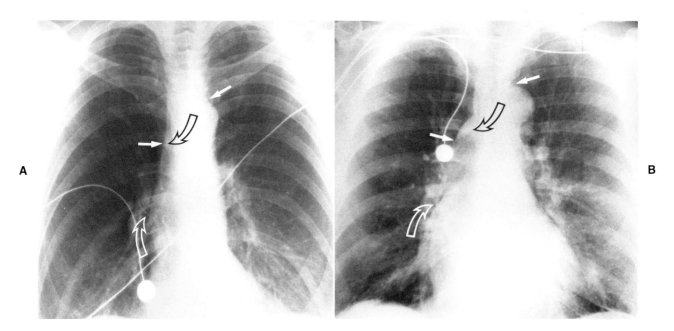

Fig. 4-27   PA erect films of a patient admitted in severe addisonian crisis, markedly dehydrated. **A,** Note the narrow pedicle *(solid white arrows)*, the barely visible azygos vein *(black arrow)*, the extremely small draining pulmonary veins *(open white arrow)*, and the oligemic upper lobes and small heart. **B,** After fluid replacement the pedicle has widened greatly to the right, the vena azygos is now large, the pulmonary veins have enlarged, the heart size has increased (much more to the right than to the left), and the upper lobe vessels are filling.

fluid) and showed only a 0.5 cm reduction in vascular pedicle width, then we would have calculated that he had lost 1 L from his *intravascular* volume and therefore only 1 L from his *extravascular* volume—the correlation between the width of soft tissues (representing the extravascular volume) and the patient's weight change would be poor. If the patient had lost the whole 2 L from the intravascular volume (a common occurrence), there would have been *no* correlation between the change in soft tissue thickness and the weight change.

Clinically a change in weight associated with an appropriate change in input and output does allow the clinician to say that a change in fluid balance has occurred, but it does not allow a statement as to how much has been lost (or gained) from the intravascular, and how much from the extravascular, compartment. Using a combination of soft tissue changes and vascular pedicle width change, the radiologist *can* give this information with a clinically valuable degree of accuracy (Fig. 4-30). It must be remembered, however, that some patients will sequester water preferentially in their ankles, lower limbs, and postsacral regions and show little change in the chest wall tissues, even though there has been a considerable gain in extravas-

cular water. In such cases it may still be possible to arrive logically at the correct diagnosis. For example a patient may have "gone ahead" 4 L in fluids. If this were entirely intravascular, it would widen the pedicle by 2 cm. If it were entirely *extravascular*, there would be no change in the pedicle but the soft tissue width should increase. If neither of these events occurred (i.e., the pedicle and soft tissues were unchanged), one could obviously deduce that the fluid had gone elsewhere and there would then be really only two choices—the soft tissues off the film or within the abdomen (Fig. 4-31).

Failure to show any change in vascular pedicle width or soft tissues despite a patient's being ahead on fluids is a not uncommon occurrence with continuous blood loss from wounds (Fig. 4-18). Similarly, actual *reduction* in VPW in patients who are far ahead on fluids is common, especially with burn patients who pour fluids into their burned tissues (third spacing). Such patients may be many liters ahead and still be in severe hypovolemic shock. The radiologist's analysis of the VPW and soft tissue thickness, integrated with the input and output data, is critical to understanding precisely what is happening to the distribution of fluid in such patients and to instituting immediately the appropriate therapy, which may be lifesaving (Figs. 4-30 and 4-31).

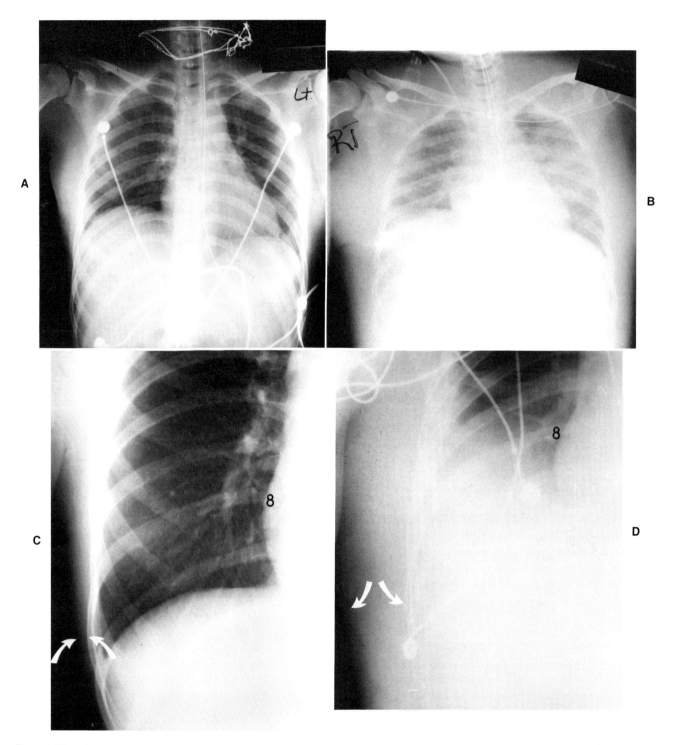

Fig. 4-28 A 27-year-old woman with systemic lupus (SLE). **A,** AP erect film. **B,** The patient has gone into florid renal failure. Note the gross changes in the soft tissues. There is very little change in width of the pedicle, indicating that the massive accumulation of fluid is almost entirely extravascular (including the development of pulmonary edema and ascites). **C,** To measure the soft tissues, the greatest point of convexity of the rib cage is found *(inner arrow)* and the distance is measured from this point to the outer edge of the skin (bright-lighted). The rib number from which the measurement was made is noted (*8* in this case) and the same point is then used on future films. **D,** The gross change in soft tissue thickness is easily seen and measured (an observation that is often neglected).

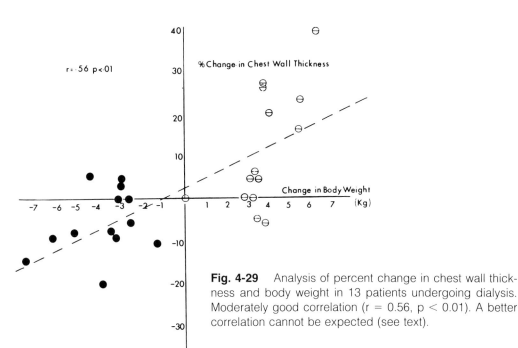

Fig. 4-29 Analysis of percent change in chest wall thickness and body weight in 13 patients undergoing dialysis. Moderately good correlation (r = 0.56, p < 0.01). A better correlation cannot be expected (see text).

Differing patterns of change in the vascular pedicle, vena azygos, and soft tissues are quite characteristic of different underlying etiologies and may lead to either a specific diagnosis or a refinement of one's knowledge of what is happening hemodynamically in a patient in whom the primary diagnosis is already known (e.g., whether the hemodynamics have improved in a patient with mitral stenosis following mitral valve replacement).

VASCULAR PEDICLE AND VENA AZYGOS IN CARDIAC DISEASE
Cardiac Failure

Cardiac failure can best be defined as "inability of the heart to respond with increased output to an increased demand." Using this definition, one can identify radiologically patients known to have cardiac disease but who are not in failure (i.e., are compensated) and those who are in failure (decompensated). For example, a patient with mitral stenosis, manifesting pulmonary venous and arterial hypertension, but showing no increase in extravascular lung water, would be described as having compensated cardiac disease; when this same patient began to manifest pulmonary edema, he would be diagnosed as having decompensated cardiac disease (i.e., as being in failure). The presence of an increased pulmonary blood volume and pulmonary edema does not in itself, however, necessarily constitute cardiac decompensation—in severe renal failure or iatrogenic overhydration the patient may have a very large pulmo-

nary blood volume and gross pulmonary edema but not be in cardiac failure, because if put on a treadmill he can increase his already large cardiac output still further and therefore does not fit the definition of cardiac failure. Despite this, the pulmonary edema seen in renal patients is still frequently erroneously referred to as cardiac failure.

Congestive Failure

Although the term "congestive failure" is almost universally employed and is a favorite in the "clinical history" box on patient requisition forms, we try to discourage its use radiologically (and whenever possible clinically) because of its nonspecificity. While it is quite true that all types of decompensated cardiac disease will cause congestion *somewhere* in the body, the anatomic region affected and whether the congestion is intravascular, extravascular, or both vary widely according to the etiology—acute left heart failure, chronic left heart failure, acute or chronic biventricular failure, acute or chronic right heart failure. A radiologic report stating that the patient has "severe congestive cardiac failure" is of limited value. Unless the correct subdivision of failure is identified, specific treatment (which may vary widely depending upon the type of cardiac failure present) cannot be instituted.

Using the vascular pedicle, vena azygos, soft tissues, pulmonary intra- and extravascular water, and cardiac shape and size, it is usually possible to decide which of the varying subdivisions of cardiac failure is present.

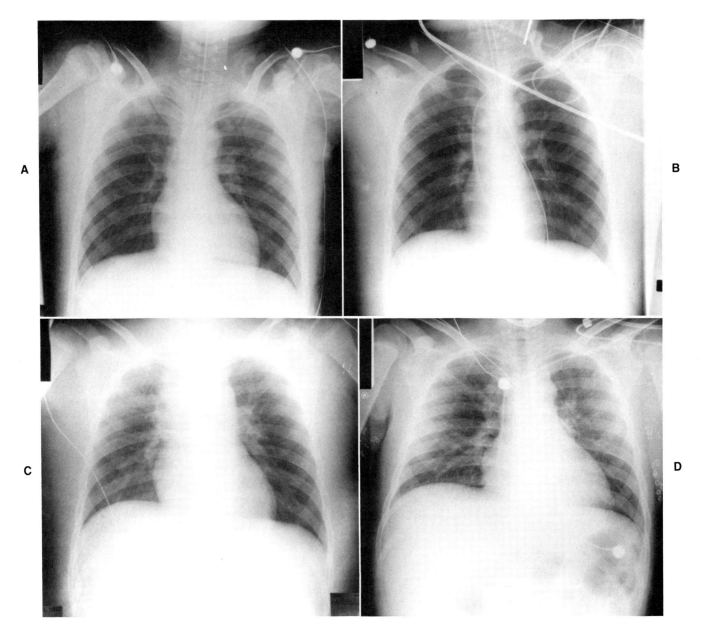

Fig. 4-30 **A,** AP supine film of a 16-year-old boy who entered a burning room to rescue a television set. The pedicle width, PBV, heart size, and soft tissues all appear normal on this initial admission film (but the mottled texture of the soft tissues and the loss of fat planes are very abnormal and indicate edema). **B,** The patient is now 10 L "ahead" on fluids, but his VPW is reduced, as are his cardiac and pulmonary blood volumes. In contrast, his soft tissue thickness (ST) has increased greatly. The patient is "third-spacing" into his burned chest wall. Even though he is 10 L ahead, this has not kept up with his fluid loss. He has lost some of his circulating blood volume and is effectively dehydrated. He was hypotensive at this stage. **C,** The VPW is markedly increased and the PBV and cardiac volume are also increased. There is no further increase in ST (i.e., the circulating blood volume has now been replenished and is increasing above normal (compare the VPW with **A**). If hydration is continued, hydrostatic pulmonary edema will develop. **D,** Three weeks later VPW, PBV, cardiac volume are all back to normal. Note the marked reduction in ST width.

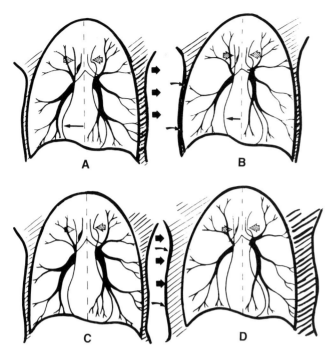

Fig. 4-31 **A** and **C** are identical and show a normal vascular pedicle, normal PBV, and normal soft tissue thickness. In **B** and **D** input and output data from the intensive care unit indicate that the patient is 10 L ahead. The question in both examples (**A** to **B** and **C** to **D**) is: What has happened to the patient's hemodynamics?

In **B** the VPW, azygos size, PBV, and cardiac volume are all reduced, indicating loss of fluid from the circulating blood volume; but there has also been a reduction in soft tissue thickness, and it is clear therefore that the excess fluid can only be in the abdomen or soft tissues other than the chest wall. **D** is identical with **B** except that the soft tissues, instead of reducing, have increased markedly, indicating that the excess fluid is third-spacing into the soft tissues. In both instances (**C** and **D**), despite the fluid overload, the patient is effectively dehydrated.

Every effort should be made by the radiologist to do this and to produce a specific diagnosis.

Acute Left Heart Failure

In true "first episode" LHF (i.e., not an acute episode superimposed on chronic heart failure) the vascular pedicle width usually does not increase, and may even narrow slightly as fluid is withdrawn from the circulating blood volume to appear in the lungs as edema.[20] In these acute cases the heart may be of normal size, there is usually no visible increase in pulmonary blood volume, and, in a high percentage, no base-to-apex redistribution of flow occurs. If the failure is severe, edema may be central in position (Fig. 4-32). (See Chapter 8.) The soft tissues will show no thickness in-

crease. This type of pattern may be seen with a massive myocardial infarct, an abrupt onset of valvular disease in subacute bacterial endocarditis, or a ruptured papillary muscle.

Chronic Left Heart Failure

In patients with long-standing CHF renal perfusion is diminished, resulting in aldosterone secretion with retention of salt and water.[20] The circulating blood volume consequently increases, and the vascular pedicle and azygos vein become enlarged. Long-standing or repeated episodes of edema lead to organic changes and deposition of fibrin in the basal microvasculature, and blood flow is therefore redistributed toward the apices—the upper lobe vessels may be "congested," but the lower lobe vessels are not (see Chapters 6 and 7). Soft tissue thickness is often not increased during periods of compensation; but when the patient decompensates, the soft tissues will usually increase in thickness as a manifestation of systemic edema (Fig. 4-33).

A comment should be made about myocardiopathies of toxic and viral origin. In these cases, although chronic failure may be present, the radiologic findings are often atypical. Whereas the vascular pedicle width *is* usually widened (because of the low cardiac output leading to renal hypoperfusion), flow inversion, usually seen in chronic left heart failure, may be missing, even in the face of severe pulmonary edema. This may be because in patients with severe myocardiopathy failure develops more rapidly than in patients with coronary artery disease, and there is not time for the organic basal lung changes to develop that are said to be the primary cause of flow inversion (Fig. 4-33). (See Chapters 6 and 7.)

Acute Right Heart Failure

Acute right heart failure is somewhat uncommon to recognize radiologically. Almost invariably it is caused by sudden elevation of pulmonary vascular resistance (e.g., from a massive pulmonary embolus, a shower of foreign body emboli in an intravenous drug addict, or an abrupt hematogenous dissemination of tumor emboli) or by acute tricuspid incompetence (Fig. 4-34). The changes seen on the radiograph are an abrupt increase in size of the vena azygos and widening of the vascular pedicle, *without* evidence of pulmonary edema. Since the obstruction to the pulmonary vascular bed is *pre*capillary, with no elevation of left atrial pressure, there is no reason for pulmonary edema to develop unless the patient has a prior cardiac abnormality (e.g., relative ischemia), in which case a large embolus could lead to abrupt *left heart* decompensation and edema.

Theoretically an abrupt elevation of right atrial pressure and the subsequent elevation of systemic venous pressure should diminish the inflow of pleural lymph

Fig. 4-32 Very abrupt first episode left heart decompensation causing classic (though rare) bats-wing pulmonary edema. Note the bronchial cuffing *(arrow)*. The VPW remains normal and can sometimes be small since fluid has been withdrawn from the circulating blood volume to "supply" the pulmonary edema. (See Chapter 2.)

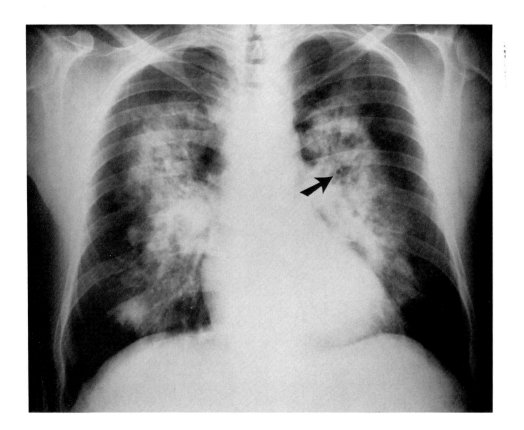

Fig. 4-33 Chronic left heart failure. Note the wide pedicle, indicating increased circulating blood volume because of renal hypoperfusion, and the inversion of flow, giving the "touchdown" appearance *(arrow)*. This inversion is partially secondary to organic change in the lung bases from recurrent episodes of failure and partially functional. It remains present even though there is no pulmonary edema. (The patient is not presently decompensated.)

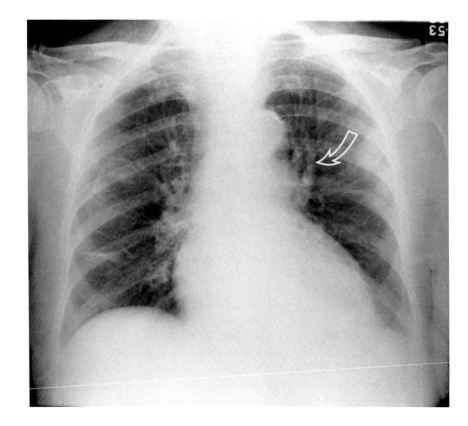

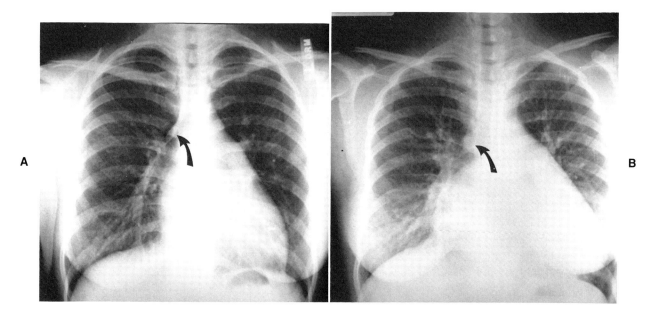

Fig. 4-34   A 28-year-old woman at term. **A,** Predelivery. The patient has a small ASD. Note the normal pedicle width and azygos vein. **B,** Postdelivery. Septic endocarditis has developed with tricuspid incompetence and neck vein distension. Note the large increase in size of the azygos vein. There is also considerable cardiac enlargement, proportionally more to the right than to the left. The picture is complicated by renal failure, causing a marked increase in circulating blood volume (with increasing size of the pulmonary blood vessels and a 1:1 flow distribution).

into systemic veins, causing an increased transudation of pleural fluid from the parietal pleural capillaries (all of this in a patient *without* pulmonary edema). In fact, we have never seen this. We *have* seen pleural effusion develop suddenly in a few young patients with an abrupt onset of tricuspid incompetence secondary to subacute bacterial endocarditis, but these patients also manifested pulmonary edema (Fig. 4-34). If the patient survives the insult that has led to the abrupt elevation of right heart pressure, the soft tissues of the chest wall will later become widened.

Note that acute elevation of right heart pressure is also a component of neurogenic edema, in which there is a gross elevation of both pulmonary arterial and systemic vascular pressures. Because the increased resistance in the pulmonary microcirculation occurs at the *venous* end of the capillaries, the very high pulmonary artery pressure is transmitted directly to the capillary bed, resulting in pulmonary edema. This is quite unlike all other causes of pulmonary arterial hypertension, which are *pre*capillary and actually protect the capillary bed from elevated pulmonary artery pressure, preventing the formation of edema. In neurogenic edema, because the tricuspid valve is usually competent, the grossly elevated right ventricular pressure may not be transmitted back into the systemic veins; also there ap-

pears to be a generalized increase in vasomotor tone and the vena azygos and vascular pedicle may not enlarge even with very high pulmonary vascular pressures.

Chronic Right Heart Failure

Chronic right heart failure (CRHF) most commonly occurs secondary to chronic left heart failure, rather than chronic pulmonary disease. While it is true that CRHF is commonly associated with chronic obstructive lung disease (cor pulmonale), the lung disease itself is almost invariably caused by smoking, which commonly also damages the coronary circulation to the entire heart so that "pure" chronic right heart failure is relatively uncommon. Even when right ventricular failure appears to be pure, radioisotope studies reveal that, on exercise, progressive dilation of the right side of the heart is occurring while the left side becomes progressively starved for blood and cannot meet the increased demand[21] (i.e., is failing).

Right heart failure is an area in which the azygos vein and vascular pedicle have proven somewhat disappointing as a means of helping the radiologist make a diagnosis. Clinically, right heart failure is diagnosed when there is neck vein distension with hepatic enlargement and soft tissue edema. Since the neck veins are in direct continuity with the intrathoracic veins, with no valves intervening from the base of the skull to the inferior vena cava, it would seem obvious that any increase in width of the veins in the neck should be *preceded* by enlargement of their intrathoracic portion (i.e., the vascular pedicle). Theoretically, therefore, the radiologist should be able to see these changes on the erect chest film, *before* they become manifest clinically. In actual fact we have often been disappointed, when we reported the pedicle and azygos vein as being normal, to have the patient's clinician inform us that the patient *does* have distended neck veins. It seemed to us that there were only two possible explanations for this discrepancy—(1) the clinician was not actually seeing distended neck veins even though they were reported as such and (2) tonic contracture of only the intrathoracic portion of the veins was occurring, in which case it might have been possible that the neck veins were distended in the face of a normal VPW. However, when we undertook to compare vascular pedicle width (measured from the midline to the right pedicular border, *MR*) with neck vein distension (confirmed by two independent observers), we actually found an excellent correlation (Table 4-4). Below an MR width of 2 cm *no*

Table 4-4 Correlation between vascular pedicle width and neck vein distension

Midline to right (MR) measurement at VPW (cm)	Distension of neck veins (clinical examination)	
	Not present	Present
1.0	√	
1.0	√	
1.1	√	
1.1	√	
1.4	√	
1.6	√	
1.7	√	
1.7	√	
1.7	√	
1.7	√	
1.75	√	
1.75	√	
1.8	√	
2.0	√	
2.0		√
2.0		√
2.25	√	
2.4		√
2.4		√
2.45		√
2.5		√
2.55		√
2.6		√
2.75		√
3.40		√
4.20		√

neck vein distension was reported clinically, but above 2.25 cm MR *all* cases were reported to have distension. In this series we found no discrepancy between the size of the vascular pedicle and the presence of neck vein distension. We also found a good correlation between circulating blood volume and such distension (Table 4-5). Despite this, we continue to hear from referring clinicians that neck vein distension is being seen even when the vascular pedicle width and azygos vein are not enlarged, and we continue to work on this apparent discrepancy between clinical and radiologic findings. Presently the soft tissues may be of greater value than the width of the pedicle in diagnosing right heart failure; they usually do increase in thickness when chronic right heart failure is present. We continue to be surprised by the relative infrequency of *radiologically* manifested right heart failure compared to the large numbers of cases of severe COPD that we see. Again, this is an observation requiring further investigation.

It is often suggested that chronic right heart failure causes pleural effusions, but this has not been confirmed and it appears to be incorrect. (See Chapter 5.)

Acute Biventricular Failure

Acute biventricular failure usually occurs because of a massive myocardial infarct or multiple valve involvement in subacute bacterial endocarditis. In both cases pulmonary edema is present—often fulminating (i.e., rapid development of severe alveolar edema)—and the vascular pedicle is widened, the azygos vein enlarged, and the soft tissue width increased (Fig. 4-34). In these acute cases the heart is frequently not enlarged and the lung may show a central distribution of edema instead of the basal (gravitational) distribution generally seen in left heart failure (90% of cases). (See Chapter 8.)

Chronic Biventricular Failure

Chronic biventricular failure usually follows the sequence of chronic left heart failure followed by the development of chronic right heart failure. If the onset of right heart failure is abrupt, there may be a sudden improvement in the patient's pulmonary edema, with some relief of subjective clinical symptoms (e.g., cessation of cardiac asthma). In our experience the exact

Table 4-5 Correlation between circulating blood volume and neck vein distension

Circulating blood volume* (ml)	Neck vein distension (%)
4000 to 6000	18
6000 to 7000	40
7000 to 10,000	80

*Not normalized for the patient's size.

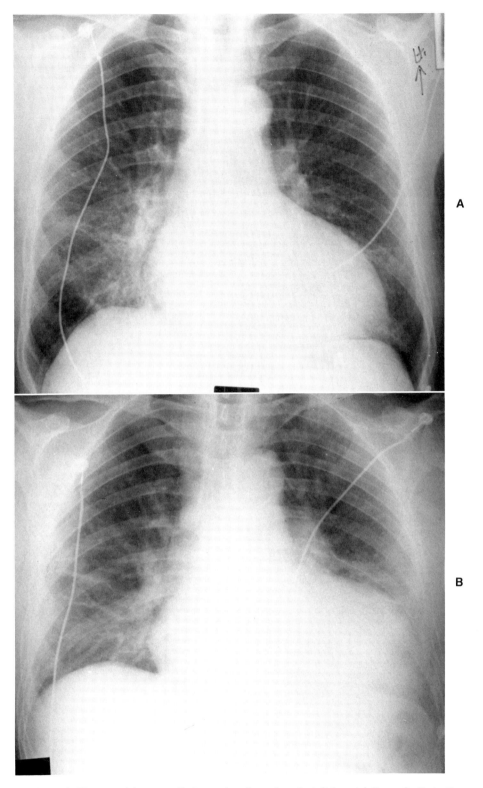

Fig. 4-35   A 58-year-old man with long-standing chronic left heart failure. **A,** Note the flow inversion, basal interstitial edema, and wide pedicle. The patient had some expiratory wheezing on auscultation, was dyspneic, and could sleep only sitting up. **B,** Note the marked enlargement of the azygos vein and VPW. Over a 36-hour period the wheezing disappeared and the dyspnea improved, but the x-ray appearance has deteriorated. The change was accompanied by neck vein swelling, ankle swelling, and liver engorgement. The patient had progressed from principally left heart failure to biventricular failure.

time at which RHF supervenes on LHF is seldom caught radiologically; but when it is, it is quite typical (i.e., on one day we see the typical changes of chronic left heart failure, with pulmonary edema and a widened pedicle but little soft tissue swelling, and then abruptly the pedicle widens further, the azygos vein enlarges, and the soft tissues increase in thickness while simultaneously the pulmonary edema *improves*). With this typical radiographic picture the clinical picture usually includes an overnight improvement in dyspnea, but this is accompanied by the onset of hepatomegaly and ankle swelling (Fig. 4-35). Subsequently the picture of chronic biventricular failure is seen—a very wide pedicle and large vena azygos, variable amounts of pulmonary edema (depending upon left heart behavior), considerable soft tissue swelling, and often ascites. When ascites develops, pleural effusions may become large and there may be a discrepancy between the large size of the effusions and the minor to moderate amount of pulmonary edema. This discrepancy is diagnostically valuable and should lead the radiologist—even in the absence of abdominal changes on the chest film—to re-port that ascites may be developing and to suggest the appropriate tests to confirm or exclude this.

In chronic biventricular failure the heart is usually enlarged (Fig. 4-35), in contrast to acute biventricular failure, in which it is initially of normal size.

Pericardial Tamponade

The radiologic appearances of pericardial tamponade are those of acute right heart failure without any of the pulmonary manifestations of massive or multiple minute emboli. Hemopericardium due to penetrating wounds or following cardiac surgery is, in our experience, the commonest cause of tamponade. Pericardial effusion is the second commonest cause. As tamponade develops, the vascular pedicle width and size of the vena azygos increase rapidly, often dramatically, while simultaneously the pulmonary blood volume diminishes (Fig. 4-36). Widening of the chest wall soft tissues is not usually seen until the tamponade has persisted for some time. Note that pericardial tamponade is one of the few instances in which there is a dissociation between the pulmonary blood volume and systemic blood

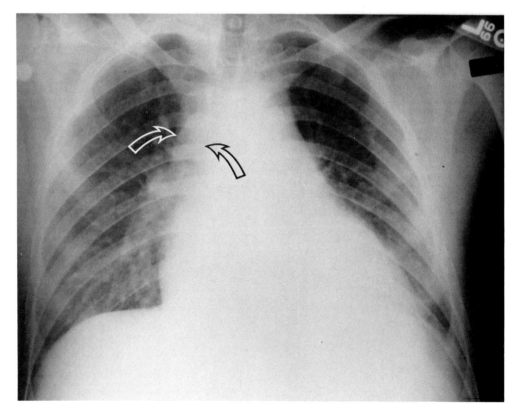

Fig. 4-36 A 36-year-old male mental patient with a Barrets ulcer of the esophagus that eroded into the pericardial cavity causing effusion and pericardial tamponade. Note the discrepancy between the huge vena azygos (between *arrows*), the very wide pedicle, and (in this case) the normovolemic lungs. The lungs are usually oligemic in association, as in this case, with pericardial tamponade.

volume (i.e., the vascular pedicle becomes wide at the same time that the lung becomes relatively oligemic). This should be contrasted with a left-to-right shunt, in which the exact reverse happens (the vascular pedicle becomes very narrow and the lungs markedly hyperemic) (Fig. 4-37). When this discrepancy between pulmonary and systemic blood volumes is seen, there is virtually no differential diagnosis in either case. A left-to-right shunt can usually be diagnosed without even having to consider cardiac size or shape.

VASCULAR PEDICLE AND VENA AZYGOS IN ACQUIRED VALVULAR DISEASE
Mitral Stenosis and Incompetence

Most of the radiologic changes of mitral stenosis and incompetence have been thoroughly described by many authors, but these descriptions rarely mention that patients with mitral stenosis and incompetence of rheumatic origin usually have a very narrow vascular pedicle and a very small vena azygos (Fig. 4-38). The very narrow pedicle, like the very small aorta seen in these patients, appears to be related to the low left ventricular output—the small left ventricular output apparently results in a smaller than normal systemic blood volume. The pulmonary blood volume is not increased[22] but is usually markedly redistributed so that the upper half of the lung appears plethoric and the lower half somewhat oligemic (flow inversion)[23-25] (Fig. 4-38). The soft tissues are normal. Even with decompensation and florid pulmonary edema, the vascular pedicle and azygos vein stay small and the soft tissues do not usually increase in thickness. If the pedicle and

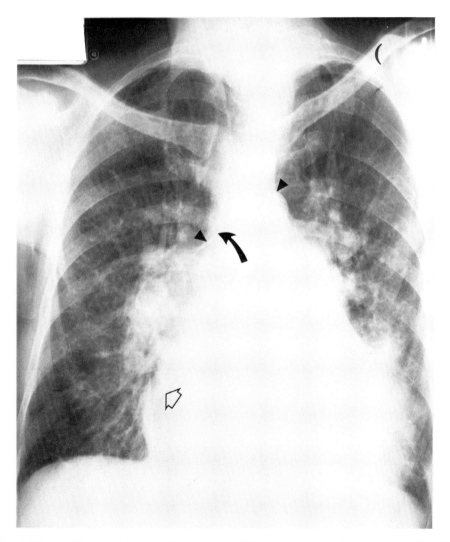

Fig. 4-37 A 40-year-old man with a large ASD and pulmonary hypertension. Despite the large heart and very large pulmonary blood volume, the vascular pedicle (between *black arrowheads*) is narrow, indicating a small circulating blood volume. The azygos vein *(curved arrow)* is also small. The open arrow indicates huge draining veins.

Fig. 4-38 A 30-year-old woman with mitral stenosis. There is some flow inversion, with larger than normal upper lobe vessels, a narrow pedicle, and large lung volumes.

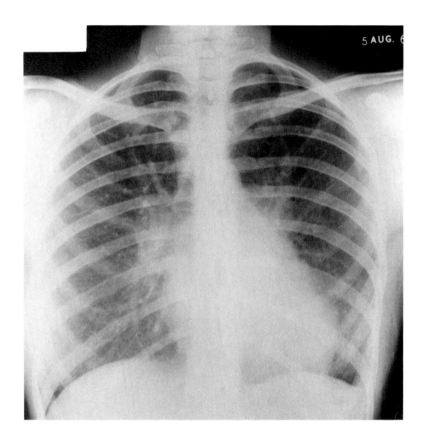

azygos vein do become enlarged, this usually means that tricuspid incompetence has developed.

Mitral valve patients do not appear to suffer from the renal hypoperfusion seen in chronic left heart failure of other etiologies. They do not therefore develop an increased CBV but instead have a *narrow* vascular pedicle. This differing behavior might be secondary to the long time it takes for MS and MI to develop, giving the kidneys time to adapt. Alternatively, the difference may lie in the fact that the musculature of the left ventricle is usually normal in mitral stenosis and, though the output is small, the ventricle's ability to contract and accelerate blood through the aorta is unimpaired.

Aortic Stenosis

The radiologic appearances of aortic stenosis (AS) have also been extensively described, but again these descriptions seldom mention that in AS both the vascular pedicle and the pulmonary blood volume are small (i.e., in compensated aortic stenosis the lungs appear slightly oligemic) (Fig. 4-39). It should be noted that this belief is not generally held—not necessarily because there is disagreement with the statement, but possibly also because the observation has not been widely disseminated in the literature. The paucity of blood within the lungs of patients with AS is more than simply a radiologic observation; it has been quantitated using radioisotopic techniques.[26]

We believe[1] that the pedicle and azygos vein are small, as in mitral stenosis, because the left ventricular output is small—which means, of course, that input to the right heart (vis a tergo) is small and the right ventricular output (matching the left) is small, leading to a small pulmonary blood volume. The pulmonary blood volume is not redistributed (inverted), because left atrial pressure is normal (Fig. 4-39). The soft tissue thickness is also normal. If the pedicle and azygos vein begin to enlarge, this usually indicates that left ventricular decompensation is taking place. Since aortic stenosis patients benefit far more from replacement of the aortic valve before they decompensate, any increase in pulmonary blood volume and VPW is an urgent sign that the patient is beginning to decompensate and requires immediate consideration for valve replacement.

Anatomic Intrathoracic Left-to-Right Shunts

As mentioned earlier, left-to-right shunts occurring within the thorax cause a size discrepancy between the pulmonary blood volume (which is increased, recruiting the upper lobe vessels and giving a 1:1 or "balanced" flow distribution) and the systemic blood volume (which is diminished, leading to a very narrow vascular

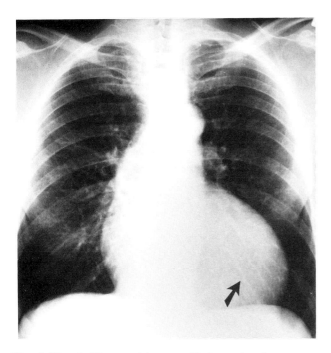

Fig. 4-39 A 38-year-old man with long-standing severe aortic stenosis. The pedicle is narrow, and the lungs markedly oligemic. Note the very narrow vessels seen through the heart *(arrow)*. The narrow pedicle and oligemic lungs indicate a very small circulating blood volume, probably secondary to very small left (and therefore right) ventricular outputs.

pedicle and small azygos vein) (Fig. 4-37). An approximate estimation of shunt size can be obtained by looking at the relative sizes of the pedicle and aorta—which reflect systemic blood volume (related to left heart output) and the size of the pulmonary vessels (related to right heart output).[27] With large left-to-right shunts the pedicle may be so narrow that it is partially concealed by the width of the thoracic vertebrae, giving the appearance that the heart is hanging like an apple from a very thin stem (Fig. 4-37). Following successful surgical closure of a large shunt, the vascular pedicle and vena azygos will enlarge and the pulmonary blood volume diminish—though if the shunt has been present for many years, these changes in the lungs will take place only gradually, over a period of months, whereas change in the pedicle and azygos will be much more immediate.

PHYSIOLOGIC INCREASE IN CBV

Initial radiologic observations suggest that small normal variations in circulating blood volume appear to take place daily (possibly diurnally) in both men and women and certainly in women during the premenstrual period. Although these can be detected by small changes in vascular pedicle width, the only normal cause of a *major* increase in CBV is pregnancy. In the midtrimester CBV increases approximately 30% and this is often readily detected by an increase in width of the vascular pedicle and increasing pulmonary blood volume, which tend to create a 1:1 flow distribution, and a slight increase in transverse diameter of the heart, particularly on the more compliant right side. Following delivery, the changes resolve within a few days to a few weeks.

RENAL FAILURE AND OVERHYDRATION

The greatest radiologic changes in vascular pedicle width and azygos vein size are seen in cases of renal failure and iatrogenic overhydration.[28] These two conditions have many similarities, but there are also important differences that can be of some diagnostic value and are of physiologic interest.

In renal cases the greatest changes in vascular pedicle width appear to occur in patients with recent onset of failure. In these acute cases the vascular pedicle and azygos vein can become huge. For example, the pedicle may increase from 5 to 10 or 12 cm and the azygos from 3 mm to 1.5 cm or more. Simultaneously the pulmonary blood volume increases markedly, recruiting all empty vessels and causing a 1:1 flow distribution. The heart will increase in size, principally to the right, even if it is not affected by uremic myocardiopathy. Enormous changes can occur in the thickness of the soft tissues. At this stage the condition is indistinguishable from gross overhydration (Figs. 4-30 and 4-40). The distribution of edema is characteristically greater in the central two thirds of the lung, tending to spare the costophrenic angles (Chapter 8) and frequently has an inhomogeneous acinar or nodular appearance (unlike that of overhydration edema) (Fig. 4-41). The amount of pulmonary edema and the size of pleural effusions vary greatly depending upon the combined levels of the oncotic and left atrial pressures (Fig. 4-18).

Unlike the lung volumes in cardiac mediated pulmonary edema, which diminish because of a decrease in compliance, the lung volumes in renal pulmonary edema and overhydration often remain large (Fig. 4-42). This may be related to the fact that all the pulmonary vessels are filled, forming a "scaffolding" for the lung (which is to a limited extent an erectile organ), overcoming the effects of edema-induced diminished compliance. It is tempting to think that filling the lung with blood will "erect" it, but the pressures required to inflate (erect) an isolated lung by filling it with blood are very high (far above normally achievable levels) in contrast to the low pressures required to erect the lung with air.

Alternatively, since these patients have a greater cardiac output than normal, they may increase their venti-

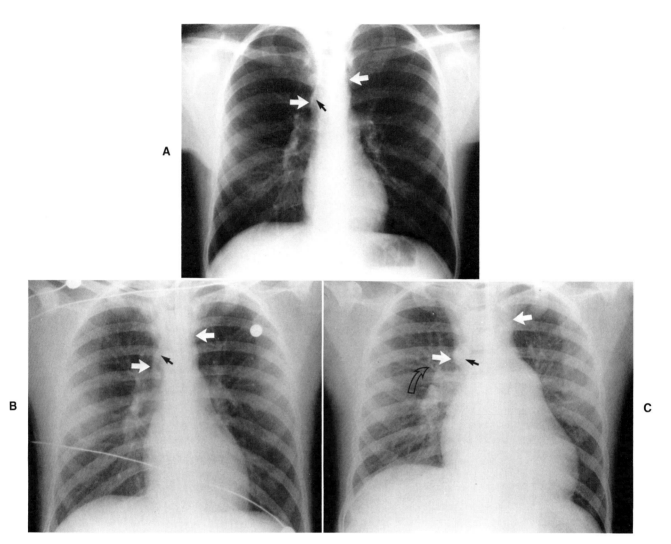

Fig. 4-40 Classic changes of progressive overhydration in a burn patient. The pedicle *(white arrows)* and azygos *black arrow)* increase in size, the PBV increases, and the distribution changes from a normal basal predominance of flow to a balanced 1:1 flow (in **C**). Developing interstitial edema produces blurring of the vessel margins, increasing whiteness of the lungs, and peribronchial cuffing *(open arrow)*.

Fig. 4-41 Young man with end-stage renal disease. **A,** No evidence of renal decompensation despite the large cardiac volume (uremic cardiomyopathy). **B,** Beginning renal decompensation. The PBV, vena azygos, and cardiac volume are increased, and interstitial edema is developing (manifested by blurred vessel margins and peribronchial cuffing). Despite all of this the vascular pedicle remains narrow. **C,** The patient is now in florid edema with the classic central distribution of renal failure. Note the curious "nodular" appearance of the edema, presumably due to acinar filling. The peribronchial cuffing is thicker, and the azygos vein still larger, but the VPW is almost unchanged.

We believe this failure of the pedicle to enlarge is due to high vasomotor tone. **D,** Spot view of film **A.** Clear vessel margins. The azygos vein is not visible, and the pedicle is very narrow. **E,** Spot view of film **B.** The vessel margins have become blurred, lung density is increasing, there is peribronchial cuffing, and the azygos is enlarged. Only slight change in the VPW. **F,** Spot view of film **C.** Further blurring of the vessels, with increasing density of the lung parenchyma. Peribronchial cuffs have become thicker, and acinar filling is seen, but the VPW remains unchanged.

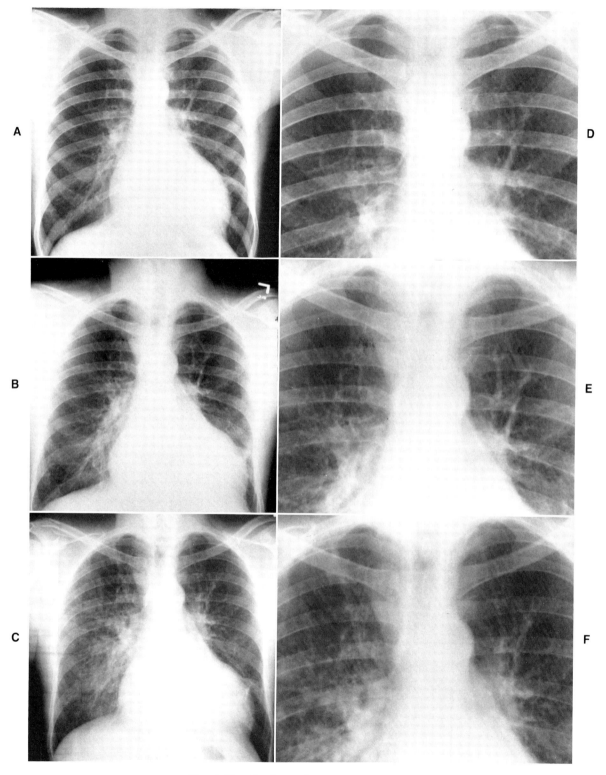

Fig. 4-41   For legend see opposite page.

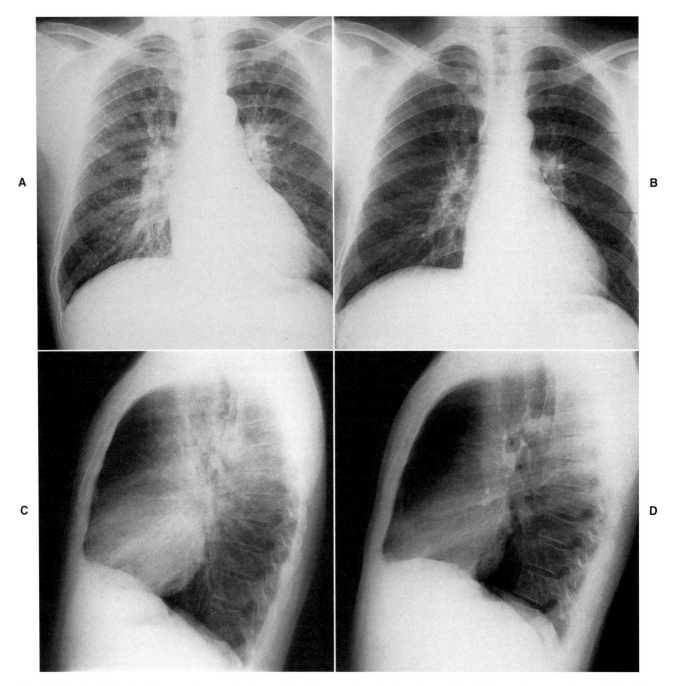

Fig. 4-42 A, Patient with recent onset of renal insufficiency. On admission, increased heart size, wide vascular pedicle (58 mm), and azygos vein (10 mm) were observed. These findings indicate an increase in circulating blood volume. Concomitant increase in pulmonary blood volume is indicated by increased density and size of the hila, pulmonary arteries, and pulmonary veins and by a balanced (1:1) distribution of flow. Early interstitial edema is present, represented by blurring of hilar vessels, Kerley B lines, and peribronchial cuffing. (Eleven ribs showing.) **B,** Lateral view showing haziness of perihilar regions, peribronchial cuffing, widening of the fissures, and large lung volume. **C,** Five days after repeated dialysis the heart size is normal, the pedicle 48 mm, and the azygos vein 5 mm. Pulmonary blood volume is markedly reduced from **A.** Interstitial edema has gone and the lung volumes have also reduced as compared to **A.** (Ten ribs showing.) **D,** After dialysis, lung volumes are reduced compared to **B.** Interstitial edema has gone.

latory volumes to match the decreased transit times of blood within the lungs. The low hemoglobin concentration in these patients may also cause this hyperdynamic circulatory condition, in order to deliver more oxygen to the peripheral tissues. The same mechanism may set the ventilatory drive to a higher level to increase the loading of oxygen in the pulmonary capillary blood causing the increase in pulmonary blood and lung volume.

In very long-standing and end-stage renal failure a curious change can take place. Although the pulmonary blood volume may remain large and the 1:1 distribution persist, the vascular pedicle width retreats back toward normal (and, even in the face of an increased CBV, is not enlarged) (Fig. 4-41). This discrepancy almost certainly results not from a decreasing circulating blood volume but from a progressive increase in vasomotor tone—presumably the same mechanism that leads to systemic hypertension. If one therefore sees a chest film with central edema, increased pulmonary blood volume, and a 1:1 flow distribution, but with a normal or narrow vascular pedicle, the diagnosis of late-stage renal failure rather than overhydration should be entertained. Patients with iatrogenic overhydration will have large vascular pedicles, in direct proportion to the degree of overhydration and size of the pulmonary blood volume. In cases of overhydration the thickness of the soft tissues will depend to some degree on the oncotic pressure of the blood (i.e., on whether the patient has been overhydrated with high or low molecular weight fluids. For example, if a patient is "overhydrated" with blood, the VPW and the PBV and the right side of the heart will all be enlarged while the soft tissues remain normal.

Table 4-6   Correlation between reduction in pulmonary blood volume and development of hypotension

X-ray grade (1 to 10) pulmonary blood volume (5 normal, 10 large)	Vascular pedicle width (cm)	Occurrence of postdialysis hypotension	
		No	Yes
7	6.8	✓	
6	4.0	✓	
6	5.1	✓	
6	4.2	✓	
6	5.0	✓	
5	5.3	✓	
5	6.0		✓
5	5.1	✓	
4	4.9		✓
4	7.0		✓
4	4.4		✓
3	6.2		✓

Hypotension Following Dialysis. It would seem logical that too rapid a reduction in CBV should be the cause for the frequently seen post dialysis hypotension; but, interestingly, in a series of patients we examined at the Italian National Research Council Renal Physiology Laboratories (Reggio Calabria), we found that there was no relationship between width of the vascular pedicle post dialysis and the occurrence of hypotension. Instead, we found a strong correlation between reduction in pulmonary blood volume and development of hypotension (Table 4-6). Note (Table 4-6) that the VPW was often large even when the PBV dropped and hypotension occurred. There is a close relationship between right ventricular output and PBV, and our findings therefore suggest inadequate right ventricular output (possibly caused by too rapid a reduction in right atrial and ventricular volume) as a cause of hypotension after dialysis. This hypothesis has not yet been tested.

DEHYDRATION

Patients who are being deliberately dehydrated (usually to reduce intracranial pressure) will have a very small vascular pedicle width and azygos vein and reduced pulmonary blood volume. If they are in the erect position, their upper lobes will be particularly oligemic, exaggerating the normal basal prominence of flow. Cardiac volume will be reduced, particularly on the right side (Fig. 4-27, A).

TRAUMA

Shock, both hypovolemic and septic, will be manifested by a reduced vascular pedicle width and azygos size and sometimes by a visible reduction in cardiac volume (Fig. 4-18), just as described for the dehydrated patient. In the initial stages the soft tissues will be normal; but, as resuscitation with IV fluid therapy continues, the soft tissues will often become wider, manifesting edema, before the circulating blood volume is restored. This effect is greatly exaggerated if the patient is losing blood at the same time as he is receiving IV fluids, particularly if the fluids are of low molecular weight. In these cases the pedicle can actually become *narrower*, even when the patient is many liters ahead on fluids—much of the fluid pouring out of the low–oncotic pressure intravascular volume into the soft tissues (Fig. 4-18). (For further discussion see Chapter 10.)

BURNS

Before discussing the soft tissue and vascular pedicle width changes in burn patients, it is useful to review the meaning of the term "third spacing." The first space is simply the intravascular volume. The second space is the total extravascular volume. The third space is the collection of extracellular fluid that is not *functionally*

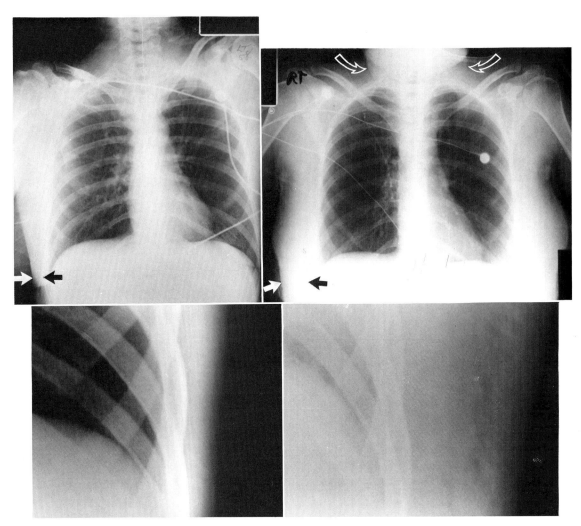

Fig. 4-43   A 32-year-old woman who was burned around the face, neck, and upper torso (55% second-degree burns). **A,** The admission AP erect chest film shows apparently normal vascular pedicle width, cardiac volume, pulmonary blood volume, and soft tissue thickness *(arrows).* **B,** Two days later she is *22 L* ahead on fluids and yet is hypotensive. Her vascular pedicle and cardiac size have decreased and her lungs have become oligemic. The reduction in width of the vascular pedicle, heart, and pulmo- nary blood volume indicate that all of the 22 L plus a com- ponent from her own circulating blood volume have passed out into the burned soft tissues of the chest wall *(solid ar- rows)* and neck *(open arrows)* (i.e., she is third-spacing enormously and, despite the huge increase in water load [22 kg] is effectively dehydrated). **C,** Spot view of the soft tissues shortly after admission. **D,** Spot view 36 hours later (17 to 19 L ahead on fluids).

available to the normal mechanisms maintaining fluid and electrolyte balance[29] (i.e., the definition is a func- tional one). Third spacing occurs almost universally into the injured tissues of burn patients, and successive ra- diographs may show VPW, cardiac volume, and PBV *decreasing* as the soft tissues increase enormously in a patient who may be 30 or more liters ahead on fluids and yet continue to be in hypovolemic shock (Fig. 4-43). While this is occurring, pulmonary edema does not usually develop; but, when fluid input begins to ex- ceed output (including third spacing) and the circulat- ing blood volume rises (manifested by increasing VPW and azygos size and by an increase in PBV), edema does develop, partially because of low oncotic pressure and partially because of an elevation in left atrial pres- sure secondary to the increased intravascular volume.[30] This is pressure edema and has relatively little deleteri- ous physiologic effect, provided it remains within the pulmonary interstitium. (See Chapter 2.) Therefore it is always much more important to restore the circulating blood volume to normal than it is to try to avoid hydrostatic pulmonary edema by reducing fluid input.

INJURY EDEMA

The many causes of injury edema are discussed in Chapter 8. In pure injury edema the circulating blood volume should not be increased. The VPW and azygos vein size will be normal, or, if the cause of the edema is septic or hypovolemic shock (as it commonly is), the pedicle and azygos may be markedly *diminished* and the soft tissues will be normal.

The picture, however, becomes more complicated if ARDS develops, accompanied by general organ failure, and increasing hydration is required to treat the patient. This is the usual course of events (i.e., the "grafting on" of the appearances of pressure edema to normal pressure injury edema), and it leads to a progressive increase in soft tissue thickness (plus peribronchial cuffing and small pleural effusions). At the same time, since lung compliance has markedly decreased (necessitating positive-pressure ventilation), the vascular pedicle is narrowed by the high intrathoracic pressure—concealing the fact that the circulating blood volume is actually large because of the forced hydration (Fig. 4-44). Without a knowledge of the pressures used to ventilate the patient, it would be impossible to distinguish between the narrow pedicle resulting from high peak pressure ventilation and that from a diminished circulating blood volume. Fortunately in such patients one is rarely dealing with a single film to be read in isolation but has a sequence of films, showing the chronology of development of soft tissue edema and increasing ventilatory pressures, to assist in the diagnosis.

SEQUENTIAL ANALYSIS OF DISTRIBUTION OF BODY WATER

It is clear that the film reader is in a unique position to evaluate the relative contributions of intra- and extravascular water volume to total body water distribution; but, in addition, the film reader is able to see and quantify (even though only approximately), from the chest film, water within the pleural space and sometimes within the abdomen. If these various compartments are quantitated from daily chest films, an excellent chronologic picture can be acquired of the sequence of development and clearance of the various compartments. This type of analysis is particularly dramatic in patients with renal failure who are on dialysis. We are uniquely able to quantitate the various "lag periods" (e.g., the delays in development of pleural effusions until edema has developed [Chapters 5 through 7] and the delays in clearing of pleural effusions after edema has reabsorbed) (Fig. 4-45). Both as a clinical and as an investigative tool, the chest radiograph is un-

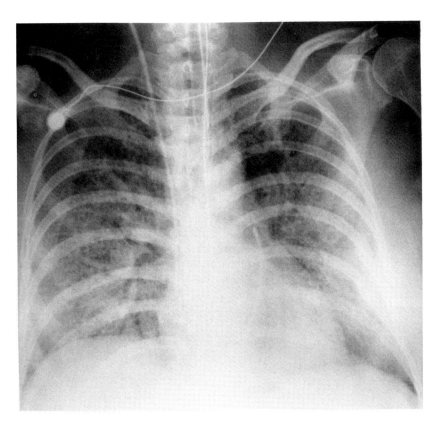

Fig. 4-44 A 31-year-old man with septicemia causing injury lung edema and ARDS. He is 6.5 L ahead on fluids and is not visibly third-spacing (either clinically or radiologically), suggesting that much of the fluid must be intravascular; but the vascular pedicle and cardiac size have not enlarged (even in the supine position). The patient is on high levels of positive-pressure ventilation (105 peak, 25 PEEP), however, and the high intrathoracic pressure makes it impossible for low-pressure vascular structures within the thorax to dilate. Note the classic air bronchograms of injury edema and the absence of peribronchial cuffing, septal lines, and effusions.

Fig. 4-45   Example of how fluid kinetics analysis can be derived from successive chest radiographs. The factors utilized in this case include soft tissue thickness, VPW, lung water, and size of effusions. On June 18 the patient receives a renal transplant. Successive films until July 14 plot her course and show how each "compartment" behaves as fluid accumulates (e.g., intravascular fluid increases initially more rapidly than pulmonary edema) and as successive dialyses are made. The patient's weight goes from 48 to 63 kg on July 5. On July 7 a dramatic fall in all compartments begins (the kidney is functioning) and all compartments return to the pretransplant level. The patient's weight drops back to 50 kg. These data would be almost impossible to obtain by any other means.

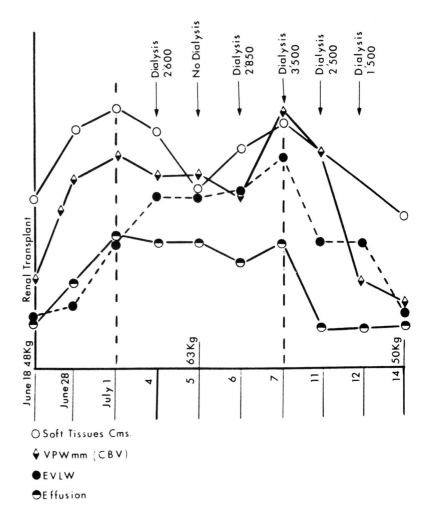

○ Soft Tissues Cms.

◊ VPW mm (CBV)

● EVLW

◒ Effusion

matched in its ability to reveal, to the informed observer, the relative speed of change and the alterations in volume of most normal and abnormal compartments of body water.[6]

REFERENCES

1. Milne ENC: Correlation of physiologic findings with chest roentgenology, *Radiol Clin North Am* 11:17, 1973.
2. Savoca CJ, Austin JHM, Goldberg HI: The right paratracheal stripe, *Radiology* 122:295, 1977.
3. Woodring JH, Pulman CM, Stevens RK: The right paratracheal stripe in blunt chest trauma, *Radiology* 143:605, 1982.
4. Milne ENC, Pistolesi M, Miniati M, Giuntini C: The vascular pedicle of the heart, and the vena azygos. I. The normal subject, *Radiology* 152:1, 1984.
5. Shratter L, Milne ENC: Unpublished data, 1989
6. Milne ENC: A physiologic approach to reading critical care unit films, *J Thorac Imaging* 1(3):60, 1986.
7. Vigran RI, Milne ENC: Unpublished data, 1989.
8. Milne ENC, Bass H: The roentgenologic diagnosis of early chronic obstructive lung disease, *J Can Assoc Radiol* 20:3, 1969.
9. Pistolesi M, Milne ENC, Miniati M, Giuntini C: The vascular pedicle of the heart and the vena azygos. II. Acquired heart disease, *Radiology* 152:9, 1984.
10. Keats TE, Lipscomb GE, Betts CS III: Mensuration of the arch of the azygos vein and its application to the study of cardiopulmonary disease, *Radiology* 90:990, 1968.
11. Heitzman ER: Radiologic appearance of the azygos vein in cardiovascular disease. *Circulation* 47:628, 1973.
12. Tori A, Garusi: Angiocardiographic demonstration of the valves of the azygos vein in tricuspid stenosis, *Acta Radiol* 56:355, 1961.
13. Poggi A, Maggiore Q: Cardiothoracic ratio as a guide to ultrafiltration therapy in dialysed patients, *Int J Artif Organs* 3:332, 1980.
14. Logue RB, Rogers JV, Gay BB: Subtle roentgenographic signs of left heart failure, *Am Heart J* 65:464, 1963.
15. Van de Water J, Sheh JM, O'Connor NE, et al: Pulmonary extravascular water volume: measurement and significance in critically ill patients, *J Trauma* 10:440, 1970.
16. Pistolesi M, Miniati M, Ravelli V, Giuntini C: Injury versus hydrostatic lung edema: detection by chest x-ray, *Ann NY Acad Sci* 384:364, 1982.
17. Milne ENC, Pistolesi M, Miniati M, Giuntini C: Assessing fluid balance from the plain chest film. [abstr.] *Invest Radiol* 19:550, 1984.
18. Pistolesi M, Miniati M, Milne ENC, Giuntini C: Measurement of lung edema: the radiographic approach, *Appl Cardiopulm Pathophysiol* 2:141, 1988.
19. Milne ENC, Pistolesi M: Pulmonary edema—cardiac and noncardiac. In Putman CE (ed): *Diagnostic imaging of the lung*, New York, 1990, Marcel Dekker, p 253.

20. Figueras J, Weil MW: Blood volume prior to and following treatment of acute cardiogenic pulmonary edema, *Circulation* 87:349, 1978.
21. Milne N: Unpublished data, personal communication.
22. Yu PN: *Pulmonary blood volume in health and disease*, Philadelphia, 1969, Lea & Febiger.
23. Milne ENC: Physiological interpretation of the plain film in mitral stenosis including a review of criteria for the estimation of pulmonary arterial and venous pressure, *Br J Radiol* 36:902, 1963.
24. Simon M: The pulmonary veins in mitral stenosis, *J Fac Radiol* 9:33, 1958.
25. Ormand E, Poznanski A: Pulmonary veins in rheumatic heart disease, *Radiology* 74:542, 1960.
26. Balbarini A, Barsotti A, Odoguardi L, Mariani M: Comportamento della vascolatura polmonare nelle valvulopathie aortiche acquisite, *Boll Soc Ital Cardiol* 18:103, 1973.
27. Fouché RF, Beck W, Schrire W: The roentgenologic assessment of the degree of left-to-right shunt in secundum type atrial septal defect, *Am J Roentgenol* 89:254, 1963.
28. Milne ENC, Pistolesi M, Miniati M, Giuntini C: The radiologic distinction of cardiogenic and non-cardiogenic edema, *AJR* 144:879, 1985.
29. Condon RE, Nyhus LM (eds): *Manual of surgical therapeutics*, ed 5, Boston, 1981, Little, Brown.
30. Haponik EF, Adelman M, Munster AM, Bleecker ER: Increased vascular pedicle width preceding burn-related pulmonary edema, *Chest* 80:649, 1986.

5 Pleural Effusions
Normal physiology, pathophysiology, and diagnosis

This book's premise is that knowledge of the normal and abnormal physiology of an organ will improve the ability of the reader to determine the cause of any particular functional or organic failure. To this end, we have tried to cover only that physiology which is important to radiologic interpretation and to avoid introducing abstruse or controversial physiology. However, both the physiologic and anatomic aspects of the pleural space are complex and controversial, and to delineate clearly the normal behavior of the pleural space, we must delve more deeply into physiology and anatomy than we have in other chapters.

Three major reviews of pleural physiology[1-3] have revealed that the classic, widely disseminated belief, that fluid is filtered by the parietal pleural capillaries and absorbed by the visceral pleural capillaries[4-7] is incorrect (Fig. 5-1), because it does not take into account several known anatomic and physiologic facts. These include the presence of stomata in the parietal pleura through which protein and fluids are absorbed into the subparietal lymphatics,[8,9] the fact that the visceral pleura may not be supplied entirely by the

pulmonary arteries,[10-13] and the role of the pleura itself in transferring pulmonary and pleural fluids.[14-16] The extensive reviews[1-3] agree with the classic view that filtration of pleural fluid occurs from the parietal pleura. In contrast with present beliefs, however, they conclude that *absorption* occurs principally via the stomata in the parietal pleura, not via the visceral pleural capillaries. The authors infer that the visceral pleural vessels filter some fluid but that, under normal conditions, little or no absorption of fluid occurs through the visceral pleura.

These comprehensive reviews provide a new, more accurate picture of the physiology of the pleural space; however, some further analysis appears to be necessary for the following reasons. First, the source of the visceral pleural circulation remains uncertain. The first review[1] states categorically that the visceral pleura is supplied not by the pulmonary circulation but by the bronchial circulation. The later, more extensive reviews[2,3] do not take a fixed position on whether the visceral pleural circulation is pulmonary, bronchial, or a mixture of the two but illustrate a slightly different scenario for each possibility. From our own injection studies of the bronchial and pulmonary circulations and from a thorough analysis of the conflicting literature reports,[10-13,17-22] we believe that the visceral pleura receives both pulmonary and bronchial vessels but that the bronchial vessels are purely nutritive, a conclusion we defend later in this chapter.

Second, in all three reviews,[1-3] as with Agostoni's original hypothesis,[4-7] the authors concentrate largely on the pleural vascular supply. They only briefly consider the pleura's role as a membrane with a large surface area, across which water (pleural or lung water) might pass in either direction without reference to the pleural vessels. We consider this later in greater detail.

Third, many other factors affect pleural fluid transudation and absorption that must also be considered more fully. These include the differing thicknesses of the parietal and visceral pleura, and the gravitational pressure gradients in the subparietal pleural and subvisceral pleural spaces.[23,24] Within the capillaries these factors include the large difference in surface area between the upper and lower parietal and visceral microvessels, the fall in pressure from arterial to venous end of both parietal and visceral capillaries, the pres-

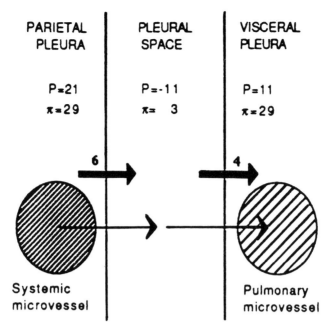

Fig. 5-1 This type of diagram is commonly used to illustrate pleural fluid formation and absorption. *P,* Hydrostatic pressure (intracapillary); *x,* oncotic pressure (intracapillary). The thick arrows indicate the result of adding the Starling forces. Fluid is said to pass out of the systemic (parietal pleural) capillaries, across the parietal pleura, and into the pleural space and is then absorbed across the visceral pleura by the pulmonary (visceral pleural) capillaries. The parietal and visceral pleural surfaces are shown simply as featureless, functionless vertical lines.

ence of clefts in the visceral mesothelium, and the large number of mast cells lying below the subvisceral pleura.[14-16] Plate 1 (p. 132 shows all these anatomic features in a semidiagrammatic form and is important for a fuller understanding of how pleural fluid is formed and absorbed.

MODELS OF PLEURAL FLUID FORMATION AND ABSORPTION

To understand how the many anatomic and physiologic factors just listed might affect the formation and absorption of pleural fluid, we have developed a model that includes the following factors (see Fig. 5-2).

1. Differing pleural pressure gradients (within the pleural space and in the subpleural interstitium, including apex to base and costal to mediastinal gradients)
2. Differing vascular pressure gradients (visceral and parietal pleural vessels)
3. Differing pressures at the arterial and venous ends of the parietal and visceral capillaries
4. Differing positions of the visceral pleural vessels (intrapleural versus subpleural)
5. Differing thickness and permeability (hydrostatic and oncotic) of the pleurae
6. Differing vascular supply to the visceral pleura (pulmonary, bronchial, or "mixed")

Table 5-1 Factors employed in model of pleural fluid formation and clearance

Anatomic/physiologic factors		Pressure	
		Hydrostatic	Oncotic
Visceral pleural (pulmonary) capillaries			
Intravascular	Arterial End	14.0[82]	25.0[82]
	Venous End	8.0[82]	25.0[82]
Extravascular	Subpleural	−5.0 to	19.0[82]
	Elsewhere	−10.0[24,82] −3.5[82]	19.0[82]
Parietal pleural (systemic) capillaries			
Intravascular	Arterial End	27.0[1]	25.0[82]
	Venous End	22.5[1]	25.0[82]
Extravascular	Subpleural	−4.5[24]	19.0[82]
Pleural space			
Costal	Inspiration	−16.0†	
	Expiration	−7.5†	
Mediastinal	Inspiration	−22.5†	3.0[1,7]
	Expiration	−12.0†	
Cranial/Caudal	Inspiration	0.75 cm H$_2$O/cm†	
Gradient	Expiration	0.66 cm H$_2$O/cm†	

* In mm Hg except where stated.
† See references 23,49,89,90.

Using this model, we have analyzed many permutations to try and determine which model is correct. The sources for our data covering pleural pressures, interstitial pressures, and oncotic pressures are detailed in Table 5-1. Since the model is somewhat complex and the computations for each permutation lengthy and somewhat tedious, we have transferred most mathematics and anatomic and physiologic arguments to Appendix A at the end of this chapter. This appendix also contains our arguments and evidence for the vascular supply of the visceral pleura and examples of the various permutations using our model. The results of all the possible permutations are displayed in Table 5-2.

From all the possible permutations considered, as the one model that fits best with observed experimental, clinical, and radiologic data, we have chosen model IIA (Table 5-2 and Fig. 5-3). This model predicts that pleural fluid is normally both filtered by the parietal pleural vessels and absorbed (including particulate material) through the parietal pleural stomata. The visceral pleura does not appear to have a significant role in the normal filtration *or* absorption of pleural fluid. This model is based on:

1. The visceral pleural vessels lying below (subpleurally) the thick visceral pleura
2. The visceral pleura being supplied by the pulmo-

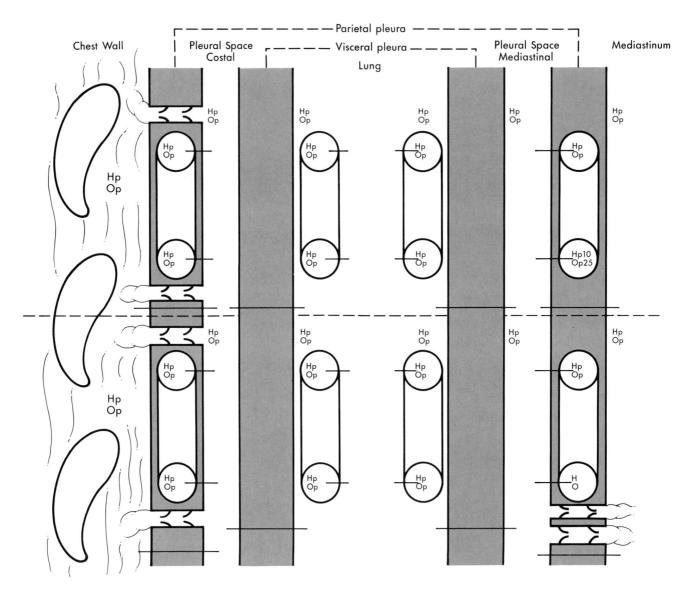

Fig. 5-2 Diagrammatic basic model of parietal and visceral pleura (visceral capillaries subpleural in location). Values for hydrostatic pressure *(Hp)* and oncotic pressure *(Op)* not yet entered. Horizontal continuous lines crossing capillary walls and pleura will have arrowheads placed to indicate flow direction when numeric values have been entered and Starling calculations have been made.

Table 5-2 Models with varying visceral pleural blood supply (see Appendix A)

I. VISCERAL CAPILLARIES SUBPLEURAL, PLEURA SEMIPERMEABLE

	Pulmonary A	Mixed B	Bronchial C
Total transudation	**42**	**42**	**42**
(1) P. caps.	42	42	42
(2) V. caps.	0	0	0
(6) P. pl.	0	0	0
(7) V. pl.	0	0	0
(3) EVLWc	26 }62	26 }79	43 }96
EVLWm	36	53	53
Total absorption	**72**	**72**	**72**
(8) P. caps.	7.5	7.5	7.5
(9) V. caps.	0	0	0
(4) P. pl.	32	32	32
(5) V. pl.	32	32	32

II. VISCERAL CAPILLARIES SUBPLEURAL, PLEURA NONSEMIPERMEABLE

	Pulmonary A	Mixed B	Bronchial C
Total transudation	**58**	**58**	**58**
(1) P. caps.	42	42	42
(2) V. caps.	0	0	0
(6) P. pl.	8	8	8
(7) V. pl.	8	8	8
(3) EVLWc	26 }62	26 }79	43 }96
EVLWm	36	53	53
Total absorption	**7.5**	**7.5**	**7.5**
(8) P. caps.	7.5	7.5	7.5
(9) V. caps.	0	0	0
(4) P. pl.	0	0	0
(5) V. pl.	0	0	0

III. VISCERAL CAPILLARIES INTRAPLEURAL, PLEURA SEMIPERMEABLE

	Pulmonary A	Mixed B	Bronchial C
Total transudation	**50**	**67**	**82**
(1) P. caps.	42	42	42
(2) V. caps.	8	25	40
(6) P. pl.	0	0	0
(7) V. pl.	0	0	0
(3) EVLWc	—	—	—
EVLWm			
Total absorption	**81**	**81**	**81**
(8) P. caps.	7.5	7.5	7.5
(9) V. caps.	9.5	9.5	9.5
(4) P. pl.	32	32	32
(5) V. pl.	32	32	32

IV. VISCERAL CAPILLARIES INTRAPLEURAL, PLEURA NONSEMIPERMEABLE

	Pulmonary A	Mixed B	Bronchial C
Total transudation	**66**	**83**	**98**
(1) P. caps.	42	42	42
(2) V. caps.	8	25	40
(6) P. pl.	8	8	8
(7) V. pl.	8	8	8
(3) EVLWc	—	—	—
EVLWm			
Total absorption	**17**	**17**	**17**
(8) P. caps.	7.5	7.5	7.5
(9) V. caps.	9.5	9.5	9.5
(4) P. pl.	0	0	0
(5) V. pl.	0	0	0

P. caps., Parietal capillaries; *V. caps.,* visceral capillaries; *P. pl.,* parietal pleura; *V. pl.,* visceral pleura; *EVLWc,* extravascular lung water, costal aspect of lung; *EVLWM,* extravascular lung water, mediastinal aspect of lung; *1,* transudation from parietal capillaries into pleural space; *2,* transudation from visceral capillaries into pleural space; *3,* transudation from visceral capillaries into the lung; *4,* absorption across parietal pleura from pleural space; *5,* absorption across visceral pleura from pleural space; *6,* transudation across parietal pleura into pleural space; *7,* transudation across visceral pleura into pleural space; *8,* absorption from pleural space into parietal capillaries; *9,* absorption from pleural space into visceral capillaries.

nary artery with nutritive twigs only from the bronchial artery

3. The visceral and parietal pleurae not behaving as semipermeable membranes but having high hydraulic conductivity

This new model has some important clinical and radiologic implications, as discussed later.

ANATOMY AND PHYSIOLOGY OF PLEURAL SPACE

The pleural space may be thought of as a thin-walled mesenchymal balloon invaginated by the lung. The outer layer of the balloon (the parietal pleura) adheres to the chest wall, and the inner layer (the visceral pleura) covers the surfaces of the lung, extending between lobes to form pleural fissures. The two pleural layers are tightly opposed along a very large surface despite being subjected to two opposite forces: the inward recoil of the lung, exerted on the visceral pleura, and the outward pull of the chest cage, exerted on the parietal pleura. Under normal physiologic circumstances the space between the pleural surfaces is only a few microns wide; its contents are limited by continuous dynamic control mechanisms to a few milliliters of fluid. These control mechanisms act to maintain the volume and pressure of the pleural space at the optimum level to hold the parietal and visceral pleura together and, consequently, to couple lung, chest wall, and diaphragm movements without friction.

The pleural space has many similarities to the lung's interstitial space and may be usefully compared to a second interstitial space placed in parallel with the

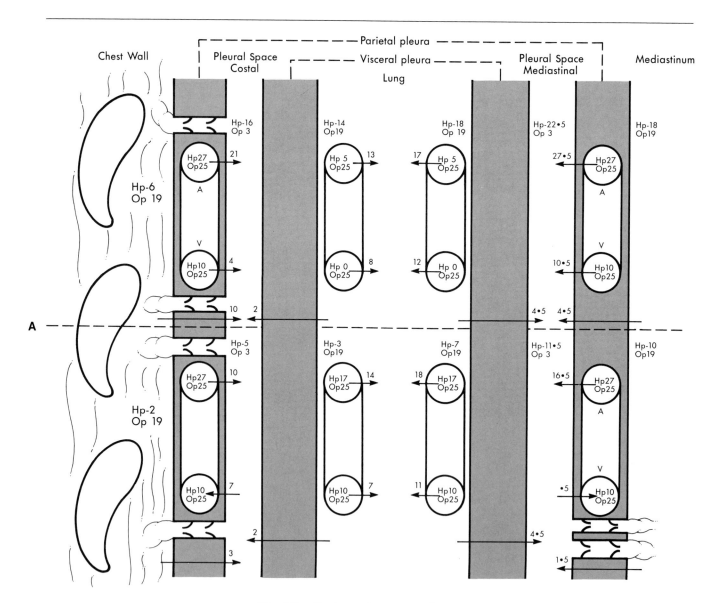

Fig. 5-3   For legend see opposite page.

lung's interstitial space, separated from it only by the visceral layer of pleura. As with the lung's interstitial space, the pleural space is designed to contain a small amount of water. In the same way that several mechanisms can cause an increase in pulmonary extravascular water (pulmonary edema), similar mechanisms can cause an increase in pleural fluid (pleural effusion). In both instances the radiologic observation of fluid increase (pulmonary edema, pleural effusion) is not itself a diagnosis but simply an indication that an underlying disease process exists whose pathophysiology must be determined.

MECHANISMS OF PLEURAL EFFUSION

Experimental studies have shown that under physiologic conditions, an equilibrium in the pleural space exists between filtration and absorption of liquid and solute.[2] The lymph flow from the pleural space, as derived by the entry rate in the plasma of albumin injected in the pleural space, is comparable to the entry rate in the pleura of albumin injected in the blood.[25-27] The estimated turnover rate of albumin in the pleural space of a 70 kg male is about 0.2 g/24 hr, corresponding to a lymph flow of 34 ml/24 hr.[2,25] Renewal rates of pleural liquid as great as 700 ml/24 hr have been calculated in patients with pleural effusions of various causes.[28,29] From these data, one can infer that the mechanisms regulating filtration and absorption of pleural liquid have great adaptive capabilities, with a large functional reserve and that a pleural effusion therefore indicates the presence of a pathophysiologic abnormality causing an imbalance between entry and egress rates of pleural liquid and protein.[30]

Fig. 5-3 **A,** In this combined anatomic and physiologic model of pleural fluid dynamics, the parietal (costal and mediastinal) pleural vessels are *intrapleural* and the visceral pleural vessels *subpleural.* Stomata, leading directly from the pleural space into subpleural lymphatic vessels, pierce the parietal pleura. The costal and mediastinal visceral pleura are shown with purely *pulmonary* circulation. The horizontal dotted line separates the upper and lower halves of the lungs and pleural space. *Hp,* Hydrostatic pressure; *Op,* oncotic pressure; *A,* arterial end of capillary; *V,* venous end of capillary. Note that the upper lobe intrapleural pressure is much more negative (Hp = −16 mm Hg) than lower lobe intrapleural pressure (Hp = −5 mm Hg). Also *sub* pleural interstitial pressure gradients exist that are smaller (Hp = −6 to −2 mm Hg) in the noncompliant subparietal pleural interstitium and larger (Hp = −14 to −3 mm Hg) in the compliant subvisceral pleural interstitium. Mediastinal pleural pressure is more negative than costal pleural pressure (Hp = −22.5 compared with −16 mm Hg), which affects the underlying lung so that a gradient courses from the costal visceral subpleural region (Hp = −14 mm Hg) to the mediastinal visceral subpleural region (Hp = −18 mm Hg). Op in the chest wall subpleural tissues and extravascular lung tissues is 19 mm Hg and in the pleural space only 3 mm Hg. Intravascular Op is 25 mm Hg. In this version of our model the pleura is regarded as being a *non*semipermeable membrane. The resultant vascular and pleural Starling calculations are represented by the arrows (*numbers* indicate flow per unit area and *arrows* the direction of flow). NOTE: we show a marked apex-to-base gradient of Hp in the visceral pleural *(pulmonary)* vessels (arterial, 5 to 17 mm Hg; venous, 0 to 10 mm Hg) but *no* gradient in the parietal pleural vessels. The reasons for this are explained in the text. The results of the Starling calculations are given in Table 5-2. (NOTE: Figures derived from the upper half of the lung and pleural space are multiplied by a factor of 0.25 to compensate [approximately] for the much smaller surface area of the upper versus lower half of the lung.) This version of our model is listed in Table 5-2 as IIA (visceral capillaries subpleural, pleura *non*semipermeable, visceral circulation pulmonary only) and is the model that most closely represents normal pleural fluid physiology. **B,** Diagram of normal pleural fluid physiology. For simplicity, only one parietal and one visceral pleural layer are shown. The arrow's thickness indicates quantity of flow, and its orientation indicates direction of flow. Granulated mast cells are shown diagrammatically below the visceral pleura, and the horizontal lines across the visceral pleura indicate closed intermesothelial cell clefts. In this normal model (visceral capillaries subpleural and supplied by pulmonary arteries, pleura nonsemipermeable, as in **A**), most pleural fluid comes from the arterial end of the parietal capillaries and is absorbed principally via the parietal stomata, although a small amount of fluid is probably also absorbed into the venous end of the parietal capillaries. Also, minimal filtration of fluid may occur from the subpleural interstitium across the parietal and visceral pleura. *Note that the visceral pleural capillaries filter into the lung, not into the pleural space.*

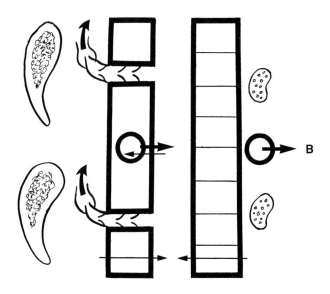

A pleural effusion may be caused by (1) increased leakage of liquid and protein resulting from altered conductivity and protein reflection of the pleura and its microcirculation, (2) reduced lymphatic drainage, (3) movement of peritoneal liquid into the pleural space, and (4) alterations in Starling forces. More than one mechanism may be operating simultaneously in certain disorders. Pleural liquid may assume the characteristics of either an exudate or a transudate according to the underlying pathophysiology.

Exudative Effusions

The pathogenesis of pleural effusion is easy to understand when the pleura and its microcirculation are directly involved pathologically, as they are in lung infections (bacterial, viral, fungal, or parasitic) and neoplasms of the lung, mediastinum, pleura, and chest wall. This group of diseases is responsible for about 80% of all exudative effusions. In these disorders the normal equilibrium, as summarized in Fig. 5-3, *B*, is completely overcome, and protein-rich pleural effusion develops despite a marked increase in pleural lymphatic outflow, as shown in Fig. 5-4, which models a subpleural pneumonic focus or abscess. Lymph flow, on the other hand, may be hindered by several mechanisms, such as lymphatic involvement in the inflammatory process, lymphatic obstruction in neoplasm, or re-

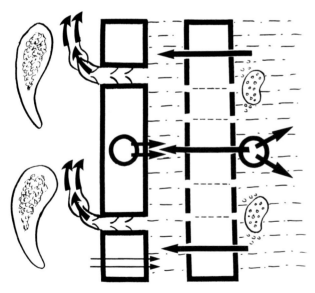

Fig. 5-4 Model of pleural or subpleural inflammation (e.g., peripheral lung abscess). Large amounts of fluid transude from subpleural visceral and intrapleural parietal capillaries and pass across the damaged pleura (probably through open intermesothelial cell clefts) into the pleural space. The transudation may be exacerbated by degranulation of mast cells. The increase in pleural fluid and protein is handled by increased flow through the parietal stomata.

duced lymphatic emptying caused by increased systemic venous pressure.* In these ways the lymphatic drainage, although partially increased, may not be adequate to balance the enormous amount of liquid and protein produced by the abnormally permeable pleura and vessels.

Other less common causes of exudative pleural effusion resulting from direct pathologic involvement of the pleura and its microcirculation are thoracic trauma, collagen vascular disease, abscesses of upper abdominal organs, esophageal perforation, pancreatitis, asbestosis, and iatrogenic conditions such as radiation or drug induction.

Additional causes of exudative pleural effusion include diseases primarily affecting the lymphatics, such as lymphangioleiomyomatosis and yellow nail syndrome.[30] Exudative pleural effusions may also result from neoplastic obstruction of the intrathoracic lymphatics or traumatic interruption of the thoracic duct.

Transudative Effusions

Most transudative effusions are caused by an alteration of the Starling forces across normal pleural mesothelium. With the exception of pleural effusions that develop because of increased negativity of the intrapleural pressure (e.g., caused by vigorous attempts to inflate a collapsed lung by negative pressure [ex vacuo effusion]), most transudative pleural effusions result from a change in hydrostatic or oncotic pressures within the systemic and pulmonary microvessels. More than 90% of all transudative effusions are caused by cardiac decompensation.[31]†

Cardiac failure. It is not completely established whether increased pulmonary or systemic venous pressure is the major determinant of pleural effusion in cardiac failure. Experimental studies performed acutely in dogs have apparently shown that for the same level of increase in hydrostatic pressure, greater pleural liquid volumes are found during *right* atrial hypertension than left atrial hypertension.[32] Furthermore, it has been reported recently that in sheep, isolated elevation of superior vena caval pressure (greater than 15 mm Hg) results in the formation of pleural effusion over 24 hours.[33] Although these animal studies suggest that acute systemic venous hypertension may hinder pleural lymphatic emptying into the systemic veins, one must remember that the lymphatics are capable of pumping against a considerable head of pressure.[27,34]

The results of these acute animal studies, however,

---

*It is still a matter of debate whether elevated systemic venous pressure does cause reduced lymphatic flow.
†This is probably not true in intensive care units, where "overhydration" is probably the most frequent cause of transudative effusion.

are in conflict with those obtained in human clinical studies. It has been demonstrated that pleural effusions are not identified in patients with isolated chronic right-sided heart failure caused by lung disease, even in those with a right atrial pressure (RAP) exceeding 15 mm Hg.[35] Similarly, we have been unable to find any relationship between the size of pleural effusions and the width of the vascular pedicle or azygos vein, both indices of RAP. Longstanding right atrial hypertension, which may be seen in patients with lung disease, may induce adaptive functional changes in lymphatics with increased drainage capabilities.[34] It remains unsettled, however, whether clinical conditions of acute right-sided cardiac failure in the human can impair lymphatic drainage from the pleura, as observed acutely in experimental animals.[32,33]

In contrast, one study[39] found that elevation of left atrial pressure (LAP) in patients with predominantly left-sided heart failure was associated significantly with the presence of pleural effusion.[36] This study, however, made no attempt to correlate actual level of wedge pressure with the size of effusions. In a series of 18 catheterized patients followed by serial radiographs throughout the course of predominantly left-sided heart failure, we were unable to show a statistically significant relationship between the level of wedge pressure and the size of effusions (Fig. 5-5). This apparent lack of relationship, however, is spurious. This stems from the fact that during the course of cardiac decompensation and recovery, the rise and fall

in wedge pressure is not immediately paralleled by an increase or decrease in pulmonary edema or pleural effusions. This "lag period" is even greater for effusions than for pulmonary edema, and the effusion lag may be as much as 1 to 2 days. If the effect of these lag periods is minimized by comparing *change* in the size of effusions versus change in wedge pressure, an excellent correlation is revealed (Fig. 5-6). We have also found a significant relationship between size of effusion and quantity of pulmonary edema. As can be seen from Fig. 5-7, however, because of a lag between change in edema and change in effusion, considerable overlap occurs so that severe edema can sometimes be accompanied by small effusions and mild edema by large effusions.

The most frequent (60%) sequence of events in our patients with cardiac failure after treatment appears to be (1) a drop in LAP followed by (2) a reduction in pulmonary edema after a lag period of 1 to 2 hours to 1 or 2 days, which in turn is followed by (3) a reduction in pleural fluid volume (Fig. 5-8). However, in 40% of patients, effusion actually cleared before (hours to days) the edema. The size of an effusion alone on a chest radiograph therefore cannot be used to decide whether cardiac failure is present or, if present, how severe it is. It remains true however, that in all patients with cardiac failure, reduction in pleural fluid volume still indicates an improvement in cardiac hemodynamics has already occurred.

Elevation of LAP clearly appears to be much more

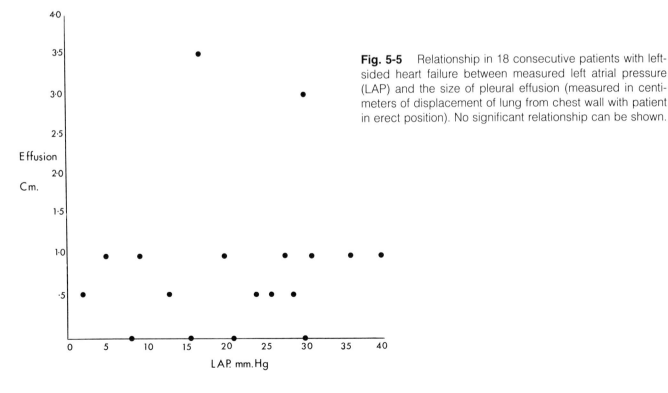

Fig. 5-5 Relationship in 18 consecutive patients with left-sided heart failure between measured left atrial pressure (LAP) and the size of pleural effusion (measured in centimeters of displacement of lung from chest wall with patient in erect position). No significant relationship can be shown.

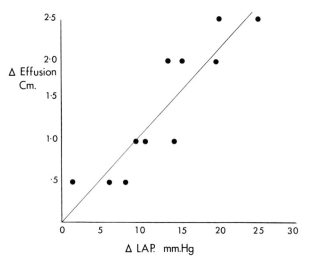

Fig. 5-6   The *difference* in left atrial pressure between two readings separated in time is graphed against the *difference* in size of pleural effusion on the same dates. An excellent relationship is shown. (See also Fig. 5-5. Same patients were studied, but only 11 had repeat studies available.)

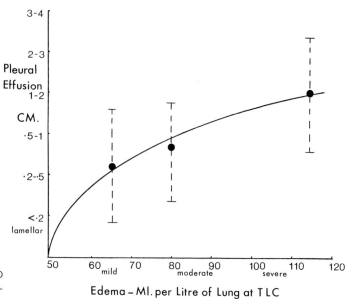

Fig. 5-7   Pleural effusion size, measured from radiographs of patients in the erect position using inward displacement of lung tissue by the effusion at the bases, is graphed against edema, quantified radiologically in 80 patients as mild, moderate, or severe. Mean values for edema correlate well with size of effusion, but a very wide deviation exists. See text for explanation.

significant in causing pleural effusions than RAP. However, in the study by Wiener-Kronish et al.,[36] although they did not mention the fact, their group of patients with left-sided heart failure and effusions contained a statistically significantly greater number of subjects with a mean RAP of 15 mm Hg or higher.

The lesser effect of raising RAP rather than LAP may be explained by taking our model and first increasing the pressure at the venous end of the *parietal* pleural capillaries to 15 mm Hg to simulate right-sided heart failure (Fig. 5-9; compare with Fig. 5-3). In this model of elevated RAP, we have included a simultaneous small passive increase in pressure at the arterial end of the capillaries, raising it from 27 to 30 mm Hg. Interestingly, and in keeping with the observed clinical absence of pleural effusions in patients with isolated elevation of RAP, this elevation of RAP has only a small effect on the total volume of fluid transuded, which increases from 58 to 73 units (Table 5-3). Even when the RAP is elevated to 15 mm Hg, some absorption can probably still occur from the pleural space into the venous end of the parietal capillaries (Fig. 5-9 and Table 5-3).

The minimal effect on pleural fluid volume of raising RAP pressure to 15 mm Hg should be compared with the effect of increasing LAP to the same level, first immediately after raising the pressure and then after the pressure increase has been allowed to persist for hours to days. The immediate effect of raising LAP (to 15 mm Hg) is an increase in subpleural extravascular lung water (from 62 to 112.5 units) but with no change in quantity of pleural fluid (Fig. 5-10 and Table 5-3). However, if the elevation of LAP is allowed to continue, pulmonary edema will increase, several Starling factors will change (see following discussion), and subpleural lung water will then pass out of the lung, through the visceral pleura, and into the pleural space (Fig. 5-11 and Table 5-3).

This transfer of water from the lung to the pleural space occurs for the following reasons. One should remember that the calculated figure of 112.5 units of fluid transuding into the subpleural space as extravascular lung water (Table 5-3) reflects only the surface area of the *single-thickness layer* of the visceral subpleural capillaries. If we take the visceral pleural surface area of an average lung as being approximately 0.25 m^2 and accept that the specialized visceral pleural capillaries have a diameter of 15 to 30 μm, and if the inner surface of each square centimeter of visceral pleura is covered approximately 50% by capillaries and 50% by intercapillary spaces, the visceral capillary surface area will be approximately 0.4 m.^{2} This contrasts greatly with the capillary surface area within the lungs of 70 m,^{2} approximately 300 times greater. Since the visceral pleural vessels are in continuity with the rest of the lung capillaries (see Plate 1, p. 132), for every 1 unit of fluid passing into the visceral subpleural space, approximately *300* units must transude into the entire lung,

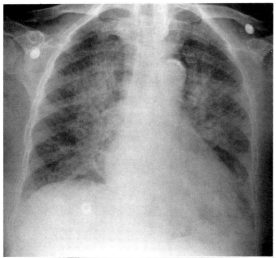

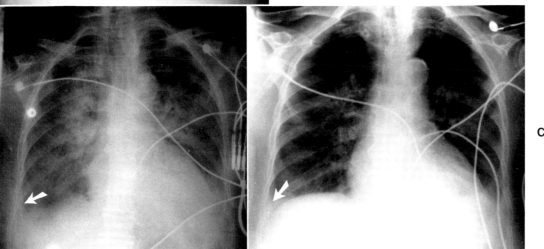

Fig. 5-8   A, Male patient 88 years of age with fulminating left-sided heart failure caused by acute myocardial infarction with edema. This shows the central distribution of edema occurring in approximately 10% of patients with cardiac failure. The central distribution usually indicates abrupt massive decompensation. No effusion is visible. **B,** After vigorous digitalis and diuretic therapy the edema is beginning to resolve 24 hours later, but a pleural effusion has now developed *(white arrow).* **C,** On day 3 of treatment, most of the edema has resolved. The pleural effusion is reduced in size *(arrow)* but is still present (i.e., lag between resolution of edema and resolution of effusion).

Table 5-3   Effects of raising right (RAP) and left atrial pressure (LAP) on total volume of fluid transuded*

	A	RAP elevated to 15 mm Hg	LAP elevated to 15 mm Hg (immediate effect)	LAP elevated to 15 mm Hg (subsequent effect)	LAP elevated to 15 mm Hg (pleural fluid) oncotic pressure, 6 mm Hg)	Low vascular oncotic pressure (15 mm Hg)
Total transudation	**58**	**71**	**58**	**159**	**109**	**102**
P. caps. (1)	42	57	42	120	70	85
V. caps. (2)	0	0	0	0	0	0
P. pl. (6)	8	8	8	10.5	10.5	8.5
V. pl. (7)	8	8	8	28	28	8.5
$EVLW_c$ (3)	26 ⎤ 62	62	112.5	77.5	77	112.5
$EVLW_m$	36 ⎦					
Total absorption	**7.5**	**2.0**	**7.5**	**0**	**0**	**0**
P. caps. (8)	7.5	2.0	7.5	0	0	0
V. caps. (9)	0	0	0	0	0	0
P. pl. (4)	0	0	0	0	0	0
V. pl. (5)	0	0	0	0	0	0

*Model IIA: visceral capillaries subpleural, pleura nonsemipermeable, pulmonary circulation. See Table 5-2.
P. caps., Parietal capillaries; *V. caps.,* visceral capillaries; *P. pl.,* parietal pleura; *V. pl.,* visceral pleura; $EVLW_C$, $EVLW_M$, extravascular lung water, costal (C) and mediastinal (M) aspects of lung.

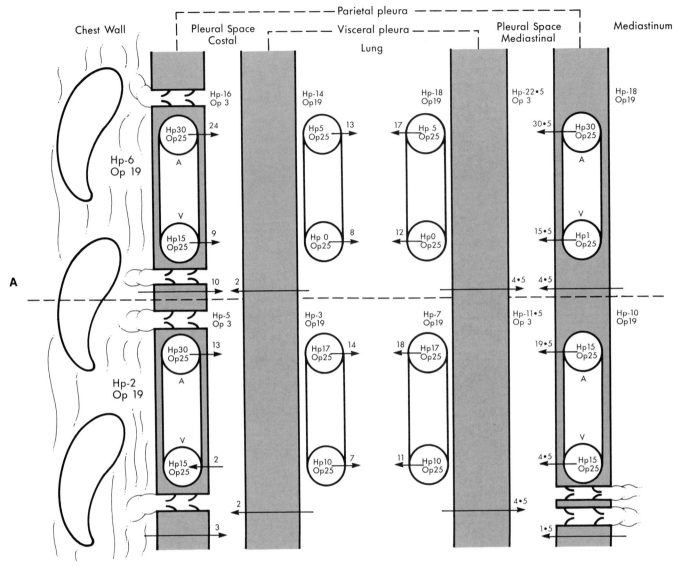

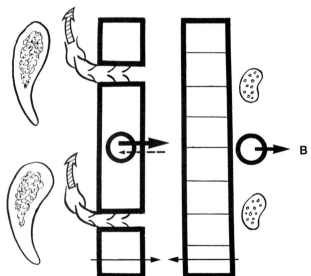

Fig. 5-9 **A,** Model with visceral capillaries subpleural, pulmonary arterial supply to visceral pleura, and nonsemipermeable pleura. The right atrial pressure (RAP) has been raised to 15.0 mm Hg (compare with Fig. 5-3, A, in which RAP is normal). The only effect is to raise transudation from 58 to 73 units and to reduce absorption from the parietal capillaries slightly (from 7.5 to 2.0 units). See Table 5-3 for comparison among normal RAP, elevated RAP, and elevated left atrial pressure. **B,** Simplified diagram of **A** showing effects of raising RAP to 15.0 mm Hg. Slight increase in transudation from the arterial end of the parietal capillaries and (questionable) slight reduction *(hatched curved arrows)* in flow through stomata to lymphatics to systemic veins to right atrium.

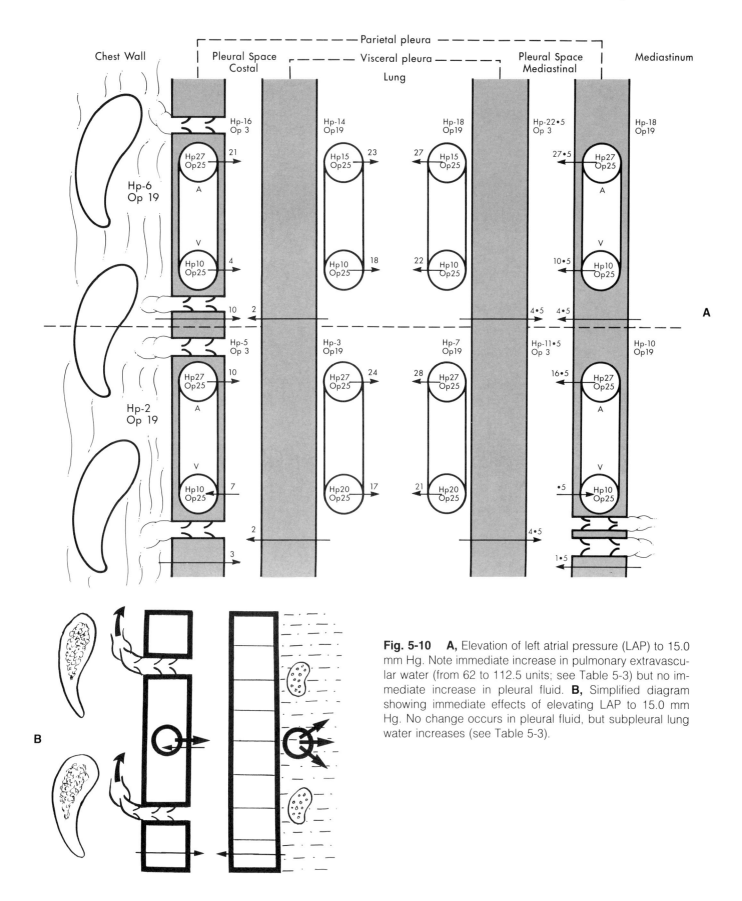

Fig. 5-10   A, Elevation of left atrial pressure (LAP) to 15.0 mm Hg. Note immediate increase in pulmonary extravascular water (from 62 to 112.5 units; see Table 5-3) but no immediate increase in pleural fluid. **B,** Simplified diagram showing immediate effects of elevating LAP to 15.0 mm Hg. No change occurs in pleural fluid, but subpleural lung water increases (see Table 5-3).

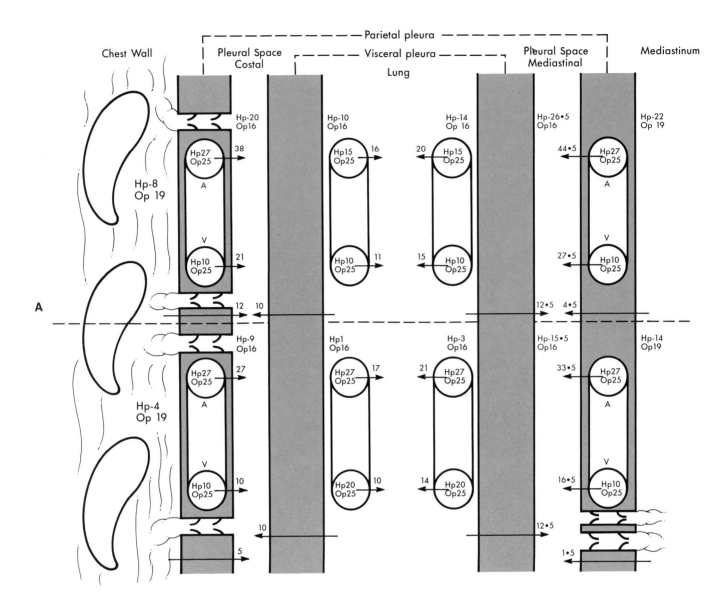

Chest Wall

Parietal pleura

Pleural Space Costal

Visceral pleura

Lung

Pleural Space Mediastinal

Mediastinum

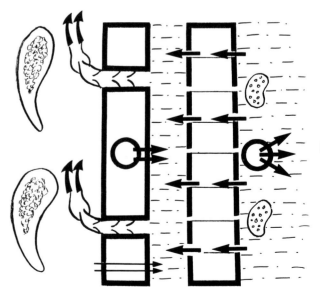

Fig. 5-11 A, *Continued* elevation of LAP to 15.0 mm Hg, causing a decrease in interpleural pressure of −4 mm Hg, an increase in lung interstitial pressure of 4 mm Hg, and a decrease in lung interstitial oncotic pressure of 3 mm Hg. Transudation into pleural space now increases (from 58 to 159 units) as fluid passes from the lung, across the visceral pleura, and into the pleural space. **B,** Simplified diagram of model in **A** (continued elevation of LAP to 15.0 mm Hg, causing changes in pleural and pulmonary interstitial pressures and lung oncotic pressure). The excess lung water now passes through the visceral pleura into the pleural space. Drainage of parietal stomata also increases (see Table 5-3).

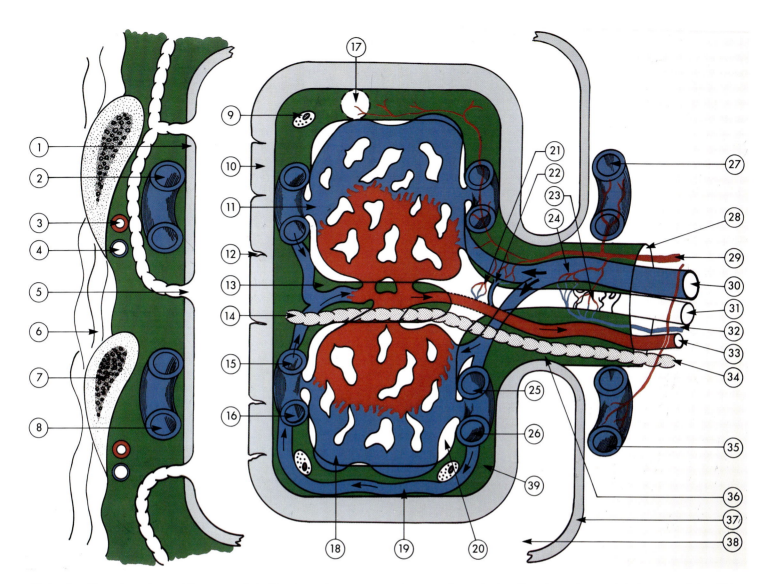

Plate 1 Pleural anatomy (diagrammatic). The lung is represented by two alveoli. *1,* Parietal pleura, costal (thin); *2,* arterial end of parietal pleural capillary supplied by intercostal arteries (systemic pressure); for clarity the pleural capillaries are drawn oversize; they actually lie *within* the thin parietal pleura; *3,* intercostal artery; *4,* intercostal vein; *5,* stomata draining from pleural space, through parietal pleura, and directly into subpleural lymphatics; these pass around chest wall to form trunks terminating in subclavian vein/internal jugular vein junctions, draining into the *right* atrium; *6,* intercostal muscles; *7,* ribs; *8,* parietal pleural capillary, venous end (drains to right atrium); *9,* mast cells; *10,* visceral pleura *(thick); 11,* anastomoses between visceral pleural capillaries, which lie *below* the pleura, and alveolar capillaries; *12,* intermesothelial cell clefts; *13,* interlobular septum; *14,* lymphatics running via septa into peribronchovascular sheaths; *15,* arterial end of pleural capillary (supplied by pulmonary circulation); *16,* venous end of visceral pleural capillary, draining to left atrium; *17,* probable anastomosis between bronchial circulation and visceral pleural capillaries; NOTE: pulmonary circulation is nonoxygenated, whereas bronchial circulation is oxygenated and may assist in nutrition/metabolism of pleura; the blank circle indicates this anatomy is still in doubt; *18,* pulmonary capillary bed ramifying around alveolus *(white).* Note hypoxic blood *(blue)* turning to oxygenated blood *(red)* as it passes over alveoli toward central draining vein; *19,* pulmonary arterial supply to visceral pleural capillaries *(arrows* indicate flow direction); *20,* alveoli *(white);* two are shown; *21,* termination of intrapulmonary bronchial arteries at level of respiratory bronchioles: anastomoses with pulmonary capillaries and drainage via pulmonary vein to left atrium; *22,* possible precapillary bronchial artery/pulmonary artery anastomosis; junction drawn incomplete because it is still in doubt whether these exist in normal lung; *23,* bronchial arterial supply to bronchi, bronchioles, and mucosa; around the hilum, venous drainage is by true bronchial veins to azygos vein or superior vena cava (and thus to *right* atrium); *24,* bronchial arteries form the vasa vasorum of the pulmonary arteries (a form of anastomosis); *25,* visceral capillaries (mediastinal aspect), arterial end, supplied by pulmonary arteries; *26,* visceral capillary, venous end, draining to left atrium; *27,* mediastinal parietal pleural capillaries, arterial end; supplied by mediastinal systemic vessels, including extrapulmonary branches of bronchial arteries; *28,* peribronchovascular sheath (source of peribronchial "cuffing" on chest radiographs; *29,* bronchial artery (oxygenated blood at systemic pressures); *30,* pulmonary artery (nonoxygenated blood at pulmonary artery pressure); *31,* bronchus, true bronchial vein, drains to *right* atrium; *33,* pulmonary vein (oxygenated blood) drains to left atrium; *34,* lymphatics exiting lung within peribronchovascular sheath and draining to systemic veins and therefore to *right* side of heart; *35,* mediastinal parietal pleural capillary, venous end, drains to right atrium; *36,* for clarity the peribronchovascular sheath is shown opening into the mediastinum, but sheath actually is *closed* around its contents and adherent to the pleura at this point, and the interstitial space of the lung does *not* therefore normally communicate with the mediastinal space; similarly the pulmonary veins are shown running within the peribronchovascular sheath, whereas in fact they drain separately (within their own sheaths) to the left atrium; *37,* parietal pleura (mediastinal), thin and containing many stomata (not shown); *38,* pleural space; *39,* subpleural interstitial space of the lung *(green)* connecting with peribronchovascular sheaths.

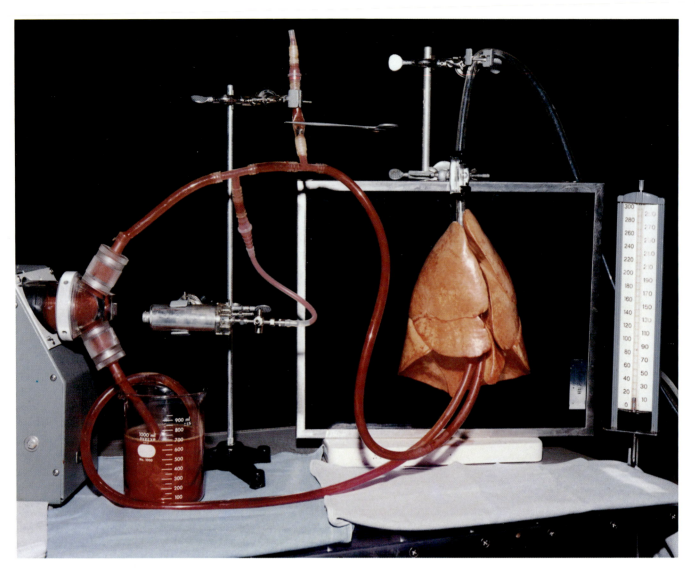

Plate 2. Isolated whole-lung preparation. The lung is inflated at a pressure of 15 mm Hg, and blood is being pumped through by a Harvard pump. The isolated lung was oxygenating the blood successfully, as evidenced by its bright-red color. (Reproduced with permission from Milne ENC: *Radiol Clin North Am* 16[3]:515, 1978.)

producing a marked increase in extravascular lung water. If the lung lymphatics cannot remove this extra fluid, pulmonary edema will develop, the interstitial pressure of the lung parenchyma will rise, the pulmonary interstitial oncotic pressure will decrease, and pleural pressure will become more negative as lung compliance drops and the work of breathing increases. A reasonable estimate for this decrease in pleural pressure would be −4 mm Hg; for the increase in lung interstitial pressure, 4 mm Hg; and for the decrease in lung interstitial oncotic pressure, 3 mm Hg. Under experimental conditions of elevated pulmonary venous pressure, pleural fluid has a protein concentration similar to that of lung interstitial fluid.[37,38]

As shown earlier, if we factor all these changes into our model, total transudation of water into the pleura would increase from 58 to 159 units (Fig. 5-11, A, and Table 5-3). However, in the clinical situation, since protein simultaneously is removed from the pleural space by the parietal stomata, we assume that only a small increase in pleural fluid oncotic pressure would occur (e.g., from a normal value of 3 to 6 mm Hg). But even this minor increase in pleural oncotic pressure would result in an increase in transudation into the pleural space from 58 to 109 units (Table 5-3). All *absorption* into the parietal capillaries would also cease.

The sequence of events illustrated in Figs. 5-10 and 5-11 (subpleural edema and an increase in lung water, with no evidence of pleural effusion, followed by the development of effusion as lung water increases) fits very well with the observed clinical sequence of development of pleural effusion in left-sided heart failure (see Fig. 5-8). This clinical sequence appears to have been observed first by Zdansky in 1929,[39] who stated, "Hydrothorax, based on radiological observations, should be considered as the *sequel* of pulmonary engorgement and edema."

Since normal pleura does not allow protein to pass through, even when the transpleural hydrostatic pressure gradient is increased,[14] we might hypothesize that the passage of proteins across the pleura occurring in left-sided heart failure[37,38] is caused by opening of the numerous intercellular clefts[14] and possibly by changes in the mast cells (see Plate 1, p. 132).

Experimental and clinical studies suggest that if LAP is elevated, a concomitant elevation of RAP may contribute to the further development of pleural effusion by interfering with pleural lymphatic drainage.[2,37,40]

The concept that pulmonary edema can pass through the visceral pleura and cause pleural effusion was initially proved by Graham[41] in 1921. He demonstrated that increasing negativity in the pleural space caused fluid to be sucked from the lung across the pleura into the pleural space. This was recently reproved experimentally by Broaddus et al.[38] The concept, however, is much older than either of these papers, having been advanced in 1633 by Bartoletti,[42] professor of logic, surgery, and anatomy at the University of Bologna. In his treatise on dyspnea, he writes, "The lung is spongy and fluid is squeezed out of it into the pleural cavity, producing hydrothorax." Bartoletti also noted, "The lung does not take up fluid but generates it."[42] Similarly, Albertini in 1746 observed, "Pulmonary dropsy easily turns into hydrothorax."[43]

In view of this transfer of fluid from lung to pleural space, the lymphatics of the parietal pleura that drain the pleural liquid may be regarded as an additional pathway for the clearance of liquid and protein from the lung interstitium during hydrostatic pulmonary edema.[37] This would be in complete accord with the behavior predicted by our model (Figs. 5-10 and 5-11). The increased ventilatory rate that often accompanies the accumulation of liquid in the lung would further enhance the lymphatic drainage of pleural liquid.[2,8,9,44-50]

In summary, in patients with left heart decompensation, pleural effusion appears to result from (1) increased back pressure in the entire pulmonary capillary vascular bed including the visceral subpleural microvessels that causes pulmonary edema leading subsequently to direct leakage of edema from the lung interstitium to the pleural space and (2) possible impairment of parietal lymphatic drainage, in which the right side of the heart and systemic venous pressures are also elevated. Table 5-3 summarizes the effects on net pleural liquid movement of elevating RAP versus LAP.

This new realization—that pleural effusion in left heart failure (LHF) is caused by pulmonary edema exiting the lung across the visceral pleura—gives a new and important diagnostic criterion; i.e., it says that pleural effusion caused by LHF must be *preceded* by the development of pulmonary edema. If an effusion develops without any evidence of preceding pulmonary edema, it was *not* caused by LHF. If it occurs *simultaneously* with the development of pulmonary edema, this is much more suggestive of oncotic edema than LHF.

Pleural effusion caused by ascites. Pleural effusion may develop because of an abnormal increase of liquid in the peritoneum. Peritoneal liquid can move into the pleural space under the influence of a pressure gradient across the diaphragm, by direct passage through congenital diaphragmatic cloacae, or by migration through transdiaphragmatic lymphatics.[30,40] In these conditions, pleural and peritoneal liquid have the same composition. (Clearly, an increase in protein in the pleural space will lead to increased filtration from the parietal capillaries.) Transudative pleural effusion may develop from cirrhosis of the liver, urinary tract obstructions, or peritoneal dialysis. Exudative pleural effusion can also occur in patients who have ovarian tumors with ascites (Meigs' syndrome).[30,40]

Reduction in colloid pressure. Considering the large functional reserve of the parietal pleural lymphatics, lowered oncotic pressure alone does not usually result in pleural effusion. However, a major decrease in intravascular oncotic pressure (e.g., from 25 to 15 mm Hg) may cause an immediate increase in parietal capillary fluid transudation from 42 to 85 units (compared with elevating LAP to 15 mm Hg, which would not cause an immediate increase in pleural fluid transudation) (Table 5-3). Both types of perturbation, oncotic or hydrostatic, would cause an immediate increase in extravascular *lung* water, which would accumulate as pulmonary edema if it could not be cleared by lung lymphatics. Therefore one would reasonably assume that in oncotic edema, pleural effusion and pulmonary edema might appear concomitantly, but in left-sided heart failure, pulmonary edema would precede development of effusion (the usual radiologic finding).

A combination of lowered oncotic pressure plus elevation of LAP frequently occurs because of overhydration, either iatrogenic or resulting from renal failure.[2] Patients with nephrotic syndrome can develop transudative pleural effusions, in which hypoalbuminemia may be a contributing factor, together with fluid overload caused by salt and water retention.

RADIOGRAPHIC EVALUATION OF PLEURAL EFFUSIONS

Pleural effusion is one of the most common radiographic abnormalities seen on the chest films of hospital patients. Keeping in mind the pathophysiologic mechanisms just reviewed, certain combinations of history, clinical findings, chest radiographic abnormalities, and chronology may allow the film reader to determine the cause of an effusion from the plain film in a large percentage of cases. Ultrasonography and computed tomography (CT) are infrequently used for the initial diagnosis of pleural effusions but are valuable adjunctive diagnostic tools to determine whether an effusion is loculated or not, to distinguish consolidation from pleural effusions, to differentiate between empyema and lung abscess, and to select the drainage site of loculated fluid.[30,31,40,51] CT scans also often reveal effusions that were unsuspected on conventional films (Fig. 5-12).

Given the pivotal role of the chest radiograph in the diagnosis and follow-up of patients with pleural effusions, one must consider how much fluid must be

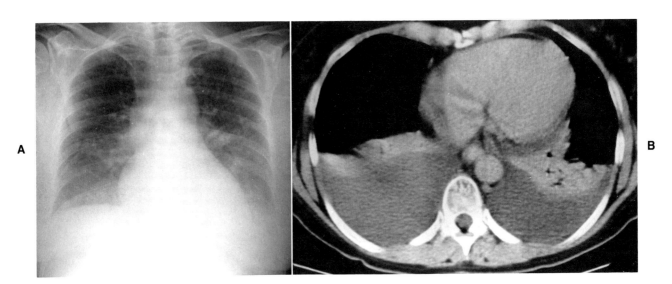

Fig. 5-12 **A,** Fifty-year-old female with left-sided heart failure. The posteroanterior (PA) view with the patient erect shows interstitial hydrostatic edema bilaterally, increasing density toward the bases, and faint densities following the curves of the greater fissures, all suggesting pleural effusions. **B,** Computed tomographic (CT) scan of the same patient reveals that massive effusions are present. Note that the lung "floats" on the pleural fluid with the patient in the supine position and extends out to the chest wall. A plain film with the patient supine therefore would not show any displacement of lung from the chest wall, despite the massive effusions. In the film with the patient erect, pressure of pleural fluid is evenly distributed all around the base of the lung, which therefore moves inward from the chest wall, revealing the pleural fluid between lung and chest wall. In the supine position the pressure is directed dorsally, and thus the lung is not peeled off the chest wall ventrally or laterally. As a result, a massive effusion may be present, with no separation of lung from chest wall seen on the plain film with the patient supine.

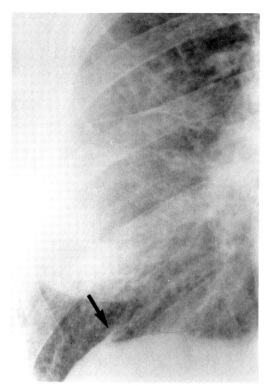

Fig. 5-13 Forty-year-old patient with renal failure and severe interstitial pulmonary edema. Small effusion and pleural fluid passing into inferior accessory fissure *(black arrow)* are seen.

present in the pleural space before it can be visualized on the plain chest film.

Excess pleural fluid gravitates to the most dependent regions of the chest cavity, and therefore one looks for the early radiographic findings of pleural effusion (in the erect patient) along the diaphragmatic surfaces. If a patient has the frequently found congenital anomaly of an inferior accessory fissure, the first findings of an effusion may be seen as the development of a minute triangle of fluid density with its base on the diaphragm and its apex entering the fissure, where it contacts the diaphragm (Fig. 5-13).

Effusions with a liquid volume of less than 100 ml may go undetected in the chest radiograph with the patient upright, since they are often located between the dome of the diaphragm and the lower lobes of the lung (subpulmonary effusions). This does not cause any blunting of the lateral costophrenic angle on the posteroanterior (PA) view or of the posterior costophrenic angle on the lateral view.[40,51] Massive amounts of fluid can accumulate in a subpulmonary location, and the only radiographic finding may be elevation of one or both hemidiaphragms, with a "squaring off" of the lateral half of the diaphragmatic contour (Fig. 5-14).

Larger amounts of liquid in the pleural space (about 200 ml) can be detected as blunting of the posterior

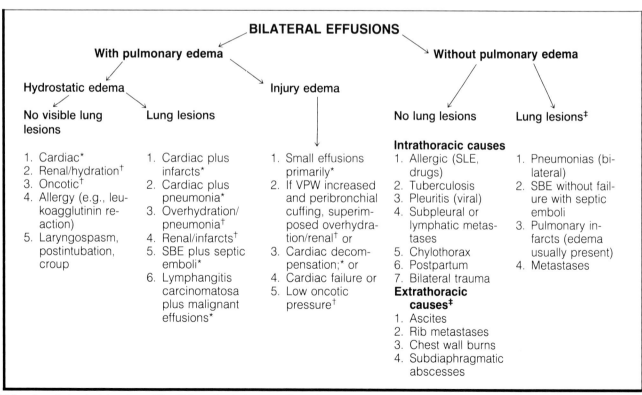

BILATERAL EFFUSIONS

With pulmonary edema → → **Without pulmonary edema**

Hydrostatic edema		Injury edema	No lung lesions	Lung lesions[‡]
No visible lung lesions	**Lung lesions**		**Intrathoracic causes**	
1. Cardiac*	1. Cardiac plus infarcts*	1. Small effusions primarily*	1. Allergic (SLE, drugs)	1. Pneumonias (bilateral)
2. Renal/hydration[†]	2. Cardiac plus pneumonia*	2. If VPW increased and peribronchial cuffing, superimposed overhydration/renal[†] or	2. Tuberculosis	2. SBE without failure with septic emboli
3. Oncotic[†]	3. Overhydration/ pneumonia[†]		3. Pleuritis (viral)	3. Pulmonary infarcts (edema usually present)
4. Allergy (e.g., leukoagglutinin reaction)	4. Renal/infarcts[†]	3. Cardiac decompensation;* or	4. Subpleural or lymphatic metastases	4. Metastases
5. Laryngospasm, postintubation, croup	5. SBE plus septic emboli*	4. Cardiac failure or	5. Chylothorax	
	6. Lymphangitis carcinomatosa plus malignant effusions*	5. Low oncotic pressure[†]	6. Postpartum	
			7. Bilateral trauma	
			Extrathoracic causes[‡]	
			1. Ascites	
			2. Rib metastases	
			3. Chest wall burns	
			4. Subdiaphragmatic abscesses	

SBE, subacute bacterial endocarditis; *SLE,* systemic lupus erythematosus.
*Effusions are usually preceded by the development of pulmonary edema.
[†]Effusions usually occur at the same time as the pulmonary edema.
[‡]These causes of effusion can usually be determined by direct inspection of the radiograph.

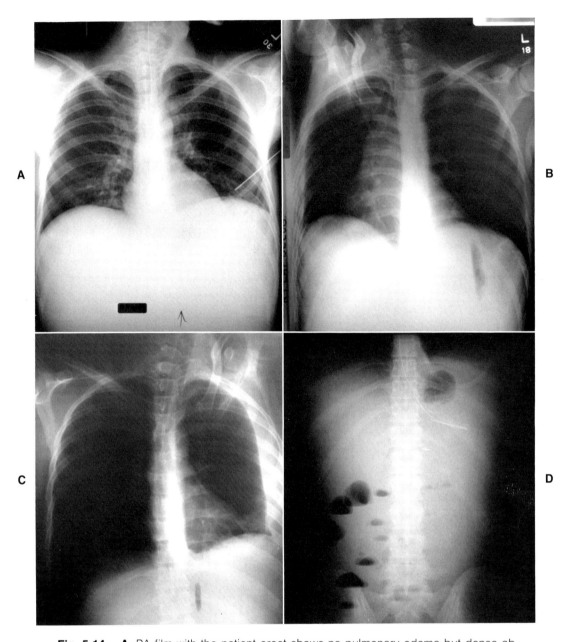

Fig. 5-14   **A,** PA film with the patient erect shows no pulmonary edema but dense abdomen and high diaphragmatic position in the face of very cachectic soft tissues (i.e., the high diaphragms and dense abdomen are clearly not caused by obesity). Note greater elevation of left hemidiaphragm, raising suspicion of left subpulmonary effusion. **B** and **C,** Decubitus views confirm that bilateral subpulmonary effusions are present. **D,** Abdominal radiograph with the patient erect reveals ascites and small bowel obstruction caused by lymphoma.

costodiaphragmatic angles on the lateral view.[31,40,51,52] Unfortunately, it is widely taught that "blunting" of the costophrenic angle on the PA view is one of the best ways of detecting (or excluding) the presence of an effusion. However, in the PA view as much as 500 ml of liquid may be necessary to cause blunting of the angle.[31,40,51,53] Frequently the observer who has not been taught to look first for subtle displacement of the aerated lung away from the inner chest wall by the effusion may mistake the sharp lower lateral lung edge floating in the effusion for a normal costophrenic angle (Fig. 5-15).

When pleural effusions are suspected, a chest film with the patient in the lateral decubitus position can re-

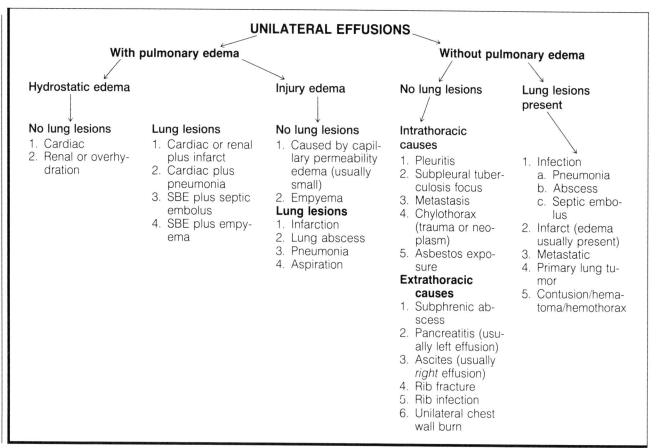

UNILATERAL EFFUSIONS

With pulmonary edema

Hydrostatic edema

No lung lesions
1. Cardiac
2. Renal or overhydration

Lung lesions
1. Cardiac or renal plus infarct
2. Cardiac plus pneumonia
3. SBE plus septic embolus
4. SBE plus empyema

Injury edema

No lung lesions
1. Caused by capillary permeability edema (usually small)
2. Empyema

Lung lesions
1. Infarction
2. Lung abscess
3. Pneumonia
4. Aspiration

Without pulmonary edema

No lung lesions

Intrathoracic causes
1. Pleuritis
2. Subpleural tuberculosis focus
3. Metastasis
4. Chylothorax (trauma or neoplasm)
5. Asbestos exposure

Extrathoracic causes
1. Subphrenic abscess
2. Pancreatitis (usually left effusion)
3. Ascites (usually *right* effusion)
4. Rib fracture
5. Rib infection
6. Unilateral chest wall burn

Lung lesions present
1. Infection
   a. Pneumonia
   b. Abscess
   c. Septic embolus
2. Infarct (edema usually present)
3. Metastatic
4. Primary lung tumor
5. Contusion/hematoma/hemothorax

SBE, Subacute bacterial endocarditis.

veal even small amounts of liquid gravitating between the lung and the chest wall.[54] An experimental study performed in cadavers showed that as little as 5 ml of injected liquid could be visualized in a properly exposed lateral decubitus chest radiograph.[55]

Differential Diagnosis of Underlying Cause of Effusions

Based on the model of pleural fluid filtration and absorption that we have developed, decision trees can be drawn (see boxes on pp. 135 and 137). These take into consideration the bilaterality or unilaterality of effusions, the presence or absence of pulmonary edema, the appearance of the heart and vascular pedicle, changes in the soft tissues and abdomen, and the chronology of appearance of edema versus effusion. Using this logical approach, certain constellations of findings often allow one to determine the specific cause of the effusion (Figs. 5-16 to 5-18).

In general, transudative effusions (e.g., cardiac, renal, overhydration), which usually reflect a generalized alteration of Starling forces within the circulation, are more often bilateral (see box on p. 135.) Exudative effusions usually result from a localized pathologic pro-

cess and are frequently unilateral (e.g., pancreatitis, pneumonia, abscess) (see box above and Fig. 5-19).

Our view that transudative effusions are usually bilateral contrasts with the deeply ingrained belief, based on the results of past papers,[56-59] that in patients with cardiac failure, pleural effusions are predominantly right sided. This belief is often repeated, unfortunately even in standard textbooks of cardiac medicine,[60,61] even though it was repudiated by Kerley[62] as early as 1962. More recent data, including our own, have shown that in the course of cardiac failure, both pleural spaces are typically involved.[63-66] In our three separate series of patients with cardiac failure studied at two different university centers in the United States and Italy on differing populations, effusion occurred most often bilaterally (108 of 202 patients) or, if unilateral (94 of 202 patients), occurred most often on the *left* side (63 patients). Effusion occurred solely on the right side in only 26 patients (16%) (Table 5-4).

The reason for the discrepancy between our findings concerning the distribution of effusion in cardiac failure and the generally taught view (i.e., that right-sided effusions are much more frequent in congestive failure may lie simply in the use of the archaic word "conges-

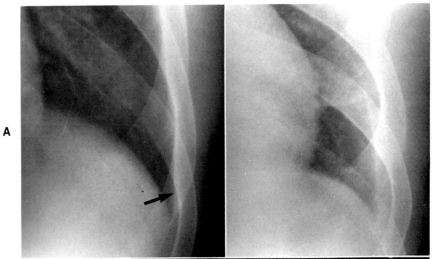

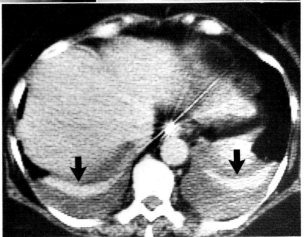

Fig. 5-15 A, "Costophrenic angle" *(arrow)* in this patient appears to be sharp. However, close inspection shows that the aerated lung has been displaced away from the chest wall by a thin layer of fluid *(arrow)* (i.e., a "lamellar" effusion is present) and that the angle is no longer costophrenic but is simply the inferior edge of the lung surrounded by fluid. **B,** The effusion (same patient as in **A**) has increased in size, further displacing the lung from the chest wall, but the "angle," caused only by the lung edge, remains sharp. **C,** CT scan in a patient with moderately large bilateral effusions shows two sharply defined, crescentic opacities at both bases *(arrows)*. These crescents are formed by the posterior costodiaphragmatic edges of the lungs surrounded anteriorly and posteriorly by pleural fluid and would be seen on a radiograph with the patient erect as sharply defined lung edges (as in **A** and **B**).

tive." This term is used very widely as if it related to all types of cardiac failure, including pure or predominant *left* heart failure, whereas it should be used correctly only to describe right-sided or biventricular failure, in which the neck veins, liver, and soft tissues are indeed "congested" (see Chapter 6). If any particular series of cardiac failure patients contained a high percentage of cases of *biventricular* ("congestive") failure, one *would* then expect to see an increased incidence of right-sided effusion because the right heart failure frequently causes ascites, which passes preferentially through the right hemidiaphragm to cause right-sided effusion. This would be the likely prevalence in *older* series of cardiac failure patients, in whom treatment was usually later and less effective. In modern series, because of earlier diagnosis and treatment, left heart failure will predominate and (as we found) there will *not* be any preponderance of right-sided effusions.

One older series (1957) of patients with cardiac failure showed at autopsy that in about one-half the pa-

tients who had unilateral effusions, either pneumonia or pulmonary embolism was underlying the effusion.[63] Therefore some have suggested that in patients with cardiac failure, whenever pleural effusion is purely unilateral, and particularly if on the left side, a localized pathologic process should be sought.[59-61] These data were based on patients who died of their disease; our patients were followed to recovery, and most unilateral effusions caused by cardiac failure resolved rapidly after treatment, with no evidence of underlying lung disease. However, if a unilateral effusion associated with cardiac failure is unusually slow in resolving, it would seem appropriate to look for an underlying cause other than the cardiac decompensation.

Clearance of Effusions

Once pleural effusions have been diagnosed on the chest radiograph, an increase or decrease in size is usually easy to detect and may sometimes correlate with the progress or regression of the underlying pathophys-

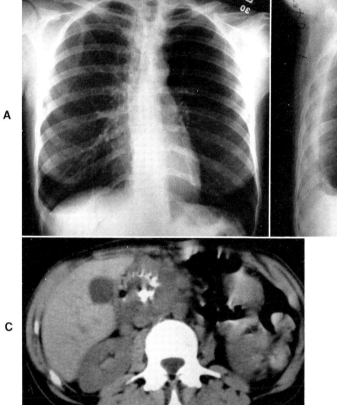
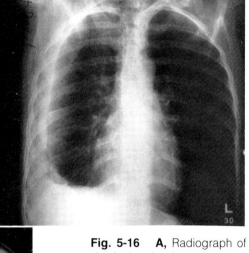

Fig. 5-16   A, Radiograph of 38-year-old female with abdominal pain shows lungs completely free of edema but unilateral effusion present, with no visible underlying abnormalities of lung or chest wall. **B,** Radiograph with patient in right decubitus position confirms the presence of a large, freely flowing effusion. At its diaphragmatic surface, however, the effusion shows some irregularity, suggesting localized adhesions and a possible inflammatory basis for the effusion. **C,** Abdominal CT scan reveals massive inflammatory enlargement of the head of the pancreas with numerous pancreatic calculi.

iology. As already discussed, however, in patients with pulmonary edema caused by cardiac failure, the radiographic findings of pulmonary edema may attenuate or disappear after adequate therapy, whereas pleural effusions remain unchanged.[66] As the astute Albertini pointed out in 1748, "The lungs are more easily freed from accumulated serum than the chest cavity [pleural space] from effused serum."[43] The delayed clearance of the pleural space may be explained by the hypothesis suggested earlier; that is, the parietal pleural lymphatics are an important adjunctive route for clearing hydrostatic pulmonary edema, and pleural fluid therefore may not be able to clear until all fluid has gone from the lung.[37]

Wiener-Kronish et al.[67] suggested recently that the pleural space may also be involved in the clearance of pulmonary edema caused by increased capillary permeability. This hypothesis is based on finding moderate pleural effusions in sheep in which the pulmonary microvessels had been acutely injured by injections of oleic acid.[67] However, the pleural effusions developed later, and their average volume was considerably less than that measured in the same type of animal with *hydrostatic* pulmonary edema.[38] This discrepancy may be explained by the different pathophysiologic mecha-

nisms occurring in the two different forms of pulmonary edema (see Chapter 2).

In hydrostatic pulmonary edema, the fluid initially begins to fill the loose interstitial connective tissue sheaths surrounding vessels and airways. Progressive distention of the interstitial space causes elevation of

Table 5-4   Most common sites of effusion in patients with cardiac failure

	Individual study			Combined studies
	1*	**2†**	**3‡**	**(1 + 2 + 3)**
No. of patients	17	73	112	202
Bilateral effusion	5	54	49	108 (53%)
Right = left	4	19	21	44 (22%)
Right > left	1	9	11	21 (11%)
Left > right	0	26	17	43 (21%)
Unilateral effusion	12	19	63	94 (47%)
Right only	5	0	26	31 (16%)
Left only	7	19	37	63 (31%)

*Milne E, Pistolesi M: University of California at Irvine study.
†Milne E, Pistolesi M, Miniati M, Giuntini C: Institute of Clinical Physiology Laboratory study, Italian National Research Council, University of Pisa.
‡Milne E, Li Chen, Bandler M: University of California at Irvine study.

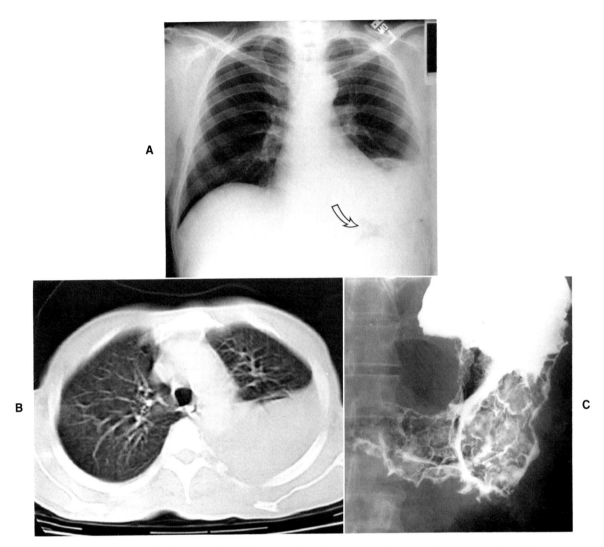

Fig. 5-17 **A,** Radiograph from 39-year-old male patient with no evidence of pulmonary edema but with a left unilateral pleural effusion. An obvious clue to the source of the effusion is given by the abnormal gastric bubble *(arrow).* **B,** CT scan shows (as it often does) a much larger effusion than suggested by the plain film. **C,** Gastrointestinal (GI) series shows massive infiltration of the stomach wall by lymphoma.

the interstitial pressure and a decrease in oncotic pressure, resulting, as described earlier, in the passage of water across the visceral pleura into the pleural space. In contrast, in lung edema caused by *injury,* disruption of the alveolar/epithelial barrier causes direct flow of *proteinaceous* edema liquid from the lung capillaries simultaneously into the alveolar air spaces (which can accommodate large amounts of liquid), and into the interstitium. Since the alveolar flooding results in the loss of fluid in the interstition, the interstitial hydrostatic pressure will not rise as much. In addotion, since this edema contains protein, the interstitial oncotic pressure may *not* fall, and the pleural space is therefore involved at a later stage and to a lesser extent than it is in hydrostatic edema. This analysis is in agreement with the

common radiologic finding that pleural effusions are detected very often in patients with interstitial pulmonary edema of hydrostatic origin (cardiogenic and overhydration) but are seldom encountered in patients with adult respiratory distress syndrome (ARDS) (Fig. 5-20).[66,68-79] (See Chapter 8.)

Small pleural effusions in patients with lung edema resulting from injury may be present but may go undetected in chest radiographs taken at the bedside with the patient supine. However, the finding of moderate or large pleural effusions in patients with ARDS[80,81] is definitely unusual and must be considered an important additional clinical finding requiring further investigation. It suggests the presence of either an exudative process (even more so if the effusion is unilateral) or the

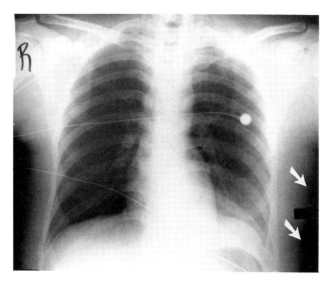

Fig. 5-18   AP radiograph of a 25-year-old patient in erect position. The lungs are oligemic, suggesting dehydration; no evidence of pulmonary edema is seen. Note reduced volume of the left hemithorax and characteristic curvature of a large, left subpulmonary effusion plus further effusion extending into the costal pleural space. Note also the sharp, so-called costophrenic angle (see text). A clue is given to the unusual etiology of this effusion by the increased density and thickness of the tissues of the left chest wall *(arrows)*. This young man was reaching into a pizza oven when the door slammed on his arm (within the oven) and the chest wall was held against the oven door, causing full thickness burns, with probable direct damage to the parietal capillaries.

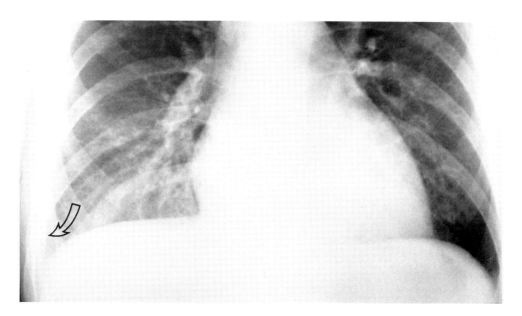

Fig. 5-19   Radiograph of 32-year-old male with fever and malaise demonstrates unilateral pulmonary edema and a unilateral effusion *(arrow)* with no visible lesions in either lung parenchyma or chest wall. The edema shows no peribronchial cuffing and did not shift with gravity; that is, it had the features of injury edema. While lying on his right side, this patient had injected minced marijuana leaves mixed with milk into a vein, which apparently caused multiple fat and marijuana microemboli in the vessels of the base of the right lung.

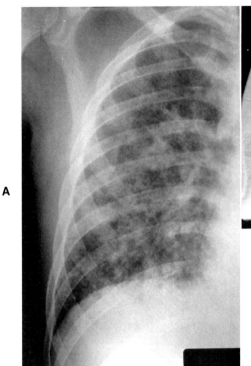

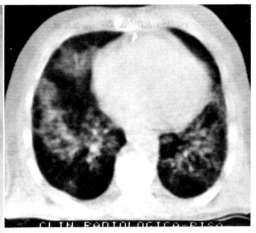

Fig. 5-20 **A,** Severe mixed alveolar and interstitial injury edema secondary to septic shock and adult respiratory distress syndrome. No evidence of pleural effusion is seen on the plain film. **B,** CT scan confirms the absence of effusions.

superimposition of hydrostatic factors such as overhydration or lowered oncotic pressure (see boxes on pp. 135 and 137). Massive liquid infusion is frequently needed to maintain adequate cardiac output and systemic blood pressure when patients with ARDS undergo positive-pressure ventilation. Overhydration may reduce the colloid osmotic pressure and increase pulmonary and systemic venous pressures simultaneously. All these factors combine to increase pleural liquid filtration and reduce its absorption (Fig. 5-21).

In patients with pleural effusion the radiologist's role in reading the plain film extends far beyond the simple detection and quantification of pleural fluid. In critically ill patients the pathophysiologically oriented reader should be able to extract from the standard chest radiograph valuable clinical information about intravascular and extravascular fluid dynamics, leading to correct diagnosis and rapid institution of the appropriate treatment.

APPENDIX A: FACTORS INVOLVED IN DEVELOPING A CORRECT MODEL OF PLEURAL FLUID FORMATION AND ABSORPTION

Parietal Pleural Capillary Pressure

In most published hypotheses concerning pleural fluid formation and absorption, Starling forces are shown at one level only in the pleural space. But clearly, pulmonary capillary pressure manifests a gradient from apex to base, as does intrapleural pressure[23]

and pulmonary interstitial pressure,[23,24,82] and these gradients should be incorporated into any model of pleural fluid dynamics. Some authors have suggested that a gradient of pressure also exists from apex to base within the *parietal* pleural capillaries.[24] Staub et al[1] state that microvascular pressure in the systemic circulation (parietal pleural capillaries) varies at the rate of 1 cm water/cm height. In their hypothetic diagrams, the authors show points in the pleura separated by a vertical height of 16 cm and add 16 cm of pressure to the parietal capillary pressure at the lowest site.[1]

If, however, we consider carefully the anatomy of the parietal pleural capillaries,[83] no good reason seems to exist to assume that there will be a gravitational gradient in these vessels, since they are supplied from apex to base by the intercostal and internal mammary arteries. Also, since these arteries maintain the same pressure from apex to base through vasomotor tone, no apex-to-base gradient should exist in the inflow pressure from these vessels into the pleural capillaries. The outflow from the capillaries will pass to the contiguous intercostal veins,[83] which are valvular and drain to the right atrium.[84] Therefore minimal variation occurs in intercostal venous pressure from apex to base. Since the influx and outflow pressures do not vary from apex to base in the lung, it is difficult to believe that a significant gravitational pressure gradient from top to bottom of the parietal pleural capillary bed can exist. In our consideration of the factors determining pleural fluid transudation and absorption, we therefore do not in-

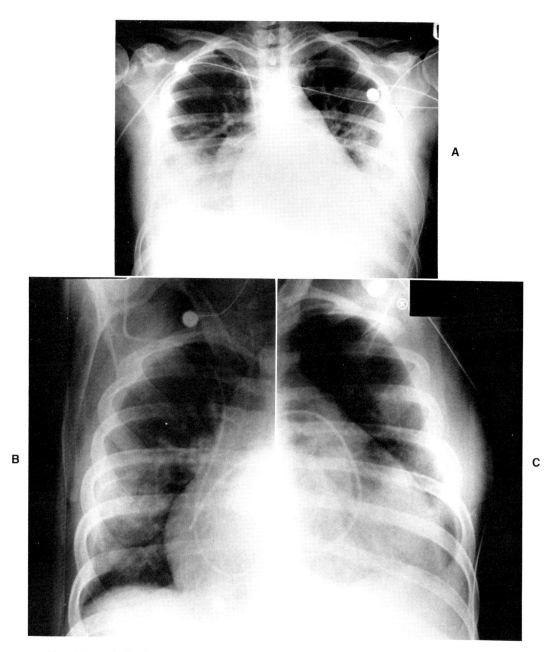

Fig. 5-21   A, Radiograph from 32-year-old female with "toxic shock" syndrome caused by bacterial contamination of vaginal tampon. She developed capillary permeability edema and required large amounts of intravenous fluid to maintain blood pressure and circulating blood volume. She has therefore developed overlying gravitationally distributed hydrostatic edema. **B** and **C,** Radiographs with the patient in the decubitus position show pleural effusions, which are rare in pure injury edema.

clude any apex-to-base pressure gradient within the parietal pleural capillaries.

Vascular Supply of Visceral Pleura

As mentioned, the vascular supply of the visceral pleura remains controversial.[2] The question is not only whether the circulation to the visceral pleura is pulmonary, bronchial, or mixed, but also whether the pleural microvessels are close enough to the surface so that the pleura itself can be disregarded in Starling calculations or are deep to the pleura and insulated from pleural space pressures.

In answer to the first part of this question, good evidence suggests that the bronchial arteries circulate to some areas of the pleura. The most convincing demonstrations are the radiologic studies of Cudkowitz,[19]

Fig. 5-22 A, Human lung from patient who died from metastatic pancreatic carcinoma. The upper arrow points to the very-fine-gauge (PE 50) catheter inserted into a bronchial artery at the hilum *(lower arrow)*. Excellent filling of the bronchial arteries surrounds lower lobe bronchi but no evidence of bronchial arteries extending out to the pleura. **B,** Section of the lung (0.5 cm thick) shown in **A.** Many small bronchial vessels ramify throughout the lung substance, but only one tortuous channel is seen *(short, straight open arrow)* extending out to the pleural surface *(black arrows)* and anastomosing directly, not passing through a capillary bed, with a large subpleural vessel *(curved open arrow)*. This subpleural vessel is identical in size and location with vessels filling much more extensively from the pulmonary circulation (see Fig. 5-23) and appears to be a bronchopulmonary anastomosis.

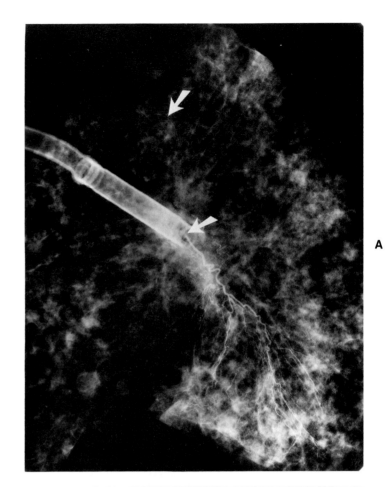

A

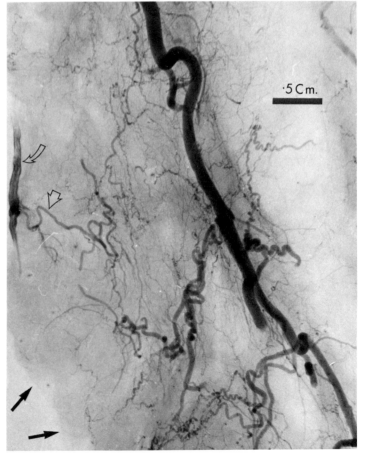

B

which show (as we have also done, Fig. 5-22) one or two very slender bronchial arteries passing over the surface of the lung below the pleural surface and ramifying sparsely. The problem with these injection studies is that they also demonstrate huge areas of pleura intervening between these vessels that show *no* evidence of a bronchial circulation. However, when one

then injects the pulmonary circulation in the same preparation, an enormous number of subpleural vessels immediately fills (Fig. 5-23). If one fills the pulmonary circulation, including the capillaries, with a vinyl injection mass, then digests the tissues away with acid leaving a cast of the circulation, the lung's surface appears completely solid to the naked eye. A microscope is needed to show that the apparently solid surface is actually made up of vast numbers of individual pulmonary capillaries with intervening spaces, where pleura overlies interstitium directly.

We have shown, as have Von Hayek[20] and Cudkowitz,[19] both bronchial and pulmonary circulation extending out to the pleura. But in our studies the bronchial circulation has been sparse and, as with Von Hayek,[20] we have not been able to show microvessels ramifying in or below the pleura from the widely separated single bronchial arterial branches. In contrast, we have shown extensive *pulmonary* microcirculation (Fig. 5-23).

A

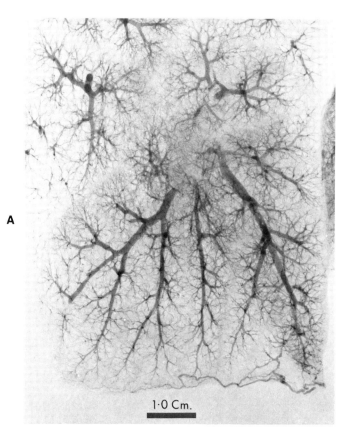

1·0 Cm.

Fig. 5-23 **A,** Human lung postmortem fixed in inflation, 3.0 mm thick section with pure pulmonary artery injection. Extensive subpleural network of vessels fills directly from the pulmonary arteries. **B,** Highly magnified view recorded on a Kodak maximum-resolution plate of the intact edge (not a section) of a human lung following pulmonary artery injection. A network of subpleural vessels *(open arrows)* is filling. The scale can be determined from the space between the two black arrows (visceral pleura), which is approximately 80 μm thick.

B

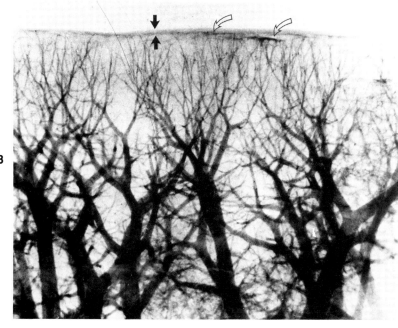

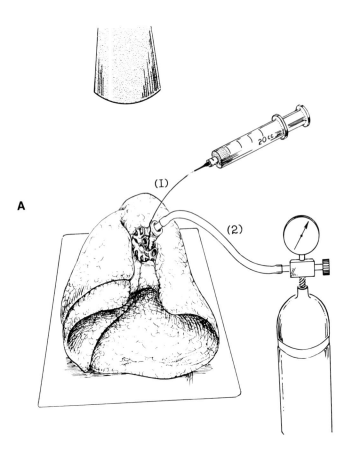

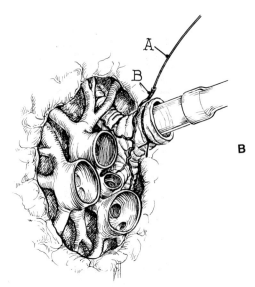

Fig. 5-24   **A,** Technique of injecting the bronchial arteries in an inflated human lung. The lung lies on a high-resolution film, and pictures are taken during filling and until filling is complete. **B,** Detailed drawing of the very slender (PE 50) catheter *(A)* tied directly into a bronchial artery *(B),* which has been dissected free at the hilum.

Our technique was to inject contrast medium first into the individually catheterized bronchial arteries (Fig. 5-24) and to take radiographs immediately at this stage, before separately injecting the pulmonary circulation and repeating the radiographic studies. As they pass deeper into the substance of the lung, some anastomoses also occur between bronchial and pulmonary vessels in the visceral subpleural vascular bed.[10-13,17-20] These appear to be direct anastomoses between bronchial arteries and subpleural vessels, which are much larger than the pulmonary capillaries (Fig. 5-25; see also Plate 1, p. 132). But with the separate injection technique and temporal filming sequence we used, one cannot confuse direct *antegrade* filling of the visceral pleural circulation by pulmonary vessels (pulmonary arteries to pleural capillaries to pulmonary veins) with filling of the pleural vessels from the bronchial circulation and *retrograde* filling of the pulmonary circulation (bronchial arteries to pleural capillaries to pulmonary veins). This is particularly true because pulmonary veins are easily distinguishable on the radiographs from pulmonary arteries by their septal position. From these studies and a careful analysis of the literature, with particular reference to the techniques used to delineate pulmonary and bronchial vessels, we conclude that the visceral pleural circulation is derived from and is continuous with the pulmonary circulation.

Since many animals have satisfactory pleural fluid formation and drainage with a purely *pulmonary* circulation to the visceral pleura, it would seem teleologically reasonable that in humans the role of the additional supply from the bronchial circulation may simply be to improve nutrition, not to cause fluid filtration. This may especially be the case because the pulmonary supply carries nonoxygenated venous blood to the pleura, whereas the bronchial blood is oxygenated. This hypothesis is further strengthened by the observation that only animals or mammals with a *thick* pleura (e.g., humans, horses, pigs, whales, elephants) show any bronchial circulation to the visceral pleura.

Some have suggested that if the visceral pleura were supplied by the bronchial circulation, we would have to perform our Starling calculations again[37] because the pressure in pleural capillaries supplied by the bronchial arteries would be much higher than in capillaries supplied by the pulmonary arteries; therefore much more fluid would transude from the visceral pleura. Again, some conceptual problems exist with this argument. First, since the bronchial arteries passing to the pleura and the lung arise from a common stem, if the bron-

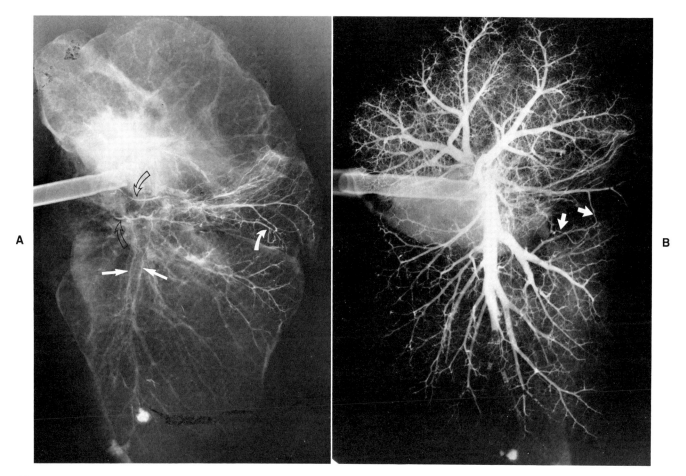

Fig. 5-25   A, Human right lung removed for carcinoma in the upper lobe. Bronchial arteries *(open arrows)* to the middle and lower lobes have been filled. Note the parallel, slender bronchial arteries following and outlining the posterior segmental bronchus *(straight white arrows).* No bronchial circulation to the pleura is seen. In the middle lobe a large bronchopulmonary anastomotic vessel is retrogradely filling the pulmonary circulation *(curved white arrow).* One or two of the retrogradely filled pulmonary artery branches do appear to extend to the pleura. **B,** Same lung now has had the pulmonary circulation filled. Many pulmonary branches extend out to the pleura. The looping bronchopulmonary anastomosis shown in **A** is very well demonstrated *(short white arrows).*

chial capillary pressure is high in the pleura, it must also be high within the lung. Also, if this high pressure were to cause fluid transudation from the pleura, it must also cause pulmonary interstitial edema. That is, if the bronchial arteries are to be credited with leaking fluid into the pleural space, they must also be credited with leaking it to a much greater extent into the pulmonary interstitium. This is because the bronchial vessels ramify to a far greater extent within the depths of the lung (see Fig. 5-22, *B*) and are subject to much the same negative extraalveolar pressures in these areas as they are in the subpleural zone. Such an excess leak of extravascular lung water (EVLW) does not appear to occur, probably because the bronchial arteries, apart from the immediate perihilar vessels,[5] anastomose at the level of the respiratory bronchiole with the pulmonary capillaries and drain through this low-resistance, low-pressure circuit into the left atrium (see Plate 1, p. 132). It would seem more sensible to believe that any visceral pleural *systemic* microvessels would have the same ability as parietal systemic vessels to regulate their pressure by controlling vasomotor tone and, as already suggested, would be simply nutritive to the pleura, as they are to the lungs.

Intrapleural Versus Subpleural Position of Visceral Pleural Circulation

In the reviews referred to previously,[1-3] some of the authors' diagrams do show the visceral pleural vessels to be *sub*pleural in location. However, the visceral

---

PROVEN AND HYPOTHESIZED ANATOMIC AND PHYSIOLOGIC FEATURES OF PLEURAL FLUID EXCHANGE

Anatomic data

PROVEN

1. Parietal pleura: thin, adherent to ribs, vascular supply systemic and located intrapleurally. Many stomata lead to subpleural lymphatics. Lymph and venous drainage occurs to right side of heart.
2. Visceral pleura: thick, can be stripped off lung, contains many intermesothelial cell clefts and many subpleural mast cells. Lymph and venous drainage occurs from costal aspect to left side of heart and from mediastinal perihilar aspect to right side of heart.

UNKNOWN OR UNPROVEN

1. Visceral pleura: vascular supply is unproven, variously quoted as pulmonary, bronchial, or mixed.
2. Visceral pleura: all authors regard vascular supply as *intra*pleural, but anatomically it appears on most studies to be *sub*pleural.

Physiologic data

PROVEN

1. Fluid transudes into pleural space from parietal capillaries according to Starling factors (a) in vessels and (b) in pleural space.
2. Intrapleural pressure increases from apex to base.
3. Subparietal and subvisceral pleural interstitial pressures increase from apex to base.
4. Intrapleural pressure decreases from costal to mediastinal aspects.
5. Subvisceral pleural interstitial pressure decreases from costal to mediastinal aspects.
6. Visceral capillaries have a hydrostatic pressure gradient increasing from apex to base.
7. Visceral pleura has high hydraulic conductivity.
8. Fluid can pass directly from lung interstitium across pleura into pleural space.

UNKNOWN OR UNPROVEN

1. Whether visceral pleura and/or visceral pleural vessels transude or absorb fluid normally is unknown.
2. Parietal capillary hydrostatic pressure is said to increase from apex to base. This is anatomically unlikely, because capillaries drain to intercostal veins, which are valvular, and all pass to the superior vena cava.
3. Parietal pleura probably has high hydraulic conductivity but is untested.
4. Whether visceral pleura normally has any characteristics of a semipermeable membrane is uncertain (literature varies).
5. Role of mesothelial clefts and mast cells is unknown.
6. Interstitial oncotic pressure in humans is only indirectly measured.

---

pleural vessels are treated as if they were definitely *intra*pleural in location, and the role of the pleura *overlying* these vessels is usually neglected. Although some controversy surrounds this in the anatomic literature, the parietal pleural capillaries apparently are intrapleural, but the *visceral* pleural vessels are consistently subpleural in position and may have a thickness of up to 80 µm of pleura overlying them.[15] Von Hayek describes "Subpleural interstitial tissue, which, owing to its rich vascularity, may be designated as the vascular layer of the pleura . . . the pleura may be readily separated from this vascular layer."[20] In this position the visceral pleural vessels would be somewhat insulated from the pleural space and would be much more likely to be affected by the *subpleural* interstitial hydrostatic and oncotic pressures rather than by the *intra*pleural pressures. This would have a major impact on whether the visceral pleural vessels filter or absorb pleural fluid (or do neither).

For clarity, the many anatomic features just listed have been shown semidiagrammatically earlier in this chapter (see Plate 1, p. 132). Some of these anatomic features and a few of the physiologic features have been proved and are not controversial, but others are only incompletely proved and still others cannot be measured and must be largely hypothesized (see box at left).

To summarize, the three most important unknown factors are:

1. Whether the visceral pleural vessels are anatomically and functionally intrapleural or subpleural
2. What is the exact source of the blood vessels supplying the visceral pleura (partially addressed earlier)
3. Whether the pleura, which is said to form (under experimental conditions with the pleura separated from the lung) a minimal barrier to the passage of water (i.e., to have a high hydraulic conductivity), has any features of a semipermeable membrane

Whether or not the pleura is a semipermeable membrane (i.e., whether the passage of water across it is affected by the oncotic pressures on either side of the pleura) will have a major effect on fluid absorption or filtration from the pleural space. Later in this appendix we calculate and illustrate what would happen to pleural fluid formation if the pleura were semipermeable, compare and contrast this with the behavior of non-semipermeable pleura, and show which situation matches best with experimental and clinical data.

We would question whether the high hydraulic conductivity demonstrated when the pleura has been forcefully stripped off the lung surface and tested as a separate membrane[14,85] would be present in the intact lung. In our experience, using an isolated dog lung with intact visceral pleura, elevating pulmonary venous pressure produces no transudation of water across the pleura until gross pulmonary edema develops (Plate 2, p. 133). Stripping the pleura may cause the numerous intercellular clefts in the visceral pleura to open, thereby increasing hydraulic conductivity (see later discussion).

So many anatomic and physiologic variables may affect the filtration and absorption of pleural fluid that many permutations are possible. To decide which permutations of the differing anatomic/physiologic factors shown in Plate 1 (p. 132) and the box (p. 148), best fit known experimental and clinical data, we developed models showing the effects of intrapleural versus subpleural positions of the visceral pleural capillaries. We evaluated the three different cases of pulmonary, bronchial, and mixed (pulmonary and bronchial) visceral pleural circulation, first with the pleura regarded as a semipermeable membrane and then as a nonsemipermeable membrane. We included the effects of pleural pressure gradients, interstitial pressure gradients, oncotic pressures, and capillary hydrostatic pressure gradients in these models. The values for the hydrostatic and oncotic factors and pressure gradients used in these calculations and their sources of derivation are shown in Table 5-1. It is important to note that the figures we quote are for an *inflated* lung at full inspiration. Our figures for pleural and interstitial pressures are therefore lower (more negative) than those usually quoted at end expiration.

The diagram we developed for this modeling is shown in Fig. 5-2 with no numeric values entered. In Fig. 5-3, *A*, we have inserted the appropriate pressure data for a pure pulmonary circulation to both the mediastinal and the costal visceral pleura, have placed the visceral capillaries subpleurally and parietal capillaries intrapleurally and have regarded the pleura as a *non*semipermeable membrane. We consider the lung's upper and lower halves (as in an erect 70 kg male adult) to be approximately 20 cm apart, yielding a pleural pressure difference between the two of approximately 11.0 mm Hg (Table 5-1).

Transudation and absorption (calculated as arbitrary flow units per unit area) for the upper and lower halves of the pleural surfaces are calculated separately. The figures derived from the upper lung are then multiplied by 0.25 to compensate approximately for the much smaller surface area of the lung's upper half compared with the lower half, which has a large diaphragmatic surface. Using this semiquantitative approach, 12 different permutations are possible.

I. Visceral capillaries in a subpleural position and the pleura semipermeable (Table 5-2, model 1), with pulmonary circulation (A), mixed circulation (B), and, bronchial circulation (C).

II. Visceral capillaries again in a subpleural position but with the pleura as a *non*semipermeable membrane. (Table 5-2, model II), with pulmonary circulation (A), mixed circulation (B), and bronchial circulation (C).

III. Visceral capillaries intrapleural and the pleura semipermeable (Table 5-2, model III), with pulmonary circulation (A), mixed circulation (B), and bronchial circulation (C).

IV. Visceral capillaries intrapleural but with the pleura *non*semipermeable (Table 5-2, model IV), with pulmonary circulation (A), mixed circulation (B), and bronchial circulation.

Fig. 5-3, *A*, shows one permutation, with pure pulmonary circulation to the pleura). Three other permutations of pure pulmonary circulation to the pleura (Table 5-2, models IA, IIIA, and IVA) are illustrated in Fig. 5-26. For the sake of brevity the other eight possible permutations, four with mixed circulation to the pleura (i.e., pulmonary to the costal visceral pleura and bronchial to the mediastinal visceral pleura) and four with pure bronchial circulation to the visceral pleura, are not shown as figures. However, the results of the Starling calculations for all 12 permutations are shown in Table 5-2. From this table, along with the anatomic diagram (see Plate 1, p. 132) and the model diagrams, several important conclusions may be drawn.

1. The parietal pleural capillaries are undoubtedly supplied by systemic arteries, and since they lie *within* the parietal pleura (intrapleural), overlaid only by a very thin layer of pleura (see Plate 1), they are therefore affected by the Starling forces of the pleural space. They are not affected by any variations in *visceral* pleural blood supply or by the permeability or nonpermeability of the pleura. As a result, the amount of transudation (calculated as 42 units[*]) from the *parietal* pleural capillaries into the pleural space (Table 5-2, models I, II, III, and IV; A, B, and C; subscript 1) and the amount of absorption (7.5 units) from the pleural space into the parietal capillaries (Table 5-2, models I, II, III, and IV; A, B, and C; subscript 8) is therefore *identical for all 12 permutations* reported in Table 5-2.

2. If the *visceral* capillaries were also held to be functionally *intra*pleural (the usual assumption) and therefore to behave as if they have only a very thin pleural layer overlying them (Fig. 5-26, *B* and *C*), they would also be affected by the hydrostatic and oncotic pressures of the pleural space (Table 5-2). Because the oncotic pressure of the pleural space is very low,[1,7] transudation from the visceral capillaries (even in an intrapleural position) into the pleural space would be very small (8 units[*]; Table 5-2, models. $IIIA_2$ and IVA_2) with normal pulmonary capillary pressures. However, this transudation would increase if the capillary hydro-

---

[*]Unit = flow per unit of area.

static pressure were high, for example, if the arterial supply to the visceral pleura were mixed (transudation increases from 8 to 25 units; Table 5-2, models $IIIB_2$ and IVB_2) or purely bronchial (transudation increases from 8 to 40 units; Table 5-2, models $IIIC_2$ and IVC_2) or if left atrial pressure were raised. With the capillaries *intra* pleural in position, little or no transudation would occur from the visceral pleural vessels into the lung, that is, no increase in EVLW.

Some authors[1,2] have recently emphasized the importance of the bronchial circulation in pleural physiology and suggested that this should change our thinking about the formation of pleural fluid; interestingly, the differences in the amount of transudation occurring whether the circulation to the visceral pleura is pulmonary, mixed, or bronchial are not very great (Table 5-2, models III and IV; A, B, and C). That is, even if the visceral pleural capillaries *were* intrapleural, whether the visceral circulation is pulmonary, bronchial, or mixed does not appear significant. If the visceral capillaries are *sub*pleural, whether their source is pulmonary or bronchial will have no effect on pleural fluid formation or absorption. Note that, regardless of the source of the visceral pleural circulation and even with

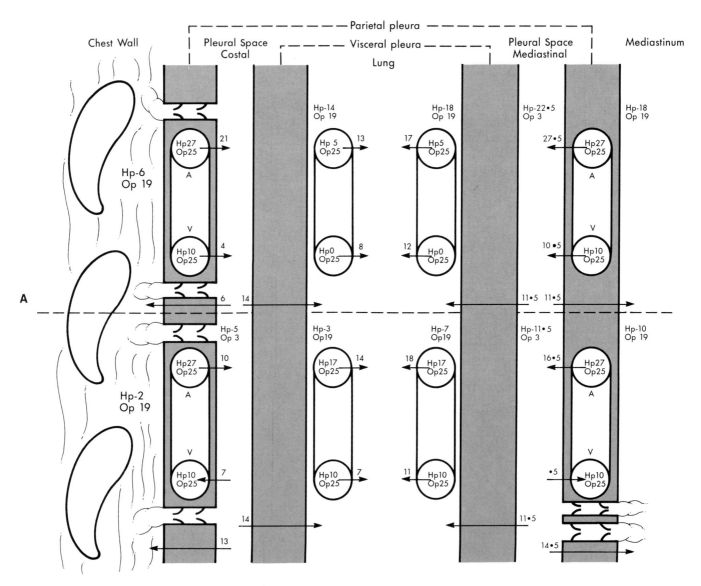

Fig. 5-26 **A,** Visceral capillaries *subpleural.* Pleural membranes considered to be *semipermeable* (compare with Fig. 5-3). Visceral pleura supplied by pure pulmonary circulation (see Table 5-2, model IA). Total transudation into pleural space is 42 units and total absorption 73 units. Transudation into lung (extravascular lung water) is 62 units. Note that this model assumes extensive absorption from the pleural space by parietal and visceral pleura.

an intrapleural capillary location, *absorption* of fluid into the visceral capillaries is minimal (calculated as 9.5 units; Table 5-2, models III and IV; A_9, B_9, and C_9).

3. If the visceral capillaries are *sub*pleural (Table 5-2, models I and II; Figs. 5-3 and 5-26, *A*) and therefore have a thick layer of pleura overlying them, they will be affected predominantly by the hydrostatic and oncotic pressures of the subpleural pulmonary interstitium. Fluid will transude into the subpleural space, not into the pleural space. Because the subpleural pulmonary interstitial oncotic pressure is normally much higher than the pleural space oncotic pressure[82] (Table

5-1), the amount of transudation for the same capillaries in a subpleural location will be much greater than in an intrapleural location (compare Fig. 5-26, *A* and *C*). But this transudation occurs into the *lung* as EVLW (Table 5-2, compare models I_3 and II_3 with III_3 and IV_3). The transudation would be even greater if the vessels were bronchial rather than pulmonary, which would cause a minor increase in subpleural EVLW, but would have no effect on the quantity of *pleural* fluid, as noted earlier. Note that because of the gradient of interstitial pressure from the costal to the mediastinal surfaces of the lung, subpleural *costal* extravascular lung water

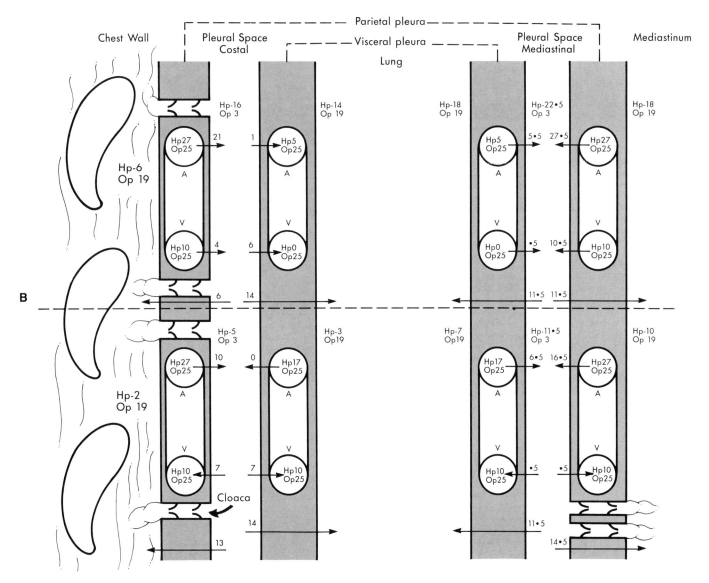

Fig. 5-26, cont'd   B, This figure differs from **A** in that the visceral capillaries are *intrapleural;* the pleura is again semipermeable, and visceral pleura is supplied by pulmonary circulation (Table 5-2, model IIIA). Total transudation into pleural space is 50 units and total absorption 81 units. Note that this model again assumes most absorption occurring through the visceral and parietal pleura.   *Continued.*

(EVLW$_C$) will be slightly less than subpleural *mediastinal* EVLW (EVLW$_M$). Although the numbers seem large (62 to 96 units), this transudation into the subpleural space is occurring (as previously discussed) from a single layer of capillaries with a very small surface area and is very small compared with the constant normal transudation occurring from the millions of layers of capillaries within the lung substance. Note also that when the visceral capillaries are anatomically and functionally subpleural in position, *no* absorption of water occurs from the pleura into the visceral capillaries (Table 5-2, models I and II; A$_9$, B$_9$, and C$_9$).

4. If the pleura were a semipermeable membrane (Table 5-2, models I and III; Fig. 5-26, *B*), because of the

balance of Starling forces, large and equal amounts of absorption of pleural fluid (32 units) would occur across both the parietal (Table 5-2, models I and III; A$_4$, B$_4$, and C$_4$) and the visceral (Table 5-2, models I and III; A$_5$, B$_5$, and C$_5$) pleura from the pleural space into the subpleural interstitium of both the chest wall and the lung. Also, *no* transudation of fluid would occur from the interstitium across the pleura into the pleural space (Table 5-2, models I and III; A$_{6,7}$, B$_{6,7}$, and C$_{6,7}$). Note that this is the only permutation in which the visceral pleura could absorb fluid in significant amounts from the pleural space, that is, *the only scenario that would agree with the popularly held Agostoni hypothesis.*[4-7]

5. In contrast, if the pleura were *not* a semiperme-

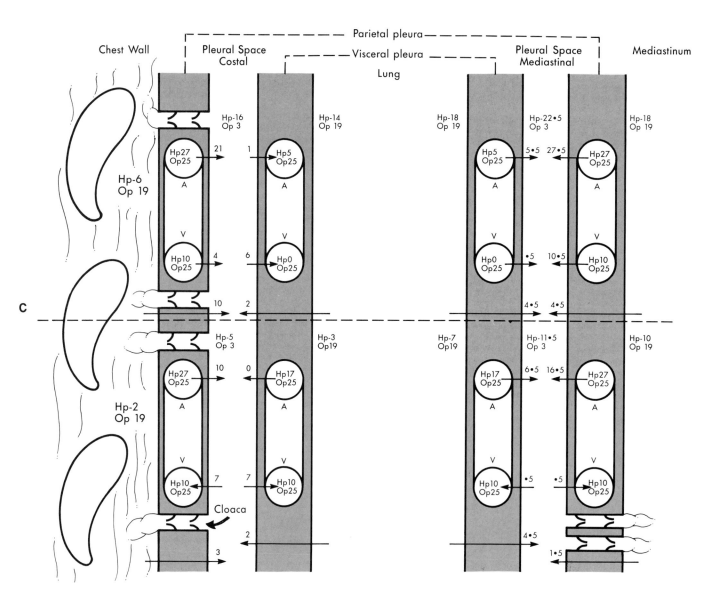

Fig. 5-26, cont'd   C, This model is the same as **B,** but the pleura is now *non*semipermeable (Table 5-2, model IVA). Total transudation is 66 units and total absorption 17 units. No absorption occurs through visceral pleura.

able membrane (Figs. 5-3 and 5-26, *C*), no absorption of pleural fluid would occur from the pleural space across the parietal and visceral pleura (Table 5-2, models II and IV; A_5, $B_{4,5}$, and $C_{4,5}$). But now some transudation would occur from the subpleural interstitium (both parietal and visceral) across the pleura into the pleural space (Table 5-2, models II and IV; $A_{6,7}$, $B_{6,7}$, and $C_{6,7}$).

Correlation of Proposed Models with Known Clinical and Experimental Data

Of the four possible groups of models just considered, models I and III, in which the pleura is considered to be a semipermeable membrane, assume the absorption of large amounts of pleural fluid through the visceral pleura into the lung. This does not fit with experimental* or clinical observations. For example, in patients with spontaneous or induced pneumothoraces, including the many thousands of pneumothoraces induced for tuberculosis in the pre-drug era, the visceral pleural surface is no longer physically available for absorption of pleural fluid, but, in the absence of complications, effusion does not normally develop.

Conversely, if the normal visceral pleural surface does filter fluid, one would reasonably expect to see, at least occasionally, in an erect patient with a large pneumothorax, droplets of fluid forming from the lung's inferior visceral pleural surface, which can be exquisitely visualized on the chest radiograph. In our experience, such transudation is not seen unless lung or pleural pathology is also present. These clinical observations and experimental data both suggest, as does our analysis of all the anatomic and physiologic factors involved in pleural fluid dynamics, that the visceral pleura and visceral capillaries, under *normal* circumstances, have little or no role in either filtration or absorption of pleural fluid.

In models II and IV the pleura is viewed as a *non-semipermeable* membrane. The difference between II and IV is that in model II the visceral pleura vessels are subpleural (Fig. 5-26, *A*) and in model IV they are intrapleural (Fig. 5-26, *B* and *C*).

The *similarities* between models II and IV are as follows:

1. In both, transudation (excluding the effects of the parietal pleural stomata) greatly exceeds absorption. The ratio between quantity of transudation (QT) and the quantity of absorption (QA) does not differ greatly if the pleural supply is pulmonary or bronchial (i.e., QT/QA of 6:1 to 9:1).
2. In both the parietal pleura and the visceral pleura do not absorb fluid from the pleural space.
3. In both the parietal pleura and visceral pleura do

transude a small amount of fluid (8.5 units) into the pleural space.

The *differences* between models II and IV are as follows:

1. In model II the visceral capillaries neither absorb nor transude fluid (Table 5-2) subscripts 2 and 9), whereas in model IV the visceral capillaries both absorb (9.5 units) and transude (8 units) small amounts of pleural fluid (Table 5-2, subscripts 2 and 9).
2. In model II, increasing visceral pleural capillary pressure causes an increase in subpleural EVLW (Table 5-2, models A_3, B_3, and C_3) from 62 to 96 but not in the quantity of pleural fluid. In model IV, however, increasing visceral capillary pressure, either pathologically or anatomically, causes an *immediate* increase in pleural fluid volume from 66 to 98 (Table 5-2, models A_2, B_2, and C_2). This does not fit with either experimental[41] or clinical observations.[31]

As discussed earlier in this chapter, of all the models considered, *IIA* (Fig. 5-3, *A* and *B*) fits best with observed experimental, anatomic, and clinical data. However, if neither the visceral pleura nor the visceral pleural capillaries absorb pleural fluid, it remains to be explained how the excess pleural fluid produced by the parietal capillaries and pleura is reabsorbed from the pleural space and why the oncotic pressure of the pleural space is so low. In this regard, the importance of the lymphatics of the parietal pleura has been very well documented.*

Stomata have been shown in the parietal pleura (Fig. 5-27) communicating directly with the pleural space and connecting this space with the parietal subpleural lymphatics,[45] which drain to the thoracic duct or the jugulomediastinal lymph trunk. These stomata, which have a diameter of several micrometers, are located in the most mobile portions of the pleura: ventrally along the sternum, dorsally beside the vertebral column, and along the retrocardiac pleural folds.[46] Respiratory and circulatory motion appears to be very important in facilitating drainage via the stomata.[2,41,44-47,49] By their action the parietal pleural lymphatics should be able to suck liquid out of the pleural space even though its pressure is less than atmospheric. The egress of albumin from the pleural space is greatest from the regions where pleural pressure is most negative.[27] From these data, one can infer that albumin absorption from the pleural space is independent of Starling factors and is caused by lymphatic clearance. This is in accord with saline or plasma injected into the pleural space having comparable rates of absorption.[8,86,87] The stomata also permit particulate material, including red blood cells,

---

*References 1,2,8,28,25,29,30,44-47,86-88.

*References 1-3,8,9,28,44,46-47,86-90.

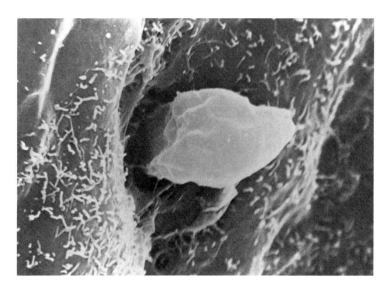

Fig. 5-27 Electron microphotograph showing stoma in parietal pleura engulfing a red blood cell. (Reproduced with permission from Kanazawa K: In Chretien J, Bignon J, Hirsch A, editors: *The pleura in health and disease,* New York, 1985, Marcel Dekker.)

to be removed from the pleural cavity (Fig. 5-27).[45,50] Ligation of the main thoracic lymph trunks at the base of the neck virtually abolishes clearance of protein injected into the pleural space.[8,25,88] Also, the most actively absorbing surface in the pleura is where the highest density of stomata exists.[27,45,46]

The bulk of experimental evidence therefore suggests that the parietal subpleural lymphatics are the major pathway for clearance of liquid and solutes from the pleural space, providing (more than Starling forces) an important control mechanism for pleural liquid volume and pressure.[2,3,25]

To reiterate, from the analyses of all the anatomic and physiologic factors affecting the formation and drainage of pleural fluid, we have concluded that model IIA (Table 5-2 and Fig. 5-3, *A* and *B*) in which the visceral capillaries are subpleural and supplied by the pulmonary arteries and the pleura is not semipermeable, comes closest to satisfying observed experimental and clinical data. This is the model we have used in this chapter to correlate radiologic and pathophysiologic changes in the pleural space. As noted, when the visceral capillaries are subpleural in position, the source of their supply, whether pulmonary or bronchial, is irrelevant to pleural fluid formation and drainage.

Although model IIA fits very well with experimental and clinical data, we do not believe that it is necessarily the final model for pleural fluid filtration and absorption. Quite possibly the visceral pleural vessels may behave as if they are partially intrapleural and partially subpleural. Also, we have not considered the many intercellular clefts in the visceral pleura,[15,16] which can open quite dramatically under certain conditions and should be regarded as a possible pathway for the passage of fluid across the visceral pleura. No study appears to have yet been done on these clefts' role or the role of the many mast cells that lie below the visceral pleura.[15]

To our knowledge, model IIA is unlike any prior model in that it takes into account all pressure gradients within the pleural space, across the pleura, within the interstitium, and across the lung, as well as all oncotic and hydrostatic pressures.

APPENDIX B: MODELS OF "MIXED" AND PURELY BRONCHIAL CIRCULATION TO THE VISCERAL PLEURA

This appendix contains models with "mixed" (bronchial and pulmonary) circulation and with purely bronchial circulation to the visceral pleura. The results of calculating the Starling equations for each of these models are given in Table 5-2.

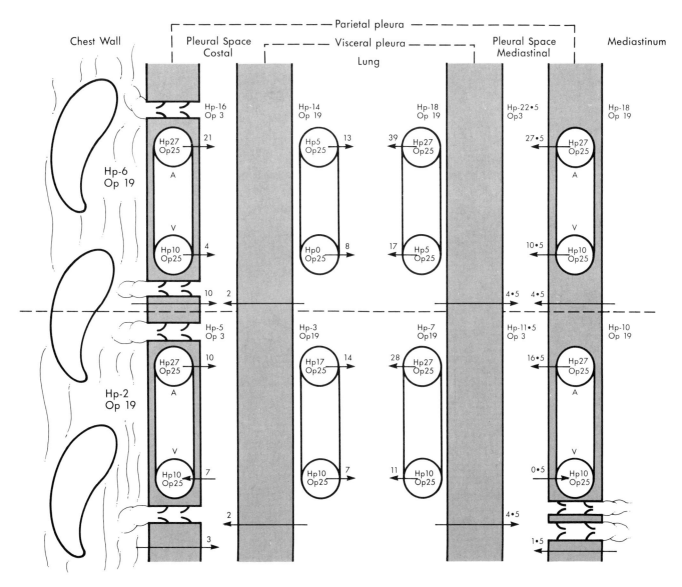

Fig. 5-28 Mixed circulation to visceral pleura, visceral vessels subpleural, and pleura nonsemipermeable (Table 5-2, model IIB).

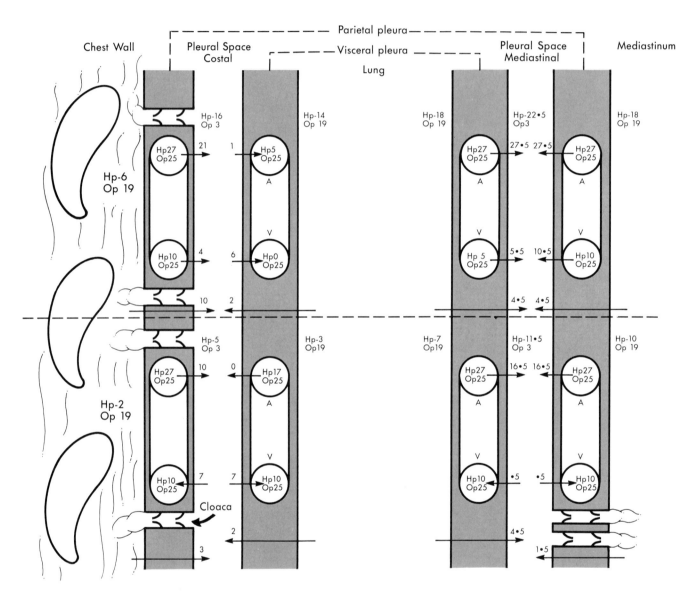

Fig. 5-29 Mixed circulation to visceral pleura, visceral vessels intrapleural, and pleura nonsemipermeable (Table 5-2, model IVB).

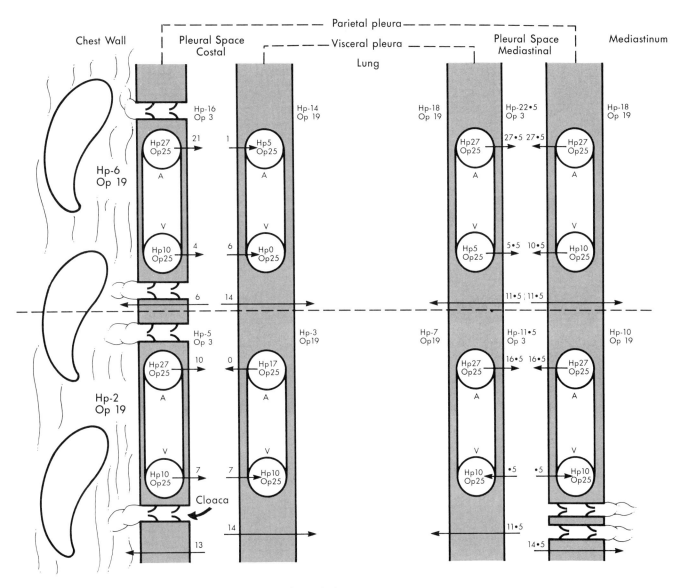

Fig. 5-30   Mixed circulation to visceral pleura, visceral vessels intrapleural, and pleura semipermeable (Table 5-2, model IIIB).

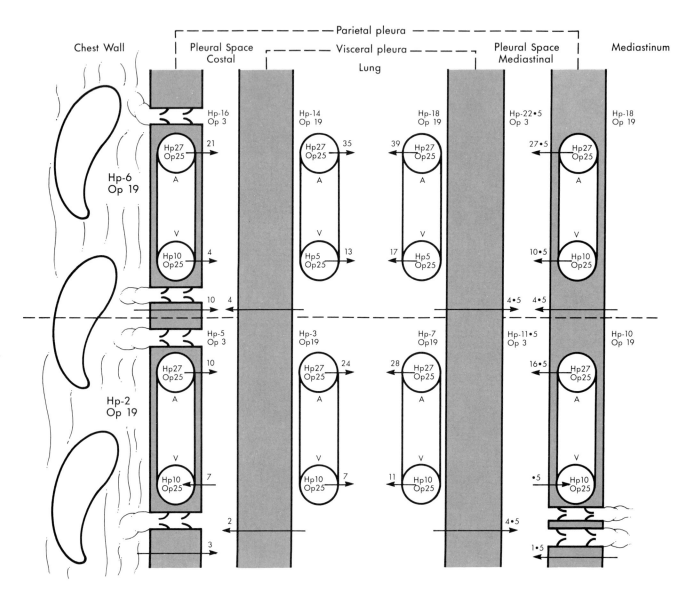

Fig. 5-31 Bronchial circulation to visceral pleura, visceral pleural vessels subpleural, and pleura nonsemipermeable (Table 5-2, model IIC).

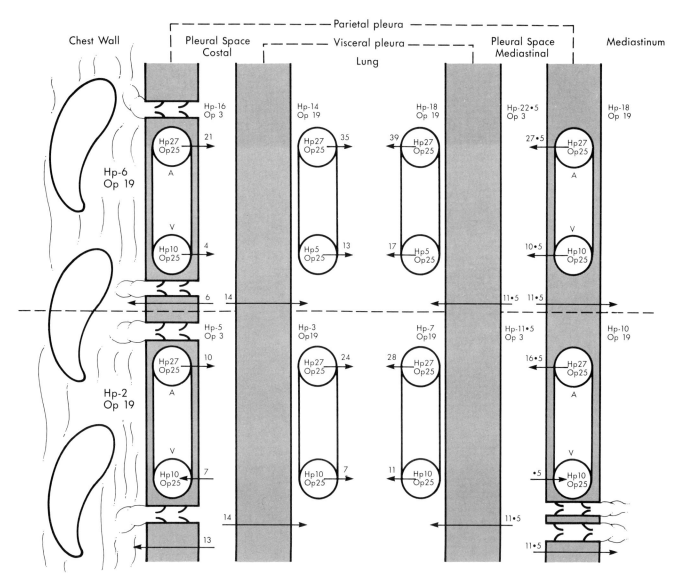

Fig. 5-32 Bronchial circulation to visceral pleura, visceral pleural vessels subpleural, and pleura semipermeable (Table 5-2, model IC).

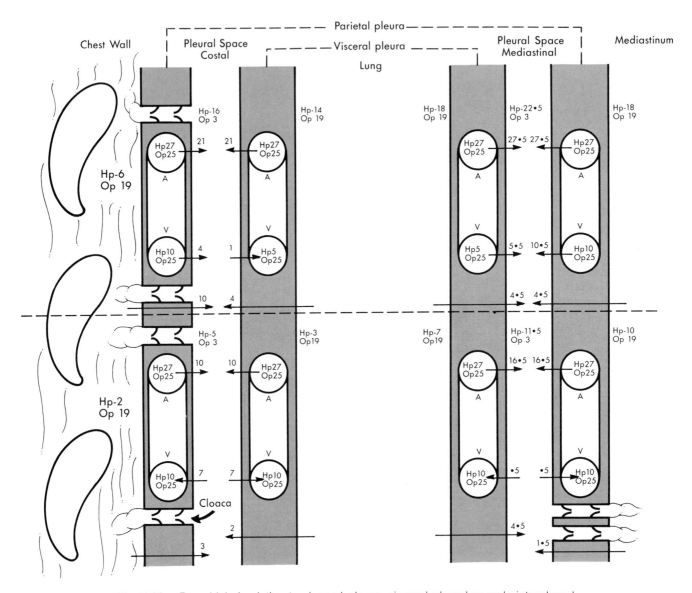

Fig. 5-33   Bronchial circulation to visceral pleura, visceral pleural vessels intrapleural, and pleura nonsemipermeable (Table 5-2, model IVC).

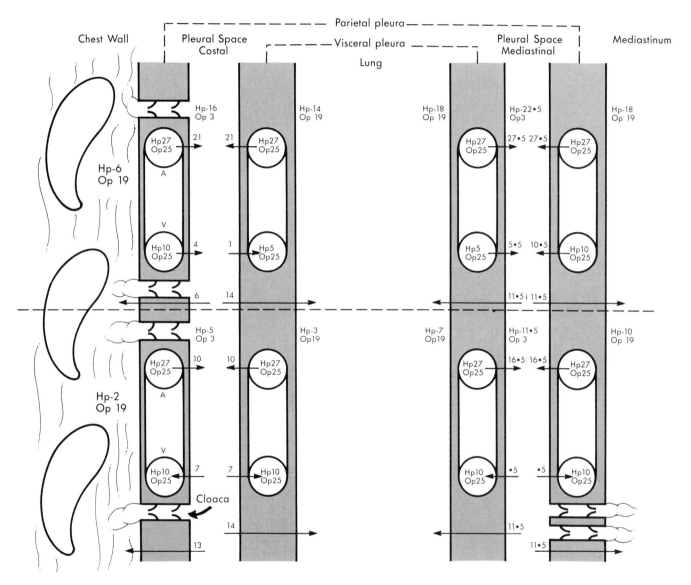

Fig. 5-34 Bronchial circulation to visceral pleura, visceral pleural vessels intrapleural, and pleura semipermeable (Table 5-2, model IIIC).

REFERENCES

1. Staub NC, Wiener-Kronish JP, Albertine KH: Transport through the pleura. In Chretien J, Bignon J, Hirsch A, editors: *The pleura in health and disease*, New York, 1985, Marcel Dekker, p 169.
2. Pistolesi M, Miniati M, Giuntini C: State of the art: pleural liquid and solute exchange, *Am Rev Respir Dis* 140:825, 1989.
3. Miserocchi G: Pleural pressures and fluid transport. In Crystal RG, West JB et al, editors: *The lung: scientific foundations*, New York, 1991, Raven Press, p 885.
4. Agostoni E, Taglietti A, Setnikar I: Absorption forces of the capillaries of the visceral pleura in determination of the intrapleural pressure, *Am J Physiol* 191:277, 1957.
5. Agostoni E, Mead J: Statics of the respiratory system. In Fenn WO, Rahn H, editors: *Handbook of physiology*, Respiration, section 3, vol 1, Washington, DC, 1964, American Physiological Society, p 387.
6. Agostoni E: Mechanics of the pleural space, *Physiol Rev* 57:128, 1972.
7. Agostoni E: Mechanics of the pleural space. In Fishman AP, Macklem PT, Mead JS, editors: *Handbook of physiology*, The respiratory system, section 3, vol III, Washington, DC, 1986, American Physiological Society, p 531.
8. Courtice FC, Simmonds WJ: Absorption of fluids from the pleural cavities of rabbits and cats, *J Physiol (London)* 109:117, 1949.
9. Cooray GH: Defensive mechanisms in the mediastinum, with special reference to the mechanisms of pleural absorption, *J Pathol Bacteriol* 61:551, 1949.
10. Verloop MC: The arteriae bronchiales and their anastomoses with the arteria pulmonalis in the human lung: a micro-anatomical study, *Acta Anat (Basel)* 5:171, 1948.
11. Bernaudin JF, Fleury J: Anatomy of the blood and lymphatic circulation of the pleural mucosa. In Chretien J, Bignon J, Hirsch A, editors: *The pleura in health and disease*, New York, 1985, Marcel Dekker, p 101.
12. McLaughlin RF, Tyler WS, Canada RO: A study of the subgross pulmonary anatomy in various mammals, *Am J Anat* 108:149, 1961.
13. McLaughlin RF, Tyler WS, Canada RO: The subgross pulmonary anatomy in various mammals and men, *JAMA* 175:694, 1961.
14. Kim KS, Critz A, Crandall E: Transport of water and solutes across sheep visceral pleura, *Am Rev Respir Dis* 120:883, 1979.
15. Gil J: Morphologic basis of exchanges across the pleura. In Chretien J, Bignon J, Hirsch A, editors: *The pleura in health and disease*, New York, 1985, Marcel Dekker, p 89.
16. Kanazawa K: Exchanges through the pleura: cells and particles, Chretien J, Bignor J, Hirsch A, editors: *The pleura in health and disease*, New York, 1985, Marcel Dekker, p 195.
17. Miller WS: The vascular supply of the pleura pulmonalis, *Am J Anat* 7:389, 1907.
18. Nagaishi C: *Functional anatomy and histology of the lung*, Baltimore, 1972, University Park Press, p 79.
19. Cudkowitz L: Bronchial arterial circulation in man: normal anatomy and response to disease. In Moser KM, editor: *Pulmonary vascular diseases*, New York, 1979, Marcel Dekker.
20. Von Hayek H: *The human lung*, New York, 1960, Hafner, p 34.
21. Milne ENC: Bronchial arteriography. In Abrams H, editor: *Angiography* ed 2, vol 2, Boston, 1971, Little Brown, p 567.
22. Pump KK: Distribution of bronchial arteries in the human lung, *Chest* 62:447, 1972.
23. Miserocchi G. Pleural liquid pressure. In Chretien J, Bignon J, Hirsch A, editors: *The pleura in health and disease*, New York, 1985, Marcel Dekker, p 151.
24. Negrini D, Capelli C, Marini M, Miserocchi G: Gravity dependent distribution of parietal sub-pleural interstitial pressure, *J Appl Physiol* 63:1912, 1987.
25. Miniati M, Parker JC, Pistolesi M et al: Reabsorption kinetics of albumin from pleural space of dogs, *Am J Physiol* 255:H375, 1988.
26. Wiener-Kronish JP, Albertine KH, Licko V, Staub NC: Protein egress and entry rates in pleural fluid and plasma in sheep, *J Appl Physiol* 56:459, 1984.
27. Negrini D, Pistolesi M, Miniati M, et al: Regional protein absorption rates from the pleural cavity in dogs, *J Appl Physiol* 58:2062, 1985.
28. Stewart PB: The rate of formation and lymphatic removal of pleural fluid in pleural effusions, *J Clin Invest* 42:258, 1963.
29. Leckie WJH, Tothill P: Albumin turnover in pleural effusions, *Clin Sci* 29:339, 1965.
30. Sahn SA: State of the art: the pleura, *Am Rev Respir Dis* 138:184, 1988.
31. Kinasewitz GT, Fishman AP: Pleural dynamics and effusions. In Fishman AP, editor: *Pulmonary diseases and disorders*, New York, 1988, McGraw-Hill, p 2117.
32. Mellins RB, Levine OR, Fishman AP: Effect of systemic and pulmonary venous hypertension on pleural and pericardial fluid accumulation, *J Appl Physiol* 29:564, 1970.
33. Allen SJ, Lane GA, Drake RE, Gabel JC: Superior vena caval pressure elevation causes pleural effusion formation in sheep, *Am J Physiol* 235:H492, 1988.
34. Uhley MN, Leeds SE, Sampson JJ, Friedman R: Role of pulmonary lymphatics in chronic pulmonary edema, *Circ Res* 11:966, 1962.
35. Wiener-Kronish JP, Goldstein R, Matthay RA et al: Lack of association of pleural effusion with chronic pulmonary arterial and right atrial hypertension, *Chest* 92:967, 1987.
36. Wiener-Kornish JP, Matthay MA, Callen PW et al: Relationship of pleural effusions to pulmonary hemodynamics in patients with congestive heart failure, *Am Rev Respir Dis* 132:1253, 1985.
37. Staub NC: New concepts about the pathophysiology of pulmonary edema, *J Thorac Imaging* 3(3):8, 1988.
38. Broaddus VC, Wiener-Kronish JP, Staub NC: Clearance of lung edema into the pleural space of volume-loaded anesthetized sheep, *J Appl Physiol* 68:2623, 1990.
39. Zdansky E: Bietrage zur Kenntnis der kardialen Lungenstraung aufgrund roentgenologischer klinischer und anatomischer Untersuchungen, *Wien Arch Inn Med* 18:461, 1929.
40. Light RW: Disorders of the pleura. General principles and diagnostic approach. In Murray JF, Nadel JA, editors: *Textbook of respiratory medicine*, Philadelphia, 1988, WB Saunders, p 1703.
41. Graham EA: Influence of respiratory movements on formation of pleural exudates, *JAMA* 76:784, 1921.
42. Bartoletti F: Pectoral dropsy or hydrothorax. In *Methods in dyspnoeam seu de respirationbus*, book 4, pt 3, University of Bologna, 1633, catalogued at the Royal Society of London.
43. Albertini IF: *The animadversiones of Ippolito Francesco Albertini on cardiac and precordial diseases which cause dyspnoea*, 1746 and 1748, catalogued at US National Library of Medicine.
44. Courtice FC, Simmonds WJ: Physiological significance of lymph drainage of the serous cavities and lungs, *Physiol Rev* 34:419, 1954.
45. Wang NS: The preformed stomas connecting the pleural cavity and the lymphatics in the parietal pleura, *Am Rev Respir Dis* 111:12, 1975.
46. Albertine KH, Wiener-Kronish JP, Staub NC: The structure of the parietal pleura and its relationship to pleural liquid dynamics in sheep, *Anat Rec* 208:401, 1984.
47. Courtice FC, Morris B: The effect of diaphragmatic movement on the absorption of protein and of red cells from the pleural cavity, *Aust J Exp Biol Med* Sci 31:227, 1953.
48. Stewart PB, Burgen ASV: The turnover of fluid in the dog's pleural cavity, *J Lab Clin Med* 52:213, 1958.

49. Miserocchi G, Nakamura T, Mariani E, Negrini D: Pleural liquid pressure over the interlobar mediastinal and diaphragmatic surfaces of the lung, *Respir Physiol* 46:61, 1981.

50. Broaddus VC, Weiner-Kronish JP, Berthiaume Y, Staub NC: Removal of pleural liquid and protein by lymphatics in awake sheep, *J Appl Physiol* 63:384, 1988.

51. Henschke CI, Davis SD, Romano MP, Yankelevitz DF: Pleural effusions: pathogenesis, radiologic evaluation, and therapy, *J Thorac Imaging* 4(1):49, 1989.

52. Vix VA: Roentgenographic manifestations of pleural disease, *Semin Roentgenol* 12:277, 1977.

53. Collins JD, Burnuell D, Furmanski S et al: Minimal detectable pleural effusions, *Radiology* 105:51, 1972.

54. Rigler LG: Roentgen diagnosis of small pleural effusions: a new roentgenographic position, *JAMA* 96:104, 1931.

55. Moskowitz H, Platt RT, Schacher R, Mellins H: Roentgen visualization of minute pleural effusions, *Radiology* 109:33, 1973.

56. Bedford DE, Lovibond JL: Hydrothorax in heart failure, *Br Heart J* 3:93, 1941.

57. McPeak EM, Levine SA: The preponderance of right hydrothorax in congestive heart failure, *Ann Intern Med* 25:916, 1946.

58. White PD, August S, Michael CR: Hydrothorax in congestive heart failure, *Am J Med Sci* 214:243, 1947.

59. Felson B: *Chest roentgenology*, Philadelphia, 1973, WB Saunders.

60. Hurst JW, Logue RB, Schlant RC, Wenger NK, editors: *The heart, arteries and veins*, New York, 1978, McGraw-Hill.

61. Braunwald E, editor: *Heart disease—a textbook of cardiovascular medicine*, Philadelphia, 1980, WB Saunders.

62. Kerley P: Cardiac failure. In Shanks SC, Kerley P, editors: *A textbook of x-ray diagnosis*, ed 3, Philadelphia, 1962, WB Saunders.

63. Race GA, Scheifley CM, Edwards JE: Hydrothorax in congestive heart failure, *Am J Med* 22:83, 1957.

64. Peterman TA, Brothers SK: Pleural effusions in congestive heart failure and pericardial disease, *N Engl J Med* 309:313, 1983.

65. Weiss JM, Spodick DM: Laterality of pleural effusions in congestive heart failure, *Am J Cardiol* 53:951, 1984.

66. Milne ENC: A physiologic approach to reading critical care unit films, *J Thorac Imaging* 1(3):60, 1986.

67. Wiener-Kronish JP, Broaddus VC, Albertine KA et al: Relationship of pleural effusions to increased permeability pulmonary edema in anesthetized sheep, *J Clin Invest* 82:1422, 1988.

68. Maruyama Y, Little JB: Roentgen manifestations of traumatic fat embolism, *Radiology* 79:945, 1962.

69. Berrigan TJ, Carsky EW, Heitzman ER: Fat embolism: roentgenographic pathologic correlation in three cases, *AJR* 96:967, 1966.

70. Joffe N: The adult respiratory distress syndrome, *AJR* 122:719, 1974.

71. Ostendorf P, Birsle M, Vogel W, Mittermayer C: Pulmonary radiographic abnormalities in shock, *Radiology* 115:257, 1975.

72. Halmagyi DFJ: Role of lymphatics in the genesis of shock lung.

In Staub NC, editor: *Lung water and solute exchange*, New York, 1978, Marcel Dekker, p 423.

73. Pistolesi M, Miniati M, Ravelli V, Giuntini C: Injury versus hydrostatic lung edema: detection by chest x-ray, *Ann NY Acad Sci* 384:364, 1982.

74. Divertie MB: The adult respiratory distress syndrome, *Mayo Clin Proc* 57:371, 1982.

75. Underwood GM, Newell JD: Pulmonary radiology in the intensive care unit, *Med Clin North Am* 67:1305, 1983.

76. Sibbald WJ, Cunningham DR, Chin DN: Non-cardiac or cardiac pulmonary edema: a practical approach in clinical differentiation of critically ill patients, *Chest* 84:452, 1983.

77. Milne ENC, Pistolesi M, Miniati M, Giuntini C: The radiologic distinction of cardiogenic and non-cardiogenic edema, *AJR* 144:879, 1985.

78. Iannuzzi M, Petty TL: The diagnosis, pathogenesis and treatment of adult respiratory distress syndrome, *J Thorac Imaging* 1(3):1, 1986.

79. Miniati M, Pistolesi M, Paoletti P et al: Objective radiographic criteria to differentiate cardiac, renal, and injury lung edema, *Invest Radiol* 23:433, 1988.

80. Smith RC, Mann M, Greenspan RH et al: Radiographic differentiation between different etiologies of pulmonary edema, *Invest Radiol* 22:859, 1987.

81. Aberle DR, Wiener-Kronish JP, Webb WR, Matthay MA: Hydrostatic versus increased permeability pulmonary edema: diagnosis based on radiographic criteria in critically ill patients, *Radiology* 168:73, 1988.

82. Murray J: *The normal lung*, Philadelphia, 1976, WB Saunders.

83. DeSousa LA: Vascularization of the parietal pleura: experimental study, *Angiology* 17:460, 1966.

84. Gray H: Anatomy, descriptive and surgical. In Gray H, Pick TP, Hamden R: *Gray's anatomy*, revised American version from the 15th English edition, 1977, Crown.

85. Payne DK, Kinasewitz GT, Gonzales E: Comparative permeability of canine visceral and parietal pleura, *J Appl Physiol* 65:2558, 1988.

86. Miserocchi G, Negrini D: Contribution of Starling and lymphatic flows to pleural liquid exchanges in anesthetized rabbits, *J Appl Physiol* 61:325, 1986.

87. Miserocchi G, Negrini D, Mariani E, Passafaro M: Reabsorption of saline or plasma induced hydrothorax, *J Appl Physiol* 54:1574, 1983.

88. Nakamura T, Tanaka Y, Fukabori T et al: The role of lymphatics in removing pleural liquid in discrete hydrothorax, *Eur Respir J* 1:826, 1988.

89. Miserocchi G, Pistolesi M, Miniati M et al: Pleural liquid pressure gradients and intrapleural distribution of injected bolus, *J Appl Physiol* 56:526, 1984.

90. Miserocchi G, Negrini D, Pistolesi M et al: Intrapleural liquid flow down a gravity dependent hydraulic pressure gradient, *J Appl Physiol* 64:577, 1988.

6 Quantification of Pulmonary Blood Volume, Flow, and Pressure: Principles

Among all the organs of the body, the lung is unique in that its capacity to hold blood (pulmonary vascular bed capacity) is normally very much greater than the amount of blood contained within it (pulmonary blood volume, PBV). Therefore from 30% to 50% of the pulmonary vascular bed is unfilled or only partially filled, from 30% to 50%, varying with the state of hydration and whether the patient is erect or supine. In the erect position, gravity causes greater filling of the lower lobe (LL) vessels, and the ratio of upper lobe (UL) to LL vessel size is normally 0.6/1.0 to 0.8/1.0 (Fig. 6-1). In the supine position the UL/LL ratio is approximately 1.0/1.0.[1,2]

The empty ("recruitable") vessels are ready at all times to accommodate either acute or chronic increases in pulmonary blood flow and volume, with little or no increase in pulmonary arterial driving pressure. This low resistance to flow is reflected in the thin walls of the readily distensible right ventricle, which is designed to handle low pressures, normally 10 to 30 mm Hg. This contrasts with the much less distensible left ventricular wall, which is about five times as thick, designed to handle systemic pressures five to six times as great. The difference in distensibility of the two cardiac chambers matches that of the right and left sides of the vascular pedicle. The heart therefore behaves very similar to the pedicle in its response to increased circulating blood volume. That is, the right ventricle responds

much more than the left, normally matching exactly the pedicle's behavior (see Figs. 4-24, 4-25, and 4-27).

A further result of the low resistance of the pulmonary microvascular bed is that even small increases in *regional* resistance cause a redistribution of flow away from that area into the lower-resistance area. Even though the increased resistance that caused the redistribution is usually at the microscopic or ultrastructural level, its existence and location can usually be deduced from the pattern of redistribution. Changes in flow distribution and PBV have considerable diagnostic significance.[3-34]

In addition to the diagnostic value of assessing flow distribution and PBV (see later discussion), regional or global changes in the appearance of the pulmonary arteries and veins give valuable diagnostic information about many different types of pulmonary and cardiac disease.[35-40] Therefore one must be familiar with the appearances of normal pulmonary arteries and veins, normal pulmonary blood flow and distribution, and the relationship between PBV and systemic blood volume (determined from vascular pedicle width). One must also understand how these parameters are controlled.

Fortunately, lungs have another unique property. The *conducting* blood vessels, down to approximately 3 to 4 mm in diameter which are the smallest vessels resolvable on the conventional chest radiograph, are outlined by air, forming a true "in vivo angiogram." The radiopaque blood within the vessels acts as a contrast medium, contrasting with the surrounding radiolucent air. This permits one to visualize the pulmonary vascular bed very easily on the plain chest radiograph.

PULMONARY ARTERIES AND VEINS
Pulmonary Arteries

An important, frequently overlooked visual property of the pulmonary arteries is their *sinuosity*.[14-16,39] The pulmonary arteries have regularly occurring, slightly alternating bends in their walls. They branch dichotomously (except for some right-angle branches too small to be seen on the radiograph), tapering gradually, with no abrupt change in caliber from the hilum to the lung's periphery, and ending (to the eye) approximately 1.0 cm from the chest wall. This leaves a "clear zone" around the periphery of the lung crammed with millions of vessels too small to resolve radiologically. This

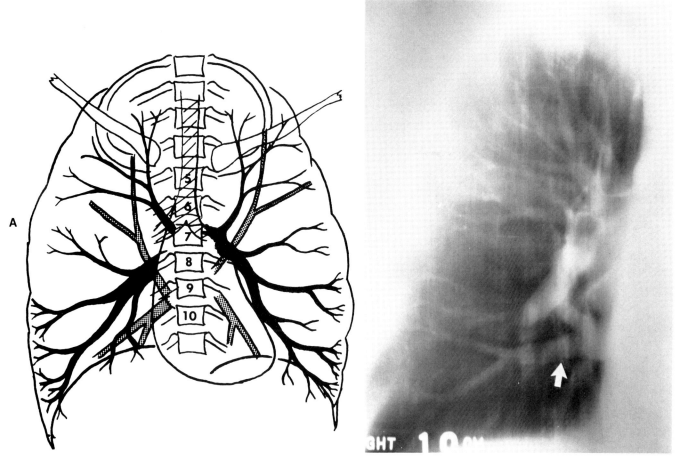

Fig. 6-1   A, Diagram of erect patient's chest. The upper lobe (UL) veins and arteries are smaller than the LL vessels; the usual UL/LL vessel size ratio is 0.6:1.0 to 0.8:1.0 in the erect position. Note the slight sinuosity of the pulmonary arteries (in *black*) and the parallel-sided appearance of the veins. **B,** Linear computed tomogram with the patient supine shows the distinctive parallel-sided appearance of normal pulmonary veins *(arrow).* LL and UL arteries and veins match approximately in size in the supine position (UL/LL 1.0:1.0).

same clear peripheral zone exists around every lobe, segment, subsegment, and lobule within the lungs (Fig. 6-2).

Normal vessels demonstrate only a narrow range of sinuosity. Any visible *decrease* in sinuosity is pathologic; the most common cause is emphysema, either true or compensatory[39] (Fig. 6-3). Any visible *increase* in sinuosity is also pathologic, with the exception that sinuosity normally increases slightly on expiratory x-ray films. The most frequent pathologic cause of increased sinuosity is the structural vascular change of pulmonary arterial hypertension, often seen in patients with chronic bronchitis, longstanding chronic heart failure, mitral valve disease, and long-standing left-to-right

shunts* (Fig. 6-4). This simple finding has useful diagnostic connotations, as discussed later.

Some have suggested that increased sinuosity ("tortuosity") of the pulmonary vessels sufficient to be readily visible radiologically occurs when the pulmonary artery pressure (PAP) reaches the 60 mm Hg level,[41-43] at which point pathologically demonstrable vascular changes are present (Fig. 6-5). However, the ability to recognize variations outside the narrow normal range of sinuosity may allow the film reader to discern beginning tortuosity at lower PAP levels than this (see later discussion).

---

*References 5,6,8-11,13,15,17,20-24,30-32.

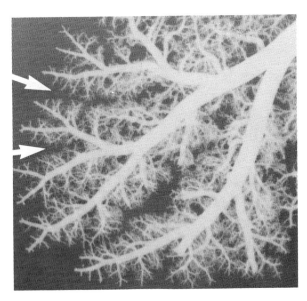

Fig. 6-2 Latex rubber cast of a lung segment, filling arteries only. Note the slight sinuosity of the vessels and the clear peripheral zone around each lobule. The clear "watershed" area between the peripheral lobules *(white arrows)* is the interlobular septum, and fluid accumulating in these septa in the lung periphery causes Kerley-B lines.

Pulmonary Veins

The pulmonary veins do not branch dichotomously and do not divide regularly and smoothly in size toward the periphery as do the pulmonary arteries. Instead, the veins increase in rather abrupt steps *from* the periphery toward the left atrium by accepting tributaries in a monopodial fashion. Where the veins are large, toward the lung's center, they have a parallel-walled appearance quite different to that of the tapering arteries (see Fig. 6-4). In addition, the course of the pulmonary veins, leading toward the left atrium and well below the level of the hilar origins of the pulmonary arteries, helps to differentiate them from the arteries. The easiest vein to recognize crosses from the right lower lobe above the cardiophrenic angle to enter the left atrium. It can be seen in 65% to 75% of all chest films (see Fig. 6-4). The upper lobe veins are much more difficult to recognize and can be confidently identified in only 35% to 50% of patients.[16] However, this difficulty gives the film reader some advantage; that is, if they are easy to visualize, this suggests that they are excessively well filled and that flow redistribution is occurring, either inversion or balanced flow.[27,28]

The differentiation between arteries and veins without angiography is virtually impossible in the periphery of the lung, but the ability to separate veins from arteries in the center of the lung is very useful diagnostically.

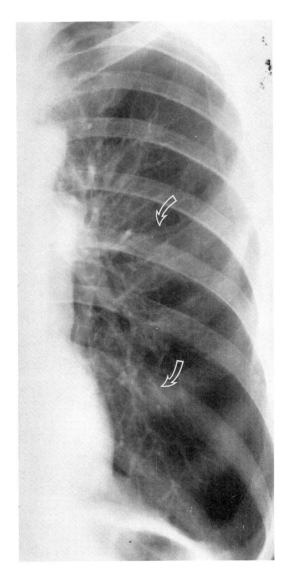

Fig. 6-3 Severe "pure" emphysema. The pulmonary arteries have lost their normal sinuosity and are now straight *(open arrows)*.

Arterial/Venous Size Ratio

At the same distance from the heart, normally the veins draining a lung region are approximately equal in size to the arteries supplying that region; that is, the arterial/venous (A/V) size ratio is approximately 1:1 (see Fig. 6-4). If circulating blood volume increases, PBV and pulmonary flow also increase, as manifested by a simultaneous global increase in the size of both arteries and veins[7] (Fig. 6-6). Similarly, if flow redistribution is present, the increased flow to the low-resistance region is also manifested by an increase in size of both the pulmonary arteries and the pulmonary veins* (Fig. 6-7). Probably the most dramatic example of arterial and venous size both increasing to reflect regional flow is a

*References 3,6,9,14,15,20.

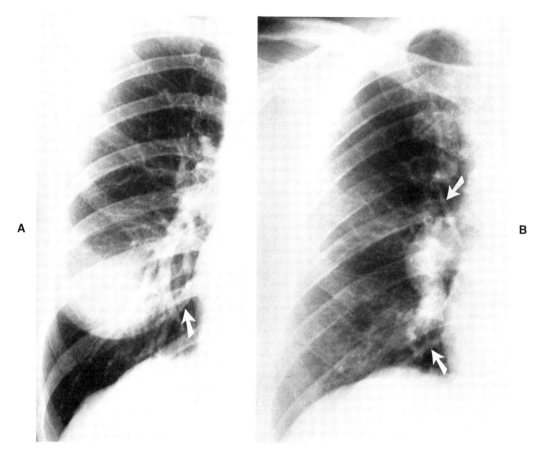

Fig. 6-4 **A,** Pulmonary vascular bed is normal. The slightly sinuous arteries should be compared with the parallel-sided vein *(white arrow).* The arterial/venous (A/V) size ratio is approximately 1:1. Contrast this with **B,** showing a patient with chronic bronchitis and far advanced pulmonary arterial hypertension. The proximal pulmonary artery is dilated and tortuous, whereas the peripheral branches are smaller than normal and are difficult to see ("pruning"). The pulmonary veins are very small *(arrows),* and the A/V ratio is approximately 5:1. Note typical thickened bronchial wall of patients with bronchitis.

large, intrathoracic arteriovenous (AV) fistula (Fig. 6-8). PBV can be increased *without* any increase in circulating blood volume in patients with a left-to-right shunt. Under these circumstances the entire pulmonary vascular bed can fill, giving a 1:1 flow distribution, and the arteries and veins both increase in size, resulting in a 1:1 A/V ratio (Fig. 6-9).

Although venous *narrowing* together with proximal arterial *enlargement* (see Fig. 6-4, *B*) almost invariably means pulmonary arterial hypertension, *absence* of narrowing does not invariably mean a normal PAP. For example, in the rather rare instance of pulmonary venous thrombosis, the veins are blocked and pulmonary arterial hypertension is present, but the caliber of the veins is not reduced.

Similarly, in association with large left-to-right intrapulmonary shunts, the pulmonary veins become very large. Then, when pathologic change develops in

the pulmonary arterioles, the veins decrease somewhat in size toward normal but may not become smaller than normal.

Precisely why the veins diminish in size in association with pulmonary arterial hypertension remains somewhat of a mystery. The usual theory is that decreased *flow* through the veins in patients with pulmonary arterial hypertension causes the veins to diminish in size, but this is probably incorrect. We believe that the decreased venous size in both pulmonary arterial hypertension and pulmonary venous hypertension is caused by functional vasoconstriction (see sections on flow redistribution).

NORMAL PULMONARY BLOOD VOLUME

As mentioned earlier, pulmonary vascular bed capacity (PVBC) normally exceeds PBV, but the physiologic literature does not clearly indicate what dictates the

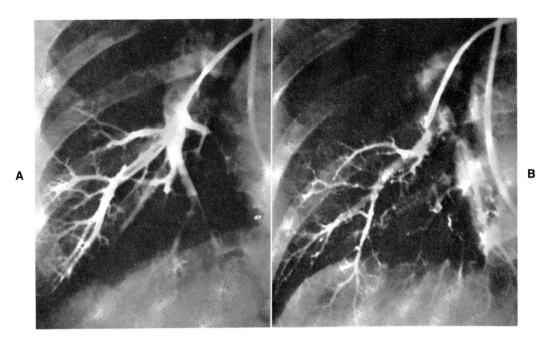

Fig. 6-5 A, Patient with mitral valve disease but *normal* pulmonary artery pressure (PAP). **B,** Patient with mitral valve disease and PAP of 65/30 mm Hg. The smaller branches are narrowed and tortuous. (From Steiner RE, Harrison CJ, Goodwin JF: In Ciba Foundation Study Group No 8; de Reuck AVS, O'Connor M, editors: *Problems of pulmonary circulation,* London, 1961, JA Churchill.)

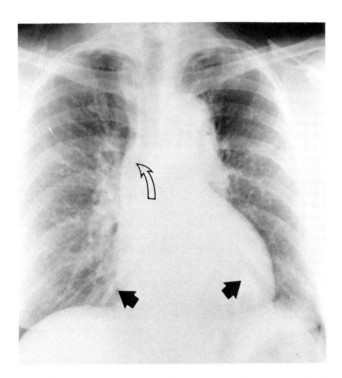

Fig. 6-6 Increased circulating blood volume in patient with renal failure manifested by wide vascular pedicle and large azygos vein *(open arrow)* and 1:1 flow distribution with vessels filled to the apices. Note large draining veins matched in size with the engorged arteries *(black arrows).*

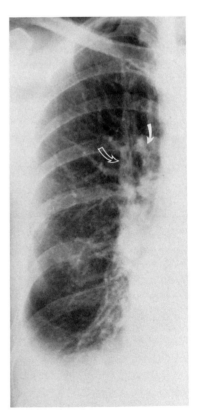

Fig. 6-7 The lung is incarcerated at the base by an organized, thickened pleura, causing a functional redistribution of flow to the upper lobes, with matching engorgement of arteries *(closed arrow)* and veins *(open arrow).*

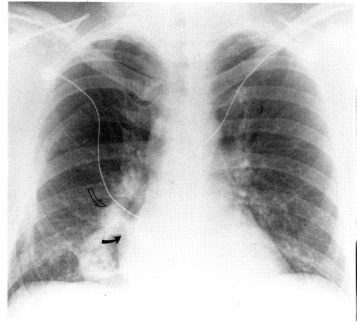

A

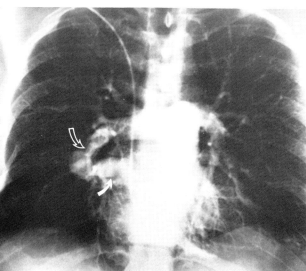

B

Fig. 6-8   A, Radiograph of 21-year-old male with traumatic pulmonary arteriovenous (AV) fistula after a stab wound 5 years previously. A dilated feeding artery *(open arrow)* and massive draining vein *(closed arrow)* are seen. **B,** Angiogram shows the artery *(open arrow)* and huge draining vein *(closed arrow)*. Note that the second loculation of the large AV fistula, seen on the plain film, has not filled because it lies anteriorly. The gravitational effect of the patient's supine position on the contrast medium has caused it to fill only the posterior (dependent) portion.

size of the normal PBV. The PBV in any individual is not fixed but varies around a mean value.[7]

Factors Affecting Normal Pulmonary Blood Volume

Alveolar and Interstitial Pressure. On inspiration, increasing negative pleural pressure is transferred across the lung to the interstitium, resulting in a "pulling open" of the conducting vessels (i.e., the vessels not involved in gas exchange), with a resultant increase in PBV[44-47] (Fig. 6-10). On expiration the interstitial pressure becomes less negative; the conducting vessels become smaller and the PBV decreases. These changes are readily seen on the plain chest radiograph. The pumping action of blood flow through the lung by this mechanism is so effective that it can maintain life for a time in the absence of a functioning heart and has therefore been called the "auxiliary heart."[48]

The conducting vessels (down to approximately 30 μm) are affected by the lung's interstitial pressure, but not directly by the alveolar pressure and are therefore

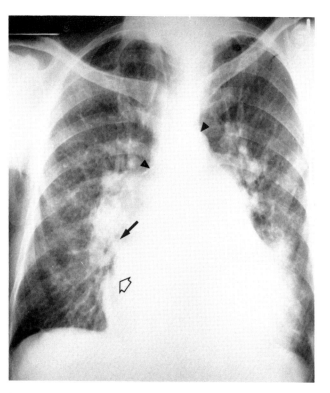

Fig. 6-9   Patient with large atrial septal defect. Note the extremely narrow pedicle *(arrowheads)* and the massive draining veins, upper *(black arrow)* and lower *(open arrow)*.

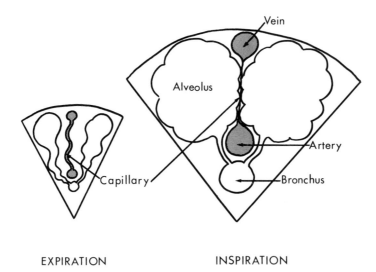

EXPIRATION   INSPIRATION

Fig. 6-10   Diagram of a portion of a lung lobule. The bronchus and artery enter centrally (within the interstitium, i.e., "extraalveolar"). The artery divides into capillaries running between the alveoli ("alveolar" vessels), and the peripheral veins lie also in an extraalveolar interstitial position. On inspiration the increasing negativity of the interstitium pulls open the artery and vein (extraalveolar vessels), making them larger, but the increase in alveolar size stretches and narrows the capillaries (alveolar vessels).

called "extraalveolar" vessels.[47] In contrast, the microvessels (invisible to the radiologist) involved in gas exchange, ramifying around and between the alveoli, are directly affected by alveolar pressure and are called "alveolar" vessels.[47]

In contrast with the visible increase in blood within the *extraalveolar* vessels that occurs on inspiration, the enlarged alveoli squeeze and elongate the *alveolar* vessels, resulting in a (radiologically invisible) reduction in microvascular volume and an increase in pulmonary vascular resistance (Fig. 6-10). This is an important phenomenon in patients who are placed on positive-pressure ventilation. The higher the ventilating pressure, the more difficult it is for blood to pass through the microvascular bed. When the intrathoracic pressure rises high enough, even the extraalveolar vessels begin to be affected, and narrowing of the larger, radiologically visible conducting vessels can be seen.

Body Habitus. Obviously a large person normally has a greater PBV and a small person a lesser PBV; that is, a relationship exists between PBV and size or, more accurately, between PBV and surface area. Therefore, in considering two persons of the same size, but with one being thin and one fat, the fat subject will have the greater PBV.[49] The film reader should therefore be prepared to accept slight hyperemia as being normal in obese patients but abnormal in thin patients.

Right Ventricular Output. PBV is clearly related to right ventricular output.[16,50,51] Radiologists are accustomed to seeing large PBVs (hyperemia) in patients with left-to-right shunts (Fig. 6-11) and large right ventricular outputs and to seeing small PBVs (oligemia) in patients with dehydration or Addison's disease (Fig. 6-12). The relationship between right-sided heart output and PBV volume is, unfortunately for the film reader, not quite linear.[16] To understand this, one should consider briefly some properties of the pulmonary vascular bed.[7]

If the pulmonary vascular bed was equivalent to a single tube with *rigid* walls (Fig. 6-13), increasing right ventricular output through this tube clearly would not cause any change in PBV. Any increase in flow would have to be mediated through a *reduction* in *transit time* of blood through the lungs. This could only be achieved by a marked increase in right ventricular driving pressure, which does not reflect the human lung's behavior. If the pulmonary vascular bed was considered again as a single tube, but now with very compliant walls, the same increase in flow would cause an increase in PBV and a lesser reduction in transit time and would require a lesser increase in right ventricular driving pressure (Fig. 6-13). This is closer to the lung's normal behavior but again requires too great an increase in right ventricular pressure to reflect this normal behavior. Instead, one could consider the lung's vascular bed to consist of a number of tubes in parallel with very compliant walls.

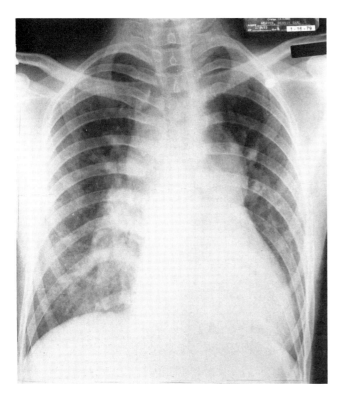

Fig. 6-11   Very large pulmonary blood volume (PBV) in a patient with total anomalous venous return and a large atrial septal defect causing a massive right ventricular output. Contrast with Fig. 6-12.

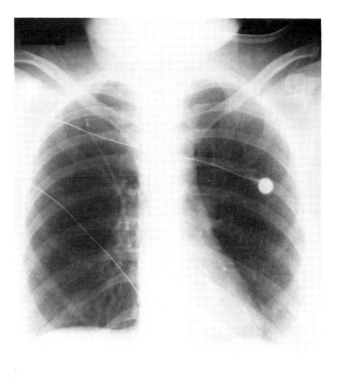

Fig. 6-12   Very small PBV (marked oligemia) in a burned patient. "Third-spacing" into his burned tissues effectively dehydrates him and causes a small right ventricular output.

The same increase in right ventricular output can now be accommodated with minimal or no change in right ventricular pressure, with a small increase in PBV and a small decrease in transit time (Fig. 6-13). This equates with the lung's normal behavior. However, the speed with which blood can be passed through the lung (transit time) has a limit; therefore, as right ventricular output increases still further, PBV must also increase. With very high right ventricular outputs, usually only resulting from massive left-to-right shunts, the pulmonary vascular bed may eventually become completely filled. That is, all the previously empty or partially filled vessels in the upper lung are recruited, and a 1:1 "balanced" distribution of flow exists (Fig. 6-14). Note that the same 1:1 balanced distribution of flow will occur with a greatly increased circulating blood volume caused by overhydration or renal failure[16,52] (see Fig. 6-6).

If one now considers that the compliance of the vascular bed may be modified pathologically or neurohormonally (i.e., that the vessel walls can "tense" and "untense"), this compliance can be functionally decreased, effectively turning the vascular bed into the stiff-walled tube originally postulated. Any attempt to increase

PBF through this stiff vascular bed would result in much higher right ventricular pressures (see Fig. 6-13). This tensing probably occurs with marked elevation of left atrial pressure, such as in severe mitral stenosis and left-sided heart failure, as discussed more fully later. Similarly, tensing of the capillaries at the venous end of the microvascular bed, resulting in gross elevation of pulmonary *arterial* pressure, would appear to be the mechanism in neurogenic pulmonary edema.[53,54]

Using an isolated lung preparation, we have shown that a good relationship exists between right ventricular output and PBV (Fig. 6-15). This same relationship has been extensively documented in normal subjects and in patients with cardiac disease.[16,50,51,55] Increasing right ventricular output in a subject with a normal heart and pulmonary vascular bed is mediated principally by decreased transit time with only minimally increased PBV; that is, one cannot recognize the increase from the chest radiograph. However, increasing right ventricular output in patients with cardiac *disease* is mediated by a lesser reduction in transit time and a greater increase in PBV, which one can recognize radiologically.

Whether a given PBV will fill only the bases of the

Fig. 6-13 **A,** Considering the lung as a single rigid tube. If the plunger in the pump is depressed to provide a flow of X liters per unit of time, the volume in the right tube is Y liters, transit time *(TT)* is 1 unit, and the pressure required to generate this flow is 1 Z unit. **B,** If flow is now doubled, the volume Y cannot increase. Therefore, to increase the flow, TT must decrease by one half, and pressure must be much higher. **C,** If the lung were a single *compliant* tube, a flow of X would cause an increase in volume and a slight increase in TT. **D,** If flow is now doubled through this compliant tube, volume will increase greatly and TT will increase slightly. **E,** If the lung is considered as a set of compliant tubes in parallel, flow can be maintained with a much lower pulmonary artery pressure. **F,** If flow is doubled in this very compliant system, the blood volume will increase greatly, but pressure will not need to increase much. The high flow state will tend to fill all the vascular bed, resulting in a 1:1 flow distribution. **G,** With a pulmonary vascular bed consisting of a set of parallel compliant tubes in which tonus can be modified neurogenically, the amount of pressure required to double flow will increase as compliance diminishes, and TT will decrease. **F** and **G** appear to reflect best the human lung's behavior. (From Milne ENC: *Radiol Clin North Am* 16:515, 1978.)

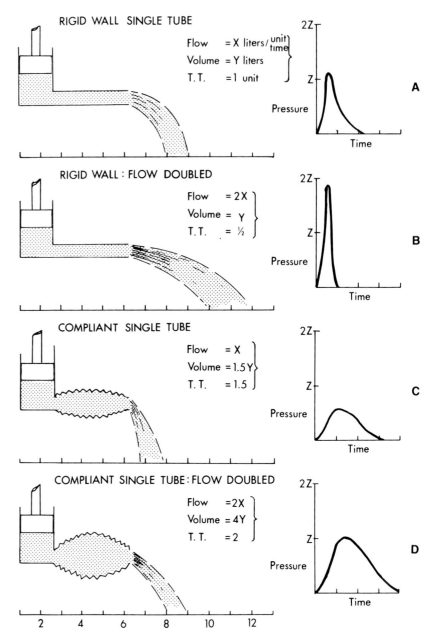

lungs, giving the usual 0.6:1.0 to 0.8:1.0 UL/LL ratio, or will fill all the lungs, giving a "balanced" 1.0:1.0 UL/LL ratio, clearly depends on the PVBC, which can be altered by many different organic and functional causes (see the box on p. 175). Conversely, if the PVBC is fixed, flow distribution will depend on the PBV, which can also be altered by several factors (see box).

Factors Causing Increased Pulmonary Blood Volume

Physiologic. In the erect position, as PBV increases, the empty (recruitable) UL vessels progressively fill and the UL arteries and veins begin to enlarge (see

Figs. 6-6 and 6-14). The oligemia of the UL disappears, changing the usual 0.6 to 0.8:1.0 flow ratio progressively to a 1.0:1.0 or balanced distribution of flow. Conversely, when PBV decreases below normal, the ULs become even more oligemic, and the UL/LL flow ratio decreases (e.g., to 0.5:1.0). Any change in PBV, whether increase or decrease, must be accompanied by some change in flow distribution.

Virtually the only physiologic cause of a global increase in PBV, besides assuming the supine position, is pregnancy. The circulating blood volume, particularly during the second trimester, may increase by as much as 33%,[56] causing the lungs to appear hyperemic and the vascular pedicle width and azygos vein to enlarge

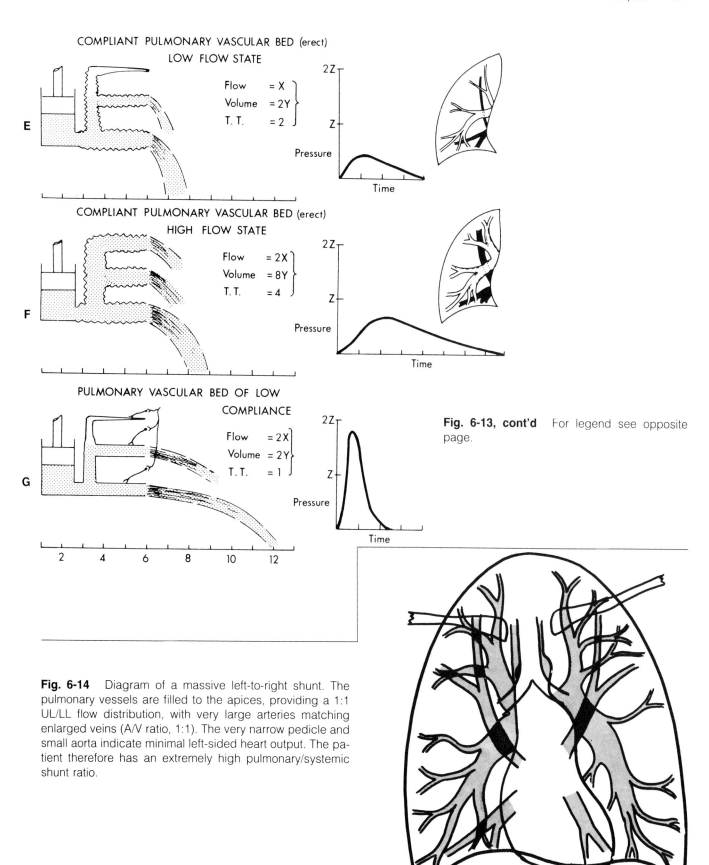

COMPLIANT PULMONARY VASCULAR BED (erect)
LOW FLOW STATE

E

Flow = X
Volume = 2Y
T. T. = 2

COMPLIANT PULMONARY VASCULAR BED (erect)
HIGH FLOW STATE

F

Flow = 2X
Volume = 8Y
T. T. = 4

PULMONARY VASCULAR BED OF LOW COMPLIANCE

G

Flow = 2X
Volume = 2Y
T. T. = 1

Fig. 6-13, cont'd For legend see opposite page.

Fig. 6-14 Diagram of a massive left-to-right shunt. The pulmonary vessels are filled to the apices, providing a 1:1 UL/LL flow distribution, with very large arteries matching enlarged veins (A/V ratio, 1:1). The very narrow pedicle and small aorta indicate minimal left-sided heart output. The patient therefore has an extremely high pulmonary/systemic shunt ratio.

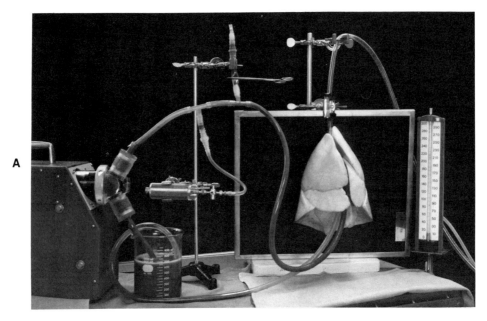

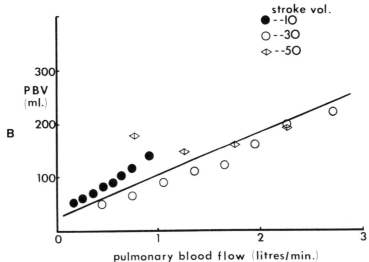

Fig. 6-15 **A,** Isolated lung preparation. A Harvard pump, which permits stroke volume and stroke rate to be varied at will, pumps blood through the inflated lung. The manometer measures lung inflation pressure. The metal transducer at the level of the left atrium measures pulmonary artery pressure. The level in the graduated beaker indicates whether PBV has increased or decreased. **B,** Result in one lung of progressively raising pulmonary blood flow at three different stroke volumes. The PBV increases progressively as pulmonary blood flow (right-sided "heart" output) is increased. No statistical difference occurs whether the stroke volume is small (10 ml) or large (50 ml).

but rarely producing a complete 1:1 redistribution of flow. This amount of redistribution would be so unusual that a 1:1 flow distribution during pregnancy should make one suspect underlying pathology, usually renal decompensation.

It has been suggested that a high salt intake might lead to increased circulating blood volume. When we gave increasing amounts of salt to healthy volunteers,

however, we found no radiologic evidence of increased circulating blood volume.

Pathologic

Global. It is widely believed that the most common pathologic cause of increased PBV is cardiac failure. However, many authors[51,57,58] have clearly shown that PBV actually *decreases* during acute cardiac failure and

REDISTRIBUTION OF PULMONARY BLOOD FLOW: FACTORS AFFECTING PULMONARY VASCULAR BED CAPACITY (PVBC) AND PULMONARY BLOOD VOLUME (PBV)

Pulmonary vascular bed capacity

A. *Functional* changes
1. Level of inflation (related to the ability to generate a negative interstitial pressure and therefore affected by chest wall pain, subdiaphragmatic pathology, and pleural pain)
2. Increased left atrial pressure, leading to functional closure (regional "loss") of lower lobe vessels
3. Alveolar pressure (increase)
   Regional
   a. Asthma
   b. Foreign body
   c. Mucous plugs
   d. Mucosal edema
   e. Postobliterative bronchiolitis
   f. Extrinsic pressure on bronchus
   General
   a. Valsalva maneuver
   b. Status asthmaticus
   c. Smoke inhalation
   d. Alveolar pressure (decrease)
   e. Müller maneuver
4. Interstitial pressure (increase: absolute or relative)
   Regional
   a. Chest wall pain or immobilization
   b. Pleural pain, thickening, or effusion
   c. Diaphragmatic paralysis or eventration
   d. Carcinoma or consolidation
   General: inability to move diaphragm (e.g., ascites, abdominal tumor, amyotrophic lateral sclerosis, pneumoperitoneum, corsets)
5. Pulmonary edema (through its effects on compliance, interstitial pressure, and oxygenation)
6. Blood gas levels (e.g., unilateral bronchial obstruction, bronchography, Carlens catheter, high-altitude hypoxia, regional hypoxia, hypercarbia)
7. Pharmacologic agents

B. *Organic* changes (general or regional)
1. Emphysema*
2. Fibrosis*
3. Embolism* (acute)
4. Sarcoidosis* (direct involvement of vessels)
5. Infiltration* or neoplasm
6. Endarteritis obliterans[†]
7. Microembolism/schistosomiasis[†]
8. Embolism (chronic)[†]
9. Venoocclusive disease[†]
10. Bodily habitus (acromegaly, pituitary dwarfism)

Note: all those entities that cause *regional* loss of PVBC also cause regional decrease in *flow.*

Pulmonary blood volume
Increased flow

A. *Functional* changes
   General
   1. Exercise
   2. Pregnancy
   3. Pyrexia
   4. Anemia
   5. Thyrotoxicosis
   6. Renal failure[‡]
   7. Overhydration with blood
   8. Overhydration with saline
   9. Hypoxia[§]
   10. Pharmacologic agents (bradykinin, isoproterenol, aminophylline)
   Regional: gravitational (e.g., increased flow to apex)
B. *Organic* changes
   General
   1. Intra- or extracardiac shunt
   2. Pulmonary and peripheral arteriovenous anomalies (including Paget's disease)
   Regional
   1. Anomalous venous return
   2. Systemic arterial supply to the lung
   3. Regional bronchial arterial hypertrophy

Decreased flow

A. *Functional* changes: general
1. Dehydration
2. Hypothyroidism
3. Addison's disease
4. Pharmacologic agents (serotonin, histamine, catecholamines, atrionatriuretic factor)
B. *Organic* changes: general
1. Cardiac failure
2. Valvular disease (aortic, mitral, pulmonary, tricuspid)
3. Myocardiopathy
4. Pericardial tamponade

---

*(In addition to organic change, these conditions also affect PVBC *functionally* by their effect on pulmonary interstitial pressure.

[†]When changes in the pulmonary vascular bed are generalized enough to cause increased pulmonary vascular resistance, the PBV may *decrease* on the venous side while increasing on the arterial and precapillary side.

[‡]Accompanied by increase in extravascular lung water and change in interstitial pressure.

[§]Radiologic effects differ greatly, depending on whether hypoxia is regional or general (e.g., high altitude).

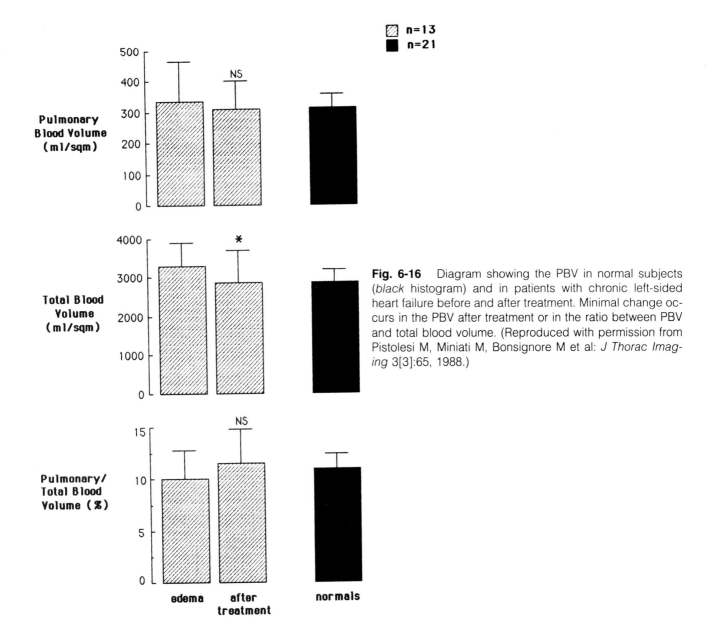

Fig. 6-16 Diagram showing the PBV in normal subjects (*black* histogram) and in patients with chronic left-sided heart failure before and after treatment. Minimal change occurs in the PBV after treatment or in the ratio between PBV and total blood volume. (Reproduced with permission from Pistolesi M, Miniati M, Bonsignore M et al: *J Thorac Imaging* 3[3]:65, 1988.)

that it remains either unchanged or increases only slightly in patients with chronic left-sided heart failure, possibly varying with the degree of renal hypoperfusion (Fig. 6-16). It is probable that the radiologist receives an *impression* that the PBV is increased in patients with chronic left-sided heart failure because inversion of flow from the bases to the apices occurs, causing hyperemia ("congestion") of the ULs. However, the *reduced* volume of the LL vessels may not be appreciated because of overlying edema. Flow inversion is discussed more fully later.

The most frequent pathologic causes of a global increase in PBV, resulting in "balanced" flow, are overhydration or renal failure (Fig. 6-17),[16,52] which do not invariably produce the same radiologic changes (see

Chapter 8). Large left-to-right shunts also cause increased PBV, reflecting the great increase in right-sided heart output. In these patients, however, a dissociation exists between the large PBV and the small systemic blood volume, which is reflected in the narrow vascular pedicle[16,59-61] (see Figs. 6-9 and 6-14 and box on p. 175).

Regional. Regional increases in PBV, besides those caused by gravity, usually occur only because of a regional reduction in PVBC elsewhere, causing blood to be redistributed from the damaged area of the lung to the "good" lung, which then becomes hyperemic. The two usual causes of a regional increase in PBV are alterations in lung structure and cardiac disease. The two frequently coexist (Fig. 6-18; see also box on p. 175).

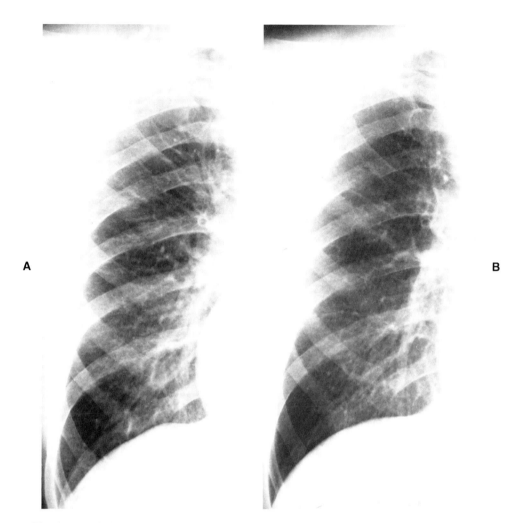

Fig. 6-17   A, Patient with renal failure before dialysis. Note filling of upper lobe vessels but no narrowing of lower lobe vessels, leading to a 1:1 flow distribution. Peribronchial cuffing indicates edema. **B,** After dialysis the flow ratio returns to normal. Bronchial cuffing is gone. (From Milne ENC, Pistolesi M: in Putnam CE: *Diagnostic imaging of the lung,* New York, 1990, Marcel Dekker; © 1989 ENC Milne.)

Factors Causing Decreased Pulmonary Blood Volume

Global. The only physiologic cause of a global reduction in PBV is dehydration. This can occur, for example, in runners and cyclists following marathons or triathlons (see Fig. 4-24).

Pathologic. The most common pathologic cause of global reduction in PBV is also dehydration, usually secondary to pyrexia, severe pneumonia, loss of blood, or Addisonian crisis (see Fig 4-27).

Iatrogenic dehydration often occurs in intensive care units (ICUs), for example, after using mannitol and similar agents to reduce circulating blood volume in patients with a head injury, intracranial bleeding, or a seizure.

In burn patients, so much third-spacing of fluids frequently occurs into the damaged tissues that the circulating blood volume becomes greatly reduced. The lungs may remain oligemic even with intravenous (IV) fluid therapy and a markedly positive fluid balance, provided the flow into the third spaces exceeds the flow into the "first" (intravascular) space.[60] Burn patients may also inhale hot gases, causing edema of their mucosa and narrowing of the bronchial lumen. This results in generalized air trapping on expiration, raising the intraalveolar pressure and causing a generalized reduction in PBV. The lungs of these patients can be startlingly oligemic for 12 to 36 hours, concealing the lung damage, which then begins to manifest itself by the development of lung edema caused by injury[60] (see box on p. 175).

Positive-pressure ventilation in the ICU is another typical cause of global reduction in PBV, caused by the increased intrathoracic pressure.[60]

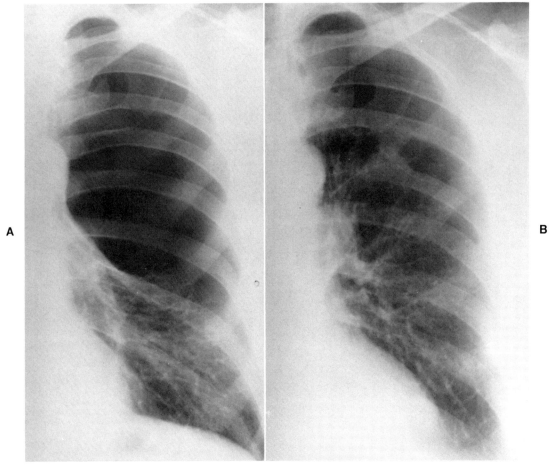

Fig. 6-18 **A,** Large bulla in left apex, which acts as a local pneumothorax, so that the remaining lung cannot be fully expanded. Flow is redistributed from the oligemic bullous upper lung into the bases. **B,** After bullectomy the negative pressure of the pleura can once again act on the lung, and it is now better expanded. Note that the basal flow is now less because some apical flow has been restored.

Table 6-1 Aortic stenosis: correlations between oligemia, cardiac chamber size, and pulmonary wedge (PWP) and pulmonary artery (PAP) pressures

	Rank order	
Correlations	*r*	*p*
Oligemia/stroke volume	0.96	0.007
PWP/mean PAP	0.90	0.0004
LV size/mean PAP	0.78	0.008
PWP/RV size	0.66	0.021
PWP/LV size	0.65	0.020
RV size/mean PAP	0.55	NS
PWP/oligemia	0.48	NS
Oligemia/RV size	0.31	NS
Oligemia/mean PAP	0.21	NS
Oligemia/LV size	0.09	NS

LV, RV, Left and right ventricles.
r, Correlation coefficient; *p*, probability.

A widely unrecognized cardiac cause of reduced blood volume is aortic valve disease (Fig. 6-19). We observed several years ago that the lungs in many patients with aortic stenosis were oligemic.[16] We hypothesized that the small PBV resulted from a low right ventricular output; this in turn was low because it had to match left ventricular output, which was reduced by the valvular obstruction to outflow.[*16] We recently completed a multicenter, multiobserver study and confirmed that most patients with aortic stenosis have radiologically identifiable lung oligemia caused by a reduced PBV.[62] Also, the oligemia correlates closely with left ventricular stroke volume: the lower the stroke volume, the greater the oligemia (Table 6-1). The left ventricle is ei-

*A second intriguing hypothesis is that the ventricular hypertrophy causes increased secretion of atrionatriuretic factor (ANF), which results in a reduction in *total* blood volume, explaining both the pulmonary oliguria and the narrow vascular pedicle.

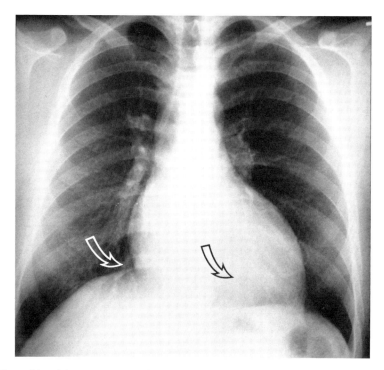

Fig. 6-19 "Classic" appearance of aortic stenosis in patient with oligemic lungs, reflecting small right ventricular output, and narrow veins *(open arrows),* reflecting venospasm to "protect" left atrial function. Narrow vascular pedicle also reflects reduced total blood volume (see text).

ther enlarged or shows increased convexity in many of these patients. The discrepant association of a large left side of the heart, small vascular pedicle, and oligemic lungs with normal flow distribution is particularly striking, since left-sided heart enlargement caused by chronic *ischemic* heart disease is usually associated with flow inversion, basal edema, a wide vascular pedicle, and relatively plethoric upper lung fields.

These new findings in patients with aortic stenosis are discussed more fully in Chapter 7. However, in general, if the film reader sees this unusual combination of oligemic lungs and enlarged left ventricle (Fig. 6-19), he or she should suggest that the diagnosis is aortic stenosis, "until proved otherwise," which in our experience rarely occurs.[33]

Regional

Physiologic. In approximately 16% of normal chest radiographs, the left lung, particularly the left UL, appears slightly oligemic compared with the right lung. This appears to be caused by a normal slight reduction in the number of vessels per cubic centimeter of lung on the left, related to a lower number of divisions of the pulmonary artery in the left than in the right lung.[63]

In addition to the usual functional oligemia of both ULs, there is an area in the right lung parallel to the upper and lower surfaces of the horizontal fissure. Here vessels to the anterior segment of the right UL diminish in size as they taper downward toward the periphery of the segment (i.e., lying above the fissure), and branches of the medial and lateral segments of the middle lobe taper similarly as they pass upward toward the horizontal fissure. The fissure therefore forms a "watershed" between the two segments, and the adjoining peripheral vessel-free clear zones of the two segments cause a relatively oligemic area. This was first described in 1969 on the plain film as the "vascular window" of the right lung[39] and was rediscovered on computed tomographic (CT) scans as the oligemic area abutting the horizontal fissure. Its particular diagnostic importance is that it should not be mistaken for oligemia distal to an embolus.

Pathologic. Probably the best publicized pathologic variety of regional oligemia is the "Westermark" sign, that is, oligemia distal to a pulmonary embolus. A remarkable aspect of this sign is its infrequent occurrence. In one large series of patients with pulmonary embolism, the Westermark sign was seen in only 6% to 7%.[64] A physical block to a vessel does not itself produce visible oligemia; for example, an entire pulmonary artery to one lung can be blocked off with an inflated balloon, with no or minimal visible reduction in the PBV distal to the balloon.[65-67] Similarly, the lung distal to a wedged catheter does not develop oligemia. The

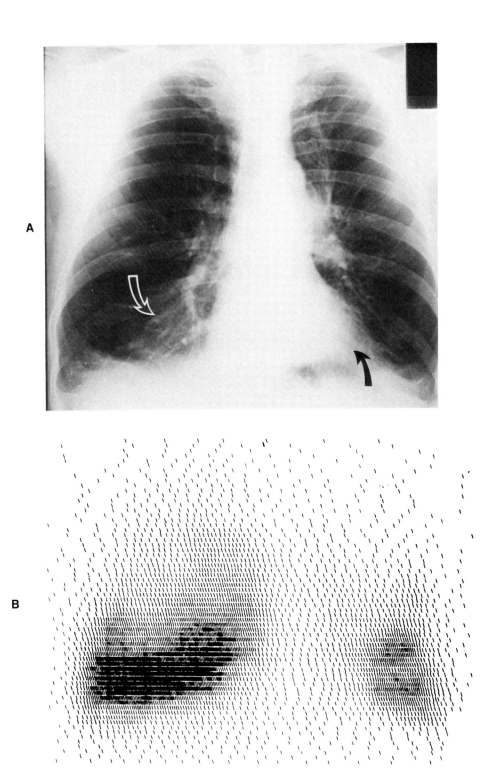

Fig. 6-20   A, This patient has extensive regional emphysema that is sparing only the right lung's base (note large vessels *[open white arrow]* and left apex). The heart's apex shows the classic elevation of right-sided heart enlargement *(closed arrow).* **B,** Radionuclide scan confirms the "organic" redistribution of flow to the only relatively normal area of the lung.

lack of oligemia distal to a block results partly because (1) the lung vessels can be held open by negative pressure whether or not active flow exists in them; (2) bronchial arterial flow occurs distal to the block, so flow does not completely cease; and (3) the veins continue to fill by reflux from the atrium during atrial systole. Oligemia distal to a blood clot is therefore not caused by the physical blockage but by vasospasm due to breakdown products of the clot, such as serotonin and 5-hydroxytryptamine.

A much more frequent cause of regional oligemia is local or randomly distributed lung disease, particularly emphysema (Fig. 6-20; see also Chapter 9).

Left UL oligemia occurring in patients with mitral stenosis (MS) was described in the 1940s and appears to be a genuine finding, although the 16% of normal patients with a slightly oligemic left lung makes it difficult to assess how often oligemia due to MS occurs. Some have hypothesized that the oligemia results from displacement or compression of left UL veins, caused by

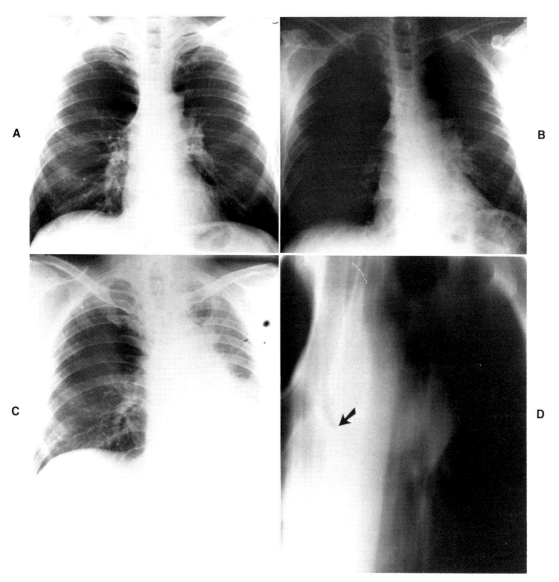

Fig. 6-21   A, Patient with cancer of left main bronchus and emphysema of left upper lobe. Despite the hyperinflation of the right lung caused by the emphysema, the *left* lung is larger and slightly oligemic, suggesting air trapping. **B,** Two hours later the left bronchus has closed off completely. Gas absorption is continuing in the left lung, which is now losing volume. **C,** Three hours later the left lung is largely collapsed. **D,** Tomogram of left main bronchus shows the extreme narrowing *(arrow)* caused by the tumor. At this time, air can pass the obstruction as the bronchus enlarges on inspiration, but is trapped as the bronchus narrows on expiration. The increasing alveolar pressure leads to the oligemia and functional redistribution of flow to the other lung.

the large left atrium, with resultant vasospasm, but no definite evidence exists for this.

A regional increase in alveolar pressure will increase pulmonary vascular resistance and decrease the blood flow and volume in the affected area (see box on p. 175). This can result from valvular air trapping (e.g., by a foreign body or a pedunculated adenoma). It has been suggested that bronchial narrowing caused by a tumor will result in absorption of air distal to the tumor and a *smaller* lung, as opposed to air trapping, which increases lung volume and oligemia within the affected area.[68] In our experience, however, the lung frequently *does* enlarge distal to a tumor, causing valvular air trapping (Fig. 6-21). When the bronchial blockage eventually causes complete obstruction, gas absorption occurs and the lung then reduces its volume (Fig. 6-21).

As mentioned, positive-pressure ventilation can cause *global* oligemia. If this ventilation is performed in a patient with a patchy distribution of disease, however, those areas of lung that are most normal and therefore most compliant with low resistance to air entry will be preferentially expanded and will become oligemic. This oligemia can reach dramatic proportions when only a single lobe or lung is normal and becomes grossly overexpanded and virtually blood free with high levels of positive-pressure ventilation (Fig. 6-22). Because of the functional closure (compression) of the capillaries in these areas, they are also "protected" from the development of pulmonary edema.

All these examples of regional oligemia also result in some redistribution of blood flow away from the affected area. In particular, in patients with *regional* emphysema, it is frequently stated that bullae "compress" the lung's normal portion, suggesting that the pressure inside the bulla is positive. However, measurement by direct puncture reveals that the pressure in the bulla is usually *not* positive. Bullae actually act like pneumo-

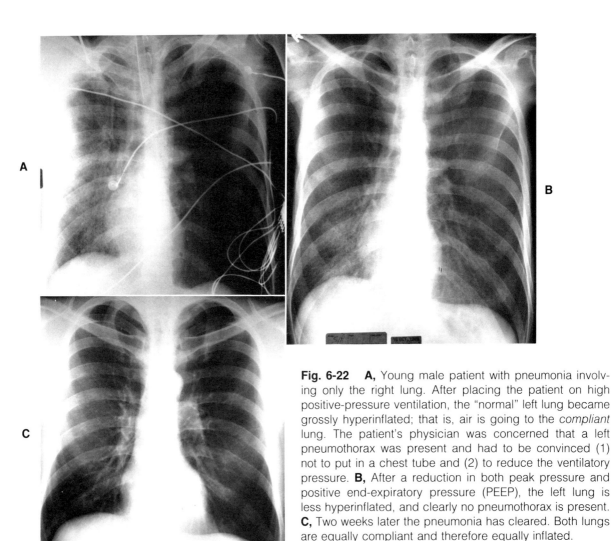

Fig. 6-22   A, Young male patient with pneumonia involving only the right lung. After placing the patient on high positive-pressure ventilation, the "normal" left lung became grossly hyperinflated; that is, air is going to the *compliant* lung. The patient's physician was concerned that a left pneumothorax was present and had to be convinced (1) not to put in a chest tube and (2) to reduce the ventilatory pressure. **B,** After a reduction in both peak pressure and positive end-expiratory pressure (PEEP), the left lung is less hyperinflated, and clearly no pneumothorax is present. **C,** Two weeks later the pneumonia has cleared. Both lungs are equally compliant and therefore equally inflated.

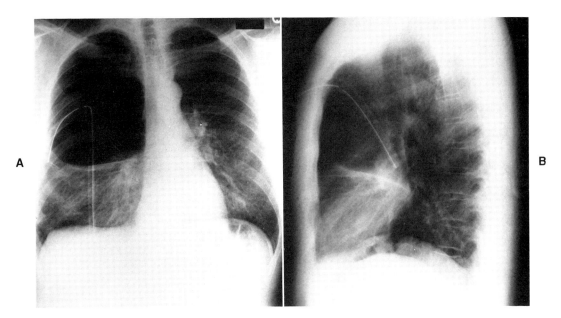

Fig. 6-23 A, Young male patient who arrived at the emergency room with mild dyspnea. The radiologist diagnosed a bulla, but the surgical service team believed it was a loculated pneumothorax "under tension" because it was "compressing" the lung at the right base. The radiologist indicated that it was a bulla and was not "compressing" the lung but simply removing it from the effects of the negative pleural pressure. This was why the vessels within the lung's base were large (they would be small if the lung was compressed). **B,** The consulting surgeon continued to believe *positive* pressure was present within the "bulla" or "tension pneumothorax" and inserted a chest tube. The large-bore tube entered the bulla directly, and, on opening the tube to atmospheric pressure, the bulla did *not* collapse.

thoraces, isolating the rest of the lung from the negative intrapleural pressure so that it is no longer fully expanded. Because the remaining normal lung is not compressed, the vessels within it remain open and freely accept blood redistributed from the emphysematous area (Fig. 6-23).

NORMAL PULMONARY BLOOD FLOW DISTRIBUTION

The lungs appear to be the only paired organs in the body where no built-in homeostatic mechanism exists to correct for the effects of gravity. For example, when one lies on one's right side all night, the left side of the brain does not become ischemic and cause early-morning paralysis! In the erect position, since the pulmonary vascular bed is not usually filled to capacity, blood gravitates to the lower zones of the lungs. As discussed earlier, the lack of any homeostatic mechanism results in the LL arteries and veins becoming larger, reflecting the increased flow through the lung bases, whereas the UL arteries and veins become smaller, again reflecting the diminished flow and volume (first described and called "orthostatic apical anemia" by Bjure and Laurell[69] in 1927).

Factors Affecting Normal Pulmonary Blood Flow Distribution

The pulmonary veins entering the left atrium have no valves within them, and blood refluxes back into the pulmonary veins every time the left atrium contracts. We demonstrated this in 1962 using magnification wedge "cine" angiography in erect patients[70] (Fig. 6-24). Since the veins have no valves, they are affected directly by the pressure within the left atrium. In particular, in the erect position the veins passing "uphill" from the LLs into the left atrium (see Figs. 6-1 and 6-4) are also affected in their distal portion by the gravitational weight of the column of venous blood extending from the base of the lungs up to the left atrium (approximately 12 cm of water).[1] Logically, this would appear to explain the larger size of LL veins versus the smaller size of UL veins on erect films. However, *flow* is also much greater at the lung bases in the erect patient, and one cannot determine in vivo how much of the vein enlargement in the bases (seen on the normal radiograph with the subject erect) is caused by blood flow and volume and how much by pressure.

Pulmonary Artery Pressure, Pulmonary Alveolar Pressure, and Pulmonary Venous Pressure. The blood

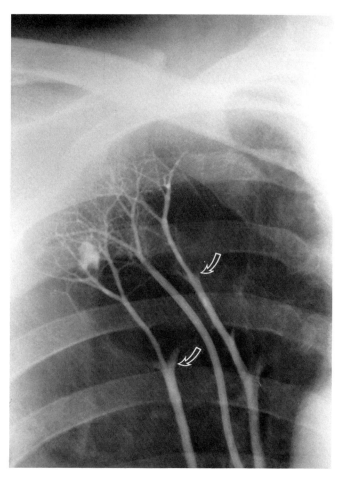

Fig. 6-24   Cardiac catheter 1.7 mm in diameter has been wedged into a small peripheral artery and 2.0 ml of contrast medium injected (a small extravasation is present). The supplying artery and the draining veins are excellently demonstrated. Note that, as the left atrium contracts, blood is forced retrogradely back up side branches of the veins *(arrow)*. A high-speed cine angiographic study showed complete reversal of the direction of flow in the veins during atrial systole.

flow/volume distribution within the *conducting* vessels, (visible on the radiograph, as described earlier) is influenced principally by gravity. However, at the *microcirculatory* level (invisible on the chest radiograph), pulmonary artery pressure (PAP), pulmonary alveolar pressure (Palv), and pulmonary venous pressure (PVP) also affect flow through the microvascular bed. These effects were initially described and demonstrated experimentally by Rodbard,[71] who used a glass and rubber model (Fig. 6-25), and were later confirmed by West and Dollery,[72] who used an isolated lung model and a radioisotopic technique to determine regional flow (Fig. 6-26).

Since blood has considerable mass, a hydrostatic pressure gradient down the lung exists, progressively adding to the pulmonary and venous pressures as one moves down the lung from apex to base. In contrast, the weight of air is so low that it does not cause any gradient of alveolar pressure from apex to base. One should recall, however, that the pressure in the lung's interstitium at the apices reflects the pleural pressure gradient and is much more negative than that at the bases (see Chapter 5). The summation of the effects of gravity, PAP, Palv, and PVP on regional flow/stroke volume distribution in the lung is shown in Fig. 6-27. In zone 1, through the apices, either no flow or minimal flow is present. In zone 2, flow is intermittent, varying with right ventricular systole. The capillaries are completely filled only in zone 3; therefore it is only in zone 3 that there is a continuous column of blood courses from the pulmonary arteries to the left atrium. This is important for the correct positioning of Swan-Ganz catheters (see Chapter 10).

Clearly, if Palv is increased (the most common physiologic cause being a Valsalva maneuver and the most common pathologic cause, positive-pressure ventilation), zones 1 and 2 will enlarge and zone 3 will diminish.

On forced inspiration (at total lung capacity) alveolar pressure rises regionally at the base of the lung, slightly narrowing the basal "alveolar" microvessels, causing a fourth zone of slightly *diminished* flow to develop at the bases. This is measurable by isotopic techniques but cannot be seen on the plain chest radiograph.

Gravity. When a normal person assumes the *supine* position, the amount of blood in the lungs is increased almost immediately by approximately 30%,[56] by blood draining upward from the body's lower half. In the supine position, this increased pulmonary blood fills the *dorsum* of the lungs, causing the zones of flow to reorient so that zone 3 now extends from apex to base posteriorly (dorsally) (Fig. 6-28). An anteroposterior (AP) radiograph with the patient supine shows that the UL and LL vessels are much the same size, resulting in a 1:1 or "balanced" distribution of flow.*

In the *prone* position, because of the shape of the thorax and the volume occupied by the heart, flow distribution is somewhat different from that seen in the supine position. UL arteries and veins enlarge even more than in the supine position, and assuming the prone position has therefore been proposed to exaggerate the UL vascular enlargement often seen in patients with chronically elevated left atrial pressure.[73] This may permit the diagnosis of incipient left-sided heart failure to be made at a stage when the UL vessels are not visibly enlarged on an erect radiograph.

---

*To be strictly accurate, because the lung is so much deeper from front to back at the bases, compared to the apices, many more vessels will be seen at the bases even in the supine position, even though the *size* of the apical vessels has increased.

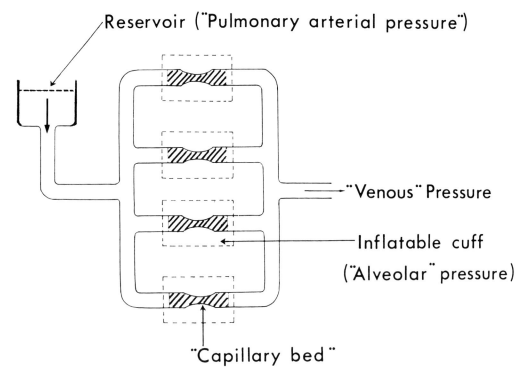

Fig. 6-25 Modified diagram of the model built by Rodbard[71] to demonstrate the effects of arterial, venous, and alveolar pressures on flow distribution in the lung.

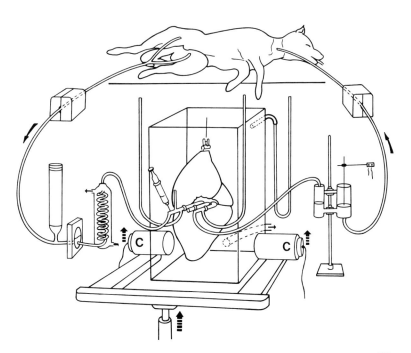

Fig. 6-26 Modified diagram of animal preparation used by West and Dollery[72] to study flow distribution in an isolated lung preparation. The recirculating blood from the live anesthetized dog is pumped through the lung, which is inflated by negative pressure. The radioisotope detectors (probes) labeled *C* can be moved upward to scan the lung.

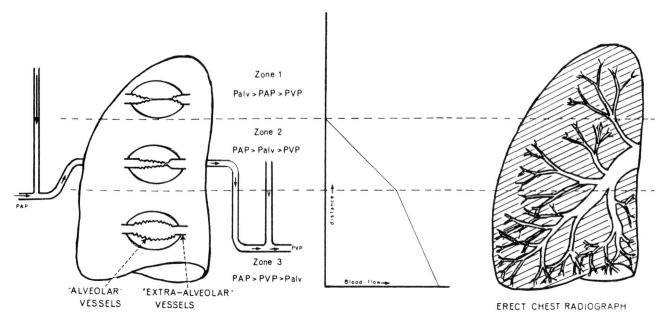

Fig. 6-27 In this diagram the capillary bed is replaced by corrugated-walled, extremely low-resistance Starling resistors, mimicking the very-low-resistance human capillary bed. The surrounding ovoids indicate alveoli. The vessels within the ovoids are "alveolar" vessels, and the supplying arteries and draining veins outside the ovoids are "extraalveolar" vessels. At the base, pulmonary artery pressure (PAP) is higher than both pulmonary venous (PVP) and alveolar (Palv) pressures. As a result, the capillaries are filled with blood. At a higher level in the lung, PVP is reduced (less gravitational effect) and PAP is greater than Palv, which is now greater than PVP. Therefore the vessels are filled, but the venous ends are opened only during right ventricular systole. In the apex, Palv exceeds both PAP and PVP and the capillaries contain very little blood. The matching flow, determined radioisotopically, is shown in the accompanying graph in the center, and the radiographic representation of this zonal distribution of flow is shown on the right.

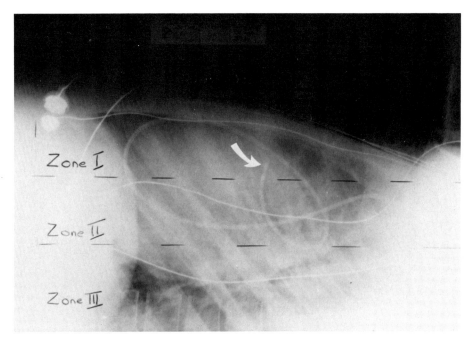

Fig. 6-28 Radiograph of supine patient made with a horizontal beam parallel to the tabletop. In this position, zone 3 lies along the lung's dorsum, and zone 1 is ventral. Note that in this patient a Swan-Ganz catheter is present and its tip is in zone 1, where it is not connected by a column of blood to the left atrium and therefore cannot measure "wedge" pressure.

When a patient assumes the *lateral decubitus* position, the pulmonary blood (including the increased volume from the lower limbs) gravitates to the lower lung, which becomes often very hyperemic, leaving the upper lung oligemic. It was once taught that the "down" lung did not function as well as the "upper" lung because ventilation of the lower lung was inadequate, but this appears to be incorrect.[2,4] The weight of the abdominal contents shifting to the down side *pulls* the upper diaphragm down, also pulling air into the upper lung. The upper diaphragm can still move upward on expiration (Fig. 6-29), so ventilation is good but the lung is relatively devoid of blood (i.e., good ventilation and diminished perfusion, so no hypoxemia occurs). In contrast, although the lower diaphragm is pushed up by the weight of the abdominal contents, it is still in a good position to contract downward, moving air satisfactorily into the lung (Fig. 6-29) and matching good perfusion with adequate ventilation.

This behavior pattern has both diagnostic and therapeutic connotations. First, the sucking of air into the upper lung allows the film reader to see any underlying pathology much more easily. This helps to distinguish between consolidation, atelectasis and masses and to determine the *compliance* of the upper lung. Clearly, if the volume of the upper lung increases greatly with

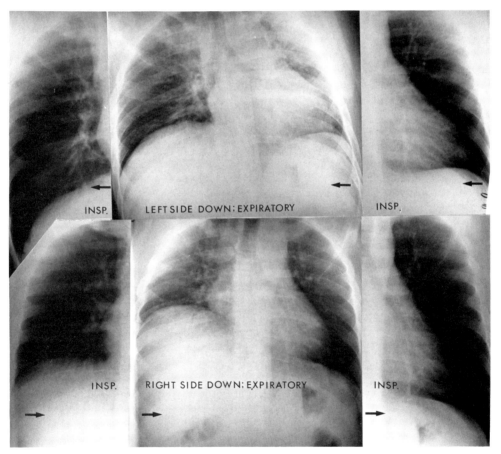

Fig. 6-29 Young male volunteer with normal lungs. With the left side down *(upper panel)*, the left diaphragm moves 3.5 cm between inspiration and expiration, whereas the upper diaphragm (right lung) moves 8.0 cm. The better excursion of the right diaphragm in the upper position appears to result from the liver's weight dropping down and away from the upper right diaphragm, causing it to move to a very low inspiratory position. Also, on expiration, since the heart is not present above the right diaphragm to prevent the diaphragm rising, the *expiratory* position is therefore very high *(upper panel)*, providing great diaphragmatic excursion.

For the same anatomic reasons, when the right diaphragm is down *(lower panel)* its excursion drops from 8.0 to 5.0 cm, which is still better than the 3.5 cm achieved by the left hemidiaphragm in the down position. When the left diaphragm is up *(lower panel)*, its excursion does increase, from 3.5 cm in the down position to 4.5 cm in the up position. Therefore both diaphragms move better in the *up* position, particularly the right diaphragm, but both move sufficiently in the down position to prevent any ventilation-perfusion mismatch. Again, the right diaphragm in the down position moves better than the left.

only the downward pull of the shifting abdominal contents, it is a very compliant lung.* Subtle areas of oligemia and air trapping can also be exaggerated by putting the suspected lung in the down position. Second, the decubitus position can be used deliberately to improve arterial oxygenation by shifting blood away from a poorly ventilated area to a better ventilated one. The effects of this can be substantial.[4] The converse is equally true; shifting blood to a poorly ventilated area decreases oxygenation.[74]

---

*Note, however, that with the same lung compliance the right diaphragm will move much more than the left because of the relative positions of the liver and heart (see Fig. 6-29).

In changing from the supine to the prone position, the shift of the abdominal contents will again affect the diaphragms, which will be at a higher level posteriorly (dorsally) in the supine position and at a lower level (dorsally) in the prone position.[75]

Flow Redistribution Caused by Pulmonary Pathology

The various organic and functional causes of redistribution are listed in the box below.

1. *Emphysema.* The most frequent organic pulmonary cause of regional flow redistribution is emphysema. As discussed in Chapter 9, emphysema is often very inhomogenous in its distribution, destroying the

---

CAUSES OF REDISTRIBUTION OF PULMONARY BLOOD FLOW

Functional changes

1. *Alveolar pressure* (Increase)
   Regional
   a. Asthma
   b. Foreign body
   c. Mucous plugs
   d. Mucosal thickening
   e. Postobliterative bronchiolitis (McLeod syndrome)
   f. Extrinsic pressure on bronchus
   General
   a. Valsalva maneuver
   b. Status asthmaticus
   c. Acute: smoke inhalation
2. *Alveolar pressure* (decrease): Müller maneuver
3. *Interstitial pressure* (increase: absolute or relative)
   Regional
   a. Chest wall pain or immobilization
   b. Pleural pain, thickening, or effusion
   c. Diaphragmatic paralysis or eventration
   d. Carcinoma or consolidation
   e. Transudation (usually caused by elevated left atrial pressure: left-sided heart failure, rheumatic valvular disease, left atrial myxoma, etc.)
   General: inability to move diaphragm (e.g., ascites, abdominal tumor, paralysis, pneumoperitoneum, corsets)
4. *Gravitational:* supine, Trendelenburg, inverted, or lateral decubitus positions

5. *Lung volumes* (related to the ability to generate negative interstitial pressure)
   a. At total lung capacy: 3 zones
   b. At functional residual capacity: 4 zones
   c. At residual volume: 1 zone
6. *Blood gases*
   a. Regional hypoxia (e.g., unilateral bronchography, bronchial obstruction, iatrogenic causes [Carlens catheter])
   b. Hypercarbia
   c. Low pH
7. *Flow states*
   High
   a. Exercise
   b. Anemia
   c. Intracardiac shunts
   d. Overtransfusion with blood, plasma, or dextran
   e. Overtransfusion with saline ⎫ Also produce edema
   f. Renal failure　　　　　　 ⎭ and interstitial
   　　　　　　　　　　　　　　　　　pressure effects
   Low
   a. Dehydration
   b. Addison's disease
   c. Arteriolar disease (pulmonary arterial hypertension)
8. *Increased pulmonary blood volume:* polycythemia

Organic changes

1. Loss of microvascular bed
   a. Emphysema (also interstitial pressure effects)
   b. Postinfective scarring (also interstitial pressure effects)
   c. Iatrogenic causes
   d. Embolic (also chemical effects)

   e. Arterioles (primary and secondary)
   f. Venoocclusive disease
2. Anomalous venous return
3. Systemic arterial supply to lung
4. Regional bronchial arterial hypertrophy

Combined functional and organic changes
(Causes bizarre "inappropriate" redistribution)

Chronic lung disease
Previous embolization
Segmental resection, etc.

With superimposed left-sided and/or right-sided heart failure or fluid overload (iatrogenic or from renal failure)

microcirculatory bed in one or more areas and causing the blood normally passing through that part of the lung to be redistributed elsewhere.[19,23,24] The most common regional distribution of emphysema is apical (bilateral), sparing the lung bases and causing them to appear extremely hyperemic and decreasing the UL/LL flow ratio from 0.8:1.0 to 0.6:1.0 or less. We refer to this as "organic" flow redistribution[39] (see box on p. 188). Bilateral *basal* emphysema occurs less frequently, but when it does, it causes flow inversion (UL/LL ratio greater than 1.0:1.0, which could be mistaken for the flow inversion of chronic left atrial pressure elevation (Fig. 6-30). Such conditions, however, can be distinguished from flow inversion caused by cardiac problems because no edema exists at the bases and there is no peribronchial cuffing.

2. *Lung resection.* Resection of one lung leads to a halving of the PVBC and a redistribution of twice its normal flow through the remaining lung, which therefore becomes hyperemic. The UL/LL ratio in this lung is usually increased but rarely 1.0:1.0 (Fig. 6-31). Shortly after resection the A/V size ratio is 1.0:1.0, but over the years the high flow through the remaining lung results in endarteritis (as occurs with left-to-right shunts), causing pulmonary arterial hypertension, en-

larging the proximal pulmonary arteries, and narrowing the draining veins (Fig. 6-32). Loss of PVBC results from the generalized endarteritis, reducing the number of recruitable vessels. Since no reduction occurs in the amount of blood to be accommodated, however, all vessels are filled and a 1.0:1.0 distribution of flow results.[16]

3. *Incarceration of the lung or part of the lung.* This is sometimes called a "poumon en cuiraisse," that is, "the lung wearing a metal breastplate." If an entire lung is incarcerated (e.g., by a healed, calcified tuberculous empyema), that lung cannot expand and therefore cannot generate the usual level of negative interstitial pressure that normally helps to hold the extraalveolar vessels open. A slight reduction in the radius of these vessels therefore occurs. Since, as Poiseuille's law demonstrates, resistance to flow is proportional to the fourth power of a vessel's radius, even this small change is enough to cause a marked increase in resistance and blood flow redistribution to the opposite side. This causes some hyperemia on that side and a tendency toward a 1.0:1.0 flow ratio (see Fig. 6-7).

4. *Obliterative bronchiolitis.* Bronchiolitis occurring in children (McLoud, Swyer-James syndrome) leads to air trapping with increased intraalveolar pressure. This can affect one lobe of a lung, causing regional redistribution within that lung, or can affect the whole lung, causing redistribution of flow to the other lung. In our experience and for no known reason, obliterative bronchiolitis appears much more frequently on the left side.

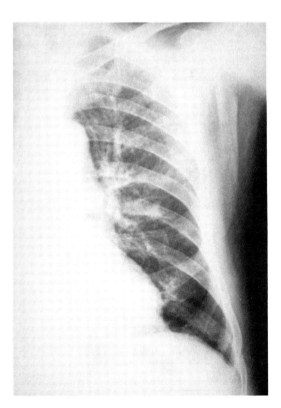

Fig. 6-30   "Organic" flow inversion caused by regional basal emphysema. Note that no evidence of basal edema is seen.

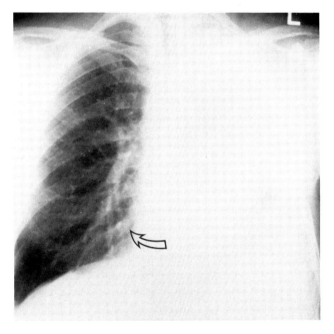

Fig. 6-31   Shortly after resection of the left lung, obligatory doubling of flow to the right lung occurs. Note the large size of the draining veins *(arrow).*

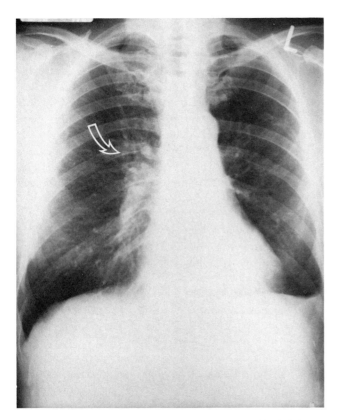

Fig. 6-32 Long standing lobar resection on the left lung. Obligatory redistribution of flow to the right lung is causing a 1:1 flow distribution (see text) and large upper lobe vessels *(arrows)*. However, *organic* endarteritis has developed because of the long-standing high flow, and the draining *veins* are becoming narrower (compare with Fig. 6-31).

The affected lung is both oligemic and *small*, presumably because the disease occurring early in childhood interferes with the lung's growth. The appearance of the redistribution to the normal lung can be exaggerated by taking an expiratory radiograph. The affected lung then traps air, deflates very little, and remains oligemic while the mediastinum bulges toward the good lung. In contrast, the opposite lung does deflate and becomes denser and more hyperemic.

5. *Hypoxemia.* This can also produce bizarre patterns of redistribution that are particularly well visualized in patients with high-altitude edema. The vasoconstrictive response of the pulmonary arterioles to hypoxemia is powerful but frequently inhomogeneous.[76-79] The hypoxia of high altitude can therefore result in patchy *regional* constriction of arterioles, with resultant redistribution of flow to the *non*constricted areas.[80] The very high flow and raised pressure within these high-flow nonconstricted areas can cause pulmonary edema. This is one of the few pulmonary edemas caused by elevated

right-sided heart pressure; others include neurogenic edema and edema of extreme effort.[53,54,81]

Because the lung appears to have limited homeostatic mechanisms to reduce PVBC to match PBV, changes in blood volume and in distribution of flow are inseparable; that is, whether the pulmonary blood volume increases or decreases, flow distribution will change.

Flow Redistribution Caused by Cardiac Disease

As mentioned earlier, cardiac failure usually does not cause an appreciable increase in PBV but may cause flow inversion. The frequency and degree of inversion depend largely on whether the failure is acute, chronic, or acute or chronic.[82-84]

Before we consider what causes flow inversion in cardiac failure and its hemodynamic significance, we should discuss the widespread practice of referring to virtually all cases of cardiac failure as "congestive" cardiac failure. One could ask legitimate questions: "Congestive as opposed to what?" or "What is the significance of the word 'congestion'?" or "Are there other varieties of cardiac failure that should be distinguished as being 'noncongestive'?" The reply might be that patients with high-output failure have "noncongestive" failure. This group of patients would presumably include those with failure following thyrotoxicosis and anemia and possibly those with cardiac failure from septic shock.

In thyrotoxicosis and anemia the cardiac output is initially unusually large, and the PBV reflects this by also being large, (i.e., hyperemic) but without evidence of failure. As the heart tires and fails, the high output drops, the left ventricular end-diastolic and left atrial pressures rise, pulmonary venous engorgement and pulmonary edema occur, and the appearances are those of simple left-sided heart failure (Fig. 6-33), that is, the lungs are "congested." In contrast, in patients with septic shock, the blood is being pumped into a vascular bed so dilated that even the large output is insufficient for adequate tissue perfusion. Therefore the heart cannot supply the body's needs and by definition is failing, even while still pumping blood at high volumes and normal pressures. Under these circumstances the PBV is *not* increased, and no pulmonary edema is seen. This would appear to be the one type of heart failure that *could* be categorized as noncongestive (Table 6-2).

One might also ask another question: "When you say 'congestion,' do you mean with water, blood, or both, and where exactly do you think this 'congestion' is occurring?" This is a relevant question that usually provokes as many different answers as the number of physicians questioned, mainly because the different stages of failure and the chamber or chambers involved cause

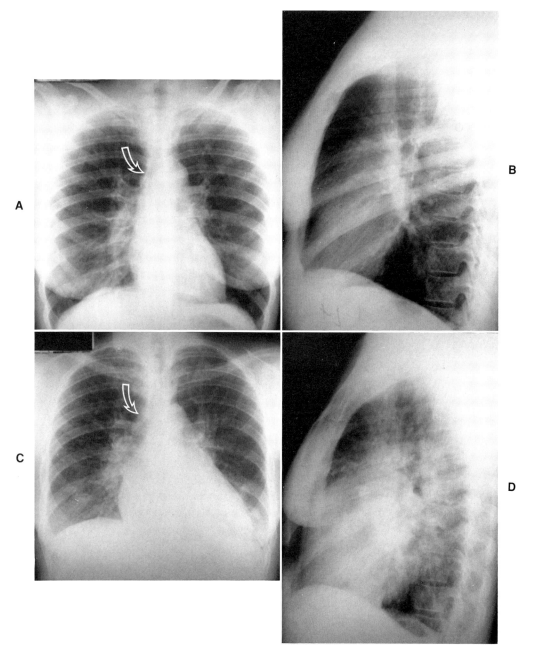

Fig. 6-33   A, Radiograph of 34-year-old woman with thyrotoxicosis. At this time the circulating blood volume, judged by the pedicle width and azygos vein *(arrow)*, appears normal. No edema is seen. **B,** Lateral view showing borderline increase in size of the right and left pulmonary arteries. The patient has a known high-flow state but has a normal PBV; that is, she is not "congested." **C,** Three years later the patient has developed heart failure. The vascular pedicle and azygos vein are now large, as is the heart, and edema is present. Output has dropped as the heart fails; some "congestion" is now present. **D,** Lateral view of the patient with heart failure. Note increased size of the pulmonary arteries.

Table 6-4 "Congestion," or vascular volume, and tissue edema in left-sided and right-sided heart decompensation

	Pulmonary arteries and veins		Pulmonary edema (interstitial and alveolar)	Systemic (VPW)	Neck veins, liver, abdomen	Soft tissues	Pleural space
	Lower	Upper					
Acute LHF	↔	↔	↑↑↑	↓	↔	↔	↔
Chronic LHF	↓	↑↑	↑↑	↑	↔	↑	↑↑
Chronic LHF and acute RHF	↓	↑↑	↑	↑↑↑	↑	↑↑	↑↑↑
Biventricular chronic	↓	↑↑	↑↑	↑↑↑	↑	↑	↑
Acute RHF ↕	↔	↔	↔	↑↑	↑	↑	↑?
Chronic RHF	↔	↔	↔	↑↑	↑↑	↑	↔
Septic shock	↓	↓	?	↓	↔	↑↑	↔

LHF, RHF, Left-sided, right-sided heart failure.
*Horizontal arrows = no increase or decrease in volume.
Upward arrows = increase in volume.
Downward arrows = decrease in volume.
Number of arrows indicates the amount of change.
Question mark indicates that there is uncertainty whether any change will occur.

different areas and organs to be congested (Table 6-2).

The time-honored phrase "congestive cardiac failure" was in use before the development of the x-ray. At that time the clinician was unable to "see" any congestion occurring within the lungs but *was* readily able to see engorged neck veins, swollen ankles, and edematous soft tissues and to palpate an enlarged ("congested") liver—all of which are of course signs of *right* heart failure. If one wishes to continue to use the phrase, it should therefore logically be confined to cases with clearly identifiable right heart failure. (See Chapter 5.)

It seems best, however, to describe cardiac failure specifically as left heart failure (LHF), acute or chronic; right heart failure (RHF) superimposed on LHF; biventricular failure, acute or chronic; or RHF, acute or chronic. Describing *all* patients with heart failure as having "congestive" heart failure does not tell the physician which chamber is failing or whether the failure is acute or chronic, and therefore does not allow him or her to plan a rational approach to therapy.

Flow Inversion in Mitral Valve Disease and Acute and Chronic Left Heart Failure

Before the worldwide burgeoning of antibiotic therapy, rheumatic heart disease occurred frequently, and radiographs of patients with longstanding severe mitral stenosis and incompetence were therefore often seen. The degree of flow inversion in these patients with advanced disease was so dramatic and easily identified (Fig. 6-34) that it stimulated a small avalanche of radiologic publications, including some of the first correlations between observed radiologic changes and mea-

sured physiologic parameters.* It was shown at that time (late 1950s and 1960s) that a very good correlation existed between the amount of inversion demonstrated radiologically and the measured left atrial pressure (LAP).[3,13]

Several authors then began to appreciate that similar although less extreme flow inversion also occurred in patients with LHF (Fig. 6-35). The degree of inversion in these patients was not as dramatic and its occurrence less constant than in those with mitral valve disease, but nonetheless it was widely believed that the most patients with LHF showed inversion of blood flow. The cause for this flow inversion has been debated for many years. Flow inversion in association with elevated LAP was first demonstrated experimentally in the isolated lung preparation developed by West and Dollery.[72] These studies were the basis for the hypothesis that flow inversion occurred because basal edema caused a loss of compliance in the lung bases, resulting in slight loss of the negative interstitial pressure that usually assists in holding the conducting (extraalveolar) vessels open.[85-88] As a result, the diameter of the LL vessels decreased, causing a major increase in pulmonary vascular resistance so that the pulmonary blood flow redirected itself into the lower-resistance recruitable vessels in the ULs, giving the appearance of flow inversion on the radiograph.

This theory initially appeared very plausible and is still frequently offered to explain flow inversion, even though it does not explain the radiologic finding that

*References 3,6,8-10,13,20,21,23,24,26,27-32.

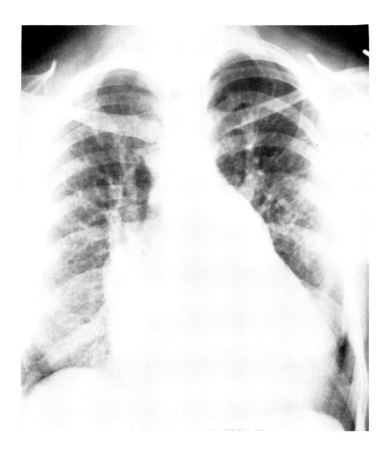

Fig. 6-34 Long-standing severe mitral stenosis and incompetence. Note abnormal fifth left rib and absence of a left atrial appendage after unsuccessful finger fracture of the mitral valve. The extremely high left atrial pressure (LAP of 38 mm Hg) is reflected in the gross (3:1 UL/LL ratio) flow inversion ("touchdown" sign). Only mild edema is seen despite the high LAP because lymphatic hypertrophy is present (deductively).

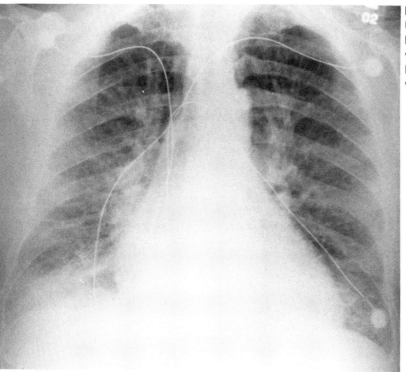

Fig. 6-35 Flow inversion (approximately 2:1 UL/LL ratio) in a patient with chronic left-sided heart failure (LAP of 30 mm Hg). Note the severe pulmonary edema. The patient has probably not had heart failure long enough to develop hypertrophied lymphatics.

the large veins draining from the bases to the left atrium (LA) are also narrowed.[6] Since there are no valves in the pulmonary veins, even where they enter the LA, the entire LA pressure (plus gravitational hydrostatic pressure in the erect position) is transferred directly to these veins, making it inconceivable that they could be narrowed (compressed) mechanically by the very small increase in pulmonary interstitial pressure, particularly since the veins become *extrapulmonary* before they enter the LA. Also it was noted early on that inversion only occurred in the isolated lung when pulmonary blood flow was reduced to very low levels, incompatible with life. Several other authors were unable to duplicate flow inversion in the isolated lung preparation when reasonable flow levels were used. Unfortunately, the validity of their findings may

have been tarnished because of the models they used, such as the sheep lung in a *supine* position and the widespread use of fluid loading and increased pressure to produce the edema.[89-91] The effect of fluid loading was to recruit all the available vessels in the lung, leaving no alternative low-resistance channels in the apices and therefore preventing the very redistribution the authors were attempting to examine. The theory that inversion results from interstitial edema-mediated functional loss of compliance in the lung bases continues to be promulgated, even though severe inversion is often present with *no* evidence of pulmonary edema.

In the 1960s one of the most astute radiologic observers and greatest proponents of physiologic reading of the chest radiograph, Leo Rigler, noted that flow inver-

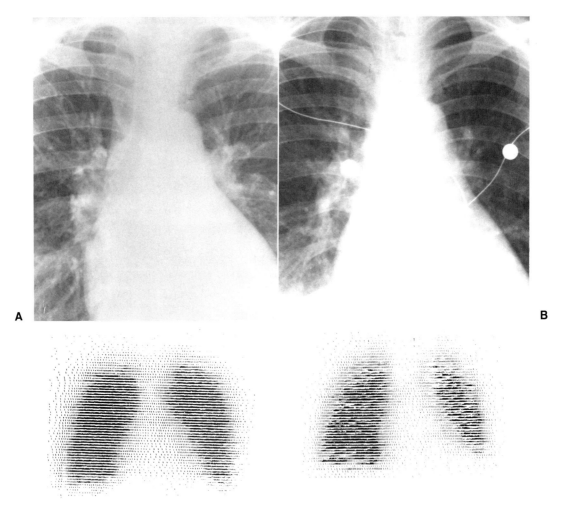

Fig. 6-36   **A,** Male patient with cardiac failure. Flow inversion is present, and the azygos vein and vascular pedicle are wide, indicating *bi*ventricular failure. The accompanying isotope scan confirms inversion of perfusion (UL/LL ratio of 1.85). **B,** After therapy, flow inversion on the radiograph has returned to normal. The azygos vein and vascular pedicle are also normal. An isotope scan confirms the improved perfusion at the lung bases and decreased apical perfusion (UL/LL ratio of 0.87).

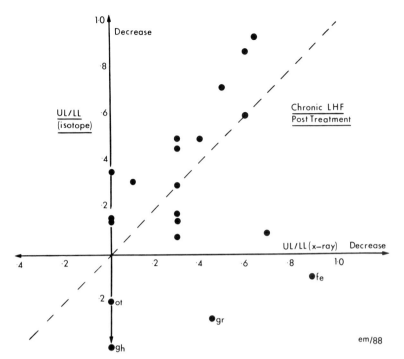

Fig. 6-37 Graph showing UL/LL flow ratio judged from the plain film (horizontal axis) versus UL/LL flow measured isotopically. The reduction in UL/LL ratio seen on the radiograph after treatment is paralleled by the reduction measured isotopically. However, the *degree* of change on the isotope scan is *less* than the change on the radiograph. That is, when distribution on the radiograph has returned to normal, it remains *abnormal* on the scan (see also Table 6-3). (The few patients in whom the UL/LL ratio *increased* after treatment did not respond to therapy and had increasing edema.)

sion was rare in patients with acute LHF, even when severe basal edema was present.[92] We therefore examined this phenomenon again, and it became clear that flow inversion was related much more to the duration of elevated left-sided heart pressure than to severity of edema. That is, inversion was virtually universal in patients with long-standing mitral valve disease, was common but not universal in those with chronic LHF, and occurred infrequently but did occur in patients with acute LHF.[22] This strongly suggested that the cause of flow inversion in response to elevated left-sided heart pressure might be organic, not functional as originally hypothesized. However, we have consistently observed that when patients with decompensated chronic LHF are treated, the amount of flow inversion greatly decreases and often appears radiologically to return to a normal distribution (Fig. 6-36).[93] This is clearly at variance with the newer hypothesis that inversion is caused by organic change. We therefore studied a group of patients with chronic LHF, before and after treatment, quantifying their flow distribution isotopically and correlating this with flow distribution, as assessed visually from chest radiographs with the patient erect.[93]

We found that in most patients, successful treatment did result in reversion to much less flow inversion or to a normal flow distribution on the chest radiograph (Fig. 6-36). The most interesting finding, however, was that although the isotopic quantification of flow always changed in the same direction as the x-ray film assessment, flow inversion measured isotopically did not change as much as in the radiograph. Also, in *all* patients, even those who appeared radiologically normal

after treatment, some isotopically demonstrable inversion of flow persisted (Fig. 6-37 and Table 6-3). Interestingly, after treatment, *pulmonary vascular resistance* decreased. In these patients, in addition to the *organic* changes,[23,41,94,95] evidently a superimposed *functional* change had occurred, suggesting a "tensing" of the pulmonary vessels during heart failure and a decrease in this tensing after treatment.[93] Some increased "stiffening" of the pulmonary vessels persisted, however, even after treatment (Fig. 6-38).

Hypothetic Explanations for Venous Narrowing in Lower Lobe Associated with Elevated Left Atrial Pressure. The question of *how* flow inversion occurs is inex-

Table 6-3   Isotopically demonstrable flow inversion before and after treatment in patients with chronic left-sided heart failure

	With heart in failure	Without heart failure*	
Mean UL/LL F (isotope)	1.77	1.34	(11 patients)
Mean UL/LL V (film)	1.26	0.85	(20 patients)

F = flow; V = volume.
UL/LL F (isotope), Ratio of upper lobe to lower lobe flow determined isotopically; UL/LL V (film), ratio of upper lobe to lower lobe vessel size (volume) on the chest radiograph with the patient erect. Note that UL/LL V (film) changes from inversion (mean ratio of 1.26:1.0) to normal (mean ratio of 0.85:1.0) after treatment. UL/LL F (isotope) parallels film change (mean of 1.77:1.0 to mean of 1.34:1.0), but some inversion of flow persists despite the normal radiograph.
*Only includes patients who improved.
(From Milne ENC: *Radiol Clin North Am* 11:17, 1973.)

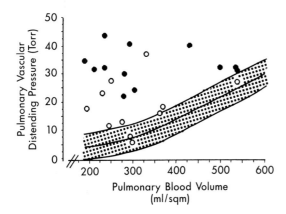

Fig. 6-38 *Patients with heart failure (black circles) and patients after treatment (open circles).* Note that although pulmonary vascular distensibility improves in most patients, with four returning to a normal pulmonary blood volume *(hatched area)* diminished distensibility persists even when visible heart failure is gone. (From Pistolesi M, Miniati M, Bonsignore M et al: J Thorac Imaging 3[3]:65, 1988.)

tricably tied to *why* it should occur. If we can answer the "why," we may be able to understand better the "how."

Leaving out the original and, we believe, untenable hypothesis that flow inversion is caused by basal edema, we have three hypotheses that have been offered to explain the narrowing of the LL veins occurring with elevated LAP:

1. Organic change occurs in the veins at the lung bases.
2. Organic change occurs in the microvascular bed at the lung bases, which reduces flow through the veins, causing them to narrow.
3. Elevated LAP causes reflexive functional narrowing of the LL veins.

Hypothesis 1 is unlikely to be the cause of venous narrowing because, even in patients with the most chronic conditions, the narrowing disappears rapidly when LAP is restored to normal (using a mitral valve prosthesis for those with mitral valve disease and medical treatment for those with chronic LHF) (see Figs. 6-36 and 6-37). Therefore, whatever the organic change present, it is evidently *not* affecting the veins themselves.

Hypothesis 2 is unlikely because flow can be blocked to a lung or portion of the lung with no evidence of reduction in size of the veins draining the blocked area. Reduced venous size as a result of decreased flow only occurs if the entire PBV is reduced (e.g., in patients with dehydration, severe blood loss, or pericardial tamponade).

This leaves only hypothesis 3: the pulmonary veins narrow reflexively in response to elevated LAP. This agrees with our earlier observations that when LAP is restored to normal, venous size also returns to nor-

mal.[93] However, the LL veins do not *invariably* narrow in response to elevated LAP; exceptions include the increased LAP in patients with renal failure, overhydration, and acute LHF. Also, in attempting to answer the question *why* inversion should occur, it would seem that, if pulmonary venous narrowing (vasospasm) were to be caused by elevated LAP, it would be teleologically a poor idea because, to function successfully, the left atrium (LA) must be able to eject a high proportion of its contents into the left ventricle (LV). The cause of an elevated LAP is usually increased resistance to outflow from the LA, either from valvular disease or elevated left ventricular end-diastolic pressure). It would seem at first sight that the LA's ability to eject blood against this resistance would not be helped by increasing pulmonary vascular resistance in the lung bases (i.e., by basal venospasm). This regional venoconstriction would not even reduce preload on the LA because blood could still flow freely through the low-resistance UL vessels.

We would suggest the following hypothesis to explain:

1. Why regional venospasm, in response to an elevated LAP, *is* appropriate when the LAP increase is caused by organic or functional resistance to outflow from the LA
2. Why venospasm does not occur with increased LAP caused by increased circulating blood volume
3. Why venospasm may not *visibly* occur in patients with acute increases in LAP

This hypothesis is based on the knowledge that no anatomic valves exist at the venoatrial junction and that retrograde flow into the pulmonary veins from the LA occurs with each LA systolic contraction[70] (Fig. 6-24).

As already indicated, the LA's vital task is to transfer pulmonary blood to the LV in adequate amounts to maintain LV output. Each time the LA contracts, however, a certain portion of its output is "wasted" by refluxing into the pulmonary veins (Fig. 6-39). If resistance to outflow from the LA into the LV increases *without* any change in the compliance of the pulmonary veins, increasing amounts of blood will reflux into the pulmonary veins during LA systole, "starving" the LV for blood.[3] Simply increasing the LA's force of contraction without changing the compliance of the pulmonary veins would simply cause increasing retrograde venous filling with no increase in LV filling. Logically, the only way to pump more blood out of the LA and into the LV would be to "stiffen" the pulmonary veins so that they cannot distend as much with LA systole, permitting more blood to pass into the LV[96] (Fig. 6-39).

Our hypothesis can therefore be stated simply: "pulmonary venospasm occurs to maintain left atrial stroke volume."

Why do the LL veins *not* narrow, therefore, when

LAP is increased because of renal failure or overhydration? In both these conditions, although the LAP is elevated, the pulmonary veins actually *increase* in size (see Fig. 6-6). This would appear to correlate with our hypothesis quite well; that is, the increased circulating blood volume increases LA diastolic volume and therefore LA systolic output but no obstruction exists to *outflow* from the LA, and therefore venospasm is not needed. Even the normal reflux of blood into the pulmonary veins occurring during LA systole will be diminished because the veins are already full from the increased circulating blood volume.

Why, therefore are the LL veins *not* usually narrowed in patients with *acute* left-sided heart decompensation with abrupt and possibly greatly increased LAP? We would suggest that in these patients an attempt *is* being made to increase pulmonary venous tone, as manifested by no *increase* in venous size even though LAP is extremely high. Also, no increase occurs in LA size, suggesting that the tonus of both the veins and the LA is increased; that is, the LA is trying to maintain its output by *both* mechanisms, and in patients with acute LHF, the LA tonus is more important.

In contrast, in patients with chronic LHF and mitral stenosis, LA size *is* increased, suggesting that the LA wall has progressively weakened with the longstanding resistance. Thus it is even more necessary for the pulmonary veins to narrow increasingly to protect LA output.

Some patients with acute LHF, however, do have venospasm. We previously suggested that this resulted from basal hypoxic arteriolar constriction causing diminished flow, resulting in smaller veins. For the reasons just discussed, however, we think this explanation is no longer tenable. We believe that in those patients

with acute LHF who do have pulmonary venospasm, the mechanism is the same as in those with chronic LHF; that is, these patients have an increased ability to contract their veins or possibly a *diminished* capacity to increase their LA tonus. It would be interesting to determine whether evidence of flow inversion in patients with acute LHF is a good or a poor prognostic sign. As far as we know, this has not been done.

The absence of venous narrowing distal to arterial block by a balloon[66,67] also agrees very well with our hypothesis. If you block off one pulmonary artery, flow immediately doubles through the other lung; the LA continues to receive its normal load of blood, and no venospasm is necessary to protect its output. (*NOTE:* vessels may sometimes narrow distal to a block if the narrowing is caused by a pulmonary embolus, in which case vasoactive breakdown products of the clot may cause active venospasm.)

One major question remains to be answered by our hypothesis: why should only the LL veins narrow to "protect" the LA output? We suggest that the explanation may simply be that this is all that is *necessary*. That is, increasing the tonus of the LL veins means that they are more difficult to distend by LA systole, while simultaneously, flow is redistributed through the low-resistance, recruitable UL vessels. The UL veins are

---

Fig. 6-39 Diagram illustrating how venospasm may be initiated by the left atrium (LA) to "protect" its output into the left ventricle (LV).

Normal: (1) During atrial diastole the LA fills from blood flowing through the pulmonary veins. (2) During atrial systole the mitral valve opens wide, and most of the atrial contents is discharged into the LV, with only a small amount refluxing into the pulmonary veins *(arrow)*.

Mitral stenosis: (3) If there was *no* venospasm, on diastole the normal venous size ratio would be present. (4) On systole, however, because of the high resistance to outflow through the stenosed mitral valve, most of the atrial contents would reflux back into the compliant veins. (5) If LL venospasm is initiated, however, and the veins are contracted, during atrial systole minimal venous reflux *(small arrows)* could occur in LL veins, with slightly greater reflux *(larger arrow)* in UL veins. Also, most of the atrial contents *will* be discharged into the LV.

NORMAL: Diastole Systole

MITRAL STENOSIS: Diastole Systole

No Venospasm.   Protective Venospasm.

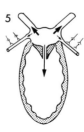

therefore more engorged than normal and are therefore also more difficult to distend by LA systole; both these mechanisms prevent wasteful reflux (see Fig. 6-39). The strength of this arrangement, as opposed to narrowing of *all* the pulmonary veins, is that minimal change occurs in pulmonary blood flow/volume, and the LA continues to receive enough blood, with no need for any active increase in PAP.

As the LA weakens with long-standing work against outflow resistance, the necessity to maintain its output results in increasing basal venospasm, with further flow redistribution to the ULs. This causes increasingly visible flow inversion on the chest radiograph, explaining the good correlation between the degree of flow inversion and the level of LAP and further indicating why this correlation improves with the chronicity of the changes.

However, investigators have also demonstrated that *organic* change in the *microvascular* bed at the lung bases increases with the chronicity of the disease.[41,43] As shown earlier, this organic change cannot be the primary cause of the reduced *size* of the LL veins resulting from elevated LAP, but it is probably the principal cause of the progressive decrease in *flow* through the lower lobes in patients with chronically increased LAP. This is better shown by radioistopic flow studies than by the plain radiograph. We have demonstrated that venous size, as seen on the plain radiograph, returns to normal after LAP is restored to normal. However, in patients with chronic disease, *flow* (as measured radioisotopically) does not return to normal. This fits perfectly with our hypothesis that the *large* vessel (venous) changes seen on the chest film are largely functional (neural or neurohormonal), *whereas the *microvascular* bed changes are largely organic (Fig. 6-40). The functional changes may be regarded teleologically as being primary and "good" in that they appear to be designed to preserve LA output and are reversible after treatment. The organic changes are secondary and undesirable because they raise PAP "unnecessarily," reduce blood flow, and are only partially reversible even when LAP is restored to normal.

These observations confirm that when the film reader sees an increase in UL/LL venous ratio (an inversion of *volume*) it can be inferred correctly that *flow* has been inverted, an important point that has been questioned by some authors.[97] When a patient with an *acute* increase in LAP is treated and the LL veins return to normal, flow has also probably been restored almost to

normal. However, when a patient with a *chronic* increase in LAP is treated and LL venous size reverts to normal radiologically, the *flow* inversion still persists, although to a lesser degree[93] (Fig. 6-40).

The teleologic hypothesis we have promulgated appears to offer a good explanation for all of the changes (or lack of changes) in pulmonary vascular distribution, seen radiologically and radioisotopically. If it is proven to be correct that changes in pulmonary blood volume and flow distribution are mediated neurohormonally from the heart, any conclusion concerning blood flow distribution drawn from previous experience and using only the isolated lung[16,17,85-91,97] would be invalid, but we would caution that further experimental work and clinical observation is now required to prove (or disprove) this hypothesis.

Fig. 6-40   *Normal:* the conducting vessels and the microcirculatory vessels at the lung bases are larger (zone 3) than those at the apices. UL/LL F ratio (flow determined isotopically) matches UL/LL V ratio (volume distribution seen radiologically). Left atrial pressure (LAP) is normal.

First-episode LHF: LAP is 30 mm Hg. No change is seen in conducting vessel size on the radiograph, with a UL/LL V of 0.8:1.0, but UL/LL F (isotope) is 1:1. Since the size of conducting veins has not *increased* despite the high LAP, this suggests that some increase in vasomotor tone *is* present (represented on the diagram by a single synapse). This may be enough to account for the discrepancy between visualized UL/LL V and measured UL/LL F.

First-episode LHF, possibly oxygen sensitive: in the fewer patients with first-episode LHF who *do* visibly invert their flow, it is unclear whether this occurs because the LA is able to reflexively vasoconstrict the LL veins to protect its output (see text) or whether the basal edema may result in regional hypoxemia, causing basal *arteriolar* and venous constriction and flow inversion on this basis. Whatever the cause, UL/LL V (film) is matched by UL/LL F (isotope).

Chronic LHF (patient does not yet have heart failure): repeated episodes of heart failure have led to organic change at the microcirculatory level *(hatch marks).* As a result, resistance to flow is increased through the lung bases and flow inversion is present, with a UL/LL F (isotope) of 1.5:1.0. However, because left ventricular end-diastolic pressure (LVEDP) is not high, outflow from the LA has minimal resistance, and therefore reflexive vasospasm of the veins is not needed. Therefore the veins are *normal* on the radiograph (UL/LL volume, 0.8:1.0), and mismatch exists between the persisting flow inversion (isotope) and the radiograph.

Chronic LHF (patient has heart failure): because the LVEDP is now high, the LA must protect itself from refluxing into the veins by venospasm (shown by multiple synapses). The LL veins are therefore narrowed on the radiograph, and the visualized UL/LL V (1.6:1.0) more closely matches the isotopic UL/LL F (2.0:1.0). That is, a combination of *organic* change in the microvasculature and *functional* change in the larger "conducting" veins is present.

---

*We have not emphasized in this chapter that VPW is usually reduced in patients with mitral valve disease, indicating a reduction in *systemic* blood volume, in addition to the reduction in PBV. There is therefore a reduction in *total* blood volume (TBU), as there is in aortic stenosis (AS). We have hypothesized earlier in this chapter that this TBU reduction in AS may be caused by increased atrionatriuretic factor and new hypotheses that the same mechanism may be operating in mitral valve disease.

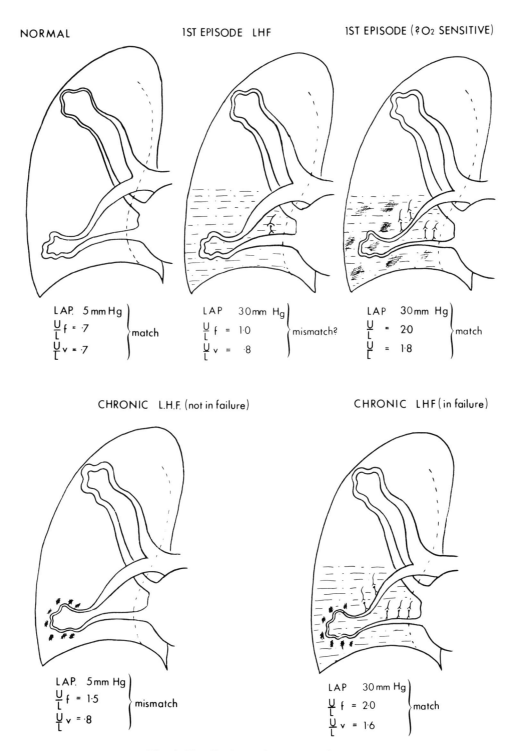

Fig. 6-40   For legend see opposite page.

REFERENCES

1. Badeer HS: Gravitational effects on the distribution of pulmonary blood flow: hemodynamic misconceptions, *Respiration* 43:408,1982.
2. Fishman AP: Down with the good lung, *N Engl J Med* 304:537, 1981 (editorial).
3. Friedman WF, Braunwald E: Alterations in regional pulmonary blood flow in mitral valve disease studied by radioisotope scanning, *Circulation* 34:363, 1966.
4. Remolina C, Khan A, Santiago TJ, Edelman NH: Positional hypoxemia in unilateral lung disease, *N Engl J Med* 304:523, 1981.
5. Ravin CE: Pulmonary vascularity: radiographic considerations, *J Thorac Imaging* 3(1):1, 1988.
6. Lavender JP, Doppman J, Shawdon H, Steiner RE: Pulmonary veins in left ventricular failure, and mitral stenosis, *Br J Radiol* 35:293, 1962.
7. Milne ENC: Some new concepts of pulmonary blood flow and volume, *Radiol Clin North Am* 16:515, 1978.
8. McMyn J: Radiological appearances of pulmonary hypertension, *J Coll Radiol Aust* 4:21, 1960.
9. Milne ENC, Carlsson E: Physiological interpretation of the plain radiograph following mitral valvotomy, valvuloplasty and prosthetic replacement, *Radiology* 92:1201, 1969.
10. Turner AF, Lau FYK, Jacobson G: A method for the estimation of pulmonary venous and arterial pressures from the routine chest roentgenogram, *AJR* 116:97, 1972.
11. Fouche RF, Beck W, Schrirer W: The roentgenological assessment of left to right shunt in secundum type atrial septal defect, *AJR* 89:254, 1963.
12. Milne ENC: Pulmonary blood flow distribution, *Invest Radiol* 12:479, 1977.
13. Milne ENC: Physiological interpretation of the plain film in mitral stenosis including a review of criteria for the estimation of pulmonary arterial and venous pressures, *Br J Radiol* 36:902, 1963.
14. Milne ENC: The physiologic basis of pulmonary radiologic changes. In Abrams HL, editor: *Angiography*, ed 2, Boston, 1971, Little, Brown.
15. Milne ENC: Radiological aspects of pulmonary mechanics (with particular reference to chronic pulmonary disease and left heart failure). In Potchen EJ, editor: *Current concepts in radiology*, St Louis, 1972, Mosby–Year Book, p 30.
16. Milne ENC: Correlation of physiological findings and chest roentgenology, *Radiol Clin North Am* 11:17, 1973.
17. Rees S: The chest radiograph in pulmonary hypertension with central shunt, *Br J Radiol* 41:172, 1968.
18. Rigler LG: Functional roentgen diagnosis: anatomical image–physiologic interpretation, *AJR* 82:3, 1959.
19. Simon G: The plain radiograph in relation to lung physiology, *Radiol Clin North Am* 11:3, 1973.
20. Simon M: The pulmonary vessels: their hemodynamic evaluation using routine radiographs, *Radiol Clin North Am* 2:363, 1963.
21. Simon M: The radiologic assessment of pulmonary hemodynamics. In Simon M et al, editors: *Frontiers of pulmonary radiology*, New York, 1969, Grune & Stratton.
22. Davies LG, Goodwin JF, Steiner RE, VanLeuven BD: Clinical and radiological assessment of pulmonary arterial pressure in mitral stenosis, *Br Heart J* 15:393, 1953.
23. Doyle AE, Goodwin JF, Harrison CV, Steiner RE: Pulmonary vascular patterns in pulmonary hypertension, *Br Heart J* 19:353, 1957.
24. Jacobson G, Schwartz LH, Sussman ML: Radiographic estimation of pulmonary artery pressure in mitral valvular disease, *Radiology* 68:15, 1957.
25. Jacobson G, Turner AF, Balchum OJ, Jung R: Vascular changes in pulmonary emphysema, *AJR* 100:374, 1967.
26. Ormond RS, Poznanski K: Pulmonary veins in rheumatic heart disease, *Radiology* 74:542, 1960.
27. Simon M: Pulmonary veins in mitral stenosis, *J Fac Radiologists* 9:25, 1958.
28. Simon M: Physiologic considerations in radiology of the pulmonary vasculature. In Abrams HL, editor: *Angiography*, St Louis, 1983, Mosby–Year Book, p 783.
29. Simon M: Pulmonary vessels in incipient left ventricular decompensation, *Circulation* 24:185, 1961.
30. Steiner RE: Radiological appearances of pulmonary vessels in pulmonary hypertension, *Br J Radiol* 31:188, 1958.
31. Steiner RE: Radiology of pulmonary circulation, *AJR* 91:249, 1964.
32. Van Epps FF: Roentgen manifestations of pulmonary hypertension, *AJR* 79:241, 1958.
33. Steiner RE, Harrison CV, Goodwin JF: Radiological assessment of pulmonary arterial and pulmonary venous pressure. In Ciba Foundation Study Group No 8; de Reuck AVS, O'Connor M, editors: *Problems of pulmonary circulation*, London, 1961, JA Churchill, p 2.
34. Dollery CT, West JB, Goodwin JF et al: Regional pulmonary blood flow in mitral and congenital heart disease. In Ciba Foundation Study Group No 8; de Reuck AVS, O'Connor M, editors: *Problems of pulmonary circulation*, London, 1961, JA Churchill, p 17.
35. Matthay RA, Schwartz MI, Ellis JH et al: Pulmonary artery hypertension in chronic obstructive pulmonary disease, determined by chest radiography, *Invest Radiol* 16:95, 1981.
36. Tikhonov KB, Bairek VG: Redistribution of pulmonary blood flow in pneumonia patients under the influence of gravitation, *Fortschr Rontgenstr* 136:660, 1982.
37. Matthay RA, Berger HJ: Non-invasive assessment of right and left ventricular function in acute and chronic respiratory failure, *Crit Care Med* 11:24, 1983.
38. Wehrmacher WH: Estimation of cardiovascular dynamics from routine radiograph of chest, *Curr Med Digest*, p 212, 1969.
39. Milne ENC, Bass H: The roentgenologic diagnosis of early chronic obstructive pulmonary disease, *J Can Assoc Radiol* 20:3, March 1969.
40. Milne ENC, Bass H: Roentgenologic and functional analysis of combined chronic obstructive pulmonary disease and congestive cardiac failure, *Invest Radiol* 4:129, 1969.
41. Heard BE, Steiner RE, Herdan A, Gleason D: Edema and fibrosis of lungs in left ventricular failure, *Br J Radiol* 41:161, 1968.
42. Short DS: Radiology of the lung in severe mitral stenosis, *Br Heart J* 17:33, 1955.
43. Heath D, Whitaker W: Hypertensive pulmonary vascular disease, *Circulation* 14:323, 1956.
44. Permutt S: Effect of interstitial pressure of the lung on pulmonary circulation, *Med Thorac* 22:118, 1965.
45. Permutt S, Howell JB, Proctor DF, Riley RL: Effect of lung inflation on static pressure-volume characteristics of pulmonary vessels, *J Appl Physiol* 16:64, 1961.
46. Bryan AC, Bentivoglio LG, Beerel F et al: Factors affecting regional distribution of ventilation and perfusion in the lung, *J Appl Physiol* 19:295, 1964.
47. Howell JBL, Permutt S, Proctor DF, Riley RL: Effect of inflation of the lung on different parts of pulmonary vascular bed, *J Appl Physiol* 16:71, 1961.
48. Wasson C: *The auxiliary heart*, Springfield, Ill, 1954, Charles C Thomas.
49. Giuntini C: Pulmonary blood volume and its relationship to total blood volume and central hemodynamics in man. In Interna-

tional Symposium on Pulmonary Circulation: *Progress in respiratory research*, vol 5, New York, 1970, Karger.

50. Bake B, Bjure J, Widimsky J: The effect of sitting and graded exercise on the distribution of pulmonary blood flow in healthy subjects studied with the 133Xe technique, *Scand J Clin Lab Invest* 22:99, 1968.

51. Yu PN: *Pulmonary blood volume in health and disease*, Philadelphia, 1969, Lea & Febiger.

52. Milne ENC, Pistolesi M, Miniati M, Giuntini C: The radiologic distinction of cardiogenic and non-cardiogenic edema, *AJR* 144:879, 1985.

53. Theodore J, Robin ED: Speculation on neurogenic pulmonary edema, *Am Rev Respir Dis* 113:405, 1976.

54. Wray NP, Nicotra B: Pathogenesis of neurogenic pulmonary edema, *Am Rev Respir Dis* 118:783, 1978.

55. Giuntini C, Maseri A, Bianchi P: Pulmonary vascular distensibility and lung compliance as modified by dextran infusion and subsequent atropine injection in normal subjects, *J Clin Invest* 45:1770, 1966.

56. Honig CR: *Modern cardiovascular physiology*, ed 2, Boston, 1988, Little, Brown.

57. Figueras J, Weil MH: Blood volume prior to and following treatment of acute cardiogenic pulmonary edema, *Circulation* 57:349, 1978.

58. Schreiber SS, Bauman A, Yalow RS, Berson SA: Blood volume alterations in congestive heart failure, *J Clin Invest* 33:578, 1954.

59. Milne ENC: Pulmonary patterns in heart disease. In Royal College of Radiologists: *A textbook of radiologic diagnosis*, vol 2, *The cardiovascular system*, London, 1985, Lewis.

60. Milne ENC: A physiologic approach to reading critical care unit films, *J Thorac Imaging* 1(3):60, 1986.

61. Pistolesi M, Milne ENC, Miniati M, Giuntini C: The vascular pedicle of the heart and the vena azygos. Part II. Acquired heart disease, *Radiology* 152:9, 1984.

62. Bruno MA, Milne ENC, Stanford WS et al: Pulmonary oligemia in chest diagnosis—film reader reliability (with special reference to a new finding in aortic stenosis), paper presented at Fleischer Society annual meeting, Montreal 1992.

63. Cumming G, Hunt LB, editors: *Form and function in the human lung*, Baltimore, 1968, Williams & Wilkins.

64. Palla A, Petruzzelli S, Donnamaria V et al: Radiographic assessment of perfusion impairment in pulmonary embolism, *Eur J Radiol* 5:252, 1985.

65. Felix R, Geisler P, Dux A: Pulmonary angiography in unilateral assessment of the pulmonary gas exchange: functional pneumectomy, *Kreislav Horsch* 56:147, 1967.

66. Felix R, Dux A, Geisler P: Angiographic examination of the pulmonary circulation during functional elimination of one lung, *Invest Radiol* 3:280, 1968.

67. Nordenstrom B: Temporary unilateral occlusion of the pulmonary artery, *Acta Radiol Suppl* 108, 1954.

68. Fraser RG, Pare JA: *Diagnosis of diseases of the chest*, Philadelphia, 1970, WB Saunders.

69. Bjure A, Laurell H: Abnormal static circulatory phenomena and their symptoms: arterial orthostatic anemia as neglected clinical picture, *Upsala Lakaref Forh* 33:1, 1927.

70. Donald KW, Milne ENC: Discussion. In Ciba Foundation Study Group No 8; de Reuck AVS, O'Connor M, editors: *Problems of pulmonary circulation*, London, 1961, JA Churchill.

71. Rodbard S: Distribution of flow through pulmonary manifold, *Am Heart J* 51:106, 1956.

72. West J, Dollery CT: Distribution of blood flow and ventilation-perfusion relationship in the lung measured with radioactive CO_2, *J Appl Physiol* 16:405, 1960.

73. Anderson G: Large upper lobe veins, *J Coll Radiol Aust* 8:214, 1965.

74. Gattinoni L, Pesenti A, Torresin A et al: Adult respiratory distress syndrome profiles by computed tomography, *J Thorac Imaging* 1(3):25 1986.

75. Simonds B, Friedman PJ, Sokoloff J: The prone chest film, *Radiology* 116:11, 1975.

76. Kato M, Staub NC: Response of small pulmonary arteries to unilobar hypoxia and hypercapnea, *Circ Res* 19:426, 1966.

77. McGregor M: Oxygen tension and the regulation of pulmonary blood flow. In *Proceedings of the International Symposium on Cardiovascular and Respiratory Effects on Hypoxia*, New York, 1966, Hafner.

78. Naeye RL: Children at high altitude pulmonary and renal abnormalities, *Circ Res* 16:53, 1965.

79. Neumann PH, Kivlen CM, Johnson A et al: Effect of alveolar hypoxia on regional pulmonary perfusion, *J Appl Physiol* 56:338, 1984.

80. Maldonado D: High altitude pulmonary edema, *Radiol Clin North Am* 16:537, 1978.

81. Bachofen H: Personal communication.

82. Pistolesi M, Miniati M, Milne ENC, Giuntini C: The chest roentgenogram in pulmonary edema, *Clin Chest Med* 6:315,1985.

83. Giuntini C, Mariani M, Barsotti A et al: Factors affecting regional pulmonary blood flow in left heart valvular disease, *Am J Med* 57:421, 1974.

84. Giuntini C, Pistolesi M, Miniati M: Pulmonary venous hypertension, mechanisms and consequences. In Wagenwort CA, Denolin H, editors: *Pulmonary circulation*, Amsterdam, 1989, Elsevier, p 131.

85. West JB, Dollery CT, Heard BE: Increased pulmonary resistance in dependent zone of isolated dog lung caused by perivascular edema, *Circ Res* 17:191, 1965.

86. Hughes JMB, Glazier JB, Maloney JE, West JB: Effect of interstitial pressure on pulmonary blood flow, *Lancet* 1:192, 1967.

87. Hughes JMB, Glazier JB, Maloney JE et al: Effect of lung volume on the distribution of pulmonary blood flow in man, *Respir Physiol* 4:58, 1968.

88. Iliff LD, Greene RE, Hughes JMB: Effect of interstitial edema on distribution of ventilation and perfusion in isolated lung, *J Appl Physiol* 33:462, 1972.

89. Ritchie BC, Schauberger G, Staub NC: Inadequacy of perivascular edema hypothesis to account for distribution of pulmonary blood flow in lung edema, *Circ Res* 24:807, 1969.

90. Maloney JE, Adamson TM, Ritchie BC, Walker A: Distribution of pulmonary blood flow during controlled perfusion of the intact lung, *Aust J Exp Biol* 51(pt5):655, 1973.

91. Muir AL, Hall DL, Despas P, Hogg JC: Distribution of blood flow in the lungs in acute pulmonary edema in dogs, *J Appl Physiol* 33:763, 1972.

92. Rigler LG: Personal communication.

93. Pistolesi M, Miniati M, Bonsignore M et al: Factors affecting regional pulmonary blood flow in chronic ischemic heart disease, *J Thorac Imaging* 3(3):65, 1988.

94. Parker F, Weiss: The nature and significance of the structural changes in the lungs in mitral stenosis, *Am J Pathol* 12:573, 1936.

95. Smith RC, Burchell HB: Pathology of the pulmonary vascular tree. IV. Structural changes in the pulmonary vessels in chronic left ventricular failure, *Circulation* 10:801, 1954.

96. Sarnoff SJ: Some physiologic considerations in the genesis of acute pulmonary edema. In Abrams W, Veith I, editors: *Pulmonary circulation*, New York, 1959, Grune & Stratton, p 273.

97. Savoca CJ, Gamsu G, Brito AC: The effect of acute pulmonary edema on pulmonary vascular resistance: significance for the interpretation of dilated upper lobe vessels on chest radiographs, *Invest Radiol* 12:488, 1977.

Quantification of Pulmonary Blood Volume, Flow, and Pressure: Practice

RADIOLOGIC CRITERIA (VARIANCE IN VALUE)

In the late 1950s and 1960s, many authors demonstrated that a trained film reader could assess arterial and venous pressures in patients with mitral valve disease with a clinically valuable level of accuracy.[1-12] However, when the same radiographic criteria (developed by correlating radiologic observations and catheterization data in mitral valve disease) were applied to a much wider spectrum of both cardiac and pulmonary disease, the "accuracy" of the estimates (again judged by correlation with catheterization data) dropped to a clinically unacceptable level. Consequently the radiologist's ability to read films physiologically fell into some disrepute.

The reason for this failure has taken time to emerge but is quite straightforward. That is, each radiologic criterion can have a quite different radiologic significance, depending on the particular pathologic and physiologic features of the disease being analyzed radiologically for abnormal hemodynamics. Therefore, when the criteria developed for mitral valve disease were applied to other widely differing pathophysiologies, the deductions were incorrect.

Consider, for example, the typically used criterion, enlargement of the main pulmonary artery (MPA). If the MPA is enlarged in a patient with chronic bronchitis, the degree of enlargement correlates well with pulmonary artery pressure (PAP),[13,14] particularly if one can see that the pulmonary arteries in the lung are larger than their draining veins (Fig. 7-1). If the pulmonary arteries enlarge in a patient with an atrial septal defect (ASD) and the pulmonary arteries and veins in the lung are enlarged equally, the size of the pulmonary artery correlates poorly with pressure and better with *flow*.[15,16] In contrast, if the MPA enlarges in a patient with renal failure and the pulmonary arteries and veins in the lungs are enlarged equally and the vascular pedicle is wide, the change in pulmonary artery size correlates best with *circulating blood volume* (Fig. 7-1).

To derive clinically useful quantitative physiologic

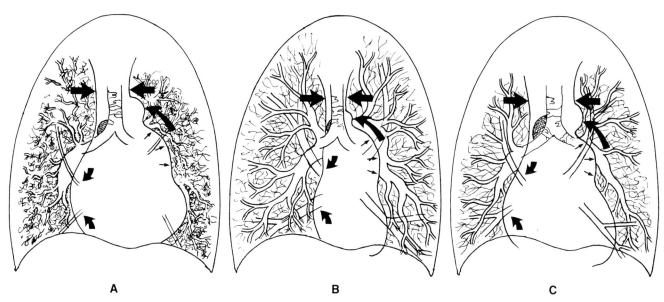

A   **B**   **C**

Fig. 7-1   The three radiographs show a similarly enlarged main pulmonary artery (MPA) *(small arrows),* but the physiologic meaning of this enlarged MPA differs in each patient because of other radiographic findings. **A,** Large comma-shaped central pulmonary arteries with tortuous, segmented, blurred peripheral branches. Arterial/venous (A/V) size ratio *(small curved arrows)* is 3:1. The cardiac apex is up, indicating right ventricular (RV) enlargement, a wide pedicle *(straight arrow),* and large azygos vein. Diagnosis: severe chronic bronchitis; meaning of large MPA: pulmonary arterial hypertension (organic). **B,** Central pulmonary arteries enlarged, extending out into peripheral branches and resulting in very hyperemic lungs. Veins equally enlarged, resulting in A/V ratio of 1:1. Very small pedicle, azygos vein, and aorta *(large curved arrow).* Diagnosis: large left-to-right shunt; meaning of large MPA: very high flow state. **C,** Large pulmonary arteries and veins, resulting in A/V ratio of 1:1. Very wide pedicle and azygos vein, indicating increased circulating blood volume. The heart is generally enlarged, slightly more to the right than the left side. Diagnosis: overhydration and/or renal failure; meaning of large MPA: increase in total blood volume and in pulmonary artery pressure (passive).

NOTE: Each example also has a 1:1 flow distribution. In **A,** this occurs because pulmonary vascular bed capacity is so reduced that the pulmonary blood volume (PBV) completely fills it; in **B** because of the huge RV output, which increases the PBV and recruits the upper lobe (UL) vessels; and in **C** because the total blood volume is increased, secondarily recruiting all vessels in the lungs.

data, the film reader must therefore learn what the different radiologic criteria (Table 7-1) mean individually, in combination, and in different pathologic settings.

In Table 7-1 the typical constellations of these radiologic observations have been displayed for normal subjects and patients with acquired valvular heart disease, ischemic cardiac disease, left-to-right shunts, renal disease, shock lung, emphysema (with and without left-sided heart failure [LHF]), and chronic bronchitis (with and without left heart failure). The most valuable radiologic observations in each disease for deriving the required physiologic data (PAP, pulmonary venous pressure [PVP], pulmonary blood flow [PBF], pulmonary vascular resistance [PVR]) have been indicated with asterisks.

Table 7-1 clearly shows that the same criteria can have widely different meanings when they occur in different diseases. Some criteria are of no value in certain diseases. For example, flow distribution is of little or no use for estimating left atrial pressure (LAP) in most patients with *acute* LHF, in whom the degree of edema is the most valuable criterion. In those with mitral stenosis, however, flow distribution is of great importance in assessing LAP, and the presence of edema adds little to this information.

Table 7-1 also illustrates that in patients with pulmonary edema, one must be able to distinguish between edema caused by pressure and that caused by injury (e.g., differentiating cardiac edema, renal edema, edema caused by overhydration, and edema from lung injury) *before* one can determine the physiologic significance of the various radiologic observations and quantify them. For example, the same amounts of pulmonary edema occurring in the three different settings of

Table 7-1 Radiologic observations and their physiologic correlates (pressure and flow)

| | Heart | | | Pulmonary vessels | | | | | Flow distribution | | |
| | | (size) | | PAs, 1st division | | | | | | | |
Disease	RV	LV	LA	MPA (size)	1st division (size)	Tor-tuosity	Prun-ing	PA/PV ratio	PBV (size)	NR	1:1 ratio
Normal	N	N	N	N	N	—	—	1:1	N	NR	—
LHF (acute)	N	N	N	N	N	—	—	1:1	N	NR	—
LHF (chronic)	0 to 3	1 to 4	N	N to 2	N to 2	—	—	1:1	N	—	—
Biventricular failure	1 to 4	1 to 4	N	N to 2	N to 2	—	—	1:1	N	—	—
MS (compensated)	1 to 4	−1 to N	1 to 4*	1 to 4*	1 to 4*	0 to 4*	0 to 4*	1 to 4/1*	N	—	—
MS (decompensated)	1 to 4	N	1 to 4*	1 to 4*	1 to 4*	0 to 4*	0 to 4*	1 to 4/1*	N	—	—
Renal	1 to 4	1 to 4	N	N to 2	N to 2	—	—	1:1	1 to 4*	—	1 to 4*
AS (compensated)	N to 4*	N to 4*	N	N to 4	N to 4	—	—	1:1	1 to 4*	NR*	—
AS (decompensated)	N to 4*	N to 4*	N to 1	N to 4	N to 4	—	—	1 to 2/1	1 to 2*	NR*	—
Shock lung	N	N	N	1 to 4*	1 to 4	1 to 4	—	1:1*	N	NR*	—
ASD	N to 3	N	N	1 to 4*	1 to 4*	—*	—*	1:1*	1 to 4	—	1 to 4*
ASD (shunt reversed)	1 to 4	N to 2	1 to 2	1 to 4*	1 to 4	1 to 4*	1 to 4*	1 to 4/1	−1 to +4*	—	1 to 2*
Emphysema (pure or predominant)	−1 to +1	−1 to −2	N	N to 4*	1 to 4*	—	1 to 4*	1:1	−1 to −4	NA	NA
Emphysema and LHF	1 to 3*	1 to 3*	N	N to 4*	1 to *4	—	—	1:1	−1 to −3	NA	NA
Chronic bronchitis (pure or predominant)	1 to 4*	1 to 4	N	1 to 4*	1 to 4*	1 to 4*	NA	1 to 4/1*	N to 2	NA	NA
Chronic bronchitis and LHF	2 to 4*	2 to 4*	N	1 to 4*	1 to 4*	1 to 4*	—	1 to 4/1*	N to 2	NA	NA

*Principal features from which alterations in hemodynamic values can be deduced. *RV*, Right ventricle; *LV*, left ventricle; *LA*, left atrium; *MPA*, main pulmonary artery; *PAs*, pulmonary arteries; *PV*, pulmonary vein; *PBV*, pulmonary blood volume; *NR*, no redistribution, *PAP*, pulmonary artery pressure; *PVR*, pulmonary vascular resistance; *PBF*, pulmonary blood flow; *LHF*, left-sided heart failure; *MS*, mitral stenosis; *AS*, aortic

cardiac failure, renal failure, and lung injury will have three quite different ranges of LAP associated with them[17] (Fig. 7-2).

Chapter 8 discusses the radiologic distinction between hydrostatic (pressure) edema and that resulting from injury.

ASSESSING PULMONARY BLOOD VOLUME

Even though severe hyperemia and severe oligemia are quite easy to recognize, film readers often appear reluctant to report them. We have found an even greater reluctance to report lesser changes in pulmonary blood volume (PBV) (Fig. 7-3), possibly because of a lack of teaching emphasis on the diagnostic value of such findings or because of the belief that this is not "hard" data, since observers assess oligemia and hyperemia differently.

In support of this, in one survey we found an inter-observer variation of 29% in assessing PBV.[18] However, this study compared only two observers with widely

Inv	Systemic vessels and tissues			Lung		Physiologic deductions			
	Aorta	VPW (size)	ST	Edema (size)	Eff	LAP (mm Hg)	PAP mean	PVR	PBF
—	N	N	N	—	—	3-10	15-25	N	N
1 to 2	N	−1 to N	N	1 to 4*	0 to 4	15-40	25-50	1 to 3	−1 to −3
1 to 3*	N	1 to 2	N	1 to 4*	1 to 4	10-25	25-35	1 to 2	−1 to −4
1 to 3*	N to 4	2 to 4*	1 to 4*	1 to 4*	1 to 4	10-25	20-30	1 to 4	−1 to −4
1 to 4*	−1 to −4*	−1 to −4*	N to 2	—	—	10-30	20-70	1 to 4	UL:1 to 2 LL:−1 to −2
1 to 4*	−1 to −4*	−1 to −4*	N to 2	1 to 4*	1 to 4	15-40	30-80	1 to 4	UL:1 to 2 LL:−1 to −2
—	N to 4	1 to 4*	1 to 4*	0 to 4*	0 to 4	10-20	20-35	1 to 4	−1 to −4
—	N to 4	−1 to −2*	N	—	—	10-30	20-50	1 to 4	−1 to −4
—	N to 4	N to 2*	N to 2*	1 to 4	1 to 4	15-35	25-60	1 to 4	−2 to −4
	−1 to N	N to 2*	N to 2x	0 to 2	0 to 2	5 to 15	20 to 70	1 to 4	1 to 4
—	1 to 4*	1 to 4*	N	—	—	3-10	25 to 40	−1 to −2	1 to 4
—	−1 to N*	−1 to N*	0 to 2	1 to 4*	—	10-30	35 to 80	1 to 4	−1 to −2
NA	1 to 4	−1 to −4	−1 to −3*	—	—	3-10	20-80	1 to 4	−1 to −4
NA	1 to 4	−1 to +2*	−1 to +2*	1 to 2*	1 to 2*	15-30	30-90	1 to 4	−1 to −4
NA	N to 4	1 to 4*	1 to 4*	—	—	3-10	25 to 85	1 to 4	−1 to −4
NA	1 to 4	1 to 4*	1 to 4*	1 to 4*	1 to 4*	15-30	30-90	1 to 4	−1 to −4

stenosis; *ASD*, atrial septal defect; *N*, normal; *ST*, soft tissue (thickness); *INV*, inverted; *Eff*, effusion; *UL, LL*, upper, lower lobes: *NA*, not applicable. Numbers from −1 to +4 refer to *amount* of change.

varying experience. We recently repeated this study using nine observers with widely differing levels of training (working in five different geographic locations) and found that the more experienced film readers had a much higher level of agreement (kappa, 0.48; standard error [SE], 0.077; probability [p] less than 0.001) than the inexperienced readers.[19] This study suggests that the more aware one is of the significance of changes in PBV and the more one looks for and compares these differences, either chronologically in the same patient or between different patients, the better one's visual memory becomes and the better one can recognize changes and factor them into the diagnosis.

Some practical observations that may assist in deciding whether PBV is normal, increased, or decreased include the following:

1. As the lungs begin to fill with blood, the usual 0.6:1.0 to 0.8:1.0 upper lobe/lower lobe (UL/LL) blood flow ratio converts to a 1:1 ratio.
2. End-on arteries and their paired bronchi usually

Fig. 7-2 For each type of edema a different relationship exists between quantity of edema and left atrial pressure (LAP). For example, if each film reader grades edema as +1 (dotted lines), in patients with injury edema the LAP is 5 (normal), with renal edema 17, and with cardiac edema 25 mm Hg.

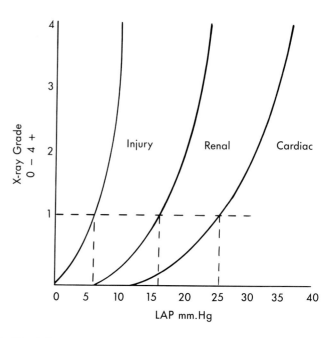

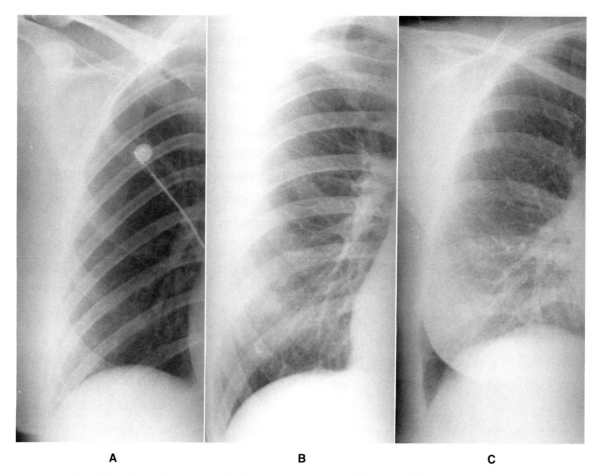

A   B   C

Fig. 7-3 These three examples have been chosen to illustrate mild, not gross, changes in vascularity. **A,** Patient with mild oligemia; **B,** normovolemic subject; **C,** patient with mild hyperemia. When seen together, the differences are quite evident. When they are seen individually, however, the quantification is more difficult and requires either experience or an available set of standard reference radiographs.

tend to be the same size. Increasing PBV increases the size and density of the end-on vessel without altering the bronchus (Fig. 7-4).

3. As PBV increases, it becomes progressively easier to see apical vessels, which increase in size and apparent number.

4. The size and number of the pulmonary vessels should correspond to the patient's physique. As PBV increases, the size and number of vessels become greater than usual relative to physique.

5. Under virtually all conditions of increasing PBV, excluding left-to-right shunts, the entire circulating blood volume is increasing and the vascular pedicle therefore becomes wider (Fig. 7-4).

6. Increased filling of the mass of nonvisualized microvessels causes a progressive increase in lung density (Fig. 7-4), which can sometimes be mistaken for edema.

However, increasing PBV alone does *not* cause the vessel margins to become blurred and does not cause peribronchial cuffing. Note also that edema lowers

lung compliance and causes a reduction in lung volume, whereas increasing PBV (particularly if it is longstanding) tends to "erect" the lung and may be associated with enlargement of the lungs (Fig. 7-5),* as in patients with large left-to-right shunts. Progressive *loss* of PBV is identifiable by reversing all the criteria given for increasing PBV. The causes for global and regional increases and decreases in PBV are discussed in Chapter 6.

ASSESSING PULMONARY BLOOD FLOW

As already indicated in our discussions of the characteristics of the pulmonary vascular bed in previous chapters, increased PBF can occur in only three ways: (1) a decrease in the transit time of blood flow through

---

*This effect is probably not large. As Fig. 7-5 shows, a major increase in PAP is needed to erect the lung, in contrast with the small change in pulmonary alveolar pressure, which erects the lung fully. Note in Fig. 7-5, *D*, that inflating the lung, even with a low PAP, "sucks" blood into the lungs, greatly increasing PAP.

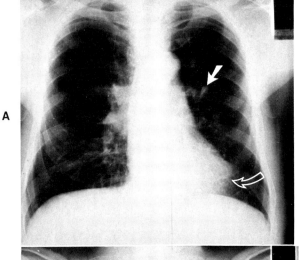
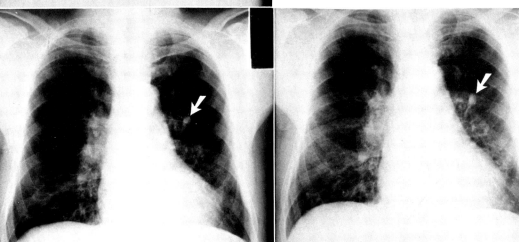

Fig. 7-4 Series of three radiographs shows the same male patient (a "blue bloater") with progressively worsening left-sided heart failure (LHF) from **A** to **C.** Note the increasing diameter of end-on vessels *(straight arrows)*, increasing lung density, and increasing cardiac volume. This patient cannot invert his flow because of UL vessel destruction. The curved arrow indicates the classic outward and upward displacement of the cardiac apex, indicating RV enlargement (see text).

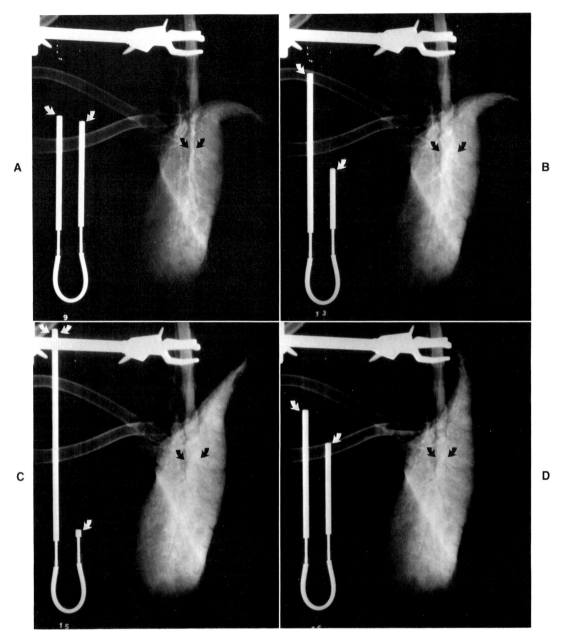

Fig. 7-5 Free-hanging single lung lobe supported only by air cannula in bronchus. Mercury manometer on the lower left indicates PAP by the difference in the levels of the two columns. **A,** PAP *(white arrows),* 5 mm Hg; pulmonary alveolar pressure (Palv), 5 cm H_2O. The lung is not erected; note drooping UL. Pulmonary artery (PA) between black arrows is very small. **B,** PAP, 50 mm Hg; Palv, 5 cm H_2O. The lung is slightly larger; note gross increase in size of PA *(black arrows)* and increased lung density caused by microvascular filling, not edema. Minimal evidence only of lung "erection" (compare UL with **A**). **C,** PAP, 95 mm Hg; Palv, 5 cm H_2O. Further increase in lung size and evidence of erection, best seen in UL. Note arteries were almost fully distended in **A** and have increased only minimally in size; that is, all vessels are fully recruited. **D,** PAP, 15 mm Hg; Palv, 20 cm H_2O. The small elevation of Palv completely erects the lung. Note that with a PAP of only 15 mm Hg the PA is large, not because it is distended by the intraluminal vascular pressure, but because it is "pulled" open by the lung's negative interstitial pressure ("auxiliary heart" effect; see Chapter 6).

the lung with *no* change in PBV, (2) an increase in PBV with *no* change in transit time, or (3) a combination of the two, (i.e., decrease in transit time, increase in PBV).[20]

Decreased Transit Time

Pure decrease in transit time with little increase in PBV results in little or no change on the chest radiograph. This type of flow increase can usually occur only when the heart is functioning normally and there is no increase in total blood volume (Fig. 7-6, *A*). For an increase in PBF of 50%, transit time would decrease 20% and PBV would increase only 25%.[21] Examples of this mechanism would occur in persons doing exercise and patients with anemia or thyrotoxicosis before heart failure (see Fig. 6-33, *A*). In all these subjects, increased microvascular filling causes an increase in film density, but this cannot usually be appreciated unless a normal radiograph of the same patient is available for comparison. (Compare *B* and *C* in Fig. 7-5.)

Two special cases of flow increase mediated largely by decreased transit time occur in patients with (1) septic shock, in whom the total blood volume may be enlarged but cannot fill the peripheral vascular bed because it is dilated, and the vascular pedicle width (VPW) is therefore not increased (Fig. 7-6, *A*), and (2) small left-to-right shunts, in whom the systemic blood volume is reduced and the VPW narrowed (Fig. 7-6, *D*).

In all these patients, flow cannot be quantified from the radiograph. However, in the patient with a left-to-right shunt the small aorta, slightly convex MPA, and the cardiac configuration may indicate that a shunt *is* present. Under these circumstances the absence of an increase in the PBV indicates that the pulmonary/systemic shunt ratio is less than 1.5:1.0 (Fig. 7-6, *D*) (i.e., if it were larger than 1.5:1, increase in PBV *would* be seen).

In patients with septic shock, the clinical history and frequently the development of lung edema caused by injury provide the diagnosis. The film reader then *knows* that a large PBF exists, even though he or she cannot *quantify* it.

Increased Blood Volume

Increased PBF through the lungs is mediated by increased PBV with *no* change in transit time. It is difficult to think of any hemodynamic circumstance that would fit this mechanism. One possibility is a long-standing left-to-right shunt in which endarteritis has begun to develop, slowing the transit time to normal levels (i.e., just before shunt reversal). An increase in the pulmonary arterial/venous (A/V) size ratio would suggest this is occurring; this indicates that precapillary arterial hypertension is developing and that the previously large PBF flow is therefore diminishing. Under these circumstances the actual flow would be very difficult to quantify (Fig. 7-7).

Decreased Transit Time/Increased Blood Volume

A simultaneous increase in PBV and decrease in transit time is the usual mechanism by which flow through the lung increases *pathologically*. In this category the most common causes are (1) overhydration and renal failure, both of which cause increased total blood volume and therefore a *wide* pedicle, and (2) moderate to large left-to-right shunts, which have a diminished systemic blood volume and therefore a *small* vascular pedicle. The difference in VPW in the two conditions simply indicates the *etiology* of the high-flow state, but the assessment of the amount of flow through the lungs is the same whether the blood volume is increased generally (i.e., increased total blood volume) or within the lungs only (see Fig. 7-6).

As PBF progressively increases, PBV will also progressively increase and the upper lobe vessels will begin to fill, causing flow distribution to change from the usual 0.6 to 0.8:1.0 to a 1:1 balanced UL/LL distribution. Simultaneously the caliber of the arteries and veins will increase equally (maintaining the normal 1:1 A/V size ratio) (see Fig. 7-6). Note that the progressive increase in flow and PBV volume will also be accompanied by a progressive elevation of PAP (Fig. 7-8).

When the signs of increased PBF are present radiologically, this virtually excludes the possibility of cardiac failure; that is, failure is defined as the inability to respond to increased demand with an increased output. One might argue that after treatment for cardiac failure, PBF increases, but the increase in cardiac output occuring after treatment is usually too small for this to be visible (Fig. 7-9). As seen on the plain film, inversion of flow disappears, apical flow diminishes, and basal flow increases, but total PBF does not change (Fig. 7-9). It is of course possible to increase PBF in patients with cardiac disease by either exercise or overhydration. Hopefully the latter will not occur.

In patients with cardiac disease, transit time at rest is usually well below normal: 23% slower than normal in patients with aortic stenosis, 38% slower in those with aortic regurgitation, 55% slower in those with ischemic cardiac disease, and 65% slower in patients with mitral stenosis and regurgitation.[21] If these patients with cardiac disease have their output (PBF) increased, as just discussed, they do decrease their transit times (by approximately 20%) but have a greater increase in PBV than normal patients. Patients with idiopathic myocardiopathy are an interesting exception to this. Their PBF increases less than one-half that of normal subjects on exercise, but their transit time decreases approxi-

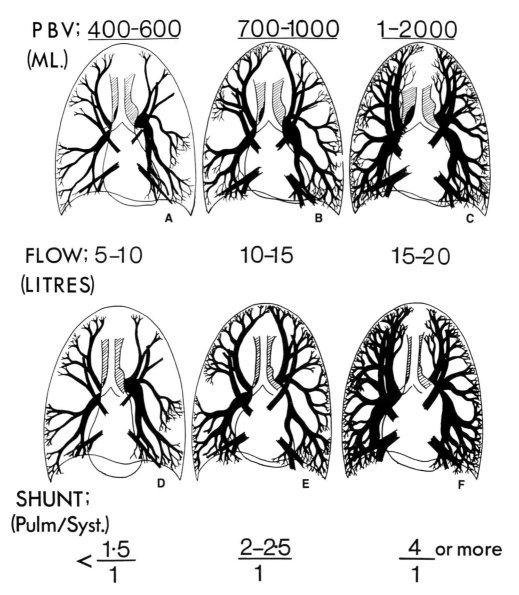

P B V; <u>400-600</u>   <u>700-1000</u>   <u>1-2000</u>
(ML.)

A   B   C

FLOW; 5-10   10-15   15-20
(LITRES)

D   E   F

SHUNT;
(Pulm/Syst.)

$< \dfrac{1 \cdot 5}{1}$ $\dfrac{2 \cdot 25}{1}$ $\dfrac{4}{1}$ or more

Fig. 7-6   Radiologic criteria used to assess PBV, pulmonary blood flow (PBF), and pulmonary/systemic (P/S) shunt ratios. Organic pulmonary arterial hypertension is *not* present in any patient (all show A/V ratios of 1:1). Note that the same radiologic appearances within the lungs have the same meaning whether a left-to-right (L-R) shunt is present (*D* to *F*) or is not present (*A* to *C*). **A,** Normal flow distribution. PBV "matches" patient size. Vascular pedicle width (VPW), azygos vein width (AW), and cardiac size match PBV. PBV varies with patient size and obesity, from 400 to 600 ml. Flow in a patient with a healthy heart can increase (e.g., on exercise) from 5 to 10 L/min, with no change in size of visible "conducting" vessel. **B,** PBV has greatly increased, and now a 1:1 flow distribution is present. The increased PBV is matched by the increased VPW and AW, indicating that the *total* blood volume (TBV) is increased. A 1.0 cm increase in VPW indicates approximately a 2.0 L increase in TBV; since PBV is approximately 10% of TBV, an increase of 2.0 L in TBV should cause an approximate increase of 200 ml in PBV. Varying with the patient's size and the degree of arterial and venous enlargement, PBV would

be assessed at 700 to 1000 ml, and flow would be 10 to 15 L/min. **C,** Massive engorgement of all arteries and veins, resulting in a 1:1 flow distribution. Massive VPW and AW. PBV assessed at 1000 to 2000 ml, varying with patient's size. Flow is 15 to 20 L/min. **D,** Same *lung* appearance as in **A.** PBV is still 400 to 600 ml, and flow will still be assessed at 5 to 10 L/min. However, note that VPW and AW are slightly *less* and that the MPA is beginning to enlarge, indicating a L-R shunt. The absence of a 1:1 flow redistribution indicates that the P/S ratio is less than 1:5:1.0. **E,** Identical radiologic appearance in the lungs as in **B;** therefore PBV and flow are assessed similarly. Note, however, progressive reduction in VPW, AW, and cardiac size. The discrepancy between VPW, cardiac size, and PA size indicates a P/S ratio of 2.0 to 2.5:1. **F,** Same lung appearance as in **C;** therefore PBV and flow are assessed similarly. VPW and AW are now extremely small, indicating a very large P/S flow ratio (4:1 or greater). Note that when the pedicle is very narrow, the heart looks as if it is hanging (similar to a pear) from a narrow stalk, an appearance sometimes called the "piccolo" syndrome in Italy.

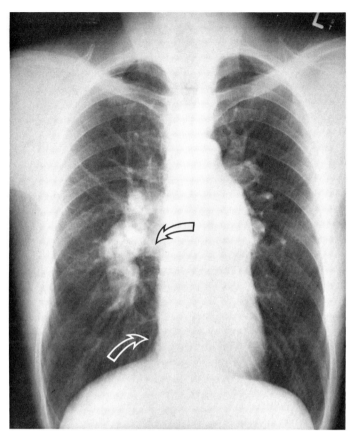

Fig. 7-7   Patient with long-standing large L-R shunt has developed organic pulmonary arterial hypertension. Note the very small size of the draining veins *(curved arrows)*, resulting in a 5:1 A/V ratio. These changes indicate that the prior high flows must be greatly reduced and indicate shunt reversal is either imminent or present. Under these circumstances the large MPA and central vessels can no longer be related to the flow.

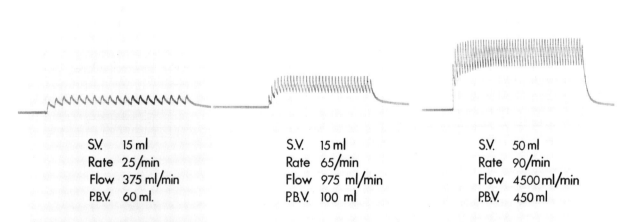

| A | B | C |

S.V.	15 ml		S.V.	15 ml		S.V.	50 ml
Rate	25/min		Rate	65/min		Rate	90/min
Flow	375 ml/min		Flow	975 ml/min		Flow	4500 ml/min
P.B.V.	60 ml.		P.B.V.	100 ml		P.B.V.	450 ml

Fig. 7-8   **A,** Pulmonary arterial pressure (PAP) tracing. Stroke volume, 15 ml; flow (RV output), 375 ml/min; PAP, 28 mm Hg. **B,** Flow increased to 975 ml/min; PBV, 100 ml; PAP has increased to 64 mm Hg. **C,** "Torrential" flow of 4500 ml/min. PBV is now 450 ml, and the PAP is 140 mm Hg. At this point, total recruitment of all the vessels has been achieved, and any attempt to increase cardiac output still further will cause instant pulmonary edema.

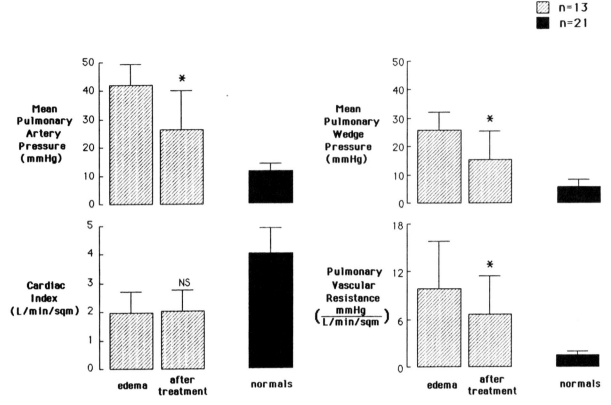

Fig. 7-9 Note that the change in cardiac index after treatment is extremely small (not statistically significant [N,S]). Also, a major increase in pulmonary vascular resistance (PVR) compared with normal subjects persists even when patients no longer have heart failure (see text).

mately 20%.[21] We state in earlier chapters that the usual "laws" of flow inversion that can be applied to patients with chronic left-sided heart failure, usually caused by ischemia or infarct, do not seem to apply to those with idiopathic myocardiopathies, in whom flow inversion is rarely seen.

One might reasonably argue, since the transit times are not known when one examines the plain chest film, that one cannot quantify flow from the plain radiograph. However, one does know that any global or regional increase in PBV (in which the arteries and the veins increase in size to the same degree) must indicate an increase in flow. Since this must be accompanied by a decrease in transit time, the flow increase is even *greater* than the increase in PBV indicates (see Fig. 6-15, *B*).

Similarly, since a decrease in PBV usually indicates diminished PBF, which is invariably accompanied by an *increase* in transit time, any decrease in the global or regional PBV (arteries and veins decreasing to the same degree) means a *greater* decrease in flow than the change in PBV alone suggests.

Transit time is usually longer in small-diameter ves-

sels and shorter in large-diameter vessels. As a result, if a regional difference of, for example, 2:1 in vessel *size* is present, the relative *flow* difference in the two areas is almost certainly *greater* than 2:1. This indicates that even small differences in vessel size are important radiologic indices of differences in flow and that it is therefore valuable to analyze the radiograph carefully for differences in vessel size. The inverse change in transit time that occurs in response to a change in cardiac output therefore lends even *more* weight to the accuracy of the film reader's ability to assess flow from the radiograph. However, film readers are probably much better at estimating proportional change in flow than at determining absolute values.[15]

ASSESSING RIGHT ATRIAL PRESSURE

For many years radiologists were frustrated by reading chest radiographs as showing no evidence of right-sided heart failure (RHF) and having the referring clinician ensure them that RHF was present. Radiologists were frequently told that neck vein distention was present, even though they could see no evidence of an enlarged superior vena cava (SVC) or azygos vein on

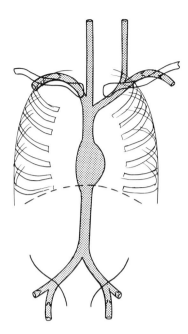

Fig. 7-10   Diagram showing that a continuous column of blood, uninterrupted by valves, courses from the base of the skull (neck veins) to the femoral veins.

the chest film. No valves exist from the base of the skull to the right atrium (RA) or from the RA down to the femoral veins, and therefore a continuous column of blood passes without interruption from the skull to the inguinal region (Fig. 7-10). Thus it seemed impossible to us that the *upper* portion of this very long column of fluid could dilate while the lower portion (in the thorax), with an even higher pressure and *not* surrounded by dense tissue, remained *normal* in width.

The only feasible explanation for this, if the clinicians were correct and the neck veins were dilated in the absence of enlargement of the vascular pedicle, seemed to be that high vasomotor tone was present in the brachiocephalic veins and SVC, causing them to constrict. If true, this would certainly explain the discrepancy between the clinical and radiologic findings, and then no relationship would exist between the VPW and the presence of neck vein dilation.

However, as discussed in Chapter 4, when we measured the VPW in a group of patients and correlated this with careful clinical examination, the venous side of the vascular pedicle measured from midline to right-hand border (MR) correlated very well with the presence or absence of neck vein dilation.[22] This satisfied us that we could predict RAP was elevated when the VPW was *increased*. However, when the VPW was *not* increased, we could not say whether right atrial pressure (RAP) was normal or not, for the simple reason (we believe) that all of the changes that could indicate to us

that RAP was elevated were occurring in the *abdomen* and *lower* limbs and were invisible to us on the chest radiograph. The clinician, seeing increasing liver size, ascites, and peripheral edema, could make a confident diagnosis of RHF without our being able to see evidence of raised RAP on the chest film. We have seen some patients with end-stage *renal* failure who have high vasomotor tone in whom the VPW has been normal on the radiograph but in whom neck vein dilation *has* been reported. (However, we have not been able to confirm the clinical findings ourselves.)

We believe the anatomic factors just discussed are also responsible for the rather poor correlation between VPW and mean RAP ($r = 0.48$; $p < 0.005$) and the better correlation between azygos vein width (AW) and mean RAP ($r = 0.74$; $p < 0.001$).[22] This latter correlation may reflect the effect of raised *intraabdominal* pressure on the tributaries making up the azygos vein. This pressure elevation within the azygos venous system would have little or no effect on the width of the SVC and therefore would have no effect on the VPW.

The regrettable conclusion is that if the VPW is not increased, the film reader cannot confidently *exclude* elevation of RAP. However, he or she may be able to derive *secondary* clues indicating that RAP is elevated, such as enlargement of the azygos vein, loss of lung volume from increasing abdominal contents, and development of effusions (particularly on the right) *without* preceding pulmonary edema from cardiac causes, indicating that the effusion is coming through the diaphragm from the abdomen. Unfortunately, since RHF typically follows LHF, cardiac edema is frequently present.

The pulmonary edema in patients with LHF frequently *improves* as the patient develops RHF, possibly because intravascular water shifts out of the circulating blood volume into the abdomen and soft tissues. Therefore a sudden increase in VPW together with a reduction in pulmonary edema and clinical improvement of "cardiac asthma" in a patient with LHF are strong evidence for an elevated RAP and the presence of RHF.

If the VPW is increased, and particularly if AW appears to be increased proportionately more than the VPW, increased RAP can be diagnosed (see Fig. 6-36). However, an enlarged VPW also means increased systemic blood volume. How can one distinguish between an increase in VPW caused by increased circulating blood volume and that primarily caused by elevated RAP? Frequently, it is impossible to make this distinction from the radiograph; however, if the VPW increase results primarily from increased *total* circulating blood volume, the PBV must also increase, yielding a *1:1 flow distribution* (see Fig. 7-1, *C*). In contrast, if the VPW increase results primarily from increased RAP following LHF, the PBV will not increase and no 1:1 flow distribution will result but flow *inversion* may be present (see Fig. 6-36). Another clear-cut example of increased VPW and large azygos vein with *normal* flow distribution occurs in patients with pericardial tamponade, in whom RAP rises and VPW progressively increases, whereas the cardiac output decreases and the PBV progressively diminishes.

RELATIONSHIP BETWEEN SYSTEMIC AND PULMONARY BLOOD FLOWS

As shown, increasing global flow through the lung is generally manifested radiologically by a progressive, simultaneous increase in size of the pulmonary arteries (including the MPA) and veins, causing a progressive change from the normal 0.6 to 0.8:1.0 UL/LL flow ratio to a 1:1 (balanced) flow. If the underlying cause of the increased flow is increased circulating blood volume,

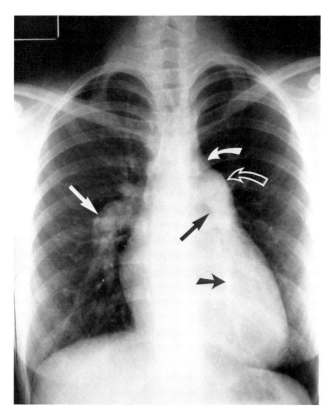

Fig. 7-11 Atrial septal defect (ASD) with narrowing of vascular pedicle. Very small aorta *(curved solid white arrow)*, large MPA *(curved open arrow)*, and central PAs *(long straight arrow)*. The veins (best seen through the heart, *short black arrow)* remain large, resulting in a 1:1 A/V ratio, indicating no organic PA hypertension is present. The P/S flow ratio can therefore be assessed, as in Fig. 7-6, and was correctly determined to be 2:1.

the VPW will increase in parallel with the increase in PBV. The VPW can therefore be of secondary value for assessing the amount of the increase in PBF.[22]

If the cause of increasing flow through the lungs is a left-to-right shunt within the thorax, the vascular pedicle will be narrow, reflecting the diminished *systemic* flow, and the aorta will be small,[23] with its reduced size reflecting the low flow through it. The relative sizes of the aorta, MPA, and central pulmonary arteries provide a good indication of the pulmonary/systemic flow ratio (Fig. 7-11; see also Fig. 7-6, *D* to *F*). The MPA's size, as seen on the frontal view just below the aortopulmonary window, is of some value as an index of flow when it enlarges in the absence of any signs of organic pulmonary arterial hypertension. When the MPA does not enlarge, however, this does not mean that flow has not increased. An MPA containing a high ratio of collagen/elastic tissue apparently enlarges much less in response to flow than an artery with a lower collagen/elastic tissue ratio.[5]

DISTINGUISHING AMONG INCREASES IN PULMONARY BLOOD VOLUME, PULMONARY BLOOD FLOW, AND PULMONARY ARTERIAL HYPERTENSION
Increase in Pulmonary Blood Volume Versus Increase in Pulmonary Blood Flow

From the discussion of the principles governing flow through the lung, it is evident that increasing PBF is most often achieved by a simultaneous decrease in transit time and increase in PBV. Because of this, increases in PBV and PBF are inseparable. The radiologic signs within the lungs for the two conditions are identical.

Is the corollary also true, that an increased PBV always or usually means an increased PBF? The answer is yes, it usually does. Cardiac decompensation might be proffered as an exception to this, but as we have already indicated, in most types of cardiac decompensation (e.g. acute LHF, mitral or aortic stenosis), PBV is not significantly increased (see Fig. 7-9).[21,24] However, in long-standing LHF, underperfusion of the kidneys usually occurs, resulting in aldosterone secretion and an increase in total blood volume, which *is* reflected by increased PBV.[25] In most patients with such chronic conditions, however, *flow inversion* occurs concomitantly (Fig. 7-12). The inversion indicates that PBV is relatively increased in the upper lobes (ULs) and decreased in the lower lobes (LLs); it also indicates that the heart is failing. Since cardiac failure is associated with a marked *slowing* in transit time, one can therefore deduce correctly that the UL flow must be traveling at a reduced rate and the LL flow at a *greatly* reduced rate; therefore the general flow through the entire lung is diminished.

Pulmonary Arterial Hypertension Versus Increased Pulmonary Blood Flow

In pulmonary arterial hypertension PBV may seem to have increased because of enlargement of the proximal pulmonary arteries. However, this can readily be distinguished from a true increase in PBV or PBF by (1) the increasing *tortuosity* of the arteries, which should be completely absent in a true PBV or PBF increase, and (2) the smaller size of the veins compared with the arteries, giving an increased A/V ratio in contrast with the 1:1 ratio seen in true PBV or PBF increase (Fig. 7-13). Further more, the cause of the pulmonary arterial hypertension is frequently seen on the chest radiograph, for example, chronic bronchitis, emphysema, chronic interstitial fibrosis, obesity (suggesting pickwickian syndrome), and kyphoscoliosis (Fig. 7-13). The special case of pulmonary arterial hypertension occurring in lungs with a high flow state is considered later.

ASSESSING CARDIAC OUTPUT

At first sight it seems improbable that, knowing nothing about the patient's heart rate or transit time, cardiac output (CO) can be quantified from a single static radiograph. However, since PBF is synonymous with right ventricular output (which in the absence of a shunt should match *left* ventricular output), the same general principles that govern the quantification of PBF also clearly govern the quantification of cardiac output. The same possibilities and the same limitations apply, and therefore, for PBF, in general one can substitute cardiac output or, in the patient with a left-to-right shunt, right-sided heart output.

At the very least, one should quite easily be able to assign cardiac output to three broad categories:

1. If a patient has a normal heart size, normal flow distribution, normal A/V ratio, no edema, and normal lung parenchyma, one can be almost certain that the cardiac output is *normal.*
2. If flow inversion and edema are present, one can be certain that cardiac output is *low.*
3. If the vascular pedicle is wide, the PBV great, the A/V ratio 1:1, and the UL/LL flow ratio 1.0, one knows that cardiac output is *increased.*

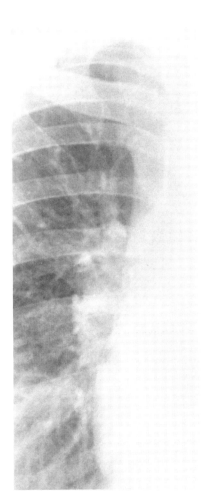

Fig. 7-12 Chronic cardiac decompensation; note 2:1 flow inversion (upper lobe/lower lobe [UL/LL] ratio). Azygos vein and vascular pedicle are also enlarged, indicating biventricular failure.

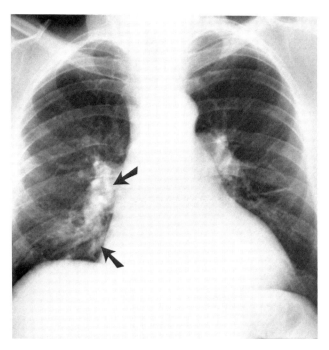

Fig. 7-13 Patient with severe chronic bronchitis ("blue bloater") and organic pulmonary arterial hypertension, manifested by greatly enlarged MPA, elevated cardiac apex, large comma-shaped central pulmonary arteries, tortuous peripheral vessels, and decreased draining vein size *(arrows),* resulting in an A/V ratio of 4:1.

By assigning grades of change to each of the criteria described, one can further subdivide these broad categories and supply more accurate estimates of cardiac output.

SPECIFIC APPLICATIONS OF PRESSURE AND FLOW ASSESSMENT

While all of the principles discussed so far can be applied in general to most patients with cardiac and pulmonary disease, modifications exist in the meanings of the radiologic criteria, both individually and as constellations, depending on the underlying specific pathophysiology. This makes it necessary to discuss more specifically how the various radiologic signs described are used in practice. Several diseases, each of which can serve as a group prototype, are considered. For each of the diseases chosen, we discuss the quantification of PVP, PAP, PBF, and RAP.

MITRAL VALVE DISEASE
Estimating Left Atrial Pressure

In patients with mitral stenosis, mitral incompetence, or chronic LHF, the LAP level is closely related to the degree of flow inversion, even in the absence of pulmonary edema.[1] For obvious reasons, we call flow inversion the "touchdown" sign of venous hypertension. Fig. 7-14 demonstrates diagrammatically the relationship between the degree of flow inversion and the LAP level (see Table 7-1). Fig. 7-15 illustrates a clinical example of how these principles are used. If pulmonary edema is present in these patients, it indicates a further rise in LAP and should push the film reader's estimate 5 to 10 mm higher.

It is frequently stated that the presence of pulmonary edema means that the LAP is more than 25 mm Hg, the logic being that it requires this amount of hydrostatic intraluminal pressure to exceed the effects of in-

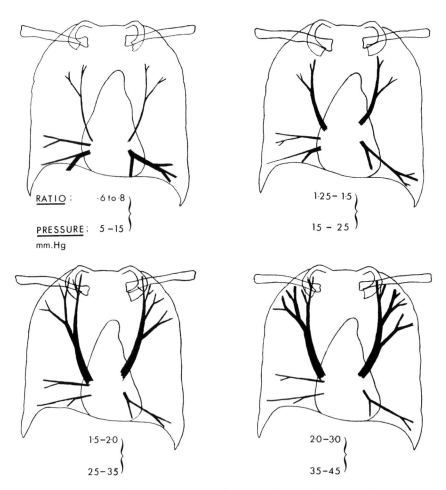

RATIO: ·6 to ·8
PRESSURE: 5 – 15 mm.Hg

1·25 – 1·5
15 – 25

1·5 – 2·0
25 – 35

2·0 – 30
35 – 45

Fig. 7-14 Diagram illustrating progressive flow inversion (pulmonary veins only shown) and the relationship between degree of flow inversion (ratio) and estimated left atrial pressure (LAP).

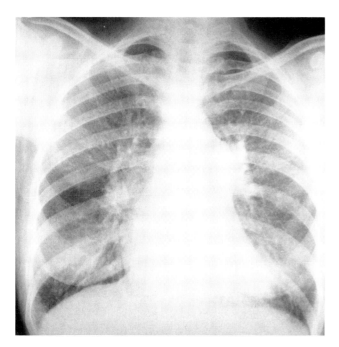

Fig. 7-15 Radiograph of 30-year-old woman with mitral stenosis. Flow inversion ratio of 1.5 to 2.0, taken alone, would indicate an LAP of 25 to 35 mm Hg. However, septal lines are present, and the very large MPA indicates some organic pulmonary arterial hypertension; both these findings push the LAP estimate to the higher end of the range. LAP was estimated radiologically at 30 mm Hg and at catheterization was 32 mm Hg. Systolic PAP was estimated at 50 mm Hg; the lack of tortuous peripheral vessels kept the estimate at a level less than 60 mm Hg. At catheterization, systolic PAP was 55 mm Hg.

traluminal oncotic pressure. The logic is incorrect, however, since fluid transudes from the pulmonary capillaries at normal LAPs. Therefore *any* increase in LAP causes an increase in pulmonary extravascular lung water, which, if it exceeds the capacity of the lymphatics to remove it, will appear as pulmonary edema, frequently with pressures much less than 25 mm Hg.[5,18] For example, if the LAP estimate based on flow inversion was 20 to 25 mm Hg and *no* edema was present, the subsequent development of edema would indicate that the estimates of LAP should be increased to 25 to 30 mm Hg. However, if the estimated level based on flow inversion was originally only 10 to 15 mm Hg, the subsequent occurrence of edema should increase the estimate only to 15 to 20 mm Hg, not to more than 25 mm Hg.

Using flow redistribution and the presence of edema only, LAP can be quantified with a clinically useful level of accuracy (Fig. 7-16); published correlations range from 0.64 to 0.9.[1,3-5,26-29] These estimates can be further improved by factoring in the estimate of PAP.[26,29]

Estimating Pulmonary Artery Pressure

The most significant radiologic criteria for assessing PAP are listed in Table 7-2. PAP increases *passively* with an elevated LAP, the mean PAP usually tracking approximately 10 mm Hg above the LAP (Fig. 7-17). This elevation can occur with no evidence of tortuous pulmonary arteries and only minimal to mild enlargement of the MPA. Nonetheless, if the LAP is estimated

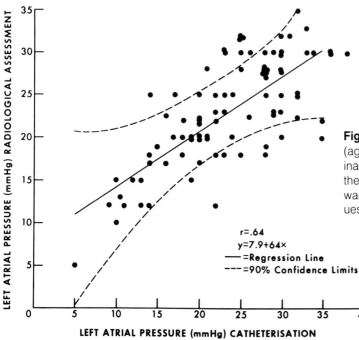

r=.64
y=7.9+64x
——— =Regression Line
- - - - =90% Confidence Limits

Fig. 7-16 LAP assessed radiologically in 85 patients (ages 16 to 80 years) with valvular heart disease (predominantly mitral valve disease). In this mixed group of patients the correlation coefficient (r) with catheterization findings was 0.64. Other authors have reported much higher r values (see text). (From Milne ENC: *Br J Radiol* 36:902, 1963.)

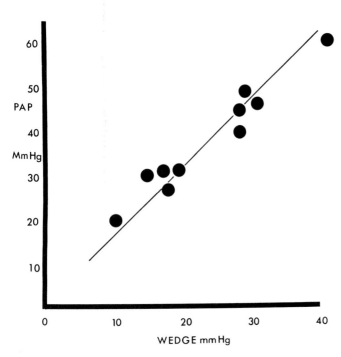

Fig. 7-17 Relationship between elevation of LAP and passive elevation of PAP.

at approximately 30 mm Hg, the mean PAP must be at least 40 mm Hg (see Fig. 7-15).

When elevated PAP has been present for some time, organic changes begin to develop in the arterioles, and a further "active" or organic increase in the PAP occurs (Fig. 7-18). As previously indicated, tortuosity of the pulmonary arteries, which is readily seen, indicates a systolic PAP of 60 mm Hg or higher[3,30-32] (see Fig. 7-7). Organic changes progressively narrow the distal arteries, causing diminished flow accompanied by lessening size of the pulmonary veins, particularly the UL veins, which were previously *enlarged*.[5] We believe the venous narrowing is caused by vasoconstriction initiated by the left atrium to maintain its output (see Chapter 6). Simultaneously the central (first and second divisions) pulmonary arteries increase in size, as does the MPA, up to a systolic PAP of 50 mm Hg[5] (Fig. 7-19). The increasing size of the central arteries associated with the decreasing size of their peripheral divisions results in comma-shaped central pulmonary arteries and progressive loss of peripheral arterioles. This leads to oligemia, described as "pruning" of the peripheral vessels (see Fig. 7-7). Pruning usually indicates a PAP of 70 mm Hg or higher.[16,31]

Note that the diminution in size of the UL veins as a result of arterial structural changes in patients with mitral stenosis must not be mistakenly read as a decrease in LAP. The presence of increasing pulmonary arterial hypertension should instead *increase* the value of the LAP estimation (see Fig. 7-18).

It has been clearly demonstrated that any one of the individual elements described (size of MPA, size and shape of central pulmonary arteries, arterial tortuosity, pruning) may be absent or insignificant, and even in the presence of pulmonary arterial hypertension, the most accurate estimations can only be given by considering *all* the features simultaneously.[4,5,28] For example, the MPA may be only minimally enlarged, but if peripheral arterial tortuosity is present, the PAP estimate will be greater than 60 mm Hg. Also, if the MPA and

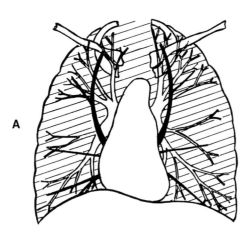
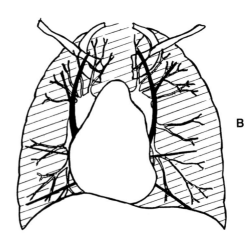

Fig. 7-18 **A,** Flow inversion (UL/LL ratio) of 1.5:1 with no evidence of organic pulmonary arterial hypertension. LAP assessed at 20 mm Hg. **B,** Exactly the same flow inversion as in **A,** but moderately severe organic pulmonary arterial hypertension is now evident, which would increase the LAP estimate to 25 to 30 mm Hg.

Table 7-2 Assessing systolic pulmonary artery pressure (mm Hg)

Vessels	Up to 20	20-40	40-60	60-80	80-100+
Main pulmonary artery*	Normal size	Questionable enlargement	Definite (+) increase in size	Moderate (++) increase in size and convexity	Gross (+++) enlargement, extremely convex
First and second divisions of pulmonary artery*	Normal size	Questionable enlargement	Definite (+) increase in size	Moderate (++) increase in size, developing "comma" appearance	Gross (+++) enlargement with "comma" shape
Peripheral branches	Normal sinuosity	Questionable increase in sinuosity	Definite (+) tortuosity present	Tortuosity (++) and questionable "pruning"	Tortuosity (++) and pruning (++)
Arterial/venous ratio†	Normal, 1:1	Normal, 1:1	Slight increase, 1.5:1.0	Marked increase, 1.5:1.0	Gross increase, 3:1

*Not applicable in patients with left-to-right shunts.
†Still applicable even in patients with left-to-right shunts.

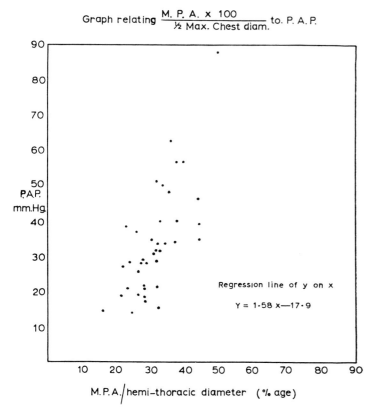

Graph relating $\dfrac{M.\,P.\,A. \times 100}{\frac{1}{2}\,Max.\,Chest\,diam.}$ to P. A. P.

Regression line of y on x

Y = 1·58 x —17·9

M.P.A./hemi-thoracic diameter (% age)

Fig. 7-19 Graph relating the ratio between *size of MPA* (measured from the midline of the thorax to the outermost convexity of the MPA) and hemithoracic diameter (measured from the midline to the maximum outer convexity of the chest wall); expressed as a percentage and the PAP (catheterization data). (From Milne ENC: *Br J Radiol* 36:902, 1963.)

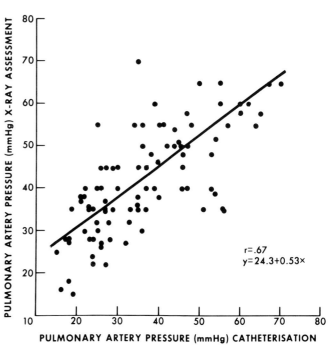

r=.67
y=24.3+0.53x

PULMONARY ARTERY PRESSURE (mmHg) CATHETERISATION

Fig. 7-20 Correlation between mean PAP assessed radiographically in 91 patients, predominantly with mitral valve disease. (Fom Milne ENC: *Br J Radiol* 36:902, 1963.)

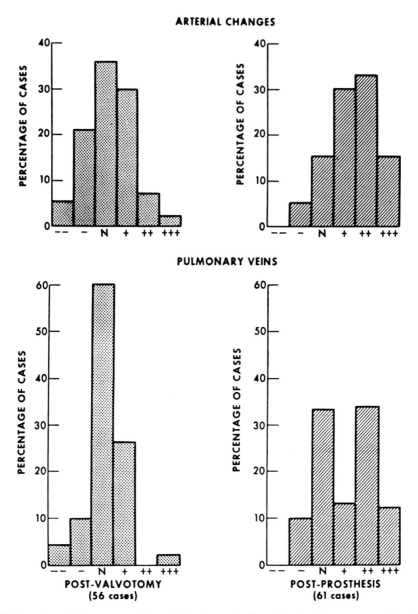

Fig. 7-21 Four histograms relate radiologic evaluation of patient improvement or deterioration after (1) valvotomy *(left-hand column)* and (2) prosthetic insertion *(right-hand column)* in the same patients. Improvement or deterioration is graded as − −, severe postoperative deterioration; −, mild postoperative deterioration; *N,* no change from preoperative status; +, slight postoperative improvement; ++, moderate postoperative improvement and + + +, major postoperative improvement.

After *valvotomy, arterial* changes indicated deterioration in 25% of patients, no change in 35%, slight improvement in 30%, and major improvement in only 10%. *Venous* changes indicated deterioration in 15% of patients, no change in 60%, slight improvement in 22%, and major improvement in only 2.5%.

After r*eplacement of the mitral valve* by prosthesis in the same patients, the radiologic results were dramatically different. Arterial changes indicated only 5% of patients deteriorated, 15% were unchanged, and 70% improved. Venous changes indicated 10% deteriorated, 35% were unchanged, and 55% improved. The summed radiologic changes correlated very well with precatheterization and postcatheterization data. (From Milne ENC, Carlsson E: *Radiology* 92:1201, 1969.)

central vessels are greatly enlarged but tortuosity is minimal or not visible, the PAP would again be estimated at more than 60 mm Hg.

Although right ventricle size is also related to the PAP level, the relationship is not linear; that is, initially, as PAP rises, the chamber walls may hypertrophy but no enlargement occurs, then dilation can occur abruptly and be much greater than the actual rise in PAP. Also, rheumatic disease may directly affect the right ventricle and cause enlargement with little increase in PAP.

Many reviews of the accuracy of PAP estimation in mitral valve disease have been made, and r ranges from 0.7 to 0.86[3,5,29-32] (Fig. 7-20).

Effects of Mitral Valve Surgery on Radiologic Estimations of Left Atrial and Pulmonary Artery Pressures

Before the development of the mitral valve prostheses, a closed approach to the stenotic valve was usually made. The stenosis was "cured" by blind finger-fracture of the valve, usually inserting the finger through the left atrial appendage, or by blindly cutting the valve using a finger knife. The results were allegedly good clinically, but usually no radiologic change was seen in flow inversion, arterial tortuosity, or cardiac chamber size. This was thought to indicate that the radiograph was insensitive (fixed) and could not be used to assess hemodynamic values postoperatively.

Preoperative and postoperative studies of a large group of patients who had had finger fracture proce-

dures, followed some years later by prosthetic valves, correlating the radiographic estimates with preoperative and postoperative catheterization studies, revealed that the radiograph was not at fault, but rather the surgery.[3] After finger fracture, few patients improved, many remained unchanged, and some deteriorated (Fig. 7-21). This was accurately reflected by the postoperative radiographs. After prosthetic replacement in the *same* patients, most improved, a few remained unchanged, and only one or two deteriorated (Fig. 7-21). The chest film was found to be slightly *more* accurate for estimating LAP after surgery than before (Fig. 7-22). In patients who had extensive organic change, manifested preoperatively by considerable arterial tortuosity, the *veins* changed readily after surgery but the arteries did not visibly change, even though catheterization showed that the PAP had greatly decreased (Fig. 7-23). Postoperatively, estimates of PAP should therefore disregard tortuosity and be calculated as being 10 to 15 mm Hg higher than the estimated LAP[3] (Fig. 7-24).

Left Atrial Size

Left atrial size is of limited value for estimating LAP in patients with mitral valve disease on preoperative radiographs. The largest left atria tend to be associated

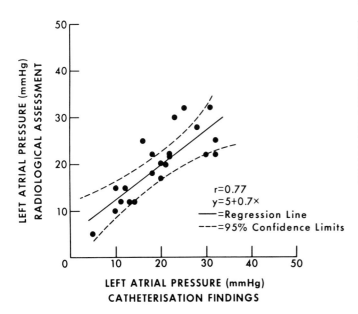

Fig. 7-22 LAP estimation after insertion of mitral valve prosthesis (*r*, 0.77). (From Milne ENC, Carlsson E: *Radiology* 92:1201, 1969.

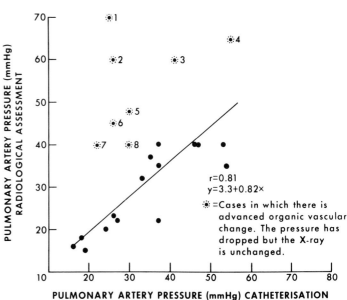

Fig. 7-23 PAP estimation following mitral valve prosthesis insertion (*r*, 0.81). Note this correlation considers only those patients in whom both arterial and venous changes occurred. When only venous change occurred, the PAs were considered to be *organically* altered and incapable of responding to altered hemodynamics. (From Milne ENC, Carlsson E: *Radiology* 92:1201, 1969.)

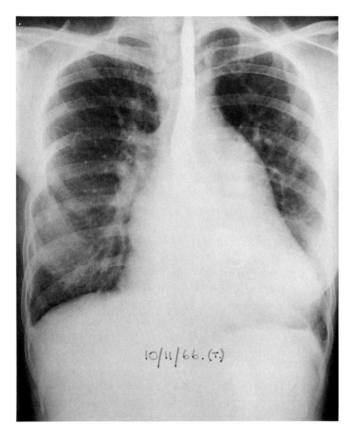

Fig. 7-24 Radiograph of 37-year-old woman after mitral valve replacement for myocardial infarction. Before surgery the PAP was assessed at 60 mm Hg (catheterization studies, 65 mm Hg) and LAP at 30 mm Hg (catheterization studies, 36 mm Hg). This patients pre-operative film is shown in Fig. 1-3. After surgery PAP was assessed at 40 mm Hg (catheterization, 46 mm Hg) and LAP at 20 mm Hg (catheterization, 20 mm Hg). (From Milne ENC, Carlsson E: *Radiology* 92[6]:1201, 1969.)

with the highest LAPs, but frequently extreme dilation can occur even with lower LAPs, presumably because of direct rheumatic involvement of the atrium. However, postoperatively a good relationship exists between the *change* in left atrial size and *change* in LAP[3] (Fig. 7-25). The one proviso is that occasionally the surgeon plicates a very dilated left atrium so that it reduces in size much more than the decrease in LAP.

Estimating Pulmonary Blood Flow

Because of the flow inversion present in most patients with mitral valve disease, flow is often greatly increased through the ULs compared with the LLs, through which flow is extremely diminished. However, because the transit time through the lungs in mitral valve disease is so slow (65% slower than normal), total PBF is *reduced*. The greater the evidence of pulmonary arterial hypertension, the more PBF will be reduced.

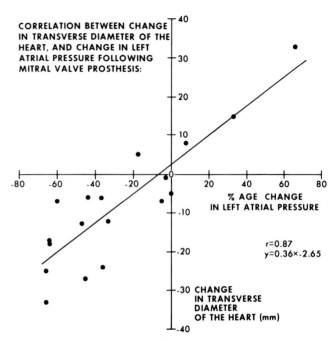

Fig. 7-25 After insertion of mitral valve prosthesis, good correlation (*r*, 0.87) exists between reduced LAP and reduced left atrial size, expressed as a percentage. (From Milne ENC, Carlsson E: *Radiology* 92:1201, 1969.)

The small output from the right side of the heart is matched to the small output from the left ventricle, which in turn appears to cause the circulating blood volume to be smaller than normal, resulting in a narrow vascular pedicle and small aorta (see Fig. 7-15).*

Estimating Right Atrial Pressure

As indicated earlier, the vascular pedicle size ranges from narrow to very narrow in pure mitral valve disease, reflecting not only a small left ventricular output but also a competent tricuspid valve and normal RAP. If the vascular pedicle and azygos vein are *normal* in size in a patient with mitral valve disease, the tricuspid valve is incompetent and the RAP elevated. Increasing enlargement of the azygos and pedicle is closely related to increasing RAP. Again, however, because increased RAP is also manifested in the abdomen and lower limbs, it is impossible to quantify RAP accurately.

AORTIC STENOSIS
Estimating Left Atrial and Pulmonary Artery Pressures

A recently completed study reveals not only that left LAP is elevated in patients with aortic valve disease, but also that the PAP is consistently increased.[19] How-

---

*As we have hypothesized previously (see Chapter 6), the reduction in circulating blood volume may be due to an increased blood level of atrionatriuretic factor.

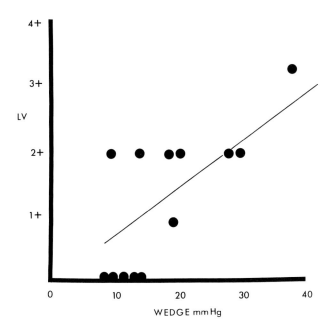

Fig. 7-26 Thirteen patients with aortic stenosis (AS). Correlation between left ventricular size assessed radiologically and wedge pressure (r, 0.65; $p < 0.02$).

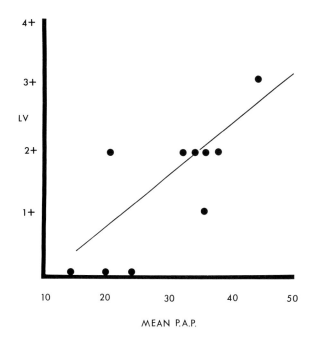

Fig. 7-27 Ten patients with AS. Correlation between left ventricular size assessed radiologically and mean PAP (r, 0.78; $p < 0.008$).

ever, since evidence of flow redistribution is rarely seen in patients with aortic valve disease and since no evidence of edema (until decompensation occurs) is seen, these two factors cannot be used as they are in patients with mitral stenosis or chronic LHF to estimate LAP. However, a correlation exists between left ventricular size and LAP (r, 0.65; $p < 0.02$) (Fig. 7-26), as well as an excellent correlation in these same patients between LAP and mean PAP (r, 0.9; $p < 0.0004$) (see Table 6-1). As a result, if the left ventricle is enlarged, even if the right is not, increased PAP will still be present. This PAP elevation is correlated with increased size of the left ventricle (r, 0.65; $p < .008$) (Fig. 7-27). Interestingly, the correlation between increase in PAP and increase in RV size is *not* significant (see Table 6-1).

As in mitral valve disease, the passive elevation of PAP that occurs secondary to elevated LAP may produce *no* evidence of arterial enlargement. Even if organic arterial hypertension begins to supervene, the radiograph will frequently show more of the classic changes of PAP, even with quite high levels of PAP. If the changes of PAP *are* present, that is, increase in size of the MPA and central divisions of the pulmonary artery, along with tortuosity and pruning of peripheral branches, these features have exactly the same significance and can be used to assess PAP as in patients with mitral valve disease, pulmonary disease, or chronic LHF. Marked elevations PAP are not uncommon in patients with aortic valve disease.[19]

Estimating Pulmonary Blood Flow

As previously noted,[19] the lungs in many patients with aortic stenosis are oligemic, reflecting low flow through the lungs secondary to a small right ventricular output and possibly to a general reduction in total blood volume from increased circulating atrionatriuretic factor. In addition to the smaller-than-normal PBV, reflecting reduced flow, the film reader should be aware that transit time in patients with aortic stenosis (AS) and AS with aortic regurgitation (AS/AR) is 23% to 38% slower than normal. The reduction in blood flow is therefore even greater in these patients than indicated by the small PBV alone. We have shown an excellent correlation between the degree of oligemia (estimated radiologically) and the stroke volume (r, 0.96; $p < 0.007$) (Tables 6-1 and 7-3).

Fig. 7-28, *A*, shows a "classic" patient with AS with oligemic lung fields and an enlarged left ventricle. Without a knowledge of the relationships between oligemia and stroke volume, the diminished transit time in AS, and the relationship between left ventricular size and PAP, it would not be possible to estimate flow, or to appreciate that pulmonary arterial hypertension *is* present and to quantify it (Table 7-3; see also Table 6-1).

As in mitral valve disease, the diminished left ventricular output is reflected in a narrow vascular pedicle. After successful insertion of an aortic valve prosthesis, the VPW and PBV both increase, reflecting the increased output from both ventricles (Fig. 7-28, *B*). The

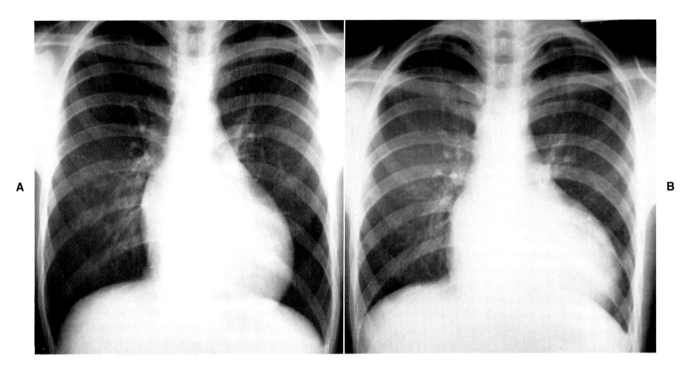

Fig. 7-28 **A,** Radiograph of 27-year-old male with aortic stenosis. Classically oligemic lung fields, very small aorta, narrow vascular pedicle, and enlarged left ventricle are seen. **B,** After insertion of an aortic valve prosthesis, the oligemia has lessened and VPW and cardiac size have increased slightly, indicating improved left ventricular output and increased circulating blood volume.

Table 7-3 Degree of correlation between oligemia and stroke volume

Patient number	Diagnosis	Oligemia* (N to +4)	LV size (N to +4)	RV size (N to +4)	Wedge pressure (mm Hg)	PAP (mean, mm Hg)	Stroke volume (ml)
25	AS	+++	+++	++	35	45 ⎫	
17	AS	+++	++	N	25	—	
1	AS	++	++	++	27	35	
14	AS	++	N	N	10	14 ⎬	31 (mean)
16	AS	++	++	N	—	—	
20	AS/AI	++	N	N	16	—	
22	AS	++	N	+	12	22 ⎭	
10	AS/AI(lupus)	+	++	++	—	— ⎫	36 (mean)
23	AS	+	++	+	21	29 ⎬	
24	AS/AI	+	+	++	—	— ⎭	
4	AS	N	+	N	22	34 ⎫	
6	AS/AI	N	++	N	9	20	
7	AS/AI	N	N	N	14	19 ⎬	88 (mean)
15	AS	N	++	N	20	36	
18	AS/AI	N	++	N	14	31 ⎭	

N, None; *LV, RV,* left, right ventricular; *PAP,* pulmonary artery pressure; *AS,* aortic stenosis, *AI,* aortic incompetence.
*Oligemia is rank ordered from most severe above to least severe below.

small aorta, reflecting the small left ventricular output and well seen in patients with mitral valve disease, may be masked in AS by dilation, resulting from turbulent blood flow distal to the AS.

Estimating Right Atrial Pressure

RAP is normal in patients with compensated AS and AS/AI. This is reflected by the narrow vascular pedicle and small azygos vein, which will only enlarge if RHF develops. Under these circumstances the combination of increased AW and VPW are of the same limited value in diagnosing elevated RAP as in straightforward cardiac decompensation.

ACUTE LEFT HEART FAILURE
Estimating Left Atrial Pressure

In acute LHF, particularly the first episode, redistribution of flow occurs in only a small percentage of patients (Fig. 7-29). In these patients this redistribution correlates with LAP and can be used for LAP estimation (Fig. 7-30). However, greater accuracy is obtained if the quantity of edema is also used in the assessment (see later discussion). We have already discussed why a few patients with acute LHF *do* show flow inversion.

Most patients with acute LHF have extensive edema *without* flow redistribution (Fig. 7-31). The correlation that must be used to assess LAP is between the quantity of edema assessed radiologically (see Chapter 3) and LAP (see Table 7-1 and Fig. 7-32). Note that in acute LHF, no increase usually occurs in cardiac size, VPW, or PBV. As previously mentioned, circulating blood volume actually *diminishes* during acute LHF failure, and the VPW may be slightly less than normal (Fig. 7-31). The estimation of LAP will be more accurate if sequential films are available. Because edema develops so abruptly in acute LHF, no appreciable lag exists between pressure elevation and development of edema. Therefore LAP estimation based on edema will be accurate, but later, when LAP *decreases* after treatment, a lag varying from hours to a day or more will occur between the reduction in LAP and quantity of edema ("posttherapeutic phase lag"). The film reader must be aware of this phenomenon and be appropriately cautious in estimating LAP at this stage of LHF. The continued presence of edema despite the LAP decrease is not a "failure" of the radiograph, but rather an accurate reflection of the efficacy of that particular patient's lymph drainage from the lungs.

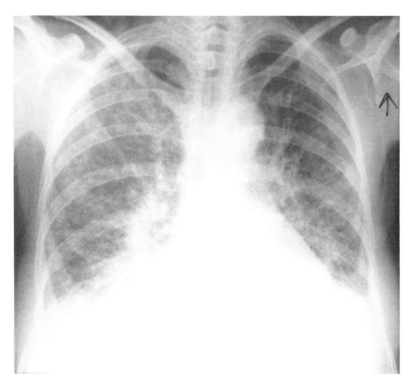

Fig. 7-29 Patient with acute LHF and severe interstitial edema. Some flow inversion (approximately 1.25 to 1.5: 1.0 UL/LL flow ratio) is present. Note that VPW and cardiac size are normal. The flow inversion in association with the edema indicates an LAP of approximately 30 mm Hg (28 mm Hg according to wedge pressure).

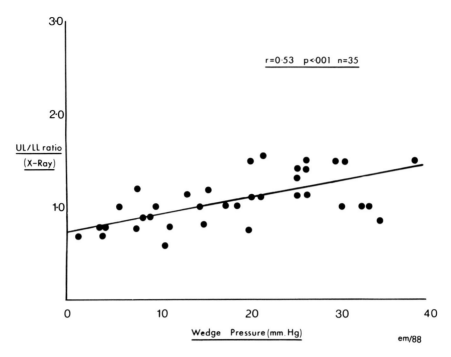

Fig. 7-30 Rather poor correlation shown between flow inversion (UL/LL ratio) and wedge pressure in LHF.

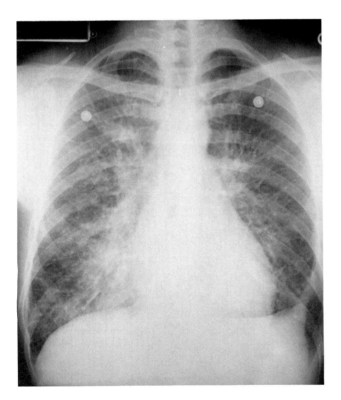

Fig. 7-31 Patient with acute left-sided heart decompensation (first episode). No flow inversion is seen, but moderately severe interstitial edema and early alveolar edema with septal lines are present. Using edema only, the assessment of LAP was 30 mm Hg (wedge pressure, 35 mm Hg).

As indicated, if flow redistribution *is* present, using the combination of flow inversion and the quantity of edema improves the accuracy of LAP assessment (Fig. 7-33).

Estimating Pulmonary Artery Pressure

As in mitral stenosis and AS, elevation of LAP causes a passive increase in PAP in patients with acute LHF. A reasonable estimate of PAP can therefore be obtained by assessing LAP (based on quantity of edema) and adding 10 mm Hg.

Estimating Pulmonary Blood Flow

Transit time through the lungs is approximately 55% slower than normal in patients with acute LHF.[21] Therefore, although no change in PBV may be seen, the film reader should be aware that PBF (cardiac output) is considerably reduced. At present we are not aware of any radiologic criteria that would allow one to quantify this flow reduction. It would seem deductively that, since edema increases pulmonary vascular resistance (PVR), the amount of *edema* present should be inversely related to the amount of flow. That is, the greater the amount of edema assessed, the lower the cardiac output. We have not, however, been able to show any great difference in cardiac output in patients with or without LHF.[33]

Estimating Right Atrial Pressure

Unless biventricular failure supervenes, the vascular pedicle and azygos vein remain normal or slightly re-

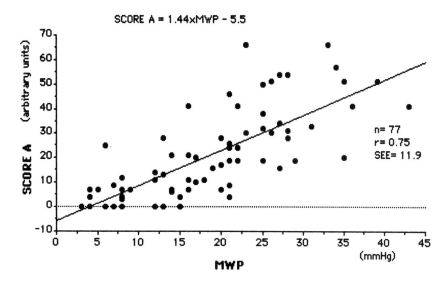

Fig. 7-32 Relationship between score *A* (pulmonary edema assessed in arbitrary units; see Table 7-4) and wedge pressure (mean). A good correlation is shown. From Balbarini A, Limbrono V, Bertoli D et al: *J Thorac Imaging* 6[2]:62, 1991.)

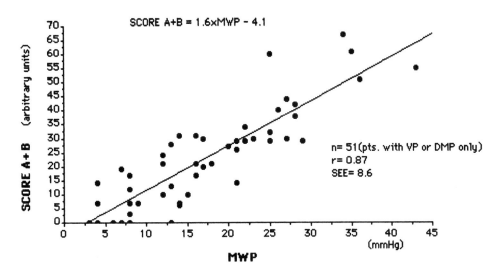

Fig. 7-33 This graph adds additional units *(score B)* derived from evaluation of *flow distribution* (see Table 7-4) to the quantification of edema. The combined data improve the correlation coefficient *r* for assessing wedge pressure from 0.75 to 0.87. (From Balbarini A, Limbrono V, Bertoli D et al: J Thorac Imaging 6[2]:62, 1991.)

duced in size in patients with acute LHF, reflecting normal RAP.

CHRONIC LEFT HEART FAILURE
Estimating Left Atrial Pressure

LAP is estimated from a combination of the presence and quantity of edema, distribution of blood flow, and certain alterations in the pulmonary vessels (Table 7-4). To improve accuracy and objectivity, Balbarini et al have assigned "scores" to each of these factors according to their statistical significance.[28] If the radiologic features *A* in Table 7-4 are "scored" for their severity a good correlation is obtained between the total score *A* and LAP (Fig. 7-32). If the score from *B* (Table 7-4) is *added* to *A* the correlation improves from 0.75 to 0.87 (Fig. 7-33). The radiologic features *C* (Table 7-4) are used to assess *PAP*. The correlation between score, *C*, and mean PAP is 0.78. If scores *A*, *B*, and *C* are *added*, the correlation between *A+B+C* and mean PAP improves to 0.89 (Fig. 7-35).

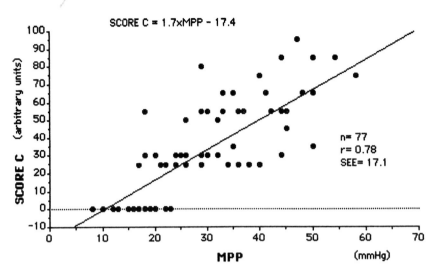

Fig. 7-34 Changes in appearance of the MPA and peripheral vessels (score C) are assessed in arbitrary units (see Table 7-4). The r between score C and mean PAP (MPP) is 0.78. (From Balbarini A, Limbrono V, Bertoli D et al: *J Thorac Imaging* 6[2]:62, 1991.)

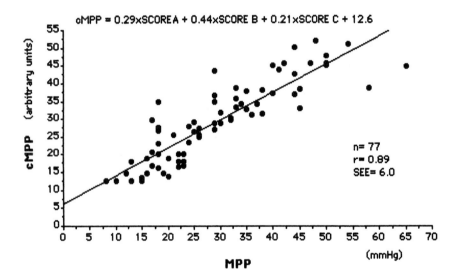

Fig. 7-35 When the scores for edema *(A)*, flow distribution *(B)*, and pulmonary arterial changes *(C)* are combined the correlation coefficient between radiologic findings and mean PAP (MPP) improves from 0.78 to 0.89. (From Balbarini A, Limbruno U, Bertoli D et al:. *J Thorac Imaging* 6[2]:62, 1991.)

If no inversion can be seen but edema *is* present, the LAP level should be assessed based on the quantity of edema alone (Fig. 7-32).

Many patients with chronic LHF, however, have flow inversion in addition to edema. This raises the LAP pressure estimate 5 to 10 mm Hg (Fig. 7-33). The greater the inversion of flow, the higher is the LAP. If inversion remains in the *absence* of edema, this indi-cates chronic elevation of LAP, suggesting that the patient has had episodes of edema over a time long enough to develop a hypertrophied lymphatic system (as in mitral stenosis), which removes edema and leaves the lung clear despite the persistently elevated LAP.

In using the quantity of edema to refine the estimate of LAP, the same warning holds true for chronic LHF as discussed for acute LHF; that is, that posttherapeu-

Table 7-4 Assessing wedge and pulmonary artery pressures

Parameter	"Score" (based on statistical importance)	
A. Radiographic findings of pulmonary interstitial edema		
Hila		
Enlarged	0, +, ++, +++	0, 8, 10, 12*
Increased density	0, +, ++	0, 6, 12
Blurred	0, +, ++	0, 8, 10
Peribronchial cuffs	0, +	0, 10
Kerley-B lines	0, +	0, 10
Micronoduli	0, +	0, 10
Widening of fissures	0, +	0, 8
Subpleural effusion	0, +	0, 6
Diffuse increase of density	0, +	0, 6
Extensive perihilar haze	0, +	0, 4
B. Pulmonary blood flow distribution		
Normal		0
Balanced		10
Inverted		14
C. Pulmonary artery abnormalities		
Right interlobar artery enlargement	0, +, ++	0, 15, 25
Main pulmonary artery dilation	0, +, ++	0, 15, 25
Pruning	0, +, ++	0, 20, 30
Tortuosity of peripheral arteries	0, +, ++	0, 15, 25

0, None; +, definite; ++, moderate +++, gross.
*These numbers are "weighted" according to their previously derived statistical importance for each radiologic feature assessed. For example, moderate hilar enlargement would be scored 10.
Modified with permission from Balbarina A, Limbruno U, Bertoli D et al: *J Thorac Imaging* 6(2): 62, 1991.

tic phase lag may permit edema to be present for many hours even when the LAP has returned to normal.

We have said little about pleural effusions in the assessment of LAP. This is because the size of pleural effusions relates very poorly to LAP (see Fig. 5-7). As shown in Chapter 5, the pleural fluid in patients with cardiac failure does not come from the parietal or visceral pleural microcirculation but from the lung interstitium, and pulmonary edema must develop *before* effusions can form. Therefore a phase lag exists between the development of pulmonary edema and the development of effusions. Similarly, the clearance mechanisms for effusions are usually considerably slower than those for pulmonary edema; therefore

edema has usually gone, while the effusions persist, sometimes for several days. The relationship between effusion size and LAP can be improved by relating *change* in the effusion's size to *change* in LAP. This is of little help when the film reader is attempting to assess LAP from a single radiograph. However, it is useful in understanding, following, and explaining the sequence of events in patients with cardiac failure and therefore in recognizing deviations from the usual sequence that herald changes in the hemodynamics.

Estimating Pulmonary Artery Pressure

Passive elevation of PAP occurs in chronic LHF as in any patient with elevated LAP. However, since smoking is one of the most frequent causes of cardiac disease, many of these patients have superimposed *organic* pulmonary arterial hypertension from the lung disease. In these patients the criteria of enlarged MPA, central vessels, tortuosity, and so on are used, as in those with mitral valve disease, to assess PAP[2,4,5,16,31-33] (Table 7-2).

Estimating Pulmonary Blood Flow

In patients with chronic LHF, as previously discussed, renal hypoperfusion frequently causes an increased circulating blood volume, a widened vascular pedicle, and an enlarged azygos vein. The lungs may appear slightly plethoric as a manifestation of the general increase in circulating blood volume. Again, however, the film reader must recall that a considerable reduction in transit time occurs with chronic LHF (mean, 55%), and the PBF (cardiac output) is therefore *reduced*, despite the apparent plethora.

As shown with mitral stenosis, accuracy of estimation of LAP in LHF can also be improved by factoring the estimated PAP into the estimated LAP. As mentioned previously, with this approach, Balbarini et al.[28] achieved correlation of *r*, 0.89; *p* less than 0.001 between radiologic and catheter estimates of mean PAP (Fig. 7-35). As with most prior studies, the authors found assessment of pressure is somewhat more accurate in patients with valvulopathies than in those with coronary artery disease.

We should reemphasize that after treatment, even when edema has gone and flow inversion has returned to normal, radiologically invisible organic changes still persist in the basal microvasculature.[33] These organic changes cause a persistent increase in resistance to flow through the LLs and a persisting flow inversion that can only be detected radioisotopically. If the film reader is aware of this, he or she will appreciate that a "normal" chest radiograph after treatment for cardiac failure does not mean that the lung vessels have been restored to complete normality. The patient, although no longer in heart failure, is not organically or physiologically normal.

LEFT-TO-RIGHT SHUNTS
Estimating Left Atrial Pressure

Unless failure supervenes, LAP is usually not elevated in patients with shunts at the atrial or ventricular level. If LHF does supervene, it usually follows the long-term gradual development of organic changes in the pulmonary arterioles, changing the initial 1:1 A/V size to a higher ratio, indicating progressive development of pulmonary artery hypertension and shunt reversal, leading to LHF. However, these organic changes do not alter the usual 1:1 flow redistribution of a left-to-right (L-R) shunt, and flow inversion is not present for LAP estimation. The estimation must therefore be made mainly on the basis of quantity of edema. The edema criteria are the same as those for LHF (Table 7-4, *A*). With increasing pulmonary arterial hypertension, increase in size of the left atrium as an ASD reverses or of the left ventricle as a ventricular septal defect (VSD) reverses also signifies increasing LAP.

Estimating Pulmonary Blood Flow

Quantification of PBF in a patient with an L-R shunt has already been discussed. However, we should emphasize that, in assessing the pulmonary-to-systemic flow ratio, the size of the aorta and vascular pedicle should be compared with the MPA and the central divisions of the pulmonary artery (see Fig. 7-6). Because of the effects of vessel diameter on resistance to flow and transit time, a ratio between aortic size (or VPW) and pulmonary artery size of, for example, 2:1 would mean a considerably higher shunt ratio, such as 4:1. If, therefore, on the basis of pulmonary vessel size a flow of 1.5 times normal was assessed (approximately 8 L/min), the left ventricular output would be only 2 L/min.

The reported correlation between radiologic assessment of PBF flow in absolute terms and indicator dilution studies is approximately 0.7.[15] Flow assessments are even less accurate in young children because of (1) their normally high cardiac output, (2) difficulties in visualizing the vascular pedicle behind the thymus, and (3) difficulties in distinguishing the mainstem, secondary, and tertiary branches of the pulmonary vessels in children.[34-36]

Estimating Pulmonary Artery Pressure

The estimation of PAP in patients with L-R shunts is complicated because the MPA and central divisions may have enlarged (because of increased flow) *before* the development of PAP, causing organic pulmonary arterial hypertension. The size of the MPA and central division on the initial film is therefore of limited value for assessing PAP. The principal factors that one must use are therefore tortuosity of the peripheral arteries, increase in the A/V size ratio, and pruning of the pe-

ripheral vessels. If sequential films are available, a further increase in the size of an already large MPA and central divisions, developing at the same time as tortuosity develops and the AV ratio increases, allows one to factor these vessels' size into the pressure estimation. Again, easily identified *tortuosity* of the peripheral arteries indicates a PAP of 60 mm Hg or greater and visible *pruning*, with even higher pressures of 70 to 90 mm Hg. The final clinical picture, with hugely dilated central vessels tapering abruptly into much smaller peripheral vessels, resulting in the comma-shaped appearance, along with severe peripheral pruning, indicates very severe pulmonary arterial hypertension, with pressures of 100 mm Hg and higher (Fig. 7-36).

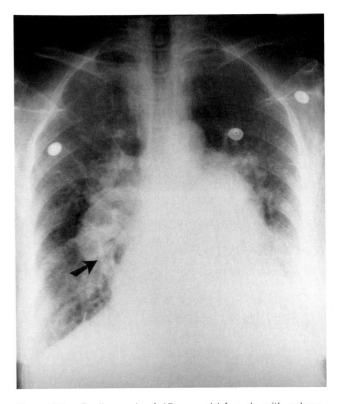

Fig. 7-36 Radiograph of 45-year-old female with a longstanding, large atrial septal defect (ASD). The patient is now becoming cyanotic. Note that although the MPA and central pulmonary arteries are huge, suggesting a very large shunt, the draining veins *(arrow)* are much smaller (A/V ratio, 6:1), and the peripheral vessels are small and difficult to see. Both changes indicate that severe pulmonary arterial hypertension is present and that flow must be greatly diminished and possibly reversed (Eisenmenger's complex). The vessel margins are blurred, a small right-sided effusion is seen entering a medial accessory fissure, and a large left-sided effusion is present. The patient is now decompensating.

Estimating Right Atrial Pressure

If tricuspid incompetence (TI) develops from high right ventricular pressure, assessment of RAP uses the same criteria as for mitral stenosis with TI, biventricular decompensation, and RHF.

PULMONARY DISEASE
Emphysema

Estimating Pulmonary Artery Pressure. Some elevation of PAP typically occurs in patients with emphysema, but those with pure or predominant emphysema rarely show the very high levels of pulmonary arterial hypertension found in patients with chronic bronchitis. This is probably because in emphysema, as alveoli are destroyed by the disease, their capillaries are also inevitably destroyed; therefore minimal ventilation/perfusion mismatch occurs, and hypoxemia is relatively absent. The relative absence of hypoxemia means that no hypoxic arteriolar constriction occurs, and any elevation in PAP is therefore anatomic, that is, principally resulting from progressive loss of recruitable vessels by the emphysematous destruction.

The vascular criteria already listed for assessing PAP in patients with cardiac disease apply equally to those with emphysema except that, since the principal characteristic of the pulmonary vessels in emphysema is a *loss* of sinuosity, tortuosity does not occur and is therefore not available for estimating PAP (see Table 7-2). Matthay et al.[13] have shown that measurement of the descending portions of the right and left pulmonary arteries does correlate, although rather poorly, (*r*, 0.56), with mean PAP. The authors concluded that this measurement alone is relatively sensitive to the presence of pulmonary artery hypertension but not specific as to its

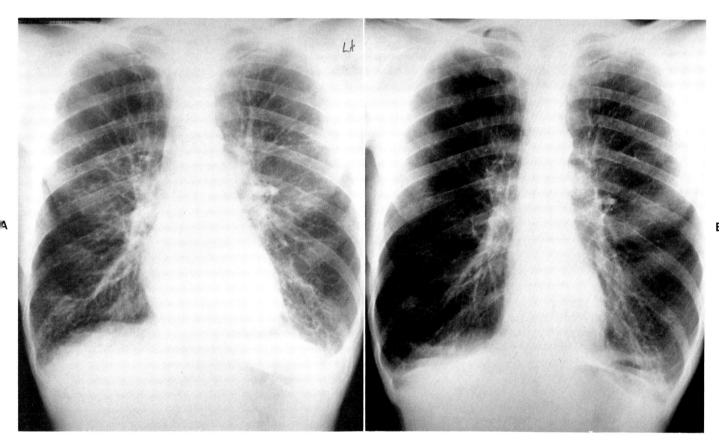

Fig. 7-37   A, The straightened pulmonary vessels, large lung volumes, and loss of background vessels suggest the diagnosis of emphysema. However, emphysematous vessels should be exquisitely and sharply defined, and these vessels are not. Also, the heart is "normal" in size, which is *abnormally* large for a patient with emphysema. These findings together indicate that LHF is present. The MPA is slightly convex, indicating a small increase in PAP. **B,** After digitalis and diuretic therapy, 24 hours later, the edema is gone and the true clinical picture is shown. The vessels are much sharper, their diameter is less, the heart has reduced in volume, and the lung volume has increased (11 ribs seen on the previous film, twelfth rib now just visible on present film). A slight reduction has even occurred in the MPA's convexity, indicating that the prior *passive* component of the elevated PAP (caused by elevated LAP) has been removed.

severity. In our experience, in emphysema the size of the *MPA* correlates better with PAP than the size of the descending branches (Fig. 7-37). Unfortunately, no significant correlation exists between right ventricular size and PAP in emphysema.

Estimating Pulmonary Blood Flow. In lung disease in general, transit time is reduced (up to 55% greater than normal), but in emphysema, great regional variation may exist. In those areas where the microvasculature has been partially destroyed, transit time is extremely slow. In the normal areas, however, through which the entire cardiac output must now pass, transit time can be extremely rapid, so rapid that transfer of oxygen may be compromised. One therefore cannot assess total PBF in patients having emphysema with any accuracy, although one can be certain that in those remaining normal areas that have large arteries and veins and a 1:1 A/V ratio, an extremely high regional flow rate exists (Fig. 7-38).

Emphysema and Left Heart Failure

LHF occurs approximately five times more often in patients with chronic lung disease than in those with normal lungs.[37] Several functional/mechanical reasons might explain this[38,39]:

1. The work of breathing is greatly increased, increasing oxygen use and the work of the heart.
2. PVR is increased, leading to elevated right-sided heart pressure and possibly to encroachment of an enlarged right ventricle on the lumen of the left ventricle.

3. The usual assistance of the "auxiliary heart" is missing, putting a greater load on the heart.
4. The heart is perfused with hypoxic blood.

However, the primary cause for the cardiac decompensation is probably none of these factors. The main cause is most likely the same one that initially caused the lung disease, smoking. Whatever the cause, despite its frequent occurrence, LHF in patients with emphysema frequently is not recognized either radiologically or clinically, being characterized simply as "an exacerbation of chronic obstructive pulmonary disease (COPD)" and attributed to infection and mucous accumulation (Fig. 7-39). Even pulmonary function studies do not help to determine the presence of LHF in emphysema and may even confuse the issue, since the presence of edema tends to *improve* many of the criteria used to diagnose COPD. That is, the greater total lung capacity and enlarged right ventricle are reduced toward normal by the loss of compliance caused by the edema (Fig. 7-40), diffusing capacity is improved by the increased capillary blood volume, and mixed expiratory flow rates are better in the stiffer edematous lung[37] (Fig. 7-41). The effects of the edema are so striking on the pulmonary function tests of patients with severe emphysema and LHF that the tests may be read as being normal (Fig. 7-41). This becomes of particular importance in patients receiving pulmonary function studies to determine their pulmonary status before cardiac transplantation. Such studies must be done with the patient *out* of cardiac failure.

The radiologic recognition of LHF in patients with

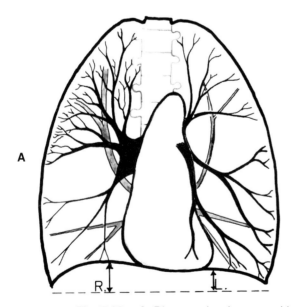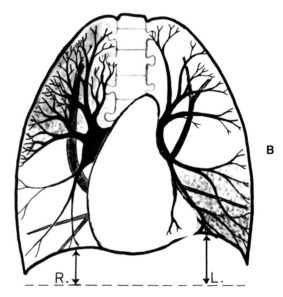

Fig. 7-38 **A,** Diagram showing normal left lung but basal emphysema on the right with organic flow redistribution to the right UL. **B,** The same patient in **A** with LHF. Edema occurs normally at the left base (the normal lung) but not at the right base, where no capillaries are present (i.e., no capillaries, no transudation possible). Instead, the edema occurs in the area to which flow has been redistributed, the right UL.

emphysema is equally difficult. Some clues to the diagnosis follow:

1. In emphysema the vessel margins should be unusually sharp; in LHF they become blurred.
2. In emphysema the bronchial walls are normal; in LHF some cuffing may develop.
3. In emphysema the vascular pedicle and heart are both small and increase in size toward normal if LHF is present.

It is very difficult to recognize these signs on a single radiograph, although they become much more evident if serial films are available for comparison (see Figs. 7-37 and 7-41). We customarily maintain a very high index of suspicion for the diagnosis (knowing its high rate of occurrence) and advocate a trial of diuretics, followed by a repeat film. The results clinically are often dramatic, and radiologically the clearing of the edema is readily recognized[37,40] (see Figs. 7-37 and 7-41).

Estimating Left Atrial Pressure. Some authors have suggested that the edema in patients with emphysema is not caused by elevated LAP but by elevated RAP.

They hypothesize that since the proximal third of the major bronchi within the perihilar area is supplied by bronchial arteries that drain back via true bronchial veins into the *right* side of the heart, increased right-sided heart pressure will cause bronchial mucosal edema and perihilar edema. However, this would not explain the presence of pulmonary edema elsewhere in the lung, and one does not see evidence of an enlarged azygos vein to indicate that RAP *is* elevated in these patients. However, catheterization studies have shown that the LAP *is* elevated.[38,39] Also, the relationship between quantity of edema and LAP applies to these patients, with the proviso that a small amount of edema in patients with emphysema has as much significance in terms of elevated LAP as a large amount of edema in a normal lung.

Chronic Bronchitis

As discussed more fully in Chapter 9, pure or predominant chronic bronchitis behaves clinically and radiologically as an entirely different disease from emphy-

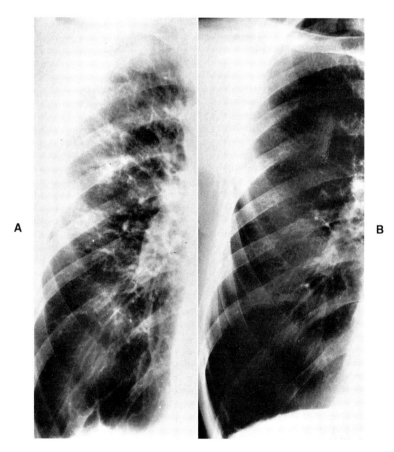

Fig. 7-39   A, Severe emphysema that is worse at the lung base. The patient's increasing dyspnea and cough were attributed to "exacerbation of chronic obstructive pulmonary disease (COPD)." The radiologic diagnosis was "LHF, superimposed on emphysema." **B,** After a diagnostic "test" of diuretics, the edema has cleared completely.

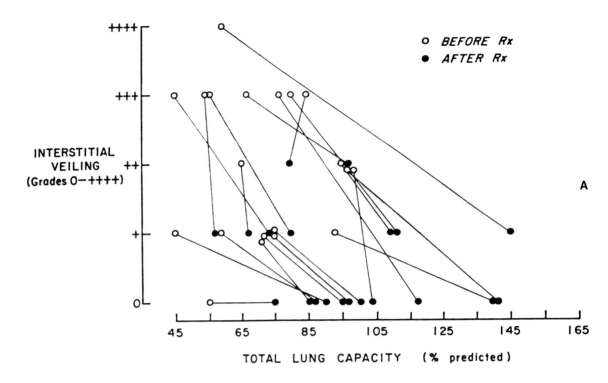

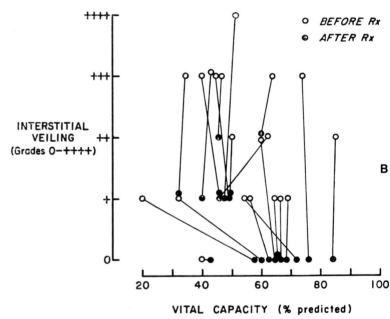

Fig. 7-40 **A,** Correlation between "interstitial veiling" seen on the chest radiograph (as a measure of lung water) and total lung capacity (TLC) in 20 patients with emphysema, chronic bronchitis, and both diseases, before *(open circles)* and after *(black circles)* treatment for LHF. The presence of edema has reduced the abnormal TLC considerably, in several patients to normal or less than normal. After digitalis and diuretic therapy, the edema is greatly reduced and the TLC is markedly increased, reflecting the *true* state of the patient's lung disease. **B,** Diagram showing that in the same 20 patients in **A,** vital capacity usually does not change after clearing of edema. As a corollary, a change in vital capacity should not be used as an index that edema is present (it has been used in renal patients to indicate whether dialysis was required).

sema. Unlike emphysema, ventilation/perfusion mismatch is very prominent in chronic bronchitis, leading to hypoxemia, arteriolar constriction, and pulmonary arterial hypertension levels that are often considerably higher than in emphysema. Also, in contrast to emphysema, the peripheral vessels in patients with chronic bronchitis are frequently tortuous, reflecting organic changes in the arterioles (Fig. 7-42). The central division of the pulmonary arteries and the MPA itself are usually large and occasionally huge (Fig. 7-43). All

these features have the same significance in estimating PAP that they have in mitral valve disease, late-stage aortic valve disease, and chronic LHF (see Table 7-2). In addition, in chronic bronchitis, right ventricular size *is* related to mean PAP. Although the radiologist's ability to recognize individual chamber enlargement on the plain radiograph has been frequently criticized, we find outward and upward displacement of the cardiac apex a consistently excellent sign of right ventricular enlargement (Fig. 7-43; see also Fig. 7-4).

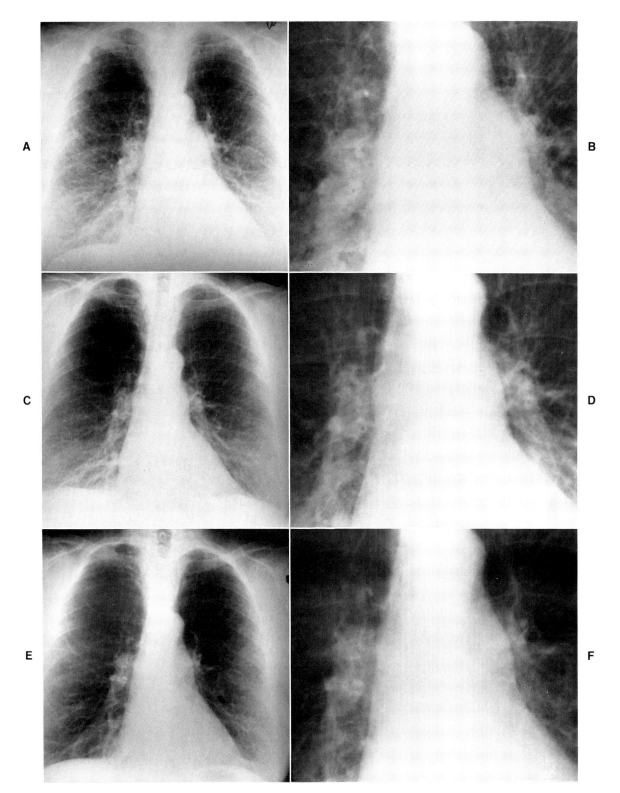

Fig. 7-41 **A,** Radiograph of 58-year-old male with chronic bronchitis and UL emphysema. Note the very convex MPA, indicating moderately severe pulmonary arterial hypertension, and the blurred vessel margins and peribronchial cuffing, indicating edema caused by elevated LAP. **B,** Spot view of the same patient in **A** to show the enlarged UL vessels and peribronchial cuffing. **C,** After treatment for LHF, 24 hours later the vessel blurring is resolving but cuffing is still present. Note slight reduction also in MPA, reflecting improvement in the passive portion of the elevated PAP. **D,** Spot view of **C** confirming the improvement in vessel blurring. Cuffing is still well seen. **E,** After treatment for LHF, 48 hours later one can see further "sharpening" in the definition of vessel margins. Cuffing is gone. Note no further reduction in MPA size, which now reflects the remaining fixed, organically caused pulmonary arterial hypertension. **F,** Spot view of **E.** Vessel margin definition is close to normal. Cuffing is no longer present.

Continued.

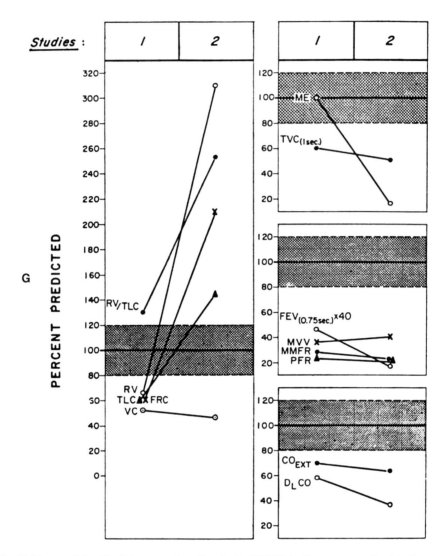

Fig. 7-41, cont'd   G, Pulmonary function tests (PFTs) in the same patient before and after treatment. The gray bands are the zones of predicted normal values (± 20%). Note that the diagnosis of COPD would have been very difficult to make by PFTs when the patient had heart failure, but it was easy to make radiologically. That is, PFTs are not the "gold standard" in patients with heart failure superimposed on emphysema or chronic bronchitis.

Estimating Pulmonary Blood Flow. Transit times through the lung are generally decreased, sometimes greatly, in patients with chronic bronchitis. Unless secondary polycythemia is present, the PBV is not usually increased. PBF is generally reduced. However, regional transit times vary too much with the severity of the disease for one to say with confidence from examination of the chest radiographs precisely what has happened to PBF.

Estimating Right Atrial Pressure. One might think that the elevated PAP that occurs so often in patients with chronic bronchitis would frequently lead to RHF. Right-sided heart enlargement certainly occurs in the majority of patients with chronic bronchitis. The vascular pedicle is usually slightly larger than normal (see Chapter 4), but in our experience it is unusual to see much enlargement of the azygos vein or progressive enlargement of the pedicle. We can seldom make the diagnosis of RHF radiologically. However, Fig. 7-44 shows a notable exception; in this patient the huge azygos vein resulted from RHF secondary to long-standing congestive heart failure. Our visual failure to detect the signs of elevated RAP may reflect a low incidence of right-sided heart decompensation in patients with chronic bronchitis. However, it may also reflect the radiologic problems of assessing RAP previously dis-

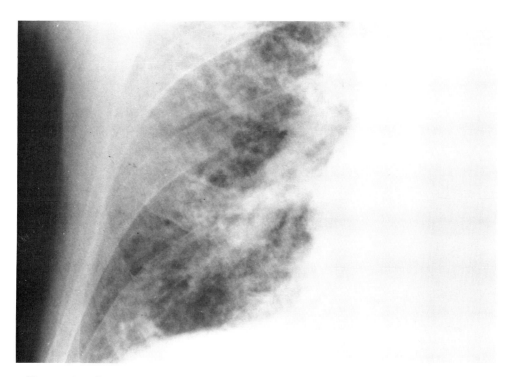

Fig. 7-42 Classic appearance of the peripheral vessels (blurred, tortuous, "segmented") in patients with severe chronic bronchitis.

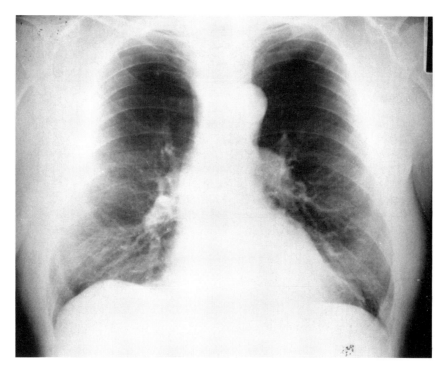

Fig. 7-43 Radiograph of 55-year-old male with severe chronic bronchitis and bilateral apical emphysema. Huge comma-shaped central PAs indicate a high level of organic pulmonary arterial hypertension. Note very small draining veins, which are very difficult to see.

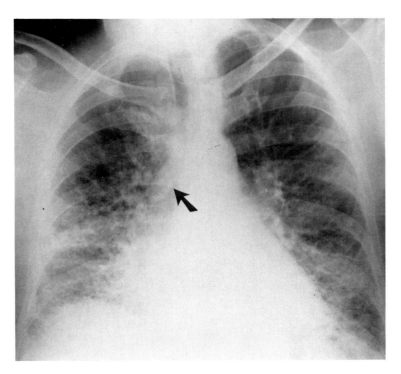

Fig. 7-44 Right-sided heart failure superimposed on LHF in a patient with severe mixed bronchitis and emphysema. The huge azygos vein *(arrow)* reflects the greatly elevated right atrial pressure.

cussed; that is, intraabdominal and lower limb changes may be occurring as manifestations of elevated RAP, and we obviously cannot see these changes on the chest film. We may therefore be underestimating the incidence of RHF in patients with chronic bronchitis.

Chronic Bronchitis and Superimposed Left Heart Failure

Estimating Left Atrial Pressure. LHF occurs as often in patients with chronic bronchitis as it does in those with emphysema, but it may be even more difficult to recognize because some of the best signs of edema are already preempted in chronic bronchitis. The vessel margins are already blurred by low-grade infection and mucous accumulation, and the bronchial walls are thickened by increased depth of the mucosal lining (see Fig. 7-42). One therefore must have a high index of suspicion to suggest the diagnosis of LHF, and the test of diuresis remains the best way of confirming or denying it.[37,40] As in emphysema, the degree of LAP elevation should be estimated from the presence and amount of edema.

Estimating Pulmonary Artery Pressure. Edema superimposed on chronic bronchitis further increases PVR and increases an already elevated PAP. One should therefore factor edema into estimates of PAP in patients with chronic bronchitis, adding 5 to 10 mm Hg.

Pulmonary Embolism

Estimating Pulmonary Artery Pressure. The general lack of sensitivity and specificity of plain-film radiologic signs for making the diagnosis of pulmonary embolism has been frequently emphasized.[41] However, Palla et al.[42] made a careful analysis of a large series of patients in whom the presence or absence of embolism had been proved by perfusion scans and pulmonary angiography. They showed that certain recognizable changes in the pulmonary vessels may be present that correlate fairly well (Fig. 7-45) with the presence and extent (number of perfusion defects) of embolization. The authors classified the radiologic changes as follows:

1. Both descending pulmonary arteries (PAs) appeared normal in size and shape.
2. One or both descending PAs appeared enlarged.
3. On one side the descending PA was greatly enlarged and abruptly tapered, giving a "sausage" appearance to the proximal vessel.
4. Both descending PAs had this sausage configuration.[42]

Patients with findings 3 and 4 had the most serious vascular obstruction (average, 56%). Patients with finding 2 had an average obstruction of 39%, and patients with finding 1 had the smallest obstruction (average, 26%).[42] As the emboli resolved, the descending PAs showed a concomitant decrease in their width.[42] In this

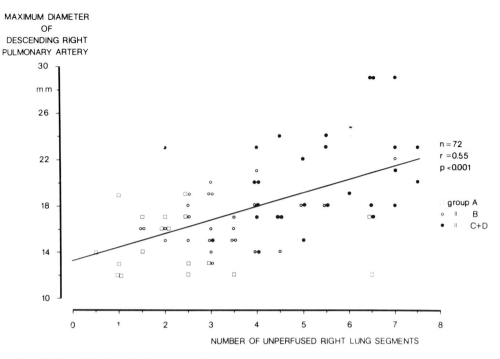

Fig. 7-45   Relationship between the maximum diameter of the descending portion of the right PA on the plain radiograph and the number of unperfused lung segments (shown by perfusion scan in 72 patients with proven emboli). *Group A,* One or both descending arteries normal; *Group B,* one or both descending arteries enlarged; *Group C,* one descending artery enlarged with "sausage" configuration; *Group D,* both descending arteries enlarged with sausage appearance. (From Palla A, Petruzzelli S, Donnamaria V et al: *AJR* 141:513, 1983.)

series (73 patients with and 85 without embolism) the features of descending PA enlargement did *not* occur in those patients without embolism. The authors did not correlate vessel size directly with PAP, but it seems unlikely that the correlation between descending PA size and mean PAP in patients with pulmonary embolism would be any better than that found in those with COPD (*r*, 0.53; *p* < 0.001).[13]

Adult Respiratory Distress Syndrome

Estimating Pulmonary Artery Pressure. In adult respiratory distress syndrome (ARDS), scattered regional vascular thromboses and pulmonary hypoxemia secondary to multiple areas of ventilation-perfusion mismatch combine to cause elevated PAP in most patients. These patients are so ill that they almost universally require positive-pressure ventilation, which alters many of the radiologic features one would normally use for physiologic assessments; for example, VPW is usually normal or narrow in patients with ARDS, even in the supine position.[18] Unfortunately, this does not automatically mean that the circulating blood volume is small because (1) many of these patients, particularly those in septic shock, have a dilated peripheral vascular bed into which a normal or even enlarged circulating blood volume may pool, leaving the VPW normal or narrowed,

and (2) the level of positive-pressure ventilation is often high enough to compress the vascular pedicle, causing it to be spuriously narrow.

The increased intrathoracic pressure caused by positive-pressure ventilation appears to have less effect, however, on the size and shape of the MPA, which is frequently enlarged in patients with ARDS, reflecting the increased PAP.[43] Because of the superimposed effects of the high ventilatory pressures, PAP level is usually underestimated. For example, when one would normally make an estimate of 40 mm Hg for the PAP based on the MPA's size, one should add 10 to 15 mm Hg to compensate for the effects of positive end-expiratory pressure (PEEP).

Estimating Left Atrial Pressure. Since the heart is not usually failing in patients with ARDS, no reason exists for the LAP to be elevated. If no overhydration is present, *no* relationship exists between the quantity of lung edema caused by injury and the LAP.

Estimating Pulmonary Blood Flow. In patients with ARDS the PBV is usually normal or slightly reduced, usually because of increased intraalveolar pressure; pulmonary A/V ratio is normal; and cardiac size and VPW are also normal. From these radiologic data, one would usually infer that the cardiac output is normal; however, in ARDS, despite these findings, cardiac output may be considerably increased, particularly in septicemic patients. Since this occurs with a normal PBV, as discussed previously, the transit time of blood through the lung must be very rapid. However, in ARDS there are usually scattered regions in which blood flow is blocked either by thrombosis[44-46] or by arterial constriction secondary to hypoxemia. Redistribution of flow occurs away from these areas into less damaged areas, and the most rapid flow must therefore occur in these least damaged portions of the lungs. When patients are on positive pressure ventilation, the least damaged portions of the lungs receive the greatest ventilatory pressures, causing compression of the "alveolar" vessels and further raising PVR. Because the heart can maintain an increased output even with this increased resistance, it is evident that the PAP must often be much more elevated than the radiograph suggests, as must the PBF.

Estimating Right Atrial Pressure. As indicated, patients with ARDS usually have normal or narrow vascular pedicles, unless they are overhydrated in treatment. Part of the narrowing results from the high ventilatory pressures, which also makes it impossible to assess RAP in these patients.

• • •

In summary, most of the features one normally uses to assess pressure and flow are either missing or concealed in patients with ARDS. Their evaluation is discussed more fully in Chapter 8.

Hypoxemia

After chronic lung disease, the next most common cause of hypoxemia is probably sleep apnea. Chest radiographs may or may not be taken routinely in assessing patients with sleep apnea, depending largely on the philosophy of the person controlling that particular sleep center. The radiologist may therefore see only a small percentage of patients with sleep apnea, even when the clinical severity warrants surgery. Since the patients most often seen tend to be those with the "pickwickian" syndrome, radiologists receive the impression that most patients with sleep apnea are obese, which in our experience is not true.

In a series of patients with sleep apnea who had been selected for surgery on the basis of altered physiologic parameters, usually including some elevation of PAP, in the nonobese patients we were unable to find a good correlation between the usual radiologic signs of PAP and the measured values.[47] However, these patients had only minor PAP elevations. In the pickwickian subgroup the correlation was much better; 60% showed MPA enlargement, the degree of which correlated well with PAP level.[47] However, we saw neither vascular tortuosity in these patients nor any increase in their A/V size ratio, suggesting that their changes were largely functional.

We have seen marked enlargement of the MPA in several patients at high altitude (10,000 feet). Two of these patients were moved to sea level, and the MPA returned to normal size almost immediately.

Damaged Lung

Lungs damaged by multiple prior infections, interstitial fibrosis, interstitial pneumonias, ARDS, AIDS, or chronic intravenous drug abuse usually have a reduced pulmonary vascular bed capacity but no reduction in PBV. The pulmonary vascular bed of these patients is therefore completely filled, and they manifest a 1:1 flow distribution and frequently develop the previously described radiologic stigmata of pulmonary arterial hypertension. In most patients a straightforward relationship exists between the level of pulmonary arterial hypertension and the severity of the radiologic changes. In some patients with more severe chronic damage, tortuosity of peripheral vessels and an increased A/V size ratio are seen.

REFERENCES

1. Friedman WF, Braunwald E: Alteration in regional pulmonary blood flow in mitral valve disease studied by radioisotope scanning, *Circulation* 34:363, 1966.
2. McMyn J: Radiological appearances of pulmonary hypertension, *J Coll Radiol Aust* 4:21, 1960.
3. Milne ENC, Carlsson E: Physiological interpretation of the plain radiograph following mitral valvotomy, valvuloplasty and prosthetic replacement, *Radiology* 92:1201, 1969.
4. Turner AF, Lauf YK, Jacobson G: A method for the estimation of pulmonary venous and arterial pressures from the routine chest roentgenogram, *AJR* 116:97, 1972.
5. Milne ENC: Physiological interpretation of the plain film in mitral stenosis including a review of criteria for the estimation of pulmonary arterial and venous pressures, *Br J Radiol* 36:902, 1963.
6. Rigler LG: Functional roentgen diagnosis: anatomical image—physiologic interpretation, *AJR* 82:1, 1959.
7. Simon M: The pulmonary vessels—their hemodynamic evaluation using routine radiographs, *Radiol Clin North Am* 2:363, 1963.
8. Lavender JP, Doppman J, Shawdon H, Steiner RE: Pulmonary veins in left ventricular failure and mitral stenosis, *Br J Radiol* 35:293, 1962.
9. Davies LG, Goodwin JF, Steiner RE, Van Leuven BD: Clinical and radiological assessment of pulmonary arterial pressures in mitral stenosis, *Br Heart J* 15:393, 1953.
10. Doyle AE, Goodwin JF, Harrison CV, Steiner RE: Pulmonary vascular patterns in pulmonary hypertension, *Br Heart J* 19:353, 1957.
11. Jackson G, Schwartz LH, Sussman ML: Radiographic estimation of pulmonary artery pressure in mitral valvular disease, *Radiology* 68:14, 1957.
12. Steiner RE: Radiology of pulmonary circulation, *AJR* 91:249, 1964.
13. Matthay RA, Schwartz ML, Ellis JH et al: Pulmonary artery hypertension in chronic obstructive pulmonary disease: determination by chest radiography, *Invest Radiol* 16:95, 1981.
14. Matthay RA, Berger HJ: Non-invasive assessment of right and left ventricular function in acute and chronic respiratory failure, *Crit Care Med* 11:24, 1983.
15. Fouché RF, Beck W, Schrirer W: The roentgenological assess-

ment of left to right shunt in secundum type atrial septal defect, *AJR* 89:254, 1963.

16. Rees S: The chest radiograph in pulmonary hypertension with central shunt, *Br J Radiol* 41:172, 1968.

17. Milne ENC: A physiologic approach to reading critical care unit chest films, *J Thorac Imaging* 1(3):60, 1986.

18. Milne ENC, Pistolesi M, Miniati M, Giuntini C: The radiologic distinction between cardiogenic and non-cardiogenic edema, *AJR* 144:879, 1985.

19. Bruno MA, Milne ENC, Stanford WS et al: Pulmonary oligemia in chest diagnosis—film reader reliability (with special reference to a new finding in aortic stenosis), 1992 preparation

20. Milne ENC: Some new concepts of pulmonary blood flow and volume, *Radiol Clin North Am* 16:515, 1978.

21. Yu PN: *Pulmonary blood volume in health and disease*, Philadelphia, 1969, Lea & Febiger.

22. Pistolesi M, Milne ENC, Miniati M, Giuntini C: The vascular pedicle of the heart and the vena azygos. Part II. In acquired heart disease, *Radiology* 152:9, 1984.

23. Milne ENC, Pistolesi M, Miniati M, Giuntini C: The vascular pedicle of the heart and the vena azygos. Part I. The normal subject, *Radiology* 152:1, 1984.

24. Figuera J, Weil MH: Blood volume prior to and following treatment of acute cardiogenic pulmonary edema, *Circulation* 57:349, 1978.

25. Cannon PJ: The kidney in heart failure: physiology in medicine, *N Engl J Med* 296:26, 1977.

26. Baumstark A, Swensson RG, Hessel SJ et al: Evaluating the radiographic assessment of pulmonary venous hypertension in chronic heart disease, *AJR* 141:877, 1984.

27. McHugh TJ, Forrester JS, Adler L et al: Pulmonary vascular congestion in acute myocardial infarction: hemodynamic and radiologic correlations, *Ann Intern Med* 76:29, 1972.

28. Balbarini A, Limbruno V, Bertoli D et al: Evaluation of pulmonary vascular pressures in cardiac patients: the role of the chest roentgenogram, *J Thorac Imaging* 6(2):62, 1991.

29. Van Epps EF: Roentgen manifestations of pulmonary hypertension, *AJR* 79:241, 1958.

30. Steiner RE, Harrison CV, Goodwin JF: Radiological assessment of pulmonary arterial and pulmonary venous pressure. In de Reuck AJS, O'Connor M, editors: Ciba Foundation Study Group No. 8; *Problems in pulmonary circulation*, London, 1961, JA Churchill.

31. Ravin CE: Pulmonary vascularity: radiographic considerations, *J Thorac Imaging* 3(1):1, 1988.

32. Short DS: Radiology of the lung in severe mitral stenosis, *Br Heart J* 17:33, 1955.

33. Pistolesi M, Miniati M, Bonsignore M et al: Factors affecting regional pulmonary blood flow in chronic ischemic heart disease, *J Thorac Imaging* 3(3):65, 1988.

34. Nitz I: Roentgenographic evaluation of pulmonary arteries in normal babies and roentgen appearance of pulmonary vascularity in young infants with congenital heart diseases, *Ann Radiol* 18:465, 1975.

35. Hislop A, Reid L: Pulmonary arterial development during childhood, branching pattern and structure, *Thorax* 28:129, 1973.

36. Leinbach L: Roentgenologic evaluation of normal pulmonary arteries in children, *AJR* 89:995, 1963.

37. Milne ENC, Bass H: Roentgenologic and functional analysis of combined chronic obstructive pulmonary disease and congestive cardiac failure, *Invest Radiol* 4:129, 1969.

38. Rao BS, Cohn KE, Eldridge FL, Hancock EW: Left ventricular failure secondary to chronic pulmonary disease, *Am J Med* 45:229, 1968.

39. Rosenow EC III, Harrison CE Jr: Congestive heart failure masquerading as primary pulmonary disease, *Chest* 58:28, 1970.

40. Milne ENC, Bass H: The roentgenologic diagnosis of early chronic obstructive pulmonary disease, *J Can Assoc Radiol* 20:3,1969.

41. Greenspan RH, Ravin CE, Polansky SM, McLoud TC: Accuracy of the chest radiograph in diagnosis of pulmonary embolism, *Invest Radiol* 17:539, 1982.

42. Palla A, Petruzzelli S, Donnamaria V, et al: Radiographic assessment of perfusion impairment in pulmonary artery in pulmonary embolism, *Eur J Radiol* 5:252, 1985.

43. Pistolesi M, Miniati M, Pravelli V, Giuntini C: Injury versus hydrostatic lung edema, detection by chest x-ray, *Ann NY Acad Sci* 384:364, 1982.

44. Pistolesi M, Miniati M, DiRicco G et al: Perfusion lung imaging in the adult respiratory distress syndrome, *J Thorac Imaging* 1(3):11, 1986.

45. Greene R, Zapol WM, Snider M, et al: Early bedside detection of pulmonary vascular occlusion during acute respiratory failure, *Am Rev Respir Dis* 124:593, 1981.

46. Tomashefski JF Jr, Davies P, Boggis C, et al: The pulmonary vascular lesions of the adult respiratory distress syndrome, *Am J Pathol* 112:112, 1983.

47. Milne ENC, Mosko S: Unpublished data.

8 Differentiating Increased Pressure from Injury Pulmonary Edema

Pulmonary edema caused by abnormal hydrostatic or oncotic pressures ("pressure edema") or by lung injury (increased permeability; "injury edema") is an extremely common condition. Pressure edema is seen more frequently than injury edema for the following reasons. First, heart disease is the leading cause of death in the United States, and during the course of progressive cardiac decompensation, a typical patient may be in and out of pulmonary edema many times. Second, with the universal use of intravenous fluid therapy for resuscitation, fluid replenishment, parenteral nutrition, and so on, pulmonary edema caused by overhydration (usually accompanied by a drop in oncotic pressure) has become the rule in hospitalized patients rather than the exception. Third, patients with

renal disease are now surviving for much longer periods; renal pulmonary edema occurring before transplantation or before dialysis, associated with rejection, is now seen very frequently.

The number of patients with pulmonary edema caused by lung injury also appears to be increasing, probably because aggressive resuscitation is prolonging the survival time of those with adult respiratory distress syndrome (ARDS). These edemas are frequently complicated by the superimposition of overhydration and cardiac or renal failure. Injury edema can also occur in association with all types of inflammatory lung disease (e.g., pneumonias, abscesses) and with many immunologically based conditions (e.g., asthma, drug allergies, transfusion reactions) (see the box on p. 243). Since more than 70 million chest radiographs are taken each year in the United States, and since approximately 25% of these are from patients with cardiac disease and other causes of pulmonary edema, the number of patients with pulmonary edema seen by radiologists is clearly enormous.

Pulmonary edema is not in itself a disease but is simply a manifestation of an underlying disease process. Detection of edema may provide the first sign that disease is present, while the amount of edema provides an index to the severity of disease and the distribution of edema a guide to its etiology and pathogenesis.

The pathogenesis of hydrostatic, oncotic, and injury edema has already been discussed in some detail, as has the effect of the sequence of development of the different edemas on their radiologic presentation. However, these differences in radiologic presentation are key to the recognition and differentiation of the various types of edema. Therefore, before discussing the differences, we must first briefly restate those features shared by all types of hydrostatic, oncotic, and injury edemas.

Objections are sometimes raised to the use of the word "hydrostatic" in discussing pulmonary edema because the system we are talking about is clearly *not* static.[1] However, when we do the "sums" for the Starling equation across the capillary endothelial wall, we are discussing only the *static* factors at that chosen point in space and time. Although many dynamic factors are also operating at that point (e.g., Venturi effect, laminar versus turbulent flow, viscosity), we do not consider these factors in our calculations. We might be more correct in our conclusions about water transfer

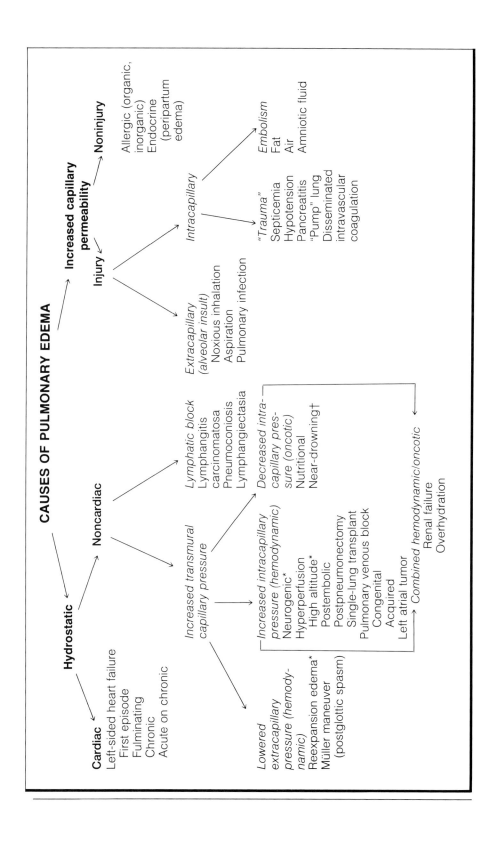

CAUSES OF PULMONARY EDEMA

Hydrostatic

Cardiac
Left-sided heart failure
First episode
Fulminating
Chronic
Acute on chronic

Noncardiac

Increased transmural capillary pressure

Lymphatic block
Lymphangitis carcinomatosa
Pneumoconiosis
Lymphangiectasia

Increased intracapillary pressure (hemodynamic)
Neurogenic*
Hyperperfusion
High altitude*
Postembolic
Postpneumonectomy
Single-lung transplant
Pulmonary venous block
Congenital
Acquired
Left atrial tumor

Lowered extracapillary pressure (hemodynamic)
Reexpansion edema*
Müller maneuver (postglottic spasm)

Decreased intracapillary pressure (oncotic)
Nutritional
Near-drowning†

Combined hemodynamic/oncotic
Renal failure
Overhydration

Increased capillary permeability

Injury

Extracapillary (alveolar insult)
Noxious inhalation
Aspiration
Pulmonary infection

Intracapillary

"Trauma"
Septicemia
Hypotension
Pancreatitis
"Pump" lung
Disseminated intravascular coagulation

Embolism
Fat
Air
Amniotic fluid

Noninjury
Allergic (organic, inorganic)
Endocrine (peripartum edema)

across capillary walls if we were able to include these factors, but they are presently beyond the scope of this book. We therefore continue to use *hydrostatic* when referring to liquid pressure and *oncotic* when referring to the transmural pressure differences generated by oncotically active molecules on opposite sides of the capillary wall (when it is functioning as a semipermeable membrane, i.e., when it is not injured).

RADIOLOGIC FEATURES OF PRESSURE EDEMA

All hydrostatic and oncotic edemas have a low viscosity and can therefore flow freely throughout the lung's interstitial continuum. These edemas are readily affected by gravity and intrathoracic pressure and are able to produce peribronchial cuffs, septal lines, and pleural effusions. The sequence in which hydrostatic and oncotic edemas occupy the interstitial and alveolar compartments of the lungs is dictated (1) by the speed with which they develop and (2) by any functional or anatomic alterations in the lung's underlying microvascular architecture. Hydrostatic edemas are usually associated radiologically with alterations in total blood volume, pulmonary blood flow (PBF) distribution, change in cardiac size, and systemic soft tissue edema.

RADIOLOGIC FEATURES OF INJURY EDEMA

Pulmonary edema caused by lung injury contains protein, cellular debris, fibrin, and hyaline material. This has a high viscosity and, in contrast to pressure edemas, cannot flow freely through the interstitium. Injury edema therefore is not able to produce peribronchial cuffing or septal lines.[2] After it is formed, injury edema cannot be affected by gravity and must remain fixed in position. Its distribution depends more on the type of lung insult (e.g., aspiration causing regional injury versus septicemia causing global injury) and much

less on any underlying functional or pathologic change in the lung itself. Pure injury edema is not associated with change in circulating blood volume (PV), cardiac size, or PBF distribution and normally produces no alteration in chest wall thickness. Because this edema occupies the alveoli but cannot flow freely into the bronchi, air-bronchograms are very common[2] (Table 8-1).

Although identifying exactly the *type* of pressure or injury edema present is desirable (see later discussion), the most important task clinically is to determine whether the edema is caused by pressure or injury. In uncomplicated cases, this is so simple, using the findings just described that one can often make the distinction as one walks past the view-box. If one sees a clear gravitational distribution of edema and bronchial cuffing, this is *pressure* edema (Fig. 8-1, *A*). If one sees a clear nongravitational distribution, air bronchograms, and no bronchial cuffing, this is *injury* edema (Fig. 8-1, *B*).

Before we discuss the practical details of differentiating between the various pressure and injury edemas, we must mention that two or more different varieties of edema often coexist. For example, a patient who enters the hospital with septicemia may first develop pure injury edema. During the course of treatment, the patient then may become overhydrated, a virtually universal occurrence because of the need to maintain cardiac output, or may develop renal or cardiac failure, sometimes with further injury to the lung caused by aspiration. If one first sees the patient at this later stage, it is difficult to distinguish the differing etiologies of edema. Even in patients with such complex conditions, however, easily identified findings (e.g., widened vascular pedicle, increased thickness of the chest wall's soft tissues) indicate that the patient has a pressure edema, while extensive air bronchograms (and lower

Table 8-1 Distinctive radiographic features of hydrostatic versus injury edema*

Feature	Cardiac edema	Renal edema	Injury edema
Heart size	Enlarged	Enlarged	Not enlarged
Vascular pedicle	Normal or enlarged	**Enlarged**	Normal or reduced
Pulmonary blood flow distribution	**Inverted**	**Balanced**	Normal or balanced
Pulmonary blood volume	Normal or increased	**Increased**	**Normal**
Septal lines	Common	Common	**Absent**
Peribronchial cuffs	Very common	Very common	**Not common**
Air bronchograms	Not common	Not common	**Very common**
Regional distribution of edema (horizontal axis)	**Even**	**Central**	**Peripheral/patchy**
Pleural effusions	Very common	Very common	**Not common**

*Each factor listed has been shown to have statistical significance in determining which type of edema is present. The boldface factors are the most significant. Note, however, that the diagnostic importance of an *individual* factor depends not only on its frequency but also on its place in a constellation of factors. Therefore, although this table does provide a simple guide to distinguishing the three varieties of edema, it must be used in conjunction with the wider knowledge of the *differing* constellations that can occur in each type of edema (see text).

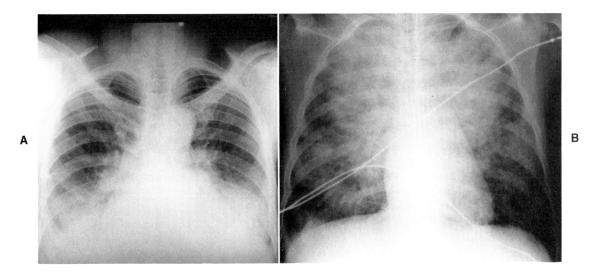

Fig. 8-1   A, Note gravitational distribution of edema, wide vascular pedicle, large heart, and effusions—all radiologically "classic" signs in patients with pulmonary edema caused by hydrostatic pressure. Diagnosis: chronic left-sided heart failure (LHF). **B,** Note *no* gravitational distribution of edema, no peribronchial cuffs, no septal lines, and no effusions, (despite edema's intensity), with normal-sized heart, normal pulmonary blood volume (PBV), and normal soft tissues—all classic signs of pulmonary edema caused by injury. Diagnosis: aspiration of gastric acid. (*NOTE:* although the margins of the vascular pedicle are obscured by the dense edema, the heart provides a cross-check that the pedicle is small. That is, a change in MR [distance from midline of heart to right side of heart border] correlates linearly with a change in vascular pedicle width [VPW]. The small MR therefore confirms that the pedicle is small.)

lung compliance) indicate the patient *also* has underlying capillary permeability edema. Clearly, the more we know about those radiologic characteristics unique to each variety of edema, the better able we will be to sort out the more complex edemas.[2]

The most common hydrostatic edemas are caused by either cardiac failure or overhydration/renal failure. These are the basic types of edema that will be contrasted with injury edema. However, several other causes of hydrostatic edema are considered elsewhere (see box on p. 243).

TECHNIQUE FOR DIFFERENTIATING CARDIAC AND RENAL/OVERHYDRATION FROM INJURY EDEMAS

In an initial study of patients with cardiac, renal/overhydration, and injury lung edemas, we identified the following 10 factors as being important for edema differentiation[2]:
1. Vascular pedicle width (VPW)
2. Distribution of pulmonary blood flow
3. Distribution of pulmonary edema

4. Pulmonary blood volume
5. Air bronchograms
6. Septal lines
7. Peribronchial cuffing
8. Pleural effusions
9. Cardiac size
10. Chest wall soft tissue thickness

Note that these features are *not* listed in any order of statistical frequency or diagnostic importance, since the level of importance of each factor will vary widely depending on the surrounding constellation of all other factors.[2] We discuss this more fully later in this chapter.

To introduce a greater degree of objectivity and to reduce interobserver variability into our assessments, we developed a checklist to which the film readers were asked to respond (see box on p. 246). Since the patient's position, (erect versus supine) and form of respiration (spontaneous versus assisted) affect VPW and perfusion and edema distribution, these data must also be recorded and factored into the assessments.[3,4] Although the checklist was essential in our initial critical

---

CHECKLIST FOR FILM READER DIFFERENTIATING PULMONARY EDEMAS

1. Patient's position: erect, partially erect, supine, (? rotated)
2. Ventilation: ?spontaneous   ?assisted→obtain peak pressure and positive end-expiratory pressure (PEEP)
3. Heart size and shape, size of main pulmonary artery (MPA)
4. Width of vascular pedicle and azygos vein (allow for patient's position, rotation)
5. Pulmonary blood volume: ?diminished, normal, increased
6. Blood flow distribution: ?normal, inverted, balanced
7. Edema distribution: ?gravitational, central, peripheral or patchy
8. Peribronchial cuffing
9. Septal lines
10. Effusions
11. Air bronchograms
12. Soft tissues: ?normal ?edematous

---

study, in which criteria were being both evaluated and developed, it is desirable but not essential in clinical practice, provided film readers have become familiar with all the factors that need to be examined and do not need a checklist to remind them.

We were initially concerned that the short-distance anteroposterior (AP) films and supine positions would have such an effect on cardiac size and VPW that we should try to correct for these factors. We proceeded to do this, using correction factors we have derived experimentally (see Chapter 10) for cardiac size and VPW.[5,6] We then compared the accuracy of our assessments of the type of edema present, comparing the corrected data with noncorrected data and found no difference. This suggests that so many factors are available to make the distinction between pressure and injury edemas that corrections for cardiac size and VPW are unnecessary (fortunately for the busy film reader).[2]

We were able to show a surprising degree of difference between the three types of edema in each of the 10 factors analyzed.[2]

Vascular Pedicle Width

The anatomy of the vascular pedicle and the effects of the patient's rotation, respiration, and supine versus vertical positions are fully discussed in Chapter 4. We have shown that the pedicle is an excellent indicator of total blood volume (TBV) and of *changes* in TBV or, more precisely, of the *systemic* component of the TBV.[6]

Three possibilities exist for change in the VPW: normal, increased, or decreased. Taking the normal VPW to be 4.3 to 5.3 cm, increase to be greater than 5.3 cm, and decrease to be less than 4.3 cm, we found a good, statistically significant separation among cardiac, renal/overhydration, and injury edemas[2] (Fig. 8-2, *A*).

The histogram (Fig. 8-2, *B*) shows that, even though most patients with injury lung edema were radiographed in the supine position, VPW was either normal or actually reduced in slightly more than 60%. In the 33% of injury edema patients with *increased* VPW, we subsequently found evidence (increase in chest soft wall tissue thickness) indicating that most of these patients were also overhydrated (i.e., they had superimposed pressure edema).

As expected, 85% of the patients with *renal* edema had an abnormally wide pedicle, indicating their increased TBV. Fifteen percent had a normal pedicle; as previously discussed, we believe these were patients with end-stage disease and with high vasomotor tone that prevented the veins of the pedicle from dilating, even though the TBV was increased.

Sixty percent of the patients with *cardiac* edema also showed a widened vascular pedicle, reflecting renal hypoperfusion that caused salt and water retention. Enlargement of the right side of the heart (midline to right border [MR]) closely paralleled enlargement of the vascular pedicle in all patients. Change in size of the heart, azygos vein, and PBV all paralleled a change in VPW and provided useful confirmation of pedicular change and added strongly to the validity of the observations.

Distribution of Pulmonary Blood Flow

Three different patterns of PBF can be distinguished: (1) normal (upper lobe/lower lobe [UL/LL] ratio of 0.6:1.0 to 0.8:1.0), (2) "balanced" (UL/LL ratio of 1.0:1.0), or (3) "inverted" (UL/LL ratio greater than 1.0:1.0). Since we have shown interobserver variation can be quite great in assessing flow distribution,[2] one might not have expected to find a particularly good separation between the three types of edema, but a useful distinction was present[2] (Fig. 8-3). Inversion of flow was common in cardiac edema, very uncommon in injury edema, and never seen in renal edema.

A balanced flow was very common in renal edema and common in both injury and cardiac edema and therefore was of little use for their separation.

Normal PBF was common in injury edema and uncommon in either renal or cardiac edema.

The presence of a balanced flow in so many patients with injury edema may be attributed to their supine position. If one insists (which we do not) on intensive care unit (ICU) patients being placed in a sitting-up position for radiography, the percentage of injury edema

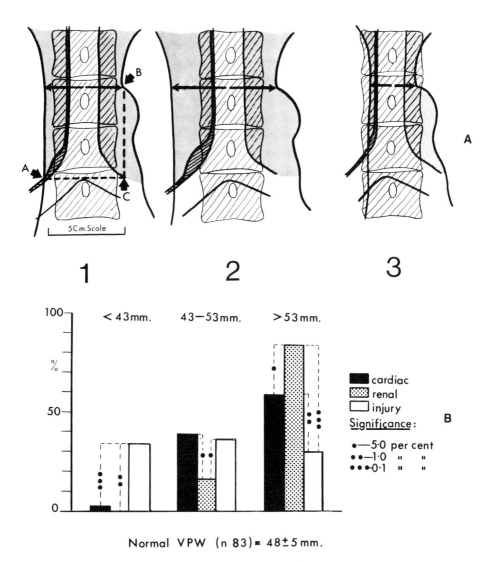

Fig. 8-2 **A,** Diagram of vascular pedicle. *1,* Normal (4.3 to 5.3 cm); *2,* enlarged (greater than 5.3 cm); *3,* narrowed (less than 4.3 cm). *Measuring points:* horizontal distance between *A,* where the right main bronchus crosses the superior vena cava, and *B,* where the left subclavian artery arises from the aorta. **B,** Percent frequency of occurrence of narrow, normal, and increased vascular pedicle width (VPW) in patients with cardiac, renal/overhydration, and injury lung edemas.

patients with balanced flow distribution would obviously decrease considerably. The effects of the supine position on PBF and edema distribution is covered more fully later.

Distribution of Pulmonary Edema

Although the distribution of edema can take many forms, particularly if the lung parenchyma has been damaged by prior disease, most patterns of edema fit into one of three categories: central, peripheral, or gravitational ("even")[2] (Fig. 8-4).

Central edema. By this we do not mean perihilar or "bat's wing," which are special cases of edema distribution discussed later. In central edema the middle two thirds of the lungs are affected most by edema, but the edema does extend down to the diaphragm. Because the peripheral third of the lungs is spared, the costophrenic angles remain clear.

Peripheral edema. Distribution is usually also very patchy, with a rather random distribution of the patches. No gravitational effect is present. The costophrenic angles are almost invariably spared.

Gravitational (even) edema. This distribution occurs principally in the lower half of the lungs in the erect patient. It becomes increasingly dense toward the bottom of the lungs and is evenly distributed from the chest wall (filling the costophrenic angles) to the heart.

In our initial study we were surprised at the wide

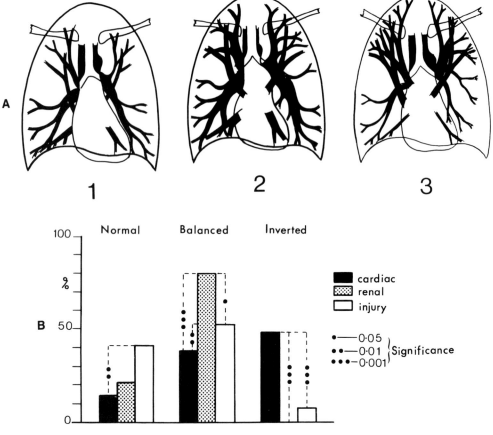

Fig. 8-3   A, Diagram showing *(1)* normal pulmonary blood flow (PBF) distribution; *(2)* "balanced" PBF, with upper lobe/lower lobe (UL/LL) ratio of 1.0:1.0; and *(3)* "inverted" flow, with UL/LL ratio greater than 1.0:1.0. **B,** Percent frequency of occurrence of normal, balanced, and inverted PBF distribution in patients with cardiac, renal/overhydration, and injury lung edemas. The statistical significance is indicated.

separation of edema distribution in the three different types of edema[2] (Fig. 8-4). In patients with cardiac edema, 96% had the gravitational (even) distribution and only 4% a central distribution. We are aware that this does not agree with the widely held belief that the most common edema in patients with cardiac failure is central. As far as we can determine, however, no previous analysis of edema distribution has been done in patients with cardiac failure to substantiate this contention. In our experience, central edema in patients with cardiac failure *does* occur and may be quite dramatic in appearance, usually accompanying very abrupt, severe left-sided heart decompensation of the type occurring with a massive myocardial infarction, papillary muscle rupture, or valve damage[7] (Fig. 8-5). Since cardiac failure occurs so often, even though the percentage of central edema is only 4%, many such central edemas will be seen. That is, if a film reader sees 100 patients with left-sided heart failure a month, four to six of these patients will have central cardiac edema. Possible causes for the rather bizarre bat's wing distribution in a few patients with cardiac failure have been discussed previously.

Pulmonary Blood Volume

PBV may be normal, increased, or diminished (Fig. 8-6). These findings are of moderate value for determining what variety of edema is present. In patients with *injury* edema, PBV is rarely increased.[2,8] When it is, it is almost certainly caused by superimposed overhydration and is accompanied by a widened vascular pedicle.

In patients with *renal* edema, 60% have an increased and 40% a normal PBV.[2] We saw no patients with renal edema who had a decreased PBV.

We previously discussed the wide spread belief that all patients with cardiac failure have an increased PBV. In our series, however, only 40% of patients with cardiac edema had recognizable increases in PBV, 48% were normovolemic, and 12% oligemic[2] (Fig. 8-6).

Air Bronchograms

We were somewhat surprised to find that air bronchograms are a very specific finding that occurs in 80% of patients with injury edema and in only 20% of those with cardiac or renal edema[2] (Fig. 8-7). The high inci-

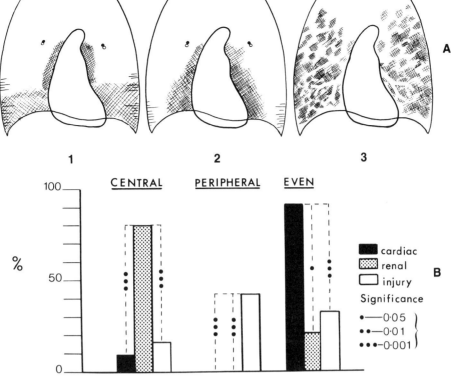

Fig. 8-4   A, Diagram of edema distribution. *1,* Gravitational or "even" (note peribronchial cuffing and septal lines); *2,* central; *3,* peripheral or random (patchy). Note air bronchogram. No cuffing or septal lines. **B,** Percent frequency of occurrence of the three main edema distribution patterns in patients with cardiac, renal/overhydration, and injury lung edemas.

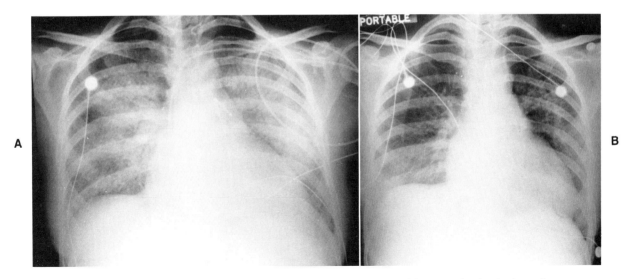

Fig. 8-5   A, Following a therapeutic abortion, this 28-year-old woman had a foul-smelling discharge. She became abruptly dyspneic and was thought clinically to have injury lung edema. The radiograph certainly shows nongravitational edema, but the distribution is central and *septal* lines are present, indicating hydrostatic edema. The wedge pressure was 19 mm Hg, still compatible with injury or overhydration, but the VPW was normal and the soft tissues were narrow. Conclusion: hydrostatic edema *not* caused by overhydration/renal failure, therefore probably cardiac failure. **B,** Same patient in **A** was found to be septicemic and to have bacterial endocarditis. The mitral and aortic valves were replaced, and the edema immediately began to improve. The film was taken 1 day after surgery.

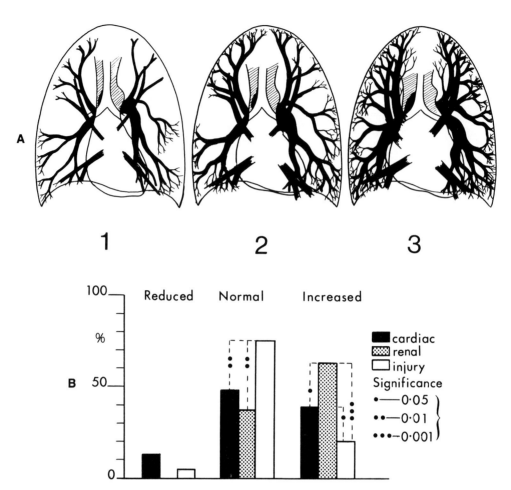

Fig. 8-6 A, Diagram illustrating *(1)* slight reduction in PBV (oligemia), *(2)* normal PBV (normovolemia), and *(3)* increased PBV (hyperemia). NOTE: the recruitment of all vessels results in a 1:1 flow redistribution. In the absence of left-to-right shunts or tamponade, the PBV and systemic blood volume must increase equally; therefore the VPW will progressively increase. **B,** Percent frequency of oligemia, normovolemia, and hyperemia in patients with cardiac, renal/overhydration, and injury lung edemas.

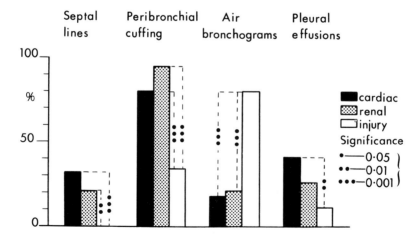

Fig. 8-7 Percent frequency of occurrence of septal lines, peribronchial cuffing, air bronchograms, and pleural effusions in patients with cardiac, renal/overhydration, and injury lung edemas.

dence of air bronchograms may occur because the viscid injury edema fills the alveoli, causing a "whiteout," but has difficulty, because of its protein/cellular content in flowing freely into the bronchi; this leaves the air column in the bronchus to stand out against the alveolar filling (in contrast to pressure edema where edema fluid can flow freely into the bronchi if alveolar filling is present).

Septal Lines

We saw no septal lines in any of the patients with injury lung edema in our initial series[2] (Fig. 8-7) and, have *never* seen septal lines in subsequent series of proven pure injury edema.[9,11] We regard the presence of septal lines as such a strong sign that, if they are present, the patient cannot have only injury edema. Hydrostatic edema must also be present. Two infrequent exceptions exist to this. First, patients with allergic lung edema, which is a variety of increased permeability edema, although without injury, *can* have septal lines.[2] Second, occasionally, if permeability edema is associated with a fulminating pneumonia, septal lines may be seen contiguous with the pneumonic consolidation.

Peribronchial Cuffing

Peribronchial cuffing is not of any value for differentiating between renal and cardiac edema but, as previously indicated, is of great value for differentiating between pressure and injury edema. Cuffing occurred in 80% to 90% of patients with cardiac and renal edema[2] (Fig. 8-7) but in only 30% of those with injury edema. Again, we believe that most of the injury edema patients who *did* show cuffing had been overhydrated and that if cuffing occurs in injury edema, it indicates that pressure edema is also present.

Pleural Effusions

On the plain film, effusions are rare in patients with injury lung edema (Fig. 8-7) (remembering that many of these patients are supine).[2] On computed tomographic (CT) scanning, a certain percentage of ARDS patients may have effusions that are too small to visualize on the supine plain film. However, it is somewhat unusual for ARDS patients to have a CT scan, and the findings we have concentrated on are those on the plain film. Even allowing for the supine position in these patients, the small effusions that may occasionally be found in ARDS are very discrepant from the much larger effusions found in 40% of patients with cardiac edema and 25% of those with renal edema.

Cardiac Size

Cardiac enlargement was found in 85% of patients with renal/overhydration, 73% of those with cardiac edema, and 32% of those with injury edema.[2] In the in-

jury patients the cardiac enlargement was usually a late finding, secondary to either overhydration or renal failure, to cardiac decompensation, or to developing septic myocardiopathy. Occasionally, we have seen the heart progressively enlarge in long-term surviving ARDS patients with no physiologic evidence of cardiac dysfunction. Such patients have usually been receiving intravenous hyperalimentation for long periods, and we suspect that a benign deposition of fat may occur.

Soft Tissue Thickness

No increase in soft tissue thickness is found in patients with pure injury edema. It is most often associated with overhydration/renal failure (85%) and biventricular or chronic left-sided heart failure (65%).[4] If soft tissue edema does develop in patients with injury edema, as it frequently does, it invariably signifies that a new pathologic change has been superimposed (Fig. 8-8). The change is usually overhydration but can sometimes be caused by third spacing from systemic capillary damage (remembering that ARDS is usually only part of a general systems failure).[4,8]

• • •

Each of the three common varieties of edema discussed can be shown to have a certain constellation of radiologic findings that characterizes it and allows it to be differentiated from the other types of edema. In our initial study[2] we published a small table that provided a brief summary of these findings (Table 8-1). This table has become quite popular and has been reproduced in several standard textbooks of pulmonary medicine and radiology.[12-14c] We have a slight regret that this table has been picked up for general use, not because the table is in any way incorrect, but because it is too simplistic. It does not include the *variations* found in the constellations of findings (published in our original article), which one needs to know beyond this table to determine correctly which type of edema is present. The table was not intended to be used as the primary method for determining what type of edema was present. We discuss later some of the unfortunate ramifications of using this simplistic table *alone* to attempt to differentiate edema etiologies.

We have now expanded the table somewhat to include the variations and cover a greater number of edema types, including complex-etiology edemas (Table 8-2).[7] However, this expanded table must still be interpreted in light not only of the relative frequency of each finding in a particular edema but also of the *importance* of that finding within a certain constellation regardless of its frequency. For example, one might have every radiologic finding indicating that injury edema is present and not one indication that hydrostatic edema is present apart from septal lines; but if

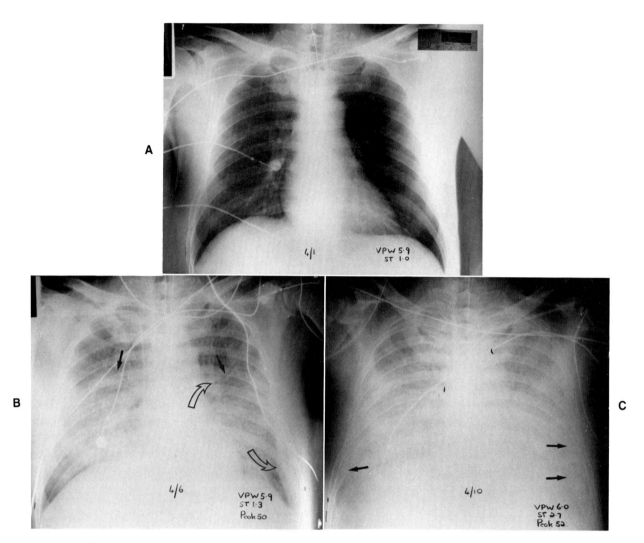

Fig. 8-8 **A,** Radiograph of 49-year-old man with alcoholic hepatitis and severe gastric bleeding. At this time slight oligemia is present, caused by hemorrhage. Note soft tissue *(ST)* thickness is only 1.0 cm. Patient is on spontaneous ventilation. **B,** Five days later the patient has severe nongravitational edema with air bronchograms *(straight arrow).* No increase has occurred in VPW or heart size, and the patient now requires positive-pressure ventilation and a peak pressure of 50 cm H_2O and is thought to have adult respiratory distress syndrome (ARDS) (wedge pressure, 16 mm Hg). However, some bronchial cuffing is present, and effusion has developed *(curved arrow).* ST thickness has increased slightly, suggesting that this is not pure injury edema and is either mixed hydrostatic and injury edema or possibly pure hydrostatic edema. Since the VPW and cardiac size have not increased, this would seem to rule out overhydration, (with the proviso that the peak pressure of 50 cm H_2O could narrow the pedicle and reduce heart size despite an increase in total blood volume). **C,** Four days later the edema is worse; this would be very unusual in pure injury edema, which stays very fixed after it has first appeared. Also, the effusions are much larger *(short arrow),* and ST thickness has increased from 1.3 to 2.7 cm. Since no radiologic evidence of overhydration/renal failure exists, the diagnosis is hydrostatic edema of oncotic origin. After treatment with albumin, the patient's edema resolves. The patient's need for high-pressure ventilation was probably related to increased intraabdominal content rather than change in lung compliance.

Table 8-2 Characteristic changes in single-etiology and combined-etiology pulmonary edema*

Type of edema	Normal	Inverted	Balanced	Even	Central	Random	Normal	Increased	Narrowed	Normal	Decreased	Increased	Normal	Increased	Peri-bron-chial cuffs	Sep-tal lines	Air bron-cho-grams	Bat's wing edema	Normal	Increased	Decreased	Normal	Increased
	Flow distribution			Edema distribution			Vascular pedicle			Heart size			Soft tissues						Lung volume			Main pulmonary artery	
Left-sided heart failure (LHF) (acute)			●	●			●		○	○		●		●	●	●	●		○		●	●	
LHF (fulminant)			●		●		○	●		●			●		●	●		●	●		○	●	
LHF (chronic)		●			●			●				●		●	●	●			●			●	
Overhydration			●	●				●				●		●	●	●			●	○		●	
Renal failure (acute)			●	●				●				●		●	●	●			●	○		●	
Renal failure (end stage)		○	●	●	○		●	○		●		○	●	○	●	●			●	○		●	
Renal failure (bat's wing)			●		●			●				●		●	●	●		●	●	○		●	
Injury	●					●	●		○	●	○		●				●		●	○			●
Noninjury permeability	●				●		●			●			●	○	●	●	●		●				●
Neurogenic	●			●	○	○	●			●			●		●	●	●		●		○		●
High altitude	●					●	●			●			●		●	●			●		○		●
Osmotic	●				●		●			●				●	●	●			●			●	
Injury and hydrostatic (over-hydration)			●		●	○	●					●		●	●	●	●		●				●
Injury and cardiac		●			●	●	●					●	●	○	●	●	●		●				●
Overhydration and osmotic			●		●			●				●		●	●	●			●			●	

*Black dots indicate the usual findings and the open circles occasional variants. The table can be used not only to determine the usual constellation of findings in a particular single-etiology or mixed-etiology edema, but also (by reading vertically) to determine under what circumstances a particular criterion will or will *not* be found. For example, enlargement of the main pulmonary artery occurs in injury, neurogenic, high-altitude, injury/hydrostatic, and injury/cardiac edemas.

septal lines *are* seen, hydrostatic edema *must* be present. Similarly, even if heart size is normal, the VPW normal, and PBF normal (all compatible with injury edema), the presence of two factors only (e.g., cuffing, central distribution of edema) would still make the diagnosis one of cardiac failure (acute), *not* of injury edema (see Fig. 8-5).

This is discussed more fully later in the next section.

"TYPICAL" CONSTELLATIONS OF FINDINGS

The typical constellations of findings that allow each type of edema to be identified are much better displayed as diagrams than as lists of data.[2,4,15] The classic appearance of chronic left-sided heart failure is illustrated in Fig. 8-9, renal failure/overhydration in Fig. 8-10, and injury edema in Fig. 8-11.[15]

Using the findings discussed earlier, we were able to differentiate pure injury edema from pure pressure edema with an accuracy of 91%.[2] The distinction be-

tween cardiac and renal edema is less accurate (81%), partially because renal decompensation is usually an inherent part of chronic left-sided heart failure and components of both types of edema are therefore present. Fortunately, it is usually quite easy to distinguish clinically between renal and cardiac edema (where our accuracy is lowest) and often difficult clinically but urgently necessary to distinguish between pressure and injury edema (where our accuracy is highest). In a subsequent study we investigated whether the subjective process of combining a number of radiographic signs in a specific pattern of lung edema could be confirmed rigorously in a more objective fashion.[11] The radiographic findings used by the readers in the process of identificaiton of the etiology of lung edema served as input variables for discriminant analysis. Discriminant analysis is a statistical technique that uses a set of variables to assign an individual or a group of individuals to one or several distinct groups. The subjective assignment of

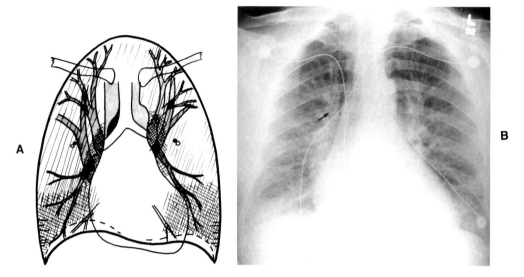

Fig. 8-9   A, Diagram of chronic left-sided heart failure. Points to note: *a,* flow inversion; *b,* wide pedicle and large azygos vein; *c,* peribronchial cuffing and septal lines; *d,* gravitational "even" distribution of edema. **B,** Left-sided heart failure. Gravitational distribution of edema in contrast to marked flow inversion is well seen. No septal lines are seen, but some peribronchial cuffing is present *(arrow).*

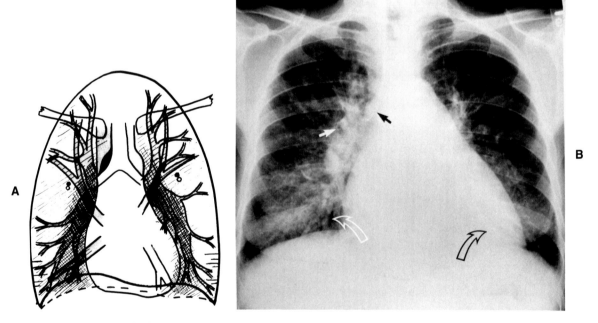

Fig. 8-10   A, Diagram of renal failure/overhydration. Points to note: *a,* 1:1 "balanced" distribution of flow; *b,* edema sparing costophrenic sulci and central in appearance; *c,* peribronchial cuffing and septal lines; *d,* wide pedicle and large azygos vein. **B,** Renal failure. Note no flow inversion (see large lower lobe vessels, *open arrows*), presence of peribronchial cuffing *(closed white arrow),* and wide pedicle and large azygos vein *(closed black arrow).* The edema also has a rather nodular appearance, which is frequently seen in renal edema.

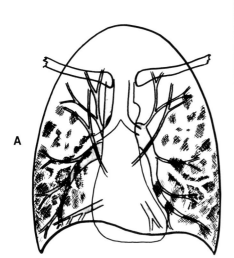
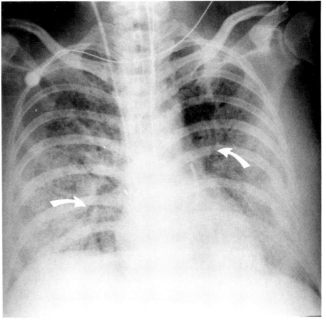

Fig. 8-11   A, Diagram of injury edema. Points to note: *a*, normal flow distribution; *b*, edema very *patchy*, often peripheral, tending to spare costophrenic angles; *c*, no peribronchial cuffing or septal lines; *d*, air bronchograms very frequent; *e*, normal VPW, azygos vein, and heart size. **B,** ARDS secondary to sepsis and hypotension. Note air bronchograms *(arrows)*, normal VPW, azygos vein, and heart size. Edema is worse peripherally but spares the left costophrenic angle. No septal lines present, and despite extensive edema, no effusions.

the chest films to the respective group of pulmonary edema etiology reached an accuracy of 86% and 90% for two different independent readers. The accuracy obtained objectively by using computer-generated classification by discriminant analysis was 88%, i.e., very similar to that of both readers. Again the lowest discriminating power was found in differentiating cardiac from renal/overhydration cases (91%), while cardiac cases were correctly discriminated from injury cases in 93% of the instances and renal cases from injury cases in all instances (100%).[37] This study offered the proof that the reader's objectivity in weighing different radiographic findings and using their combined patterns to differentiate pressure and injury edema is indeed very high.

Once the characteristic appearances of the three "pure" basic types of edema are familiar to the film reader, he or she can recognize variations from the patterns to suggest or specifically identify other varieties of edema and mixtures of edema of different etiologies.[4,7] Many of these variations are listed in Table 8-2.

Variant and Mixed-Etiology Edemas

The most common variant that makes it difficult to identify what edema is present or indeed if edema is present at all is the combination of edema and lung disease.[16] This has been fully discussed for emphysema and chronic bronchitis in Chapter 7. One special case of this variant is bilateral upper lobe emphysema. In such patients, because the apical vessels are destroyed, it is impossible for flow inversion to occur even with longstanding chronic left-sided heart failure. Also, the heart is small because of the emphysema, and when it enlarges as a result of the failure, it may become only normal in size (see Fig. 9-21).

Bilateral upper lobe emphysema is particularly important in patients with mitral stenosis. Since no redistribution of flow can occur to the upper lobes, the lower lobes are chronically hyperemic and develop much more organic damage than usual in mitral stenosis. If the patient then has surgery and a mitral valve prosthesis is inserted, the instant improvement in

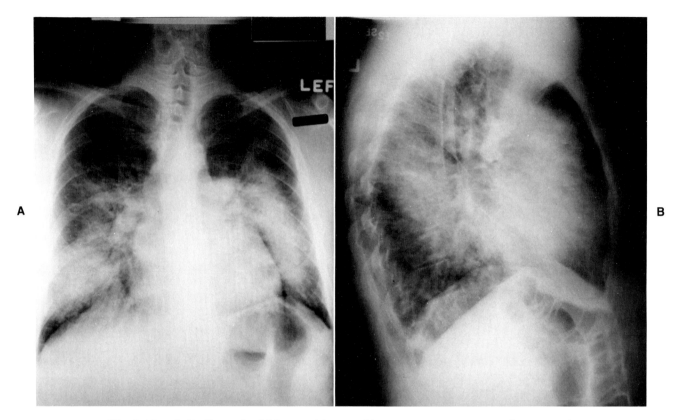

Fig. 8-12 **A,** Radiograph of 33-year-old man with severe coronary artery disease and prior myocardial infarcts showing the "bat's wing" distribution of edema seen in a small percentage of patients with abrupt, severe left-sided heart decompensation (see text). Note that although intense alveolar edema is seen centrally, minimal edema is present in the periphery of the lungs. Also, despite the severity of the edema, only lamellar effusions are present. **B,** Lateral view shows that this is a true bat's wing edema completely sparing the dorsum of the lungs and showing no tendency toward gravitational distribution. This suggests, as discussed previously, that the lung's interstitial space has been "closed off" peripherally. (Courtesy Denise Aberle.)

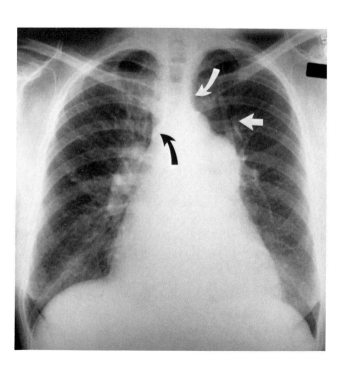

Fig. 8-13 Severe mitral stenosis with approximately 2:1 flow inversion *(straight arrow)* indicating very high left atrial pressure and greatly dilated main pulmonary artery indicating that some organic pulmonary arterial hypertension is present in addition to the passive hypertension. Very small aorta is accompanied as usual by a very narrow vascular pedicle and very small azygos vein *(curved arrows)*.

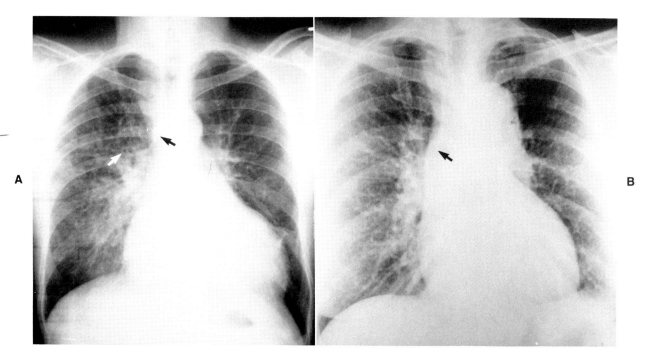

Fig. 8-14   A, End-stage renal failure with classic centrally located edema, 1:1 flow distribution, and peribronchial cuffing *(white arrow)* but a normal to narrow vascular pedicle and azygos vein *(black arrow)*. This would usually imply the systemic blood volume is normal or reduced, but in end-stage renal disease the narrowing is probably caused by increased systemic vasomotor tone. Although moderately severe interstitial and alveolar edema is present in the lungs, the soft tissues of the chest wall are virtually cachectic. Why patients with end-stage renal failure can have severe pulmonary edema without any visible systemic edema is not clear but may also be related to increased systemic vasomotor tone. Note also that the edema does not extend into the periphery of the lungs, and therefore no pleural effusions exist. **B,** Usual picture of renal failure or overhydration: increased PBV and 1:1 flow distribution and matching increased systemic blood volume manifested by a wide pedicle and large azygos vein *(black arrow)*.

cardiac output means that the right ventricle must immediately pump more blood but since the upper lobes are destroyed, the ventricle can do this only through the already organically damaged lower lobes, which have a high pulmonary vascular resistance, and thus the right ventricle may abruptly fail. In a series of patients with chronic obstructive pulmonary disease (COPD) and mitral valve disease examined by Milne and Bass,[16] those with upper lobe emphysema had a much worse survival rate than those with normal upper lobes.

First Episode: Acute Left-Sided Heart Failure

Patients with acute left-sided failure may differ considerably from those with chronic left-sided heart failure. As discussed in Chapter 7, the pedicle is normal or even narrowed, the heart often normal in size, and if the failure is very acute, the edema may take a central or bat's wing distribution. Since the pulmonary edema in these patients frequently does not extend to the periphery of the lung, no subpleural edema exists and pleural effusions therefore will not develop (Fig. 8-12). That is, pleural effusions from heart failure are caused

by pulmonary edema passing from the lung into the pleural space; therefore, if the periphery of the lung does not contain edema, effusion cannot develop. Interestingly, these acutely developing central edemas usually become alveolar very rapidly, apparently bypassing the interstitial "sump filling" phase. As a result, despite the presence of florid edema, peribronchial cuffing may be minimal or even absent.

Chronic Mitral Valve Disease

In addition to the expected marked flow inversion of high left atrial pressures, patients with chronic mitral valve disease differ from those with chronic left-sided heart failure by having an unusually narrow vascular pedicle (Fig. 8-13). We believe this is caused by a smaller-than-normal TBV caused probably by the low left ventricular output[15] and resulting also in a very small aorta.* In addition, the lung volumes are usually large (unlike in patients with chronic left-sided heart failure), possibly because of recurrent infection and de-

---

*The low TBV may also be caused by increased circulating atrionatriuretic factor.

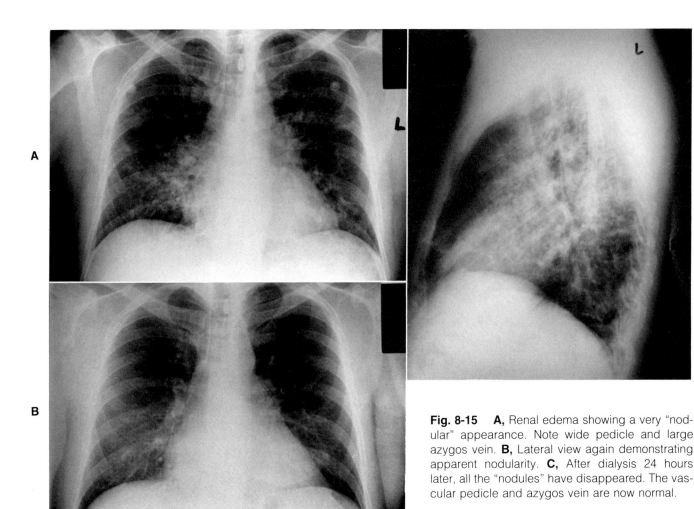

Fig. 8-15 **A,** Renal edema showing a very "nodular" appearance. Note wide pedicle and large azygos vein. **B,** Lateral view again demonstrating apparent nodularity. **C,** After dialysis 24 hours later, all the "nodules" have disappeared. The vascular pedicle and azygos vein are now normal.

velopment of COPD in lungs that are continuously moist from the persistent transudation of fluid.

Variants in Renal Edema

Edema occurring as a result of renal disease is usually accompanied by a wide vascular pedicle. In end-stage renal disease, however, the vascular pedicle is often *narrow* even with an increased TBV. As stated earlier, we believe this narrowing results from high vasomotor tone (Fig. 8-14). The PBV, however, remains large, reflecting the increased TBV. This discrepant combination of findings can help to differentiate renal failure from simple overhydration, in which the VPW is invariably enlarged. Another differentiating point between renal edema and simple overhydration occasionally seen is the *texture* of the edema. In patients with renal edema, particularly uremic ones, this may have a curious nodular appearance (Fig. 8-15). This nodularity can be so intense that it can be mistaken for metastases, but it disappears abruptly after dialysis.

Variants in Injury Edema

The most common variation is in the distribution of injury edema.[17] This depends largely on the original cause of the injury. For example, if it results from aspiration, it may be extremely regional, even completely unilateral. Another variant can occur in elderly patients, who may have tortuous ectatic great vessels arising from the aorta. This causes a spurious widening of the vascular pedicle.[6] If such patients then develop injury edema, they will not manifest the normal or narrow VPW usually seen in patients with ARDS.

Combined-Etiology Edema

In patients with injury edema, overhydration during treatment occurs so frequently that it is the rule rather than the exception. In such patients the classic changes of injury edema are submerged by those of overhydration (Table 8-2). That is, the usually normal pedicle widens, the normal PBV increases, cuffing and septal lines may be present, and the chest wall's soft tissues

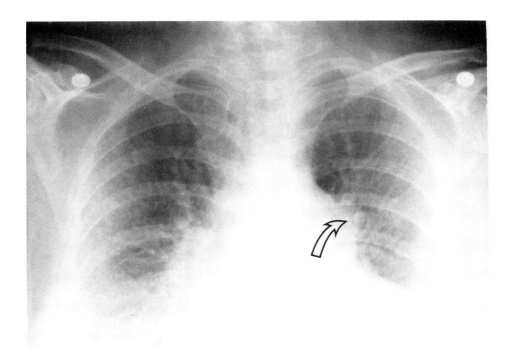

Fig. 8-16   Radiograph of 35-year-old male diabetic who developed coma abruptly. The main pulmonary artery has enlarged massively *(arrow)*. No specific "classic" distribution of neurogenic edema exists, although a whiteout is often seen.

increase in thickness (see Fig. 8-8). Very frequently the *chronology* allows one to make the diagnosis of injury and overhydration. The appearances of overhydration will *not* be present at the inception of injury edema, and injury edema, once it has formed, will *not* change in its appearance and distribution from day to day. Any change that does occur must result from a different etiology; this is usually overhydration but frequently aspiration, nosocomial pneumonia, or renal failure may also be causes.

Neurogenic Edema

As discussed in Chapter 2, neurogenic edema results from the transference of a very high right ventricular pressure directly into the capillary bed. This causes extensive transudation and pushes apart the endothelial cell junctions so that some protein molecules can emerge, giving neurogenic edema some physiologic and radiologic characteristics of injury edema.[2,7,18] Radiologically, the edema does not have a specific general or regional distribution. Its classic manifestation is said to be a "whiteout," and certainly this does occur, but the edema can also be very patchy. One outstanding feature that may suggest the diagnosis is an abrupt increase in size of the main pulmonary artery (Fig.

8-16).[4,9,10] If this is seen with an abrupt whiteout, and if the VPW or cardiac size is not increased, neurogenic edema should be strongly suspected.

High-Altitude Edema

As with neurogenic edema, high-altitude edema is caused by an abrupt elevation in right ventricular pressure, but this is secondary to hypoxemia, which causes arteriolar vasoconstriction. In the areas subserved by the constricted arterioles, the elevated right ventricular pressure cannot be transferred directly to the capillary bed; however, in those regions *unaffected* by the hypoxemia, torrential (redistributed) blood flow may occur. In these areas the force of the elevated right ventricular pressure is transferred directly to the capillaries, and edema will develop in these "normal" but hyperperfused areas of the lung (Fig. 8-17). At times, if such patients stay at or return to high altitudes (usually above 8000 feet), the edema can recur and often does so in exactly the same regional distribution.[20,21]

Near-Drowning, Postglottic Obstruction, and Croup

Patients with edema due to these etiologies all have an episode of greatly increased negativity of the inter-

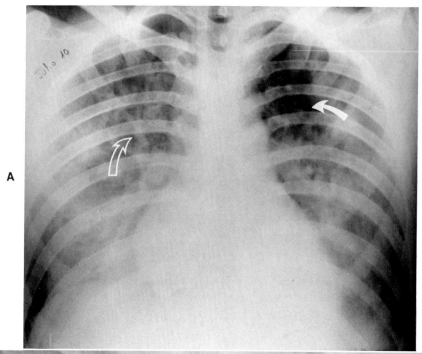

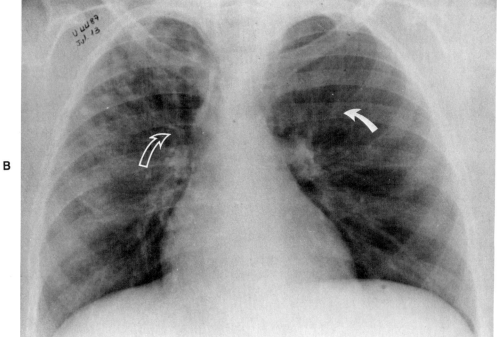

Fig. 8-17   **A,** Young male patient from Bogota (elevation, 8000 feet) with high-altitude edema. Note that the *non*edematous left upper lobe area *(closed arrow)* appears to contain very few visible blood vessels. In contrast, the edematous right upper lobe area contains unusually large vessels *(open arrow)*. Thus edema does not appear to occur in those areas that have developed arteriolar constriction in response to the hypoxemia but does occur in those areas where flow redistribution and *hyperemia* are present. **B,** Three days later the edema has largely cleared but with some residuum in the right upper lobe, where the vessels have decreased in size back to normal *(open arrow)*. On the left *(closed arrow),* however, they have *increased* in size back to normal.

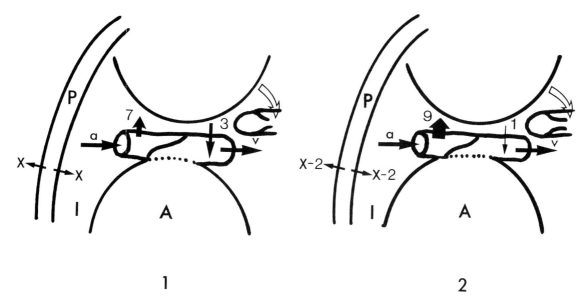

Fig. 8-18 *P,* Pleural space; *I,* interstitium; *A,* alveolus; *a,* arterial end of capillary; *v,* venous end of capillary. **1,** The outward pull *(x)* of the chest wall on the pleura is opposed by the elastic recoil of the lung *(x),* and the interstitial pressure is slightly negative. Liquid will exchange with an outward force of 7 mm Hg (arterial end) and an inward force of 3 mm Hg (venous end) *(arrow thickness* indicates amount of flow). The difference between transudation and reabsorption is *4 mm Hg,* taken up by the lymphatics *(open arrow).* **2,** If the patient now inspires against a closed glottis, the interstitial pressure will drop *(x − 2).* The Starling sums indicate that transudation (at *a*) will increase to 9 mm Hg (indicated in quantity and direction by *thick black arrow*), and at the venous end *(v)* reabsorption will decrease to 1 mm Hg *(thin black arrow).* The difference between transudation and reabsorption is now *8 mm Hg* (i.e., 100% increase in transudation) leading to pulmonary edema. Increasing negativity of interstitial pressure *(x − 2)* must be matched by increasing negativity of pleural pressure *(x − 2).*

stitial space of the lung caused by violent attempts to inspire against a partially closed or obstructed glottis (i.e., prolonged Müller maneuver) (Fig. 8-18). VPW, cardiac size, and PBV do not increase and flow distribution is normal, but peribronchial cuffing is usually seen and septal lines may occur. This combination of findings clearly indicates that this is a pressure edema but that it is *not* caused by overhydration or cardiac failure and is some variant of hydrostatic edema. This should raise the question of glottic obstruction or near-drowning. Various literature reports suggest that edema caused by glottic spasm secondary to difficult intubation for anesthesia may occur, particularly in young vigorous patients capable of making forceful inspiratory efforts and generating high negative interstitial pressures.[22-25]

CORRELATION BETWEEN TYPE OF EDEMA AND PHYSIOLOGIC CHANGES

Three patients with exactly the same amount of edema but with three different etiologies (cardiac, re-

nal/overhydration, injury) will have entirely different left atrial pressures[4,26] (see Fig. 7-2) and manifest extremely different symptoms and severity of disease, not because of the edema but because of the mechanism of edema production.[26] In a patient with cardiac edema, left atrial pressure is high (probably in the 20s to 30s) because of the progressive elevation of left ventricular end-diastolic pressure. Such a patient has a small cardiac output, and the blood reaching the body's periphery is extremely hypoxemic. The patient manifests the severe symptoms of poor oxygenation of the brain, intestines, and peripheral tissues.

In contrast, a patient with renal failure and the same amount of edema has a "supernormal" cardiac output.[27] The lungs are slightly "erected" with blood; they are usually quite large and of *normal* compliance. This patient has a much greater respiratory excursion than the patient with cardiac edema (see Fig. 4-42). The oxygenation of blood in the lungs is much better than in the patient with cardiac edema, and an ample supply of

Table 8-3 Interobserver variability (mean) in assessing nine different parameters (216 chest radiographs, two observers)

	Percent disagreement
Heart size	11
Vascular pedicle	2%
Pulmonary blood flow distribution	29
Pulmonary blood volume	26
Septal lines	8
Peribronchial cuffs	8
Air bronchogram	19
Lung density increase	6
Lung edema (regional distribution)	8

(From Milne ENC, Pistolesi M: in Putman CE: *Diagnostic imaging of the lung,* New York, 1990, Marcel Dekker; © 1989 ENC Milne.)

blood travels to the periphery. Part of the edema in a patient with the renal type is caused by low oncotic pressure, and left atrial pressure is only mildly elevated (15 to 25 mm Hg), caused by the large circulating blood volume.[28] Such patients can have severe pulmonary edema but show so little symptomatology that they are able to walk comfortably to the radiology department, stand, and hold their breaths readily to have a PA film taken. This would be so unusual in a patient with cardiac or injury edema of this degree that seeing a PA film in an erect patient with severe pulmonary edema should immediately suggest renal edema.

Patients with the same amount of *injury* edema usually have severe physiologic problems, with extremely stiff lungs, multiple areas of diminished perfusion, severe ventilation/perfusion mismatch, and pulmonary arterial hypertension. The hypertension is often manifested by an enlarged main pulmonary artery segment and enlargement of the heart's right side.[4,9,10] These patients may have a large cardiac output if they are septicemic, but they are extremely hypoxemic, have poor peripheral oxygenation, and require positive-pressure ventilation. They usually have a normal left atrial pressure.

EFFECTIVENESS OF RADIOGRAPHIC TECHNIQUE FOR DIFFERENTIATING CARDIAC, RENAL/OVERHYDRATION, AND INJURY EDEMA

Several of the radiologic features used to determine what type of edema is present are subject to considerable interobserver variation (Table 8-3). This variation is reduced considerably as film readers gain expertise. It is of less importance than one might initially think, however, because so many factors must be considered to make the diagnosis that different observers may disagree on several findings and still come to the same final conclusion about the type of edema present. Table 8-4 is an analysis of agreement and disagreement between two observers analyzing 216 chest films. The first seven and the last (no. 216), films have been shown as examples. One readily sees that there is only one radiograph in which the two observers agreed on every feature, but they did agree on so many features that they made the *same* final diagnosis in each patient.

Although our method of determining edema etiology has been widely adopted, it has also attracted some criticism concerning its validity. Aberle et al.[29] studied a group of ICU patients with very severe edema. Their study, according to the authors, was designed to test our criteria. However, the criteria we published were formulated for widespread use in patients with widely varying severities of disease whereas the study by Aberle et al. was deliberately designed to test the criteria *only* in acutely ill ICU patients. Furthermore, these authors did not use our separate criteria for renal, overhydration, and cardiac edema as published but lumped them into a "combined" set of criteria for the general diagnosis of hydrostatic edema. Departing still further from our methodology, they attached "weighting factors" to each criterion, according to the statistical frequency with which it occurred in our original article, overlooking the fact that some features may occur frequently and be of limited importance in diagnosis, whereas others occurring less frequently have much greater diagnostic significance (see following discussion).

Table 8-4 Interobserver variability in assessing 9 different parameters (216 chest radiographs, two observers)*

	Case number							
	1	2	3	4	5	6	7.	216
Heart size	+	+	+	−	+	+	+	+
Vascular pedicle	+	+	+	+	+	+	+	+
Hilar abnormalities	+	+	+	+	+	+	+	+
Pulmonary blood flow distribution	+	+	+	+	−	+	+	+
Pulmonary blood volume	−	+	+	+	+	+	−	+
Septal lines	+	+	−	+	+	+	+	+
Peribronchial cuffs	+	+	+	+	+	+	+	+
Air bronchogram	+	−	+	+	−	+	+	+
Lung density increase	+	+	+	+	+	+	+	+
Lung edema (regional distribution)	+	+	+	+	+	+	+	−

*First seven radiographs and film no. 216 shown as representative examples. +, Agreement; −, disagreement.

Even with these departures from our methodology, Aberle et al.[29] did make the correct diagnosis of hydrostatic edema in 80% of patients but were correct in only 60% of patients with injury edema. They concluded from this that "chest radiography is limited in the differentiation of type of edema in *severe* cases" (our italics). We do agree that the complex edemas seen in the ICU are much more difficult to assess than simple "pure" edemas and therefore the percent accuracy decreases somewhat from the accuracies we achieved in our study, although *all* our patients with injury edema *were* in the ICU.

However, we believe Aberle et al.[29] have somewhat exaggerated the difficulties because of the way in which their study was designed. First, they based their diagnosis of injury edema on alveolar/serum protein ratios, but considerable overlap occurs in the ratios found in cardiac failure and injury edema,[30-32] and the accuracy of the protein ratio as a "gold standard" for separating injury versus severe cardiac edema is very debatable. Second, when they found widened vascular pedicles and septal lines (which we believe are good evidence of hydrostatic edema) in those patients whom they believed from the protein ratio had pure injury edema, they made no attempt to prove that these patients did not *also* have hydrostatic edema. That is, they did not study fluid input/output data, patients' weights, or soft tissue changes nor did they apparently compare with previous films to determine radiologically whether the changes of hydrostatic edema had developed after those of injury edema (see Fig. 8-8). Since their patients (by preselection) were seriously ill, they would (almost inevitably) have been treated by extensive fluid replacement, which strongly suggests that the authors' failure to diagnose injury edema in some patients radiologically was because the injury edema was overlaid by hydrostatic edema. If the authors had used our criteria for dual-etiology edema, their results, even in these patients with very acute conditions, would have been very close to ours.

A somewhat similar study by Smith et al.[33] begins by saying that the authors' aim is "to confirm the results reported by Milne et al." These authors point out that in our initial study[2] we asked our readers to give a specific diagnosis of cardiac, renal/overhydration, or injury edema but "without the criteria used to make these diagnoses clearly stated." We would accept this as a valid criticism; we did not emphasize sufficiently in our original paper that simple statistically significant differences in *frequency* of occurrence of the various criteria between the three types of edema were often not enough to make a specific diagnosis. One's knowledge of the pathophysiology of each type of edema and the variants that occur in their presentation also has to be taken into account (see following discussion).

The film readers in the Smith et al.[33] study were asked to record their observations but *not* to make a diagnosis, unlike in our study. Furthermore, the condition was made that all patients admitted to the study had to have alveolar edema. This, as in the Aberle et al.[29] study, immediately skews the data and is quite unrealistic, since most patients do not enter the ICU with full-blown ARDS but develop it subsequently. Therefore one usually has a chronology of change to refer to, and relatively few patients are seen for whom the only films to study are those in the late alveolar phase. Making alveolar edema an absolute condition of the study means that some useful criteria are much more difficult to assess, as we explained in our original article.[2] For example, PBV, flow distribution, peribronchial cuffing, and even VPW would be difficult or impossible to assess, whereas others (e.g., air bronchograms) may be easier to see.

With this in mind, we converted Smith et al.'s numeric data[33] into histograms so that we could make a direct visual comparison with our own data. We discovered that the findings of both studies were quite similar (Fig. 8-19), except that, as anticipated, air bronchograms were easier to see and peribronchial cuffing much more difficult. The similarities in the two studies are clear, but one of the most valuable diagnostic features for distinguishing between pressure and injury edema (peribronchial cuffing) has been lost because of the experimental condition in the Smith et al.[33] study that all patients must have alveolar edema. This article contains other differences, however, that we cannot explain. For example, a high proportion (60%) of *injury* patients were reported as having radiologically increased PBVs and a mean VPW of 6.1 cm. This is entirely at variance with the findings *in the same patients* that 95% had normal-sized hearts, even though 26 of the 33 patients were supine. We know of no physiologic explanation for a simultaneous increase in systemic blood volume and PBV with no accompanying change in cardiac volume.

Since the film readers were not asked to make a diagnosis, one cannot determine from the Smith et al.[33] paper what level of success they might have achieved in distinguishing the three types of edema. However, the authors do point out, as discussed at the beginning of this chapter, that hydrostatic edema can often be readily distinguished from injury edema using such simple criteria as cardiac size and the presence or absence of septal lines.

A third paper, published by Rocker et al.,[34] contains similar design problems. The authors begin by saying they intend to duplicate our initial study, but in fact they have used a different approach, which refers back to our Table 8-1. We indicated this is a very simple table, containing simply statistically significant *frequen-*

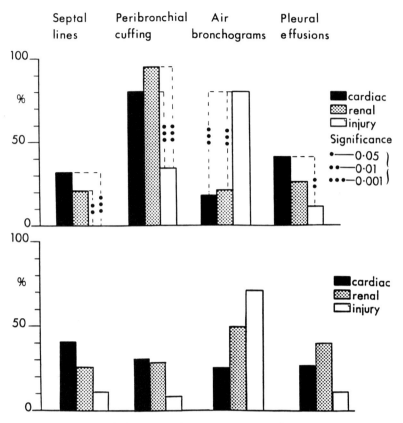

Fig. 8-19 The upper set of histograms is our original data,[2] as already displayed in Fig. 8-7. The histograms are redisplayed to contrast them with the data of Smith et al,[33] which we converted to histogram form for ease of comparison. The strong similarity can be seen, with the only major difference being the marked percentage reduction of peribronchial cuffing in all patients. This has occurred presumably because a condition of the Smith et al. study was that *alveolar* edema must be present, which would make cuffing increasingly difficult to see but would increase the ability to see air bronchograms (as it has). Interestingly, despite the requirement (not in our study) that severe edema be present, the incidence of effusions in patients with injury edema is exactly the same as in our study.

cies of appearance of the various radiologic findings with no attempt to state the diagnostic importance or unimportance of any finding. Unfortunately, Rocker et al. chose to attach weighting numbers to each of these radiologic features based principally on their statistical frequency, but with some change in the weighting according to a feature's degree of discrimination. The approach sounds reasonable, but some of its problems surface if we consider, for example, the presence or absence of septal lines. If these authors saw septal lines, they simply added the value of minus 3 to their "score" for that patient, and using their approach, one could still make the diagnosis of injury edema. As we have pointed out, septal lines virtually never occur in injury edema; therefore "weighting" the finding is inappropriate.

Similarly, since centrally located pulmonary edema has entirely different values depending on whether the TBV is increased or not, assigning it the same weighting number under both circumstances is of limited value. That is, if central edema is present with a narrow VPW and normal PBV, the diagnosis is acute left-sided heart failure (Fig. 8-20, *A*). If central edema is present with a wide VPW and increased PBV, the diagnosis is renal failure or overhydration (Fig. 8-20, *B*). Rocker et al.,[34] using their own scoring method, achieved an accuracy of 75% for cardiac edema, 78% for renal edema, and 77% for injury edema. This was a carefully conducted study, but the accuracies achieved are considerably less than those found in our original study. Their scoring system failed to distinguish between cardiac and renal edema. Using this type of scoring also requires much added work for the film reader and does not appear to have much virtue.

For the reasons given, we do not think that any of the three studies[29,33,34] just discussed is completely valid.

Another frequent criticism concerns the value of flow distribution in determining which type of edema is

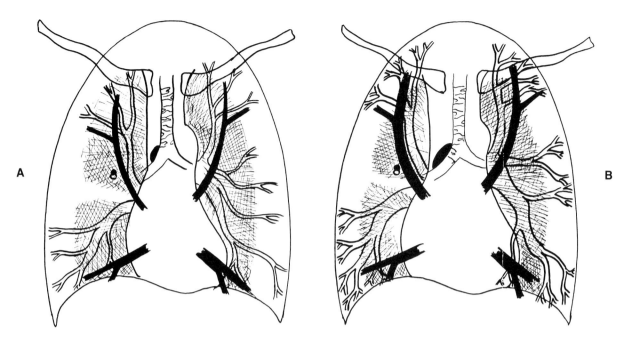

Fig. 8-20 **A,** "Central" edema with peribronchial cuffing, normal VPW, normal PBV, and normal flow distribution. Diagnosis: acute left-sided heart failure with the rarer (4% to 10%) presentation of central, or bat's wing, edema. **B,** Central edema with peribronchial cuffing, wide pedicle, increased PBV, and 1.0:1.0 flow distribution. Diagnosis: renal failure or overhydration.

present. The objection is that many patients in the ICU are supine and therefore manifest a 1:1 flow distribution, not an inverted one. However, we are not aware of any work that proves that an inverted flow distribution *does* disappear in the supine position. Inversion may actually be exaggerated by the supine position.[35] Inverted flow does not disappear in patients with mitral stenosis, and in our experience it does not do so in patients with chronic left-sided heart failure.[36] If our hypothesis in Chapter 10 is true, that basal venospasm occurs in these patients to protect left atrial output, it would not appear to be reasonable teleologically for the venospasm to disappear in the supine position. During the pre-CT era, study of the pulmonary veins by conventional linear tomography and supine angiograms confirmed that in patients with high left atrial pressure who have flow inversion in the erect position, narrowing of the lower lobe veins remains present on supine films.[36]

Another objection has been offered that distribution of edema must also change in the supine position.[37] This is true, but only for patients with *hydrostatic* edema; injury edema is not affected by gravity. One might still object that the central edema characteristic of renal failure or overhydration might disappear in the supine position. We have not had the opportunity to test this because, as discussed earlier, most patients with renal failure have minimal physiologic effects from

their edema, and therefore it is rarely necessary to care for them in a supine position.

SUMMARY

Pulmonary edema is a very common and clinically important feature of cardiac, pulmonary, and systemic disease. If the film reader is unable to detect and quantify edema and determine its cause, he or she is at a professional disadvantage. The simple skills of detecting and quantifying edema can easily be taught. However, in the past some have thought that it is almost impossible to distinguish between hydrostatic and nonhydrostatic edema radiologically.[38-42] Certainly this is somewhat more difficult than simply quantifying edema, but, as we have shown, such differentiation can be done with considerable accuracy.

Success in differentiating edemas, particularly when they have a compound etiology, must be based on a greater depth of knowledge of the relationships between radiologic changes and their causative pathophysiology than is usually necessary for conventional chest radiographic interpretation. However, once this knowledge has been acquired, the film reader will have gained a new, very useful diagnostic tool. As discussed in Chapter 7, the ability to determine what type of edema is present also permits the film reader to be more accurate in assessing left atrial pressure (see Chapter 10).

REFERENCES

1. Badeer HS: Gravitational effects on the distribution of pulmonary blood flow: hemodynamic misconceptions, *Respiration* 43:408, 1982.
2. Milne ENC, Pistolesi M, Miniati M, Giuntini C: The radiologic distinction of cardiogenic and non-cardiogenic edema, *AJR* 144:879, 1985.
3. Milne ENC: Correlation of physiologic findings with chest roentgenology, *Radiol Clin North Am* 11:17, 1973.
4. Milne ENC: A physiologic approach to reading critical care unit films, *J Thorac Imaging* 1(3):60, 1986.
5. Milne ENC, Burnett HK, Aufrichtig D et al: Assessment of cardiac size on portable chest films, *J Thorac Imaging* 3(2):64, 1988.
6. Milne ENC, Pistolesi M, Miniati M, Giuntini C: The vascular pedicle of the heart and the vena azygos. Part I. The normal subject, *Radiology* 152:1, 1984.
7. Milne ENC, Pistolesi M: Pulmonary edema—cardiac and noncardiac. In Putnam CE, editor: *Diagnostic imaging of the lung*, New York, 1990, Marcel Dekker, p 253.
8. Iannuzzi M, Petty TL: The diagnosis, pathogenesis and treatment of adult respiratory distress syndrome, *J Thorac Imaging* 1(3):1, 1986.
9. Pistolesi M, Miniati M, Ravelli V, Giuntini C. Injury versus hydrostatic lung edema: detection by chest x-ray, *NY Acad Sci* 384:364, 1982.
10. Pistolesi M, Miniati M, Milne ENC, Giuntini C: The chest roentgenogram in pulmonary edema, *Clin Chest Med* 6:315, 1985.
11. Miniati M, Pistolesi M, Paoletti P et al: Objective radiographic criteria to differentiate cardiac, renal, and injury lung edema, *Invest Radiol* 23:433, 1988.
12. Fraser RG, Par *Diagnosis of diseases of the chest*, ed 3, Philadelphia, 1942, WB Saunders.
13. Goodman L, Putman C: *Critical care unit radiology*, Baltimore, 1989, Williams & Wilkins.
14. Elliot L: In Taveras J, Ferrucci J, editors: *Cardiac radiology*, vol 5, 1989.
14a. Fishman AP: *Pulmonary diseases and disorders*, ed 2, vol 2, New York, 1988, McGraw-Hill, p 191.
14b. Murray JF: *Disorders of the pulmonary circulation*. In Murray JF, Nadel JA, editors: *Textbook of respiratory medicine*, Philadelphia, 1988, WB Saunders, p 1294.
14c. Elick MR: Pulmonary edema and acute lung injury. In Murray JF, Nadel JA, editors: *Textbook of respiratory medicine*, Philadelphia, 1988, WB Saunders, p 1380.
15. Milne ENC: Pulmonary patterns in heart disease. In Royal College of Radiologists: *A textbook of radiological diagnosis*, vol 2, Partridge J, editor: *The cardiovascular system*, London, 1985, Lewis.
16. Milne ENC, Bass H: Roentgenological and functional analysis of combined chronic obstructive pulmonary disease and cardiac failure, *Invest Radiol* 4:129, 1969.
17. Pistolesi M, Miniati M, DiRicco G et al: Perfusion lung imaging in the adult respiratory distress syndrome, *J Thorac Imaging* 1(3):11, 1986.
18. Theodore J, Robin ED: Speculations on neurogenic pulmonary edema, *Am Rev Respir Dis* 113:405, 1976.
19. Wray NP, Nicotra B: Pathogenesis of neurogenic pulmonary edema, *Am Rev Respir Dis* 118:783, 1978.
20. Maldonado D: High altitude pulmonary edema, *Radiol Clin North Am* 16:537, 1978.
21. Maggiorini M, Buhler B, Walter M, Oelz O: Prevalence of acute mountain sickness in the Swiss Alps, *Br Med J* 301:853, 1990.
22. DeFranco M: Negative-pressure pulmonary edema following laryngospasm, *Crit Care Nurse* 9:20, 1989.
23. DeDio RM, Hendrix RA: Postobstructive pulmonary edema, *Otolaryngol Head Neck Surg* 101:698, 1989.
24. Bonadio WA, Losek JD: The characteristics of children with epiglottitis who develop the complication of pulmonary edema, *Arch Otolaryngol Head Neck Surg* 117:205, 1991.
25. Guinard JP: Laryngospasm-induced pulmonary edema, *Int J Pediatr Otorhinolaryngol* 20:163, 1990.
26. Overland ES, Severinghaus JW: Noncardiac pulmonary edema, *Adv Intern Med* 23:307, 1976.
27. Guz A, Moble MIM, Trenchard D: The significance of a raised central venous pressure during sodium and water retention, *Clin Sci* 30:295, 1966.
28. Stein L, Beraud JJ, Cavanilles J et al: Pulmonary edema during fluid infusion in the absence of heart failure, *JAMA* 229:65, 1974.
29. Aberle DR, Wiener-Kronish JP, Webb WR, Matthay MA: Hydrostatic versus increased permeability pulmonary edema: diagnosis based on radiographic criteria in critically ill patients, *Radiology* 168:73, 1988.
30. Sprung CL, Rockow EC, Fein IA et al: The spectrum of pulmonary edema: differentiation of cardiogenic, intermediate and noncardiogenic forms of pulmonary edema, *Am Rev Respir Dis* 124:718, 1981.
31. Carlson RW, Schaffer JR, Michaels SG, Weil MH: Pulmonary edema fluid: spectrum of features in 37 patients, *Circulation* 60:1101, 1979.
32. Matthay MA, Wiener-Kronish JP: Intact epithelial barrier function is critical for the resolution of alveolar edema in humans, *Am Rev Respir Dis* 142:1250, 1990.
33. Smith RC, Mann H, Greenspan RH et al: Radiographic differentiation between different etiologies of pulmonary edema, *Invest Radiol* 22:859, 1987.
34. Rocker GM, Rose DH, Manhire AR et al: The radiographic differentiation of pulmonary edema, *Br J Radiol* 62:582, 1989.
35. Anderson G: Large upper lobe veins, *J Coll Radiol Aust* 8:214, 1965.
36. Lavender JP, Doppman J, Shawdon H, Steiner RE: Pulmonary veins in left ventricular failure and mitral stenosis, *Br J Radiol* 35:293, 1962.
37. Aberle DR, Wiener-Kronish JP, Matthay MA: *Radiology* 170:892, 1989 (letter).
38. Petty TL: Adult respiratory distress syndrome: definition and historical perspective, *Clin Chest Med* 3:3, 1982.
39. Sibbald WJ, Warshawski FJ, Short AK et al: Clinical studies of measuring extravascular lung water by the thermal dilution technique in critically ill patients, *Chest* 83:725, 1983.
40. Staub NC, Hogg JC: Conference report of a workshop on the measurement of lung water, *Crit Care Med* 8:752, 1980.
41. Unger KM, Shibel EM, Moser KM: Detection of left heart failure in patients with adult respiratory distress syndrome, *Chest* 67:8, 1975.
42. Loyd JE, Newman JH, Brigham KL: Permeability pulmonary edema, *Arch Intern Med* 144:143, 1984.

9 Detecting and Quantifying Chronic Bronchitis and Emphysema

The blanket term "chronic obstructive pulmonary disease" (COPD) was originally adopted to encompass a spectrum of different diseases, often occurring simultaneously and difficult to separate clinically, with the common denominator of increased airway resistance to expiration. COPD includes such diseases as asthma and chronic bronchitis, in which the obstructive mechanism arises from intrinsic airway disease (reversible in asthma, irreversible in chronic bronchitis), and emphysema, in which the obstruction is caused by destruction of alveolar walls with loss of lung recoil. A small percentage of patients may have no functionally detectable evidence of air trapping, which has caused some authors to suggest that the term "obstructive" is misleading. However, even these apparently nonobstructed patients may show air trapping when imaging techniques are used,[1] and it is probably appropriate to continue to use COPD *clinically*.

The difficulties of distinguishing among chronic bronchitis, emphysema, and asthma clinically (which necessitated the use of this blanket term) are much less evident on chest radiography, which can usually identify each of these entities separately. Suggesting that the plain chest film is of value in diagnosing COPD is equivalent to putting one's hand in a hornets nest or, possibly more appropriately, entering the lists of a battle between knights in armor. Both sides are well armed (with different data), but both see only narrow (and differently directed) views through the visors of their helmets, while riding into battle on ground that may contain quicksands. In other words, the plain chest film's role in the diagnosis of emphysema, chronic bronchitis, and asthma has been and continues to be a topic of great controversy and occasional acrimony. Although some authors, including ourselves, believe that the chest radiograph can reliably detect emphysema and chronic bronchitis,[2-9] other authors state that the plain chest film can only detect these diseases at a fairly advanced stage.[10-12]

Highly reputable authors continue to make statements such as, "In chronic bronchitis, even if fatal, and in asthma the radiograph is usually normal. The same is true of emphysema with a few important exceptions."[11] This statement is at *complete* variance with our experience. Although we would agree that a patient with severe status asthmaticus can have a chest radiograph that is close to normal, we have not, in a lifetime of chest radiology, seen a single patient dying of emphysema who had a normal chest film. We have seen several patients with chronic bronchitis who were severely ill but did not have the usually described radiographic parenchymal changes. However, the changes they *did* have, including a large main pulmonary artery, enlarged right ventricle, and thickened bronchial walls, along with the minor parenchymal changes (a very revealing discrepancy), were quite characteristic of this particular variant of chronic bronchitis. The principal changes occur within the bronchi, and little visible change occurs in the lung parenchyma.[12] At bronchoscopy the mucosa of such patients usually is grossly inflamed and friable. Even these infrequent patients have radiographs that are far from normal and should be diagnostic to the trained interpreter (Fig. 9-1).

In two separate large studies, we have correlated the radiologic changes of COPD with the patient's clinical history (including smoking history), lung compliance, and pulmonary function tests (PFTs).[7,8] We have shown that the plain chest film can detect COPD at an early stage and that the disease's severity on the radiograph,

267

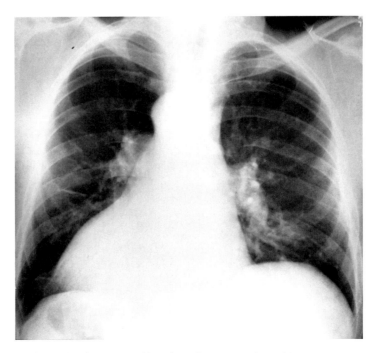

Fig. 9-1 Radiograph of 45-year-old male, a heavy smoker with severe exacerbation of chronic bronchitis. Small patch of consolidation is seen at right lung base; minor lung changes only, but gross evidence of severe pulmonary arterial hypertension. Bronchoscopy revealed red, "beefy," edematous bronchial mucosa.

based on both extent and regional distribution, correlates well with the clinical symptomatology. Our findings are supported by carefully controlled studies by other authors.[2-4,9] However, as already stated, many other papers appear to show that the chest radiograph *cannot* pick up COPD at an early stage and correlates poorly with PFTs and pathology.[10-12]

The considerable discrepancy between our findings and these authors requires analysis and exploration. Recently, Pratt carefully analyzed the more significant papers in the literature dealing with the radiologic diagnosis of COPD and concluded that the chest film is an excellent method for detecting emphysema.[2,3] He stated that the discrepancies in other papers that disagree with this conclusion result from (1) differing *criteria* (both radiologic and pathologic) between studies, (2) different uses of the criteria, and (3) differing *intentions* (study goals), which are often not even stated.

This critique, although extensive, deals only with radiologic/*pathologic* correlations. As Pratt noted, "Few of the reported studies are directly comparable to each other, and the lack of success in one study does not imply that the diagnostic reliability reported in another study should be disregarded."[2] Pratt specifically analyzes "one particular study [Thurlbeck and Simon[10]] that commonly receives the primary role in support of the conclusion . . . that radiography can only detect severe disease and that inconsistently." This study[10] has

been shown to have severe flaws in its experimental design, including films of poor quality and use of only one radiologic observer. Although very skilled, this interpreter appears to have been instructed to be extremely conservative. In addition, the pathologist involved in the study decided to classify mild emphysema as "normal," so when the radiologist *correctly* read the film as mild emphysema, his answer was recorded as being a false positive! Curiously, although Pratt points this out as a serious design fault, the same methodology reappears in a much more recent study,[13] of which Pratt is a coauthor.)

In the past, we have also pointed out some of the flaws in the Thurlbeck and Simon[10] study. As an example, we took from the article a radiograph that had been read as showing *no* emphysema (Fig. 9-2). Using our own criteria, we would have read this film as showing a mixture of severe emphysema and chronic bronchitis, which it was pathologically. We showed this figure, with no clinical information and no hint of what we were trying to establish, to 15 persons, including five board-certified radiologists, two computed tomography (CT) fellows, five residents at various stages of training, and three medical students. All 15 readers reported the film as showing emphysema, and two experienced chest radiologists correctly graded its severity.

If 15 people of widely varying radiologic training were all able to make the correct diagnosis, why did the

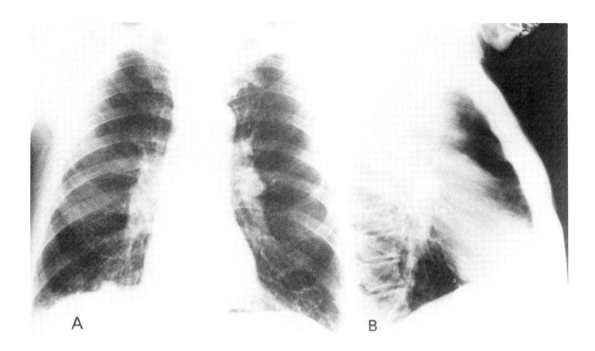

Fig. 9-2 The original interpreter of these posteroanterior (PA) and lateral films reported the patient as having no emphysema.[10] By our criteria, the films show a mixture of severe emphysema and chronic bronchitis, evidenced by the severe pulmonary hypertension. This patient died of chronic airflow obstruction with the "blue bloater" syndrome. (From Thurlbeck WM, Simon G: *AJR* 130:429, 1978.)

skilled chest radiologist in this study fail to detect emphysema? The experimental design apparently constrained him to using limited criteria and required him to be excessively conservative in his readings.

In addition to the design problems that Pratt has identified, there are other causes that explain the discrepant results between those authors who have found radiology to be useful in the diagnosis of COPD and those who have not. First, most papers that conclude that radiology is of limited value in COPD do not deal with all the diseases encompassed by COPD but confine their analysis to emphysema.[2-6,10,12] In our studies we have defined very specifically the differing diagnostic criteria for chronic bronchitis, emphysema, and asthma and have diagnosed each entity separately. If the criteria for chronic bronchitis were present but no emphysema was seen, we nevertheless made the diagnosis of COPD. Many studies appear to have accepted that all patients with COPD must have some emphysema (we disagree; see later discussion) and therefore have concluded that if no radiologic criteria of emphysema were seen, COPD could not be present.

Second, there are problems using either pathology or PFTs alone as gold standards for the presence of emphysema and chronic bronchitis. Pratt has delineated

some of these,[2,3] but we believe additional problems exist in correlating the chest film with pathology.

CORRELATION OF RADIOLOGIC DIAGNOSIS WITH PATHOLOGY

One might intuitively believe that pathology should be the final gold standard against which we must compare the accuracy of radiologic diagnosis. However, it is not necessarily correct to believe that radiographic findings, particularly those involving the lung, must correlate exactly with pathologic findings before they can be accepted. Both pathologists and radiologists study tissue by transmitting electromagnetic radiation through it and recording the resultant image. However, x-rays have the inestimable advantage of being able to visualize the lung exactly as it is in life and therefore to record many characteristics that are lost to the pathologist in the examination of the dead organ.

For example, abnormalities in the quantity or distribution of air within the thorax are easy to see radiologically but may be very difficult to see, or even totally absent, in the pathologic specimen. As another example, although a pneumothorax may be defined in pathologic terms, the diagnosis is invariably made from the radiograph and could not be made pathologically unless a very complex procedure were employed of instantly freezing the entire thorax and then bandsawing it from apex to base. The gold standard for diagnosing and quantifying a pneumothorax is therefore the radiologic image, not pathology.

The use of pathology as the gold standard for emphysema shares some of the same problems. Much diagnostic information depends on the radiologist's ability to see the pulmonary vessels in their entirety, their size, their definition, their tortuosity, and degree of taper; the relative sizes of arteries and veins; and most importantly the distribution of blood flow within the lungs (Fig. 9-3). All this information is lost to the pathologist, who takes a lung that is drained of blood, fixes it, often without prior inflation, and rarely sections it from apex to base in the coronal plane viewed by the radiologist, which is the ideal plane for seeing the vessels in profile. Even when the lung is fixed in inflation, positive pressure is almost invariably used for inflation and the lung is rarely, if ever, inflated to the same total lung capacity (TLC) that it occupied in life (which would incidentally have to be determined from the radiograph). The additional information that the pathologist can gain from sectioning, staining, and magnifying may not compensate for the *loss* of diagnostic information available to the radiologist, particularly with emphysema.

Furthermore, if the definition of a disease is to be made only in pathologic terms, then the pathologic description, to be of any value, must relate closely to the disease's behavior in the live patient in order that one may diagnose and treat it. If the pathologic classification of the disease's severity correlates poorly with its in vivo manifestations,[14] it is of little value. This can unfortunately be true with emphysema, in which pathologic classification of severity relies heavily on the total quantity of lung destroyed and not at all on its regional distribution. The *quantity* of emphysema alone, disregarding its *distribution*, has been shown to correlate poorly with PFTs (Fig. 9-4). For example, it is rarely pointed out that severe destruction from emphysema affecting the *upper* lobes has little physiologic effect, whereas the same amount of destruction involving the *lower* lobes has a major physiologic effect (Fig. 9-5). In these two instances, although the amount (severity) of emphysema defined pathologically may be the same, the clinical picture is quite different.[7]

The simple, atraumatic, inexpensive, and insufficiently used *expiratory* film may also reveal why a discrepancy exists between the apparent severity of emphysema on the chest radiograph and the patient's clinical/physiologic status.[7] The patient in Fig. 9-6 would be classified from the radiograph as having severe emphysema but clinically had only minor dyspnea. The ex-

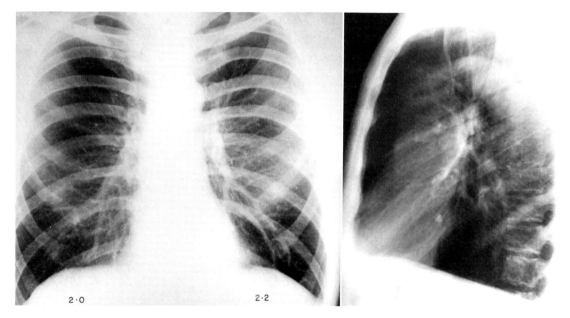

Fig. 9-3   Radiographs of 55-year-old male smoker. Pulmonary function tests (PFTs) revealed a total lung capacity (TLC) of 8.11 L (106% of predicted normal), which falls within the normal range, but the radiographs are clearly abnormal. The diaphragm is at the level of the twelfth rib and on expiration moves only 2.0 cm on the right and 2.2 cm on the left (normal, 3.5 cm). The pulmonary vessels are attenuated and sharply defined. The appearance is that of moderately severe, generalized, pure emphysema, as confirmed by the diffusing capacity, which was only 71% of predicted normal value.

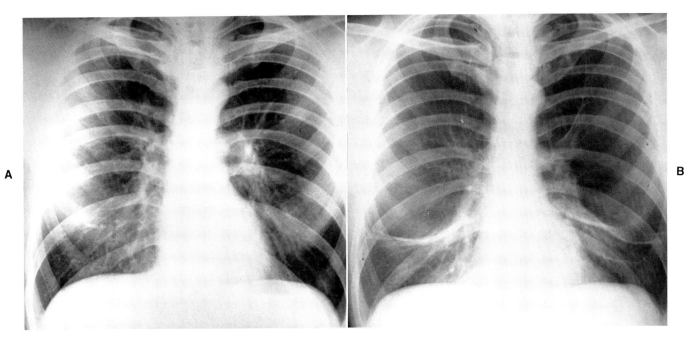

Fig. 9-4 **A,** Radiograph of 32-year-old male patient with mild to moderate but progressing dyspnea. Minimal vascular attenuation and loss of background vessels in upper lobes indicate mild upper lobe emphysema. **B,** Three years later, huge bullae have developed because of alpha-1-antitrypsin deficiency, probably heterozygous. Despite these gross changes, the patient was able to complete a 20-minute treadmill exercise test with only mild discomfort.

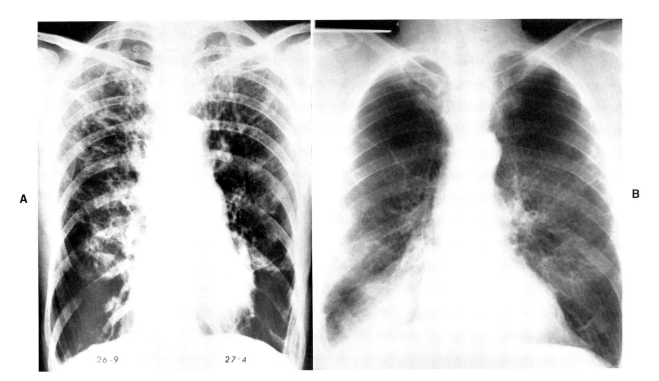

Fig. 9-5 **A,** Extremely severe emphysema of lower lobes with organic redistribution of flow to upper lobes. Evidence of moderate pulmonary arterial hypertension. Diaphragms moved only 1.2 cm on expiration. This patient had severe dyspnea at rest and minimal exercise tolerance. **B,** Severe upper lobe emphysema with massive apical bullae. Chronic bronchitic changes are seen at both lung bases with superimposed acute right lower lobe pneumonia. Moderately severe pulmonary arterial hypertension is present. The combination of the cardiac size/shape (a sign of chronic bronchitis) and the large lung volumes is typical of dual disease. This patient had no dyspnea at rest but a considerable reduction in exercise tolerance.

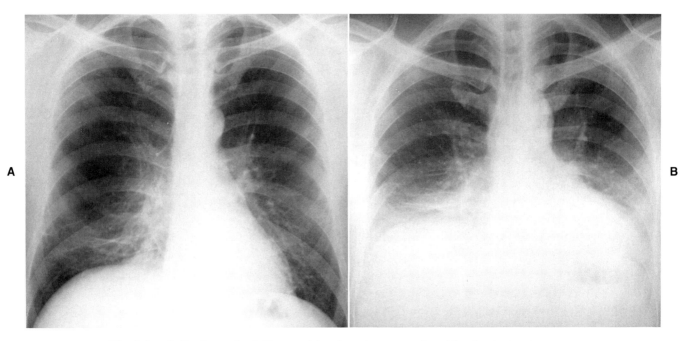

Fig. 9-6 **A,** Radiograph of 47-year-old male, a heavy smoker. Massive bullae in upper two thirds of right lung and moderate to severe emphysema of left upper lobe are seen. Radiologically, the patient would be classified as having severe emphysema, but he had little symptomatology. **B,** Same patient in **A.** On expiration, no evidence of air trapping is seen, explaining the lack of symptoms.

piratory film shows that much less air trapping is present than one would have anticipated from the inspiratory film alone. The inability to detect functional air trapping is another reason why the present pathologic quantification of emphysema does not constitute the ideal standard against which the accuracy of the in vivo roentgenogram can be compared.

CORRELATION OF RADIOLOGIC DIAGNOSIS WITH FUNCTION STUDIES

Pulmonary function data in general are regarded as being objective and absolute, whereas the radiologic image is viewed as being too subjective to be acceptable as the gold standard. A radiograph, however, is simply a detailed photograph of the patient's interior. The visual data provided are admittedly affected by the recording technique, but if the technique is erroneous, this is obvious to the experienced reader and can be factored into his or her reading of the film. Radiographic data are therefore quite objective, and only the interpretation of the data injects subjectivity.

In contrast, PFT data are very subject to the recording technique used and may be quite variable even when repeated on the same patient in the same laboratory.[15] Furthermore, once the data have been obtained, they must then be compared with a range of

"normal" values measured at a different time, usually by a different laboratory, on a different population to determine whether the data are abnormal. Finally, once one has established whether the data are abnormal, they then become subject to an observer's interpretation before a clinical diagnosis can be made. This introduces into the analysis of PFTs the same subjectivity complained of in radiologic interpretation.

The accepted range of normal in PFTs is so wide $(\pm 25\%)^{15}$ that studies of lung volumes become quite insensitive. Postmortem studies, for example, have well documented[16] that a good relationship exists between TLC and the amount of emphysema present in the lung. However, in many patients with mild to moderate emphysema (less than 30% destruction), even though the TLCs are abnormally large for these individuals (average, 117% of predicted), they still fall within the accepted wide range of "normal" and cannot therefore be read by PFTs as being abnormal.[6,15] In contrast, an increase of 15% to 20% in volume is *readily* detectable on the chest radiograph (see Fig. 9-3), but PFTs have too wide a range of normality to detect it, hardly a characteristic of a "gold standard." Yet it is from such PFTs that it has been inferred that it is the radiograph which is inaccurate.

With so much overlap between the accepted range of

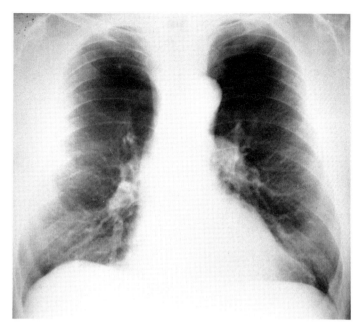

Fig. 9-7 Upper lobe emphysema ("pure") with mild to moderate changes of pure chronic bronchitis at the bases. The cardiac shape, with slightly elevated apex and the large comma-shaped central pulmonary arteries, is typical of patients with chronic bronchitis, but the heart is not enlarged. This is the typical appearance of a heart midway between the small vertical heart of pure emphysema and the large transverse heart of pure chronic bronchitis.

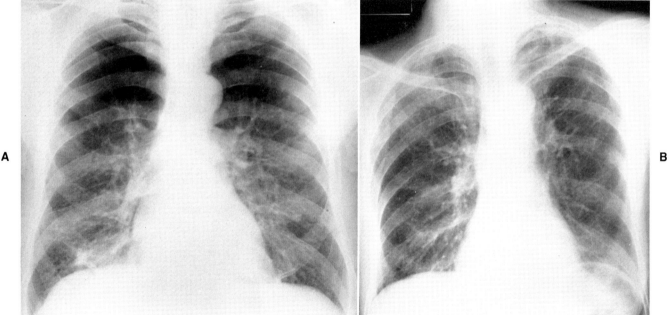

Fig. 9-8 **A,** Male 48-year-old smoker with changes of both chronic bronchitis (mild to moderate), principally basal, and upper lobe emphysema, most severe in the right upper lobe. Prevalence of the two diseases assessed as emphysema, 40%; chronic bronchitis, 60%. **B,** Male 60-year-old smoker with a combination of attenuation of vessels (indicating emphysema) and thickened bronchial walls, slightly blurred vessels, and increased background pattern (indicating interspersed chronic bronchitis). This patient has no areas of pure emphysema or chronic bronchitis. Prevalence of the two diseases assessed as emphysema, 50%; chronic bronchitis, 50%.

values in normal subjects and in patients with emphysema and chronic bronchitis, few physiologists will claim they can characterize either emphysema or chronic bronchitis from PFTs alone.[15] Some investigators even state that no criteria have been agreed on for making the diagnosis of emphysema during life.[16] This lack of specificity may be a contributing factor to the belief that "pure" emphysema and "pure" chronic bronchitis rarely exist clinically (i.e., that the two diseases are always admixed), and yet the radiologist often sees pure (or predominant) emphysema or pure chronic bronchitis. These often occur regionally in the same patient, for example "pure" upper lobe emphysema and "pure" lower lobe chronic bronchitis (Fig. 9-7). In such patients, although the two diseases are pure in the sense that they are not anatomically admixed, PFTs would integrate the changes from both diseases and would certainly be interpreted as showing mixed disease.

In any patient the two diseases may be generally admixed, but with a more or less accentuated prevalence of one or the other disorder (Fig. 9-8).

From clinical findings and pulmonary function data alone, admixed emphysema/chronic bronchitis would appear to occur much more often than "pure" disease. In a rigorous, independent, three-observer blind study of the radiographs of 71 patients with proven COPD, however, we found "pure" emphysema in 49%, "pure" chronic bronchitis in 21%, and mixed emphysema and chronic bronchitis in 30% (Table 9-1). However, 50% of the patients with pure emphysema showed only mild to moderate upper lobe or apical destruction, with normal lung elsewhere, and had no detectible *clinical* abnormality at rest. Therefore a discrepancy would exist in these patients between the radiologic findings and the clinical findings (but the radiograph would be correct). Clinically, these patients would not have been suspected of having COPD and thus would not have been investigated, leaving only 75% of the patients with clinical symptoms. In this *clinically* detectable group, 39% had mixed emphysema and chronic bronchitis, a greater apparent swing toward mixed disease.

To summarize, the discrepancies between those authors whose work shows that the chest film is sensitive for the detection of COPD and those who apparently show that it is not appear to arise from the following causes:

1. Differing criteria for diagnosis
2. Different uses of the same criteria
3. Different study goals
4. Consideration of only emphysema and not the full spectrum of COPD (failure to record COPD if emphysema is not present)
5. Insensitivity of PFTs and inability to distinguish between emphysema and chronic bronchitis
6. Lack of correlation between pathologic and functional severity (due partially to a disregard of distribution of disease)
7. Inability of fixed pathologic specimens to reflect in vivo radiologic changes
8. Faulty experimental design
9. Possible lack of distribution of knowledge of the differing vascular changes characterizing chronic bronchitis and emphysema on the chest radiograph

Patients are never biopsied in practice to make the diagnosis of either emphysema or chronic bronchitis, and PFTs have limited sensitivity. Therefore one should place greater emphasis on a very careful history and informed reading of the patient's chest film, realizing that the radiograph may become the best gold standard, as it has for pulmonary edema.[17]

RADIOLOGIC DIAGNOSIS

The radiologist's task is (1) to detect the presence of COPD as early as possible, (2) to differentiate between patients with pure or predominant emphysema and those with pure or predominant chronic bronchitis, and (3) when mixed disease is present, to estimate with clinically useful accuracy the relative proportions of each disease present. This differentiation is important because the etiology, prognosis, and treatment involved with each disease are different.

Many of the radiologic signs have been known for more than 40 years. In 1950 Kerley[5] stated that for the diagnosis of emphysema, "the most important radio-

Table 9-1 Radiologic distribution of emphysema (E) and chronic bronchitis (CB) in 71 cases of COPD

Emphysema (pure)		
Regional:		
Upper lobes	18	
Lower lobes	2	35
Generalized:	15	
Chronic bronchitis (pure)		
Regional:		
Upper lobes	3	
Lower lobes	1	15
Generalized:	11	
Emphysema and chronic bronchitis in the same patient		
Regional:		
Pure lobe E: lower lobes mixed E and CB	3	
Pure upper lobe CB: upper lobes mixed E and CB	3	
Upper lobes E and CB mixed: lower normal	2	21
Generalized:		
Mixed E and CB	3	

logic appearances are in the blood vessels" and gave an excellent description of these changes. Since that time, many other authors have added to the vascular criteria,[4,7,8,18] but they are still not widely known or used. We believe this is largely because of erroneous teaching that the chest film is not of much value for the diagnosis of COPD. Our radiologic criteria for identifying and grading the severity of emphysema and chronic bronchitis are given shortly, and since these data are all visual, carefully chosen, typical radiologic examples of each disease process and the grading method are supplied, followed by examples of mixed disease. Before describing the radiographic criteria, it is necessary to define emphysema and chronic bronchitis as accurately as possible.

Emphysema

In this book we use the term "emphysema" to mean a permanent dilatation of the air spaces distal to the terminal bronchioles, accompanied by destruction of alveolar walls.[19,20] In so-called compensatory and obstructive emphysema, neither destruction nor permanent dilatation occurs, and these terms should be replaced by "compensatory" or "obstructive hyperinflation" (Fig. 9-9).

Chronic Bronchitis

Several well-recognized problems exist with the term "chronic bronchitis."[16] First, the disease process is seldom confined to the bronchi alone. Second, the disease may be recurrent rather than chronic. Third, one cannot "officially" make the diagnosis without certain highly specific clinical findings, such as cough and expectoration on most days for at least 3 months of the year over 2 successive years. However, many patients who clearly have chronic bronchitis, both developing and more advanced, do not always meet these criteria. In such patients, since we apparently cannot use the term "chronic bronchitis," what diagnosis can we give to the manifestly abnormal radiograph?

In Europe the term "dirty lung" has been used for many years to describe the radiologic appearances of such patients and alert the clinician to a disease process, even though it cannot be "officially" named "chronic bronchitis." Presently, no satisfactory alternative has been devised to apply to these patients. Clearly the term "dirty lung" is not satisfactory, since it conveys no idea of what particular pathology is present although it does have some value in that it excludes pure or predominant emphysema, in which the lung is conspicuously "clean."

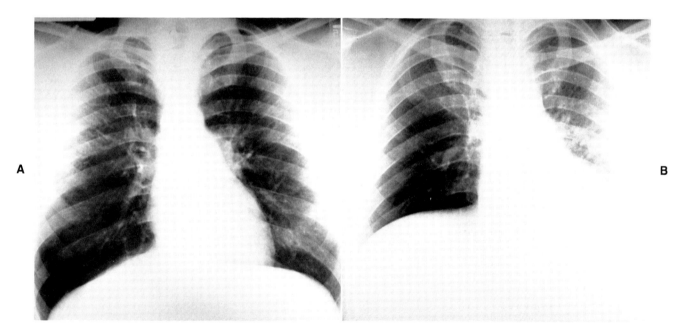

A   **B**

Fig. 9-9 A, Radiograph of 32-year-old male who arrived at emergency room with moderate dyspnea. Film shows relative oligemia of the right lung base with depression of the right diaphragm, strongly suggesting air trapping. Functional redistribution of blood flow to the right upper lobe is seen. **B,** Expiratory film confirms the presence of right lower lobe air trapping (obstructive hyperinflation). At bronchoscopy a pedunculated adenoma was found causing a valvular obstruction of the right lower lobe bronchus. It was successfully removed by a snare through the bronchoscope.

Some years ago, on the basis of the pathologic changes present, we suggested the term "recurrent bronchopneumonitis" (RBP) to describe these patients and replace the term "dirty lung."[7] However, the phrase is too similar to recurrent bronchopneumonia (which it is not) to be satisfactory. The words chronic bronchitis are hallowed by use, despite their descriptive flaws, and it is widely understood that the disease is seldom purely bronchial and that the full clinical spectrum may not always be present. Therefore it is probably best to retain the term and to use the phrase "chronic bronchitis forme fruste" (CBF) to describe those patients who have the radiographic findings but not the full spectrum of clinical findings of chronic bronchitis. In this book we use the words chronic bronchitis as an umbrella term to include both "classic" chronic bronchitis and CBF ("dirty lung" or RBP).

RADIOLOGIC CRITERIA FOR EARLY DIAGNOSIS

Up to the present the literature has placed much more emphasis on the diagnosis of emphysema than on chronic bronchitis. Also, much importance in the radiologic diagnosis of emphysema has been placed on abnormal lung volumes, diaphragmatic flattening, and a widened retrosternal space. Unfortunately, when all these findings are present, the diagnosis has usually been made long ago by the patient's next-door neighbor, watching him walk painfully up his front path, blowing out his pink cheeks, and puffing.

Many years ago, during the daily reading of many chest films, it became evident that patients with pure or predominant emphysema and pure chronic bronchitis had characteristic and consistent changes in their pulmonary vessels that allowed us to differentiate them correctly.[7] Logically, if we could consistently diagnose patients with *advanced* disease from these pulmonary vascular changes, with developing skill it seemed we should be able to find the same changes, although less evident, in patients with less severe disease and possibly only in their beginning phase.

Our descriptions of the differing vascular changes in emphysema and chronic bronchitis were first published in the study just quoted,[7] in which we analyzed inspiratory and expiratory radiographs in a series of 700 patients suspected of having early chronic lung disease. In each of these patients, inspiratory and expiratory films were made and PFTs performed within 1 hour of the radiographs. The expiratory films confirmed the relationship between air trapping and the vascular changes of emphysema so consistently that we eventually stopped using them and came to rely on the inspiratory film alone. Using our vascular criteria, we were able to diagnose emphysema, chronic bronchitis and mixed disease consistently in their early and often preclinical phase. These results may be criticized because the ra-

diologic findings were correlated with the only "gold standard" available at the time, PFTs, with the inherent problems already discussed. However, the PFTs were performed rigorously and always by the same personnel within 1 hour of the films. They included the swallowing of an esophageal balloon in more than 200 patients for compliance studies and, within the limitations, were as accurate as possible.

In this study we confirmed that we were able to detect and grade the severity of emphysema and chronic bronchitis early in their clinical stages.[7] Other authors have been more successful in using criteria of hyperinflation and have found the vascular criteria to have

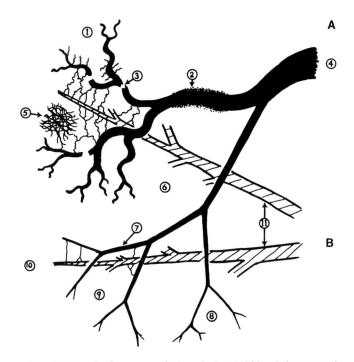

Fig. 9-10   **A,** Changes of chronic bronchitis: *1,* increased tortuosity of vessels; *2,* blurred vessel margins caused by infection; *3,* apparent breaks or "segmentation" of vessels so that they cannot be followed to the periphery; *4,* enlargement of the central vessels, indicating pulmonary hypertension—often these vessels assume a comma shape, narrowing abruptly at the lobar vessel level; *5,* small irregular densities caused by "cherry stones" of fibrosis (subsegmental atelectases) or mucus-filled acini; *6,* draining vein is reduced in size when compared with the supplying artery, a manifestation of pulmonary arterial hypertension. In addition to these changes, bronchial wall thickening is almost invariably seen. **B,** Classic vascular changes of emphysema: *7,* loss of normal sinuosity and reduction in caliber of vessels, which appear attenuated and excessively sharply defined; *8,* increased branching angles; *9,* loss of side branches with loss of normal background pattern and increasing lucency of the lung; *10,* peripheral normal clear zone of the lung becomes progressively wider, with vessel loss; *11,* draining veins become reduced in caliber.

more interobserver and intraobserver variation,[2-4] but again, these authors studied only emphysema and not chronic bronchitis. We also use lung lucency, volume, and diaphragmatic contour as *part* of our criteria for the diagnosis of emphysema. However, we believe that because our descriptions of the vascular changes include both emphysema *and* chronic bronchitis and are more detailed and specific than those published elsewhere,[12,21,22] this may account for our better results in diagnosing *early* emphysema and chronic bronchitis, in which we believe the vascular criteria are more valuable than changes in lung volume. Our interobserver and intraobserver variation is quite small, and the technique is easily learned.[7,8]

We tested our criteria again in 1986 using three independent observers, this time correlating the radiologic findings with, in addition to the PFTs, clinical findings, a rigorous history, and the number of pack-years of smoking. We found again an excellent correlation between our radiographic gradings of COPD and the clinical grading.[8] This study is discussed more fully later.

Our criteria for the diagnosis of chronic bronchitis and of emphysema are illustrated in Fig. 9-10.

The upper portion of Fig. 9-10 *(A, numbers 1 to 6)* shows the vascular findings in "pure" chronic bronchitis, contrasted with the lower portion of the diagram *(B, numbers 7 to 11)*, which shows the classic changes in "pure" emphysema.

As we attempt to show, the chest radiograph has a primary role to play in the clinical process of defining the prevalent underlying pathophysiologic mechanisms of airway obstruction.

Chronic Bronchitis

The criteria for diagnosing chronic bronchitis include increased tortuosity of the pulmonary arteries, patchy blurring of the normally clearly defined vessel margins, apparent breaking up or "segmentation" of the vessels, and inability to follow them from the center of the lung to the periphery (Fig. 9-11). Further criteria are enlarged central arteries, with a discrepancy in size between the large central and smaller peripheral

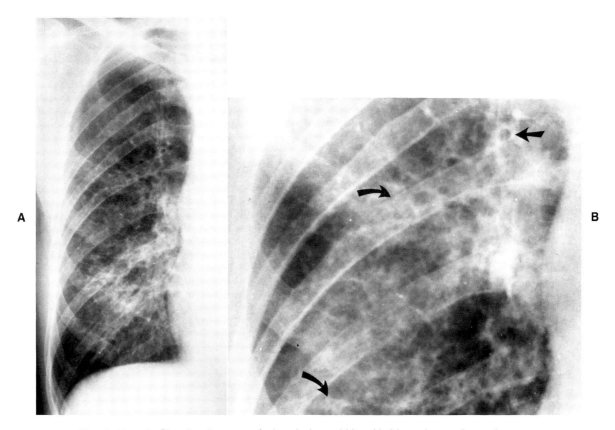

Fig. 9-11   A, Classic changes of chronic bronchitis with blurred vessel margins, segmentation and tortuosity of vessels, and increased background pattern. **B,** Enlarged spot view of the right lung base showing the bronchial wall thickening *(straight arrow)* and scattered, small, poorly defined nodules (mucus-filled acini or areas of subsegmental atelectasis and fibrosis, *curved arrows*). Note the impossibility of following any vessel from center to periphery.

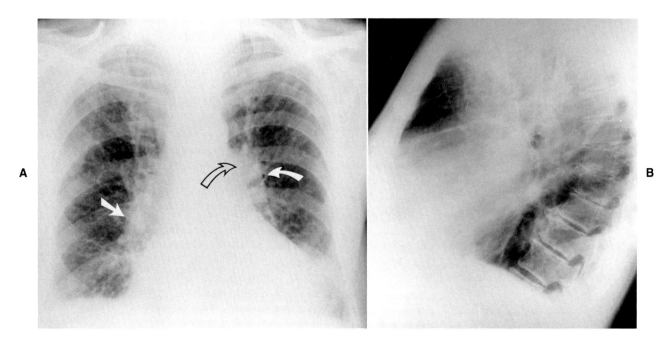

Fig. 9-12 **A,** Radiograph of 65-year-old male, heavy smoker with chronic bronchitis. Tortuous, poorly defined peripheral vessels, increased background pattern, thickened bronchi *(curved white arrow),* enlarged heart with transverse lie, enlarged pulmonary outflow tract *(open arrow)* and central vessels *(straight white arrow),* but no visible increase in lung volume. **B,** Lateral view showing no increase in lung volumes.

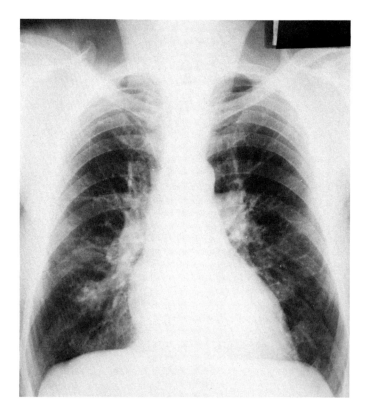

Fig. 9-13 Radiograph of 59-year-old male, heavy smoker with persistent cough and sputum production (oxygen tension [Po$_2$], 51 mm Hg; carbon dioxide tension [Pco$_2$], 50 mm Hg). Radiologically typical chronic bronchitis with pulmonary arterial hypertension; clinically the patient was a typical "blue bloater."

branches; increased interstitial markings, consisting of a coarse reticular arteriolar pattern; and poorly defined nodules caused by fibrosis, lobular atelectasis, or acini filled with mucus. A discrepancy in size also is seen between the arteries, which are unusually large, to a lung region, and the veins draining the same region, which are unusually small, indicating precapillary pulmonary arterial hypertension. These chronic bronchitic patients almost invariably have thickened bronchial walls (Fig. 9-11).[23]

The configuration of the chest and heart in patients with pure or predominant chronic bronchitis differs greatly from that in patients with emphysema. No flattening of the diaphragms and no increase in retrosternal width occur, and the transverse diameter of the chest tends to be wide in contrast with its vertical diameter (Fig. 9-12). The heart is usually enlarged, showing an apex deviated outward and upward, a convex main pulmonary artery associated with pulmonary hypertension, and a somewhat transverse lie in the thorax. The left ventricle also often appears enlarged, and these patients have a marked increase in the incidence of pulmonary edema compared with patients with normal lungs.[24,25]

Radiologic/Physiologic/Clinical Correlation. Patients with all these radiologic findings are usually heavy smokers in their 50s who are overweight and *cyanotic.* This combination of findings and their frequent cardiac failure, with an increase in intravascular and extravascular water, has given rise to the term "blue bloaters."[26] Their main complaint is a productive cough and dyspnea. Recurrent episodes of respiratory infection and right-sided heart failure are the salient clinical features (Fig. 9-13). Because of the patchy atelectasis and mucous accumulation, these patients have a ventilation/perfusion (V/Q) mismatch and are chronically hypoxemic. As a result, they develop pulmonary arterial vasoconstriction and manifest pulmonary arterial hypertension to a much greater degree than patients with emphysema. The poor oxygenation gives the blue appearance, and bloating results from cardiac decompensation, although some suggest that heavier-set patients are initially more likely to develop chronic bronchitis than emphysema. In many of these patients, PFTs show only slightly or moderately increased lung volumes accompanying the obstruction to airflow during expiration.

Pathologically, definite inflammatory changes are

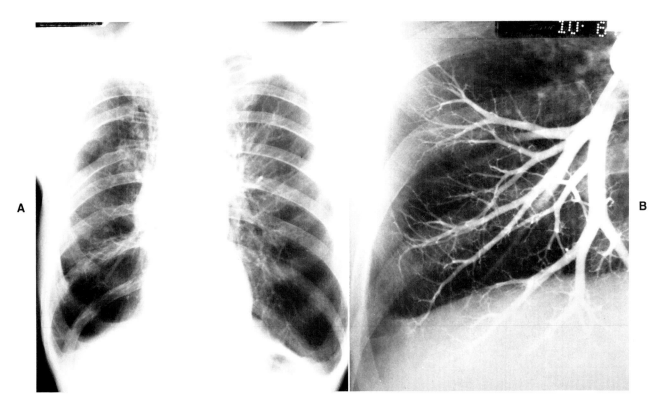

Fig. 9-14 A, Radiograph of 52-year-old male "pink puffer." Marked straightening of all vessels with sharply defined margins and reduction in caliber (besides the large discrepant central vessels), indicating pulmonary arterial hypertension. Complete loss of vessels at the right lung base and in the peripheral one third of the left lung (central sequestration of blood). Previous right upper lobe bullectomy. Classic small vertical heart. Note typical, very thin tissues of chest wall. **B,** Arteriogram performed after inflating a balloon in the right pulmonary artery (balloon arteriogram) shows the gross loss of background vessels, straightening and narrowing of the segmental and subsegmental vessels, and increased branching angles.

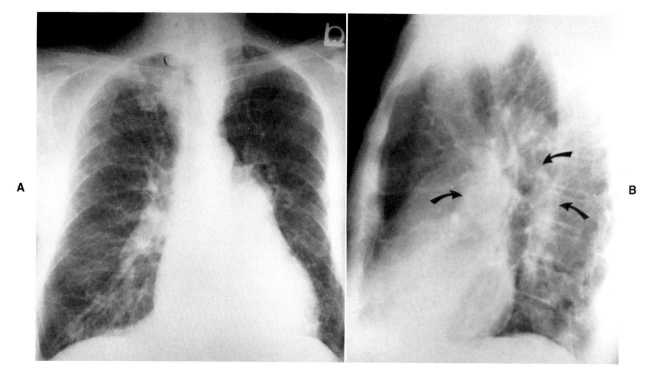

Fig. 9-15 A, Radiograph of 60-year-old male, heavy smoker. The pulmonary vessels are so well filled that they resemble a left-to-right shunt, an appearance sometimes called "increased markings emphysema" (IME). Note, however, that the vessels maintain a slight sinuosity and are *not* sharply demarcated. The background pattern is increased rather than diminished, and vessels are seen well out to the lung's periphery. Despite the large lung volumes, these are the appearances of chronic bronchitis, not emphysema. The enlarged heart and severe pulmonary arterial hypertension are also typical of chronic bronchitis. This patient was a "blue bloater" with predominant chronic bronchitis and only minor emphysema. **B,** Left lateral view of same patient in **A.** Note that the retrosternal space has not increased and the diaphragm is not flattened. The pulmonary arteries show the massive enlargement *(arrows)* of severe pulmonary hypertension, again much more typical of chronic bronchitis than emphysema.

seen in the airways, with a pathognomonic increase in the ratio of the width of the mucous glands to the thickness of the bronchial wall—the Reid index.[27] If emphysema coexists, as it frequently does, it is usually the centrilobular type.[11,14] Centrilobular emphysema in these patients is caused by inflammatory damage to the walls of the respiratory bronchioles, involving adjacent peribronchiolar alveoli.

We have found a very good correlation between the classic radiologic picture of pure or predominant chronic bronchitis and the clinical picture of the "blue bloater." A great contrast exists between all these findings in chronic bronchitis (pulmonary vessels, cardiac configuration, thoracic configuration, diaphragmatic curvature, chest wall thickness) and those seen in pure or predominant emphysema (compare Figs. 9-14 and 9-15).

Emphysema

The criteria for the diagnosis of emphysema include a regional or diffuse progressive loss of vessel tortuosity (vessels appear attenuated), with loss of side branches and unusually sharp definition of the vessel walls (Fig. 9-14). The lungs look "dry," and emphysema patients do have less extravascular lung water than normal, in contrast to patients with chronic bronchitis who have more extravascular lung water than normal. Emphysema causes an increase in branching angles between dichotomous branches and a loss of the background arteriolar pattern, causing the lung to become progressively blacker on the radiograph. This leads to a progressive increase in the lung's peripheral clear zone, which is normally only about 1 cm wide. Sometimes this widening of the peripheral zone may progress so far that all the blood appears to be sequestered in the central third of the lungs (Fig. 9-14).

If the emphysema is *generalized*, lung volumes will increase proportional to the area involved as the lung's elastic recoil progressively reduces and the dynamic compliance diminishes. If the emphysema is *regional*, redistribution of blood flow to *normal* areas with lower vascular resistance will make them appear hyperemic

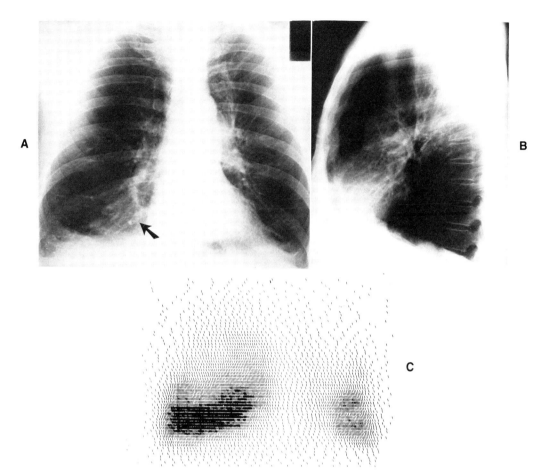

Fig. 9-16   A and **B,** PA and lateral views of a 53-year-old male smoker (50 to 60 cigarettes per day). The films show severe emphysema sparing only portions of the left upper lobe and the right lower lobe. Blood flow has been redistributed into these remaining more normal areas, which are now hyperemic. Note massive draining vein at the right base *(arrow).* Radiologically this is almost pure emphysema, and one would predict that this patient was a "pink puffer." PFTs revealed a forced vital capacity (FVC) of 41% of the predicted value, forced expiratory volume in 1 second (FEV$_1$) of 20%, residual volume (RV) of 289%, functional residual capacity (FRC) of 215%, and RV/total lung capacity ratio (RV/TLC) of 200%. There was no evidence of respiratory infection. Clinically the patient was a pink puffer who had severe dyspnea on minimal effort. Treatment was unsuccessful, and the patient died a few days after this film was taken. **C,** Anteroposterior (AP) radioisotope scan confirms the organic redistribution of blood flow to a portion of the right lower lobe.

and radiodense (Fig. 9-16). This has been described by Milne and Bass[7,24] as "organic redistribution" of blood flow and by Simon[28] as "marker vessels." This is a valuable radiologic sign that draws the observer's attention to the abnormal, more oligemic (lucent) areas from which the blood flow has been redistributed.

All these features give the classic appearance of "pure" emphysema, with large black lungs, flattened diaphragms, and a narrow vertical heart. This is the advanced stage of emphysema, but using the vascular criteria described, one can diagnose it at a much earlier stage, before any diaphragmatic flattening or increase in retrosternal space can be seen.

As we have shown, one often sees radiologically a re-

gional distribution of emphysema (e.g., involving both upper lobes). In such patients, even when the regional destruction is severe, no diaphragmatic flattening will occur and the heart size, usually reduced in emphysema, may be normal (Fig. 9-17). The recognition that emphysematous destruction of the lung is often regional is important for an understanding of the resulting physiologic changes and for the realization that such areas, largely devoid of microcirculation, cannot produce edema. These areas will have a bizarre radiographic appearance when the patient is in heart failure, renal failure, or is overhydrated.[7,24,29,30] This is discussed more fully later.

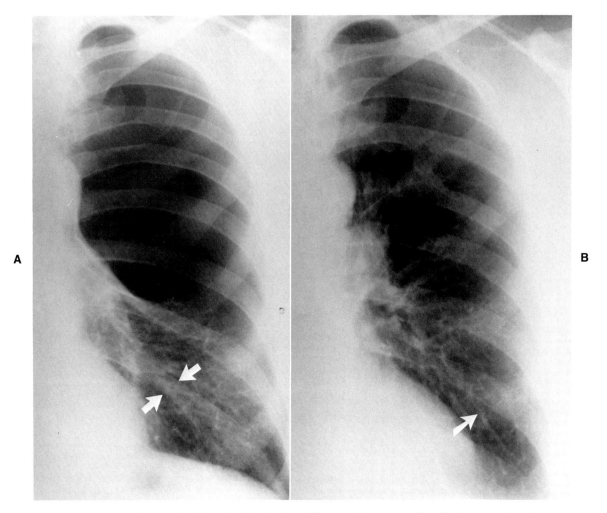

Fig. 9-17 **A,** Massive left apical bullae in a 49-year-old smoker. Despite the severity of the upper lobe emphysema, the diaphragm maintains its normal curvature. Note the large size of the vessels in the normal base *(arrows)*. These are often erroneously referred to as "compressed" vessels, but in fact the normal lung is not compressed; the reduced volume is caused by loss of the negative traction that normally keeps the lung inflated. If the normal lung *were* compressed, it would be very difficult for blood to redistribute into it and for the vessels within it to be large. **B,** Same patient following upper lobe bullectomy. The tractive force of the normal pleural negative pressure has been restored, and the basal lung volume has increased. Organic redistribution of flow no longer is occurring, and vessel size is now normal *(arrow)*.

Radiologic/Physiologic/Clinical Correlation. The typical patient with emphysema is usually thin, and this paucity of chest wall tissues can be seen on the chest radiograph (see Figs. 9-4, 9-5, and 9-14). Because of loss of elastic recoil, the usual inward pull on the chest wall and diaphragm diminishes; the chest wall moves outward, giving the classic "barrel-shaped" chest; and the diaphragm moves downward, causing diminished diaphragmatic excursion (normal, 2.5 to 3.5 cm; with emphysema, 0.5 to 1.5 cm). This same loss of elastic support (diminishing negativity of interstitial pressure) causes both the bronchi and the vessels to narrow. On breathing out, the emphysematous patient's bronchi tend to collapse because of their lack of elastic support.

To prevent this, patients tend to purse their lips and breathe out against the resistance, effectively giving themselves positive end-expiratory pressure and keeping the bronchi open, thus the expression "pink puffer."[26] As a result of the decrease in interstitial pressure and the loss of elastic recoil, the pulmonary vessels become smaller, and their resistance to flow increases. Also, venous return into the thorax diminishes, causing the vascular pedicle to become narrower than normal and the cardiac volume to decrease (see Figs. 9-4, 9-5, and 9-14).

In addition to this functional loss of vascular bed capacity, organic destruction of the alveoli occurs, but because the associated microcirculation is destroyed simultaneously, the V/Q ratio is not reduced. The total quantity of the vascular bed is reduced but may still be sufficient to serve the patient's needs when he or she is at rest, and the skin will remain pink because the patient has no marked hypoxemia. When such patients exert themselves, however, the small area of surviving microvascular bed is insufficient to oxygenate the increased cardiac output, and the patient will very rapidly become severely hypoxemic. Since the required increase in cardiac output cannot be mediated through increased pulmonary blood volume, it must be mediated through *increased speed of flow* through the remaining vascular bed. Very rapid transit times can result, and the transfer of oxygen may become diffusion limited because of the brief time the red cells are exposed to oxygen within the alveoli.

Since such patients develop pulmonary edema only in those areas of microcirculation that remain intact and have no other microcirculatory reserve, they are much more severely affected physiologically by an amount of edema that would be barely noticeable in a patient with normal lungs.[24,30] A further interesting but presently unexplained finding in patients with emphysema is that they frequently have a greatly enlarged aortic knob, despite the small size of the heart.[31]

It is often stated that the heart in patients with emphysema is not really small but simply appears small because the diaphragm is so low.[10,32] This can easily be disproved by calculating cardiac volume from posteroanterior (PA) and lateral views. One finds that the cardiac volume is reduced from the normal, even though it has been shown that the right ventricular wall is often hypertrophied. Also, although the heart's transverse diameter seen on the frontal view *is* diminished, the anteroposterior (AP) diameter seen on the lateral view may be somewhat larger.[5,10,29] Clearly, since the heart is small and the right ventricular wall thick, the right ventricle's internal volume is small and the stroke volume less than normal.

The radiologic differences between "pure" emphysema and "pure" chronic bronchitis are very great and match very well the clinical appearances of the pink puffer and the blue bloater.

"Increased Markings Emphysema"

A variant of COPD has been described in which, although the lung volumes are large, as in emphysema, the pulmonary vessels are also enlarged rather than being narrowed and attenuated.[23] In patients with so-called increased markings emphysema (IME) the enlargement of the vessels may be so great that the chest film has the appearance of a left-to-right shunt (see Fig. 9-15). The cause for this aberration has not yet been fully determined. The pulmonary blood volume undoubtedly is enlarged in these patients, but the vascular pedicle remains small, indicating that no *generalized*

increase occurs in blood volume, even though polycythemia may be present. In most patients with IME the heart is enlarged, unlike in classic emphysema; there is much greater radiologic evidence of pulmonary arterial hypertension than is usually seen in emphysema alone; and they frequently have pulmonary edema. In addition, the vessels have many of the typical characteristics of chronic bronchitis. We believe that these patients with IME principally have *chronic bronchitis* intermixed with emphysema and often with superimposed cardiac decompensation. The term "IME" may therefore be somewhat of a misnomer.

Mixed Emphysema and Chronic Bronchitis

As discussed earlier, mixtures of emphysema and chronic bronchitis are frequently seen, and we believe one can determine radiologically, with reasonable accuracy in each patient, what percentage of each disease is present and how it is distributed regionally (see Figs. 9-5 and 9-8). As already indicated, the regionality of the disease plays a large part in determining its physiologic consequences in that particular patient. The most common distribution of mixed disease that we see is bilateral upper lobe emphysema with bilateral basal chronic bronchitis (Table 9-1). These patients have no diaphragmatic flattening, and the heart is midway between the small vertical heart of patients with pure emphysema and the enlarged transverse heart of those with chronic bronchitis (see Fig. 9-8).

Physiologically, this mixture of diseases has a much greater effect than either separately. For example, if a patient simply has *upper* lobe emphysema, there is no hypoxemia, probably no clinical symptomatology at rest, and little or no pulmonary hypertension. If the patient has only basal chronic bronchitis with normal upper lobes, the basal V/Q mismatch causes regional hypoxemia, resulting in vasoconstriction and increased basal vascular resistance. This causes blood to be redistributed into the normal upper lobe vessels, reducing the hypoxemia and vascular resistance and ameliorating the effects of the basal disease. Because recruitable vessels remain open in the upper lobes, the patient is still able to increase cardiac output on exercise without grossly elevating pulmonary artery pressure. However, when both diseases occur together (i.e., basal chronic bronchitis and apical emphysema), this redistribution from base to apex cannot take place, hypoxemia at rest is greater, and pulmonary arterial hypertension more severe. Also, no vessels are available for recruitment to accommodate the increased cardiac output of exercise, causing a marked reduction in the patient's exercise tolerance.

Asthma

The third major disease under the umbrella of COPD is asthma, which is often believed to cause no

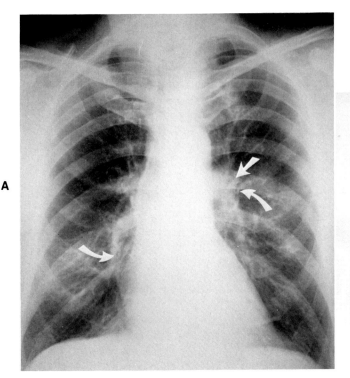

A

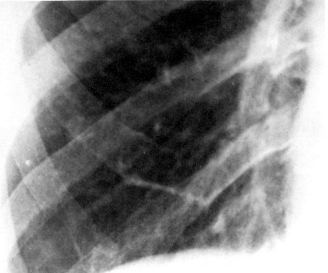

B

Fig. 9-18 **A,** Asthmatic 48-year-old male. Despite the large lung volumes, slight sinuosity of the peripheral vessels persists, and the vessel margins, particularly at the bases, are not sharp, as they would be in emphysema. No loss of background vessels has occurred at the bases; however, both apices do show some loss, suggesting that mild emphysema is developing at the apices. The hila are slightly blurred *(straight arrow),* a common finding in asthma, and some bronchial wall thickening *(curved arrow)* is seen, which never occurs in pure emphysema. Diaphragmatic curvature is maintained, and cardiac size is normal. **B,** Spot view of the base confirms that no loss of background pattern has occurred (i.e., loss of microvasculature) and that the vessel margins are not clear-cut, as they would be in emphysema. **C,** PFTs concur with the clinical and radiologic diagnosis of asthma. Note there is no loss of diffusing capacity, which suggests that the upper lobe emphysema suspected on the chest film, if present, is very minor.

C

SYMBOL	UNIT	MEASURED	% PREDICTED
VC	L	3.74	114
FRC	L	3.48	103
RV	L	2.17	110
TLC	L	5.91	112
RV/TLC	%	36.	99
ME	%	51.	101
$FEV_{0.75} \times 40$	L/min	76.	84
MVV	L/min	99.	103
PFR	L/sec	6.6	78
MMFR	L/sec	1.8	60
TVC (1 sec)	%	56.	
$D_L CO$	mlCO/min/mlHg	14.3	104
CO_{EXT}	%	.35	88

radiologic changes unless complications are present, such as bronchitis, mucous plugging, atelectasis, or pneumonia.[33] However, this very absence of signs in association with the clinical findings can be of considerable value in differentiating the large "black" lungs that sometimes accompany an asthmatic attack from the lungs of patients with emphysema. Although narrowing of the conducting vessels and apparent loss of background microvasculature (a functional loss from high intraalveolar pressure) will occur, the visualized vessels will *not* completely lose their sinuosity and will not increase their branching angles (Fig. 9-18). Also, although in small children with asthma the diaphragms may flatten or even invert during severe bronchospasm, in the adult this is much rarer. Some diaphragmatic curvature usually persists, unlike generalized emphysema, and inspiratory/expiratory films show a diaphragmatic excursion of 2.0 to 2.5 cm, in contrast with the 0.5 to 1.0 cm excursion of patients with emphysema. The vessel margins in a patient with an asthmatic attack are often *more* blurred than normal (Fig. 9-18), particularly in the perihilar region, unlike patients with emphysema, in whom they are unusually sharp. The bronchial walls are *frequently* thickened in asthmatic patients but should never be thickened in those with pure emphysema.[33,34]

Usually, one can make such a distinction easily because the clinical picture is so different in the two patients. However, the clinical distinction becomes much less easy to make in a patient who has both emphysema *and* heart failure or has a mixture of emphysema and chronic bronchitis with associated bronchospasm. In such patients the vessel margins may be blurred by either infection or edema, obscuring the usual sharp margins of emphysema. It may be impossible to be certain whether the patient has asthmatic bronchitis or a mixture of chronic bronchitis and emphysema with superimposed active infection or heart failure (Fig. 9-19).

Left Heart Failure on COPD

From our observations the incidence of heart failure in patients with COPD is very much higher, approximately five times, than in patients with normal lungs.[7,23-25] (Since pulmonary edema is present, this appears to be *left*-sided rather than right-sided heart failure.) Initially, we had reasoned that this higher incidence resulted from several physiologic factors: (1) increased work of breathing using more oxygen and rendering the heart hypoxemic, (2) increased resistance to blood flow through the lungs and diminished blood return to the heart, (3) hypoxemic perfusion of the myocardium from lowered V/Q ratios, and (4) loss of the normal "auxiliary heart" action of the lungs that assists in pumping blood in and out of the lungs.[35] Although these all appear to be viable reasons for the higher incidence of left-sided heart failure (LHF) in COPD patients, a better reason is probably that most are smokers and have damaged their hearts as well as their lungs. It is intriguing to speculate whether this evidence of vascular damage caused by smoking could be extrapolated to explain the large aorta[31] seen in most patients with emphysema. Similarly, it would be interesting to see whether patients who are able to smoke heavily *without* sustaining lung damage have the same "protective" mechanisms preventing them from sustaining *cardiac* damage.

The radiologic importance of this high incidence of pulmonary edema (? LHF) in COPD patients is that one must have a very high index of suspicion for it, since it may be very difficult to detect, particularly in those with chronic bronchitis. In patients with pure emphysema, LHF is a little less difficult to detect, since the vessel margins are usually very sharp and the bronchial walls are normal; but when edema develops, the vessels become blurred and peribronchial cuffing can be seen (Fig. 9-20). In patients with chronic bronchitis, however, the vessel margins are *already* blurred and the bronchial walls are thickened because of mucosal hypertrophy. The superimposed changes of edema may therefore be impossible to detect unless one is fortunate enough to have a previous film for comparison.

Another cause of difficulty in recognizing edema and distinguishing it from infection in patients with COPD is the frequently bizarre distribution of the edema. Edema can only develop where capillary vessels are intact.[7,24,29,30] Wherever regional emphysema occurs, with its accompanying capillary destruction, this area remains free of edema. If the lower lobes only are affected by emphysema, *organic redistribution* of flow to the upper lobes occurs, and all the edema appears in the upper halves of the lungs. Similarly, if only the upper lobes are affected by emphysema, organic redistribution of flow to the lung bases occurs, with increased capillary filling and therefore exaggeration of basal edema (Figs. 9-19 and 9-20). At times one lung may be much more emphysematous than the other, and the superimposed edema is predominantly unilateral. The oligemic lungs of patients with postobstructive bronchiolitis (Swyer-James syndrome) are similarly "protected" from developing edema.

Frequently the patient's deteriorating clinical status is referred to as an "exacerbation" of COPD and is usually attributed to infection, which it often is. A trial of diuretics in such equivocal patients is often very revealing. If the exacerbation was actually caused by edema, the next morning the patient will feel much better, the chest film will show abrupt disappearance of the blood vessel blurring and peribronchial cuffs (Fig. 9-21), and cardiac volume may be reduced. If these changes do not occur, one should strongly presume that the exacerbation did result from infection and not from edema.

Some suggest that the increased extravascular water frequently seen in patients with COPD may not be caused by left-sided heart failure but by elevated right-sided heart pressure causing increased pressure in the bronchial veins.[36] This theory has some logical attraction and has certainly not been disproved. If it is correct, one would expect to see edema distributed in a localized perihilar region (the zone of drainage of the true bronchial veins). However, we have never seen this particular distribution of edema in COPD patients, and the vascular pedicle is not widened as one would expect if right atrial pressure ever elevated.

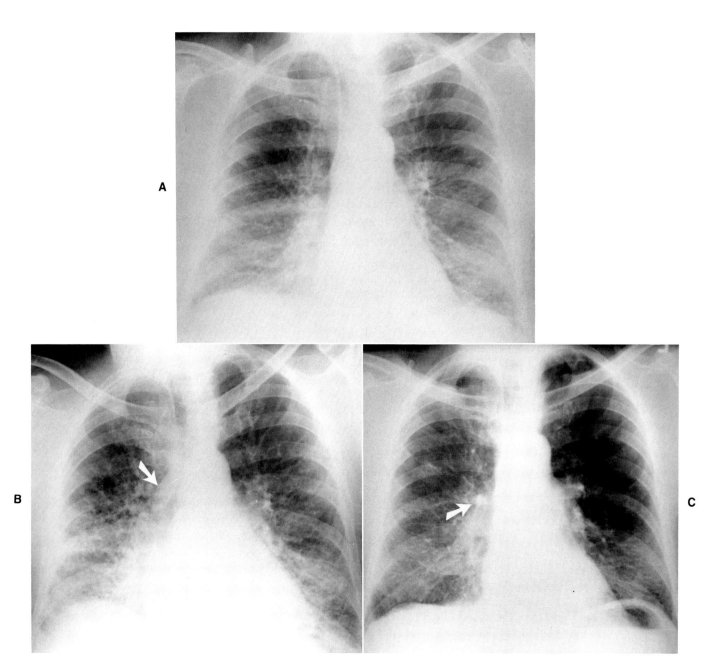

Fig. 9-19   A, Elderly male patient with known chronic bronchitis of many years' duration. Typical appearances of chronic bronchitis and mild pulmonary arterial hypertension. The blurring of lower lobe vessels was thought to be caused by the chronic bronchitis. **B,** Patient was admitted 2 years after the first film **(A),** with increasing severe dyspnea and what was called an "exacerbation of chronic bronchitis." The film was read as showing "progressive fibrosis." Note, however, the increase in cardiac size, the massive increase in size of the azygos vein *(arrow),* and increased pulmonary blood volume, all suggesting cardiac decompensation. The honeycomb appearance is typical of edema superimposed on damaged lung. **C,** After vigorous diuresis the lungs have cleared of the patchy edema (which occurs only where the microvessels are intact). The azygos vein has returned to normal. The treatment for heart failure had a major effect on this patient, who had been previously labeled a "respiratory cripple," and he was able to return to work. Compare films **A** and **C.** Note that in **C,** the film after cardiac treatment, although the bronchial wall thickening persists *(arrow),* the basal vessel margins are now clear, indicating that the thickening is *not* caused by edema but by chronic bronchitis.

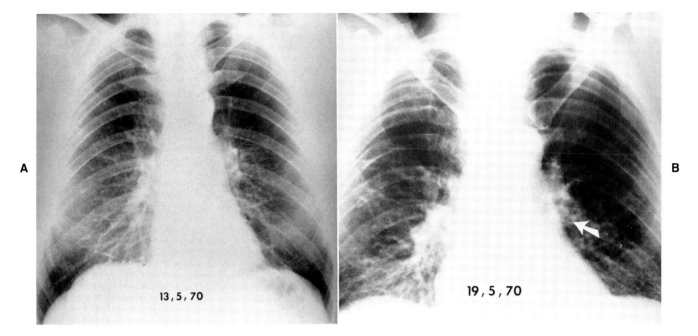

Fig. 9-20   A, Radiograph of 52-year-old male with mild generalized emphysema and slight organic redistribution of flow to the right lung base. In this region the microvasculature is intact, and slight hyperperfusion is seen. Vessel walls show normal definition. The left upper lobe shows the greatest changes of emphysema. **B,** Six days later the patient has become very dyspneic. The film shows marked blurring of the margins of the vessels at the right lung base (edema following the intact microcirculation), some peribronchial cuffing *(arrow),* and reduced lung volume caused by diminished compliance from the edema. However, no edema is seen in the area of greatest emphysematous change, the left upper lobe. After diuresis the radiograph returned to its appearance before cardiac failure, and the patient's dyspnea disappeared. (Film supplied by the late Dr. George Genereux.)

COMPUTED TOMOGRAPHY FOR DIAGNOSIS OF CHRONIC OBSTRUCTIVE PULMONARY DISEASE

Up to this point, we have only discussed the use of *plain* chest films in the diagnosis of COPD. Recently, however, several authors have hypothesized and others have categorically stated that CT is "better" than the plain film for the diagnosis of COPD.[37-43] Interestingly, only two of these articles contain any examples of the plain films on which the diagnosis allegedly could not be made; the authors[37,39] stated that these films were normal or close to normal, but they were clearly abnormal by our vascular criteria.

Many authors appear to have simply *assumed* that CT must be better than the plain film (1) because of the widely disseminated (and we believe erroneous) belief that the plain film can detect only severe COPD and (2) because the better density resolution and lack of overlying lung detail on the CT section compared with the plain film should *theoretically* improve one's ability to see the changes of COPD, specifically those of emphysema and chronic bronchitis. Although this would seem intuitively to be correct, some problems may cause artifacts and loss of useful data on CT scans, including the necessity to take axial views and the problems of correct windowing without a priori knowledge that COPD exists or is suspected. To determine the effects of such variables on CT's ability to detect emphysema and chronic bronchitis, we performed an experimental CT study on a fixed, inflated, blood-containing human lung (Fig. 9-22).

As discussed earlier, we and others have shown that the best criteria for the plain film diagnosis of emphysema and chronic bronchitis are changes in the blood vessels.[5,7,21-23] The criteria used for the CT diagnosis of emphysema and chronic bronchitis are virtually identical to those used for the plain film diagnosis, with the addition on CT of regional changes in attenuation coefficient (lucency) of the lungs.[13] Changes in the vessels are most easily observed when the vessel's whole length is parallel to the plane of cut (e.g., in the midzone) and are unfortunately lost in those CT sections axial to the vessels (e.g., at the apices and bases of the lungs and lobes). In these cranial and caudad sections, vessels appear as dots and ovoids, and an actual *loss* of

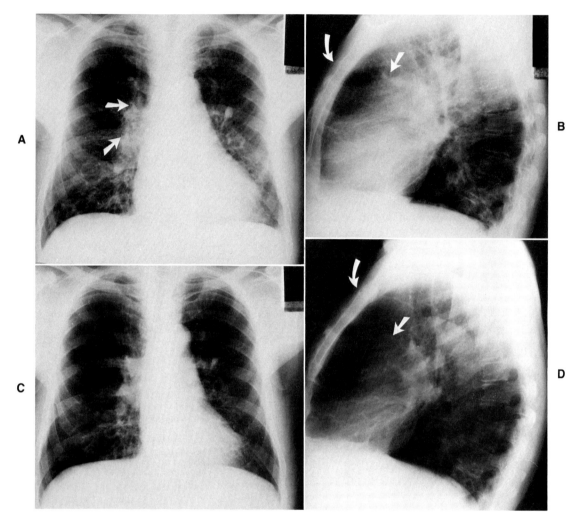

Fig. 9-21   A, Radiograph of 55-year-old male smoker (40 cigarettes daily). On the day of this film the patient had respiratory insufficiency (pH, 7.30; Po_2, 37 mm Hg; Pco_2, 61 mm Hg) and biventricular cardiac failure. His condition was critical. The film demonstrates mixed emphysema and chronic bronchitis with considerable cardiomegaly (biventricular) and severe pulmonary arterial hypertension. Many thickened bronchial walls are seen *(arrows),* but it is impossible at this stage to say whether they are caused by thickened mucosa from chronic bronchitis or peribronchial cuffing from cardiac failure. **B,** Lateral view shows slight blurring of vessel margins, which would not occur in emphysema, suggesting that edema may be present superimposed on the pulmonary disease. Base-to-apex redistribution of blood flow is present, with enlarged upper lobe vessels *(straight arrow).* Compare the soft tissues *(curved arrow)* with film **D. C,** The patient was treated with diuretics, digitalis, bronchodilators, and antibiotics. He lost 5 kg in weight and improved greatly physiologically (pH, 7.38; Po_2, 71 mm Hg; Pco_2, 41 mm Hg). PA film shows marked reduction in cardiac volume and almost complete disappearance of all peribronchial cuffs. **D,** Note change in the soft tissues *(curved arrow).* The increased lucency of this film compared with **B** is not a technical problem but is caused by the removal of large amounts of water from the soft tissues and lungs. This is a common finding in postdiuresis and postdialysis films. Compared with the pretreatment film **(B),** reversal of the redistribution of blood flow is evident *(straight arrow).*

diagnostic information occurs compared with the plain film (Fig. 9-23). Although reducing the thickness of the CT cut improves the visibility of the interstitium, it makes the vascular criteria even more difficult to pick up (Figs. 9-23 and 9-24). Varying window width also introduces artifactual changes in vessel thickness, which further decrease the accuracy of the diagnosis (Fig. 9-25). It is apparent from this experimental study[8] that the gain in diagnostic information from using CT over plain films might not be as great as anticipated. The one new and valuable diagnostic feature that *can* be seen much more easily on CT than on plain films is regional decrease in attenuation.[44]

Miller et al.,[44] in a study of 38 patients, correlated pathology with the CT scan, using both 10.0 and 1.5 mm cuts, and concluded that CT was insensitive in detecting the earliest lesions of emphysema. Similarly, Sider et al.[40] found that although CT was accurate for

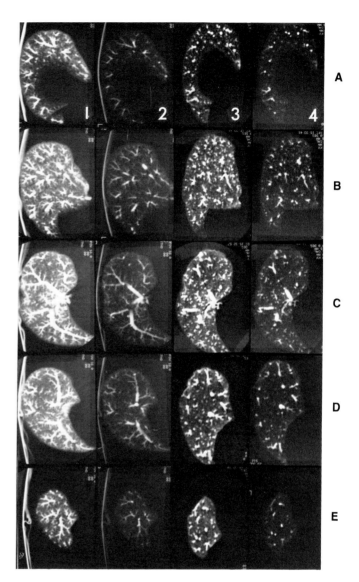

Fig. 9-23 Each of the four vertical columns contains the same five sections of lung from the base *(top row)* to the apex *(bottom row)*. Each transverse column *(A to E)* contains the same slice with different image manipulations. From left to right: *1,* 10.0 mm section, window width 1000; *2,* 10.0 mm section, window width 2000; *3,* 2.0 mm section, window width 1000; *4,* 2.0 mm section, window width 2000. Section *C1* (10.0 mm section, window width 1000) is made parallel to the line of the vessels and provides the greatest amount of information about vessel changes. Changing the window width to 2000 *(C2)* changes the vessel characteristics in a major way, making the vessels appear thinner and more sparse. Reducing the thickness of the section to 2.0 mm *(C3:* 2.0 mm section, window width 1000) reduces the vessels to a constellation of dots. The vascular information content is further reduced by increasing window width to 2000 *(C4).* These changes are even more exaggerated at the base *(a)* and apex *(e).*

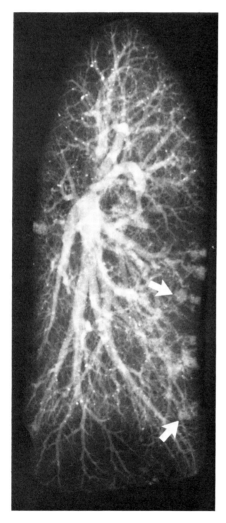

Fig. 9-22 Human lung fixed in inflation. Pulmonary circulation filled with gelatin/blood/barium mixture. Some leakage has provided acinar densities *(arrows).*

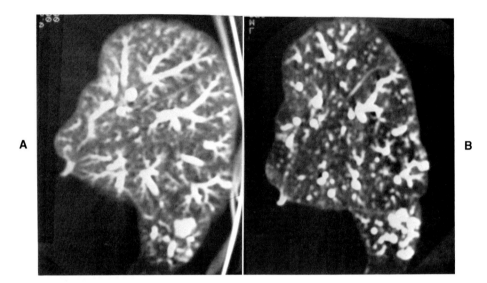

Fig. 9-24 **A,** Slice thickness, 10.0 mm. **B,** Slice thickness, 2.0 mm. Interstitial detail is better seen, but information about vessel sinuosity, number of branches, and branching angles is lost.

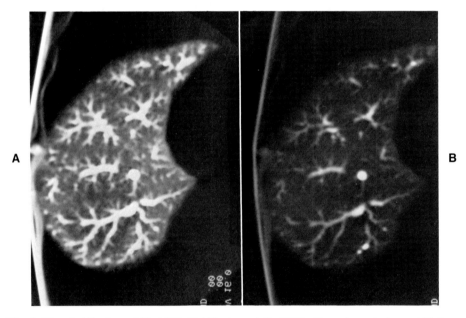

Fig. 9-25 **A,** Window width 1000. **B,** Window width 2000. Changing window width has a major effect on the appearance of the vessels. **A** could be mistaken for chronic bronchitic change and **B** for emphysema.

detecting interstitial disease, it was less successful in detecting or quantifying COPD. Foster et al.[13] believe that even though centrilobular emphysema can be "reliably identified" on CT, panlobular emphysema cannot. Bergin et al.[39] appear to disagree with this view and state that each type of emphysema has specific characteristics that can be recognized. They show an illustrative case of moderately severe panlobular emphysema, comparing the plain chest film to the CT scans, and conclude that the vascular changes are better seen on the CT scan. In our view, however, the changes on the chest film shown are quite evident and much easier to see than those on the CT scan. Goddard et al.[37] found that they could detect emphysema on the CT scan when it could not be seen radiologically. However, we have some problems with accepting the conclusions of their study. Again, the one example the author gives of a plain chest film, described as being "normal apart from hyperinflation," would be read as showing emphysema by our vascular criteria.

We were not satisfied that any of the papers quoted adequately proved that CT was better than the plain film for diagnosing COPD. Therefore we decided to determine for ourselves whether radiologists trained both in the vascular changes of COPD on the plain film and in the interpretation of CT scans could see COPD better on the plain films or on the CT scans. We set up a study in which three radiologists—an experienced specialist in chest radiology, a fellow in chest radiology, and a senior resident who had completed training in

chest radiology and CT—independently read the plain films and CT scans of the same 200 patients. The scans were taken not more than 7 days from the plain films but were not read by the researchers until several months after they had read the plain films. All patient names were obliterated to minimize the risk of recognizing that the CT scans correlated with any particular plain chest film. We used nonselected patients referred for chest CT, listed sequentially in our register, and had no knowledge of the clinical history or diagnosis of these patients until after all the plain films and chest CT scans had been read.

The first part of the study was designed to retest the ability of our criteria to detect and quantify COPD and the second part to determine whether we could do this as well, better, or possibly less well using CT.

To make the reading as objective as possible, each observer used the same reading table (Fig. 9-26), incor-

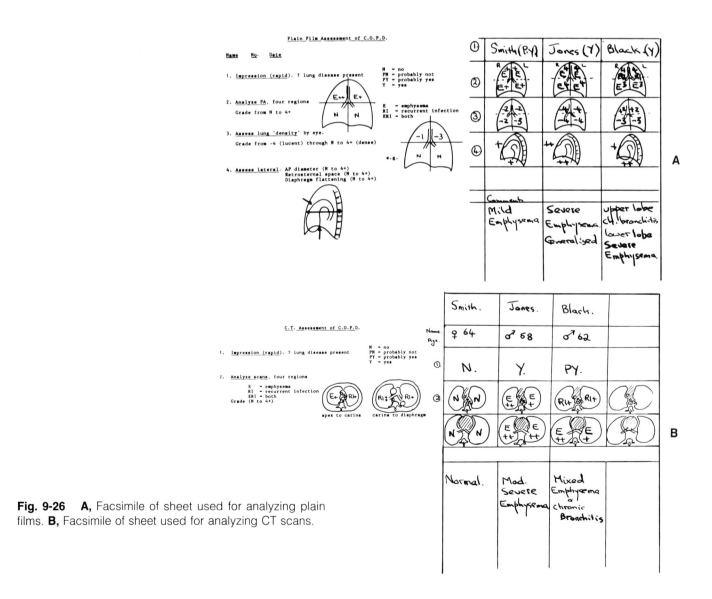

Fig. 9-26 **A,** Facsimile of sheet used for analyzing plain films. **B,** Facsimile of sheet used for analyzing CT scans.

porating our criteria for the diagnosis of both emphysema and chronic bronchitis. On the basis of these criteria, observers were required to state whether emphysema and/or chronic bronchitis was present and if so, in which of four lung areas and to what degree of severity (from normal to 4+). Regional lung lucency was also assessed and graded, as well as the AP depth of the chest, the retrosternal air space, and the diaphragmatic curvature. An identical approach was used for the same four areas of the lung (both upper lung fields, both lower lung fields) on the CT scans. Criteria for the diagnosis of emphysema and chronic bronchitis on the plain films and on the CT scans are given in Fig. 9-11. Criteria for grading severity are given in the following sections.

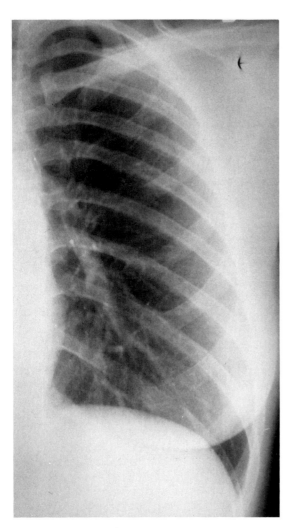

Fig. 9-27   Normal lung (see text).

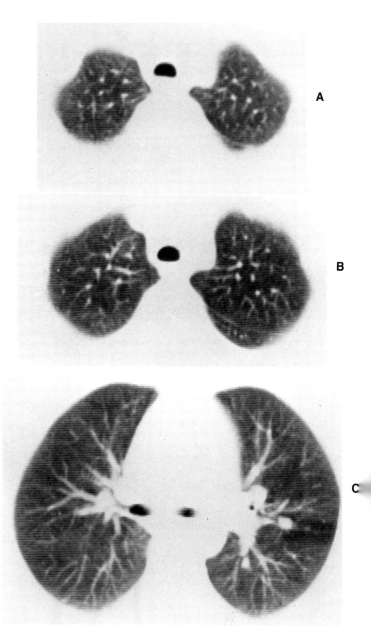

Fig. 9-28   **A** to **C**, Normal CT scans (see text).

Emphysema

Grade N (Normal)

Plain Film (Fig. 9-27). Vessels slightly sinuous in all lung areas. Normal flow distribution. Margins easy to see but not excessively sharp on lobar vessels. Lung background between vessels gray rather than black, with a faint pattern of poorly defined small vessels. Normal acute branching angles.

CT (Fig. 9-28). Vessels well defined down to lobular level, slightly sinuous; not as evident as on plain films. Many side branches with normal acute bifurcation angles. Between vessels, faint background pattern of small microvasculature. Almost homogeneous attenuation, increasing slightly from ventral to dorsal surface.

Grade 1 (Mild)

Plain Film (Fig. 9-29) (compare with normal Fig. 9-27). Early loss of sinuosity of vessels and unusually well-defined vessel margins (seen down to segmental vessels). Background arteriolar pattern less evident, and lung parenchymal lucency increased, giving black rather than gray background. Changes may be general or more often regional. Normal lung volume.

CT (Fig. 9-30). A suggestion of early loss of side branches and some attenuation of larger vessels. Loss of attenuation gradient from ventral to dorsal surfaces.

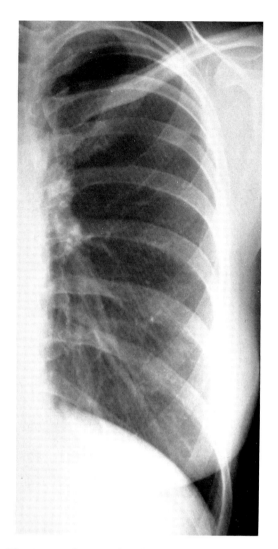

Fig. 9-29   Grade 1 (mild) emphysema (see text).

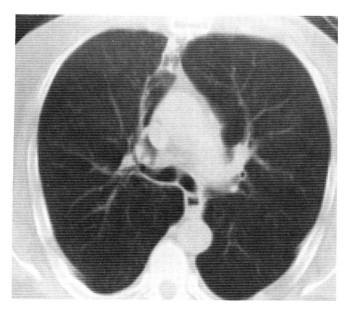

Fig. 9-30   CT scan of grade 1 (mild) emphysema (see text).

Grade 2 (Moderate)

Plain Film (Fig. 9-31). Definite attenuation of pulmonary vessels. Marked increase in sharpness of vessel margins down to subsegmental vessels. Definite pruning with loss of vessel branches. Lucent black background with very little arteriolar pattern remaining. Increasing lung volumes, occasional bulla. Heart size usually below normal. Diaphragm may lose curvature.

CT (Fig. 9-32). Loss of sinuosity with some distortion of normal vessel pathways and loss of side branches. Irregular patchy increase in attenuation with one or more circumscribed lucencies ("black cherry" appearance) per slice. Some branching angles increased. Increased retrosternal space often well shown.

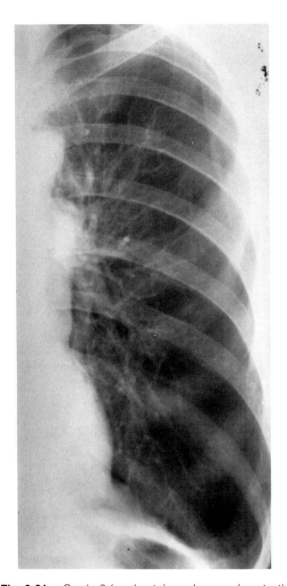

Fig. 9-31   Grade 2 (moderate) emphysema (see text).

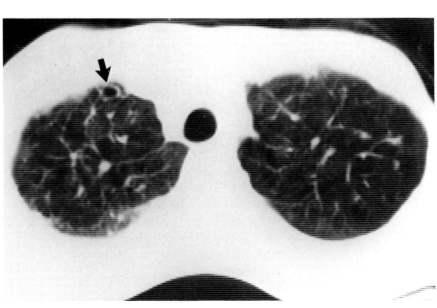

Fig. 9-32   CT scan of grade 2 (moderate) emphysema (see text). Note "black cherry" appearance *(arrow)*.

Grade 3 (Severe)

Plain Film (Fig. 9-33). Extremely attenuated, sharply defined, narrowed vessels with gross loss of background vascular markings causing featureless black lung, bullae, and often complete loss of peripheral lung vessels. If destruction is principally in the upper lobes, as often occurs, diaphragm may not be flattened. Heart usually very small. Soft tissues cachectic. Narrow vascular pedicle.

CT (Fig. 9-34). Very marked, often patchy localized areas of diminished attenuation, often with arcades of vessels curving around the lucent areas. Vessels distorted around bullae.

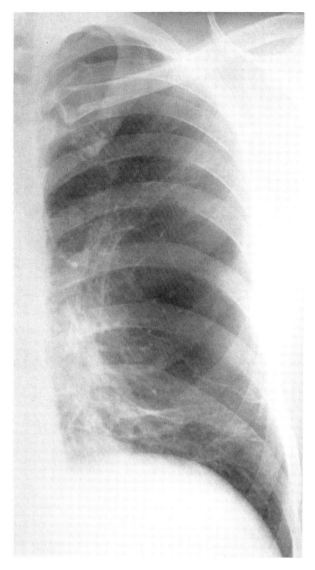

Fig. 9-33   Grade 3 (severe) emphysema (see text).

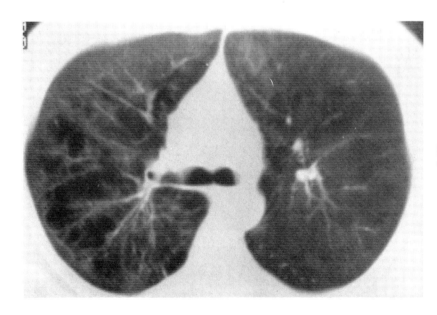

Fig. 9-34   CT scan of grade 3 (severe) emphysema (see text).

Grade 4 (Gross)

Plain Film (Fig. 9-35). Almost complete replacement of normal vessels by black, featureless lung. Multiple bullae, flattened diaphragms, and large retrosternal space. Few remaining vessels in emphysematous areas are very slender and attenuated, but in remaining "normal" areas, organic redistribution of flow causes vessels to be unusually large and crowded together.

CT (Fig. 9-36). Little or no normal attenuation areas remaining. Severe vascular pruning and distorted vessels draped around numerous bullae.

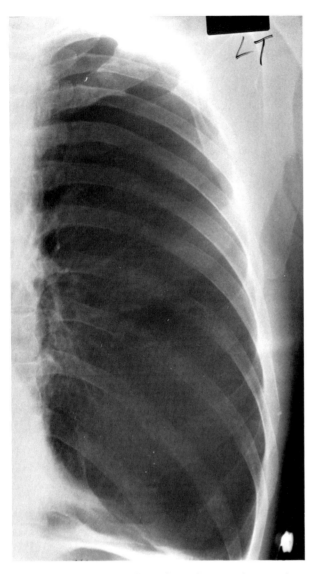

Fig. 9-35   Grade 4 (gross) emphysema (see text).

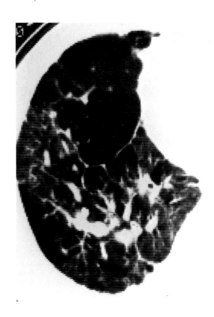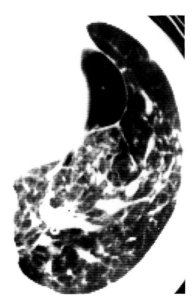

Fig. 9-36   CT scan of grade 4 (gross) emphysema (see text).

Chronic Bronchitis

Grade N (Normal) (Fig. 9-37)

Grade 1 (Mild)

Plain Film (Fig. 9-38). Definite but slight increase in vessel tortuosity with blurred vessel margins. Slight increase in background pattern reticulation and occasional faint, poorly defined nodules. Slight thickening of bronchial walls. Heart size normal to slightly increased.

(CT) (Fig. 9-39). Borderline increase in vessel tortuosity. Slight increase in background markings. Slight thickening of bronchial walls. Normal ventral-to-dorsal attenuation gradient maintained. No increase in lung volume.

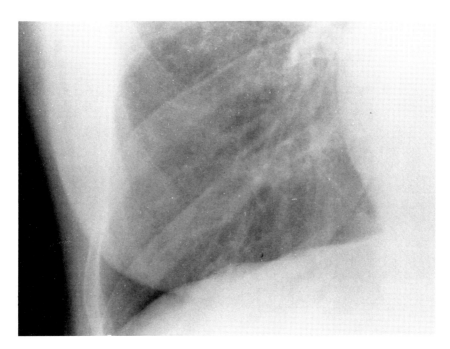

Fig. 9-37   Normal lung parenchyma.

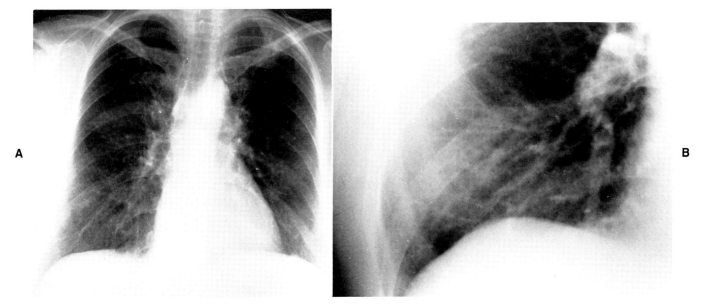

A

B

Fig. 9-38   A, Grade 1 (mild) chronic bronchitic change (see text). **B,** Spot view for better demonstration of lung detail (see text).

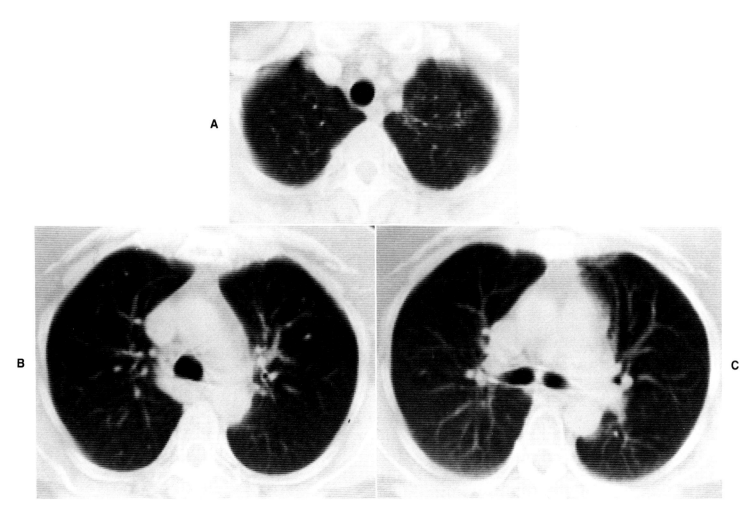

Fig. 9-39 **A** to **C,** CT scans of grade 1 chronic bronchitis (see text).

Grade 2 (Moderate)

Plain Film (Fig. 9-40). Tortuosity of peripheral arteries with blurred margins and increased size of central arteries. Increased background pattern with poorly defined nodules of acinar size. Arteries difficult to follow to the periphery, apparently "segmented." Cardiac size increased with tendency toward transverse orientation of heart. Thickened bronchial walls. No increase in lung volume. Normal diaphragmatic curvature.

CT (Fig. 9-41). Considerable increase in vessel tortuosity with blurring of vessel margins. Thickened bronchi, marked increase in background markings, and poorly defined acinar densities. Interspersed areas of decreased attenuation often present, but ventral-to-dorsal gradient usually maintained.

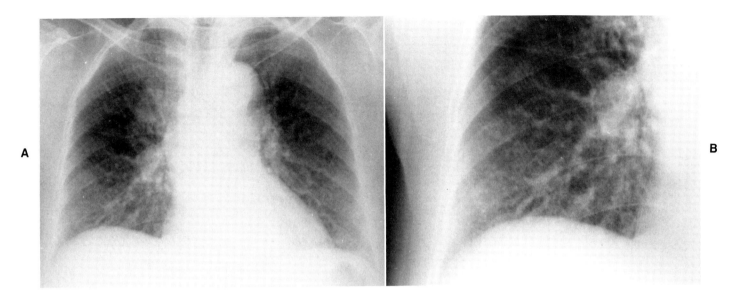

Fig. 9-40   A and **B,** Grade 2 (moderate) chronic bronchitis.

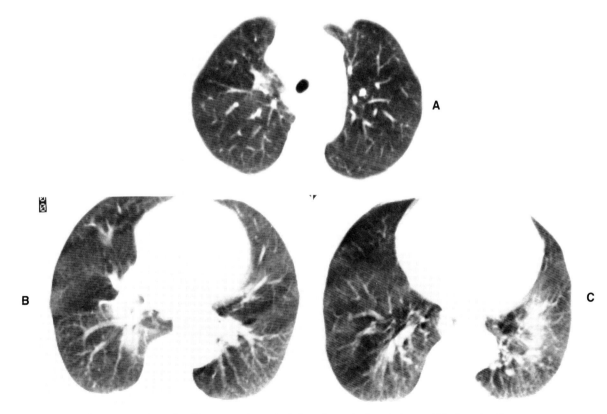

Fig. 9-41   A to **C,** CT scans of grade 2 (moderate) chronic bronchitis (see text).

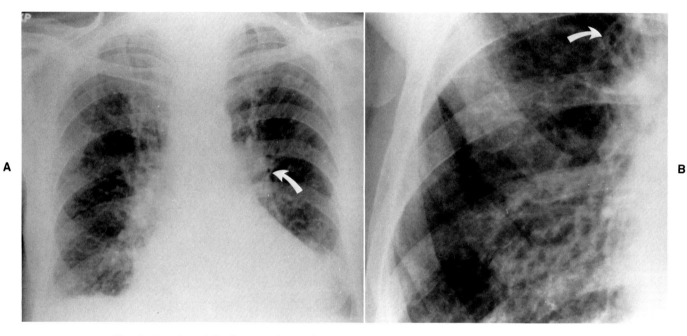

Fig. 9-42 **A** and **B,** Grade 3 (severe) chronic bronchitis (see text). Note on spot view the greatly thickened bronchial walls on frontal view (**A,** *arrow*) and in profile (**B,** "tramlines," *arrow*).

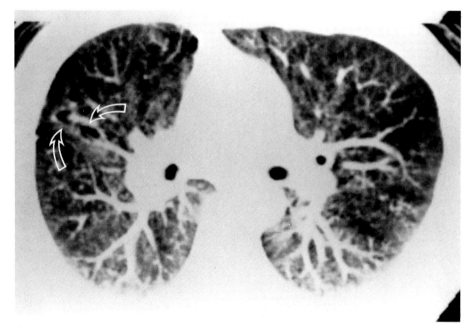

Fig. 9-43 CT scan of grade 3 (severe) chronic bronchitis (see text). Note area of bronchiectasis *(arrows).*

Grade 3 (Severe)

Plain Film (Fig. 9-42). Gross tortuosity and apparent segmentation of peripheral arteries with extremely blurred vessel margins. Impossible to follow vessels from center to periphery. Marked increase in coarse, irregular background pattern. Multiple poorly defined acinar-sized shadows. Extreme bronchial wall thickening. Large comma-shaped central pulmonary arteries and enlarged convex main pulmonary outflow tract. Enlarged heart with evidence of right ventricular enlargement; 1:1 (balanced) blood flow distribution typically seen in pulmonary arterial hypertension secondary to lung disease. Lung volume usually normal. No loss of diaphragmatic curvature.

CT (Fig. 9-43). Tortuous thickened vessels, particularly evident at subsegmental level. Extreme increase in background pattern. Greatly thickened bronchi with bronchiectasis often present. Patchy random loss of attenuation mixed with general increase in attenuation. Ventral-to-dorsal gradient persists.

CLINICAL/FUNCTIONAL GRADING OF CHRONIC OBSTRUCTIVE PULMONARY DISEASE

Using the previous criteria, numeric grades from 0 to 8 were established by combining the severity of the COPD with the number of lung regions involved (see box above).

Correlation of Plain Film and Clinical Findings

In the earlier part of this chapter we discussed the problems of using only PFTs or pathology for the gold standard to establish whether one is correct in radiologic diagnoses. Few of the patients we examined in this series died, and lung pathology was therefore absent, as it would usually be in making the clinical diagnosis of COPD. However, most patients did have PFTs and had a full pulmonary history, which included information on their smoking habits. We elected to correlate the radiographic findings with all three of these features: PFTs, clinical history, and smoking history. We did so on the statistical principles that:

1. Severity of each disease type is not accurately reflected by a single test. In emphysema, for example, clinical findings may be minimal with major changes in PFTs. In chronic bronchitis, on the other hand, PFTs may be only minimally affected, whereas clinical findings may be severe.

2. Any individual standard may be too low or too high because of measurement error or inherent variation, but the likelihood that all three standards could vary simultaneously in the wrong direction is minimal.

The value of using the three different nonradiologic standards is shown in Table 9-2, in which three cases of COPD of *similar* moderate severity—"pure" chronic bronchitis, "pure" emphysema, and mixed emphysema and chronic bronchitis—are compared with PFTs alone, pack-years of smoking alone, clinical findings and history alone, and then with all three combined.

Using the combined criteria, case 1 (chronic bronchitis) is graded 14, case 2 (emphysema) 14, and case 3 (mixed emphysema and chronic bronchitis) 14. This is a correct result. If PFTs alone had been used, case 1 would be graded 2, case 2 graded 6, and case 3 graded

---

NUMERIC GRADING OF COPD FROM RADIOGRAPHS	
No disease	0
Questionable emphysema and/or chronic bronchitis	1
Definite but mild emphysema and/or chronic bronchitis in one or two regions	2
Definite but mild emphysema and/or chronic bronchitis in three or four regions	3
Moderately severe emphysema and/or chronic bronchitis in one or two regions	4
Moderately severe emphysema and/or chronic bronchitis in three or four regions	5
Severe emphysema and/or chronic bronchitis in one region	6
Severe emphysema and/or chronic bronchitis in two regions	7
Severe emphysema and/or chronic bronchitis in three to four regions	8

Table 9-2 Use of three different nonradiologic standards for diagnosis of chronic obstructive pulmonary disease (COPD)

Radiographic grading (moderately severe COPD)	Functional/clinical grading			
	PFTs (including DLco)	Smoking (pack-years)	Clinical history	Combined
Case 1: pure chronic bronchitis	2	6	6	14
Case 2: pure emphysema	6	6	2	14
Case 3: mixed emphysema and chronic bronchitis	4	6	4	14

PFTs, Pulmonary function tests; *DLco*, diffusing lung capacity for carbon monoxide

4. If clinical findings alone had been used, case 1 would be graded 6, case 2 graded 2, and case 3 graded 4. The correlations we have used are clinically realistic, since these are the data usually available on such patients, whereas pulmonary pathology is not. We have been repeatedly impressed by the value of a rigorous, detailed clinical history in these patients.

The clinical grading of each patient was not made until all films had been read so that there could be no inadvertent effect of the clinical grading on the film readers. Each of the three features (PFTs, clinical history, smoking) was graded from 0 to 8 (see boxes below). A maximum score combining all three would therefore be 24.

GRADING SYSTEM FOR SMOKING HISTORY (PACK-YEARS)

Nonsmokers	0
5-10	1
10-20	2
20-30	3
30-40	4
40-50	5
50-60	6
60-70	7
70+	8

GRADING SYSTEM FOR CLINICAL SIGNS AND SYMPTOMS

None	0
Mild cough and/or dyspnea	2
Moderately severe cough and/or dyspnea	4
Severe cough and/or dyspnea	6
Evidence of pulmonary arterial hypertension and/or hypoxemia, add 2 to above	8

GRADING SYSTEM FOR PULMONARY FUNCTION TESTS

No evidence of disease	0
Mild COPD	2
Moderate	4
Severe	6
Very severe	8

As an example, a patient with a 15 to 20 pack-year history, moderate cough, and mild COPD on PFTs would be graded $2 + 4 + 2 = 8$. Note that even if the PFTs had been read as negative, this patient would still have been graded 6 on the basis of his clinical history.

From our reading of the plain films, we again demonstrated, as in our previous work in 1969,[7] that we were able to diagnose COPD and estimate its clinical severity with considerable accuracy (Fig. 9-44). An excellent correlation also existed between our radiographic grading of COPD (emphysema, chronic bronchitis, or mixture of both) and pack-years of smoking. We were unable to detect any changes on the chest film until approximately 20 pack-years had accumulated; thereafter, we found a steeply rising relationship (Fig. 9-45), which began to flatten off at 40 pack-years. That is, between 20 and 40 pack-years, severity of COPD increased to only grade 2 (out of 8), but between 40 and 50 pack-years, it increased to grade 6 and between 50 and 60, to grade 8. This was an in-hospital study of patients who either had or were suspected of having lung disease, and we saw no patients who had normal lungs after 10 pack-years of smoking. In this series a good correlation

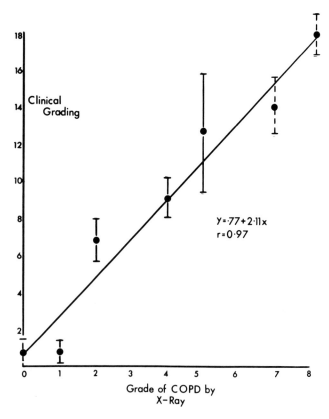

Fig. 9-44 Correlation between radiographic grading of chronic obstructive pulmonary disease (COPD) (emphysema and chronic bronchitis) using the plain film and clinical grading using history, PFTs, and smoking history.

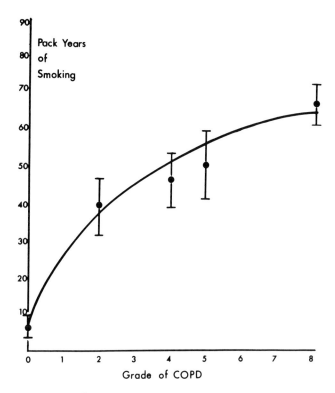

Fig. 9-45 Correlation between radiographic grading of COPD (emphysema and chronic bronchitis) using the plain film and pack-years of smoking.

existed between lung damage and pack-years of smoking, but a general population is likely to include many patients with more than 20 pack-years of smoking who do *not* show radiologic changes. We believe we can conclude, however, that in patients whose smoking *does* damage their lungs, a good correlation is present between the amount of smoking and the amount of damage.

Comparison of Plain Film and Computed Tomographic Findings

The results of our comparison between plain films and CT in diagnosing COPD are shown in Table 9-3 for all three observers. For all observers, sensitivity, specificity, and accuracy were somewhat better using the

plain film than the thick-section CT. However, observer 3 had a much greater sensitivity (without loss of specificity) in reading the CT scans than observers 1 and 2, suggesting that if we had used the services of a true "expert" in chest CT, the results from CT might be better. This seemed a reasonable criticism, so we asked a distinguished colleague, a leader in CT investigation of the lungs, to read the CT scans for us, again with no knowledge of the patient's clinical signs and symptoms. The result was a major increase in sensitivity (96%), but this was unfortunately accompanied by a great decrease in specificity (to 36%). We therefore believe that our readings of the CT scans were correct. Fig. 9-46 illustrates a case typifying the discrepancy between the plain film and CT. Grade 3 (severe) mixed emphysema and chronic bronchitis was read by all three observers on the plain film. The CT scans were read as normal by two observers and as 1+ emphysema by the third. The patient had end-stage oxygen-dependent COPD.

An occasional case was found in which the usual pattern was reversed and the CT showed *more* evidence of COPD than the plain film (Fig. 9-47). This occurred more often when the patient had chronic bronchitic changes. These are very evident on CT scans, particularly when they are exaggerated by window widths of 1000 or less (Fig. 9-48).

As many other authors have documented, interstitial disease that may be virtually undetectable on plain films may be readily shown on CT (Fig. 9-49).

Somewhat ironically, we have decried the use of such features as an enlarged retrosternal space on lateral chest films for diagnosing emphysema on plain films, on the basis that these changes are too late to be useful. On the CT scan, however, we found increased retrosternal space to be a sensitive finding that was often positive when the lung parenchyma on the scan was read as normal. Another feature that is much easier to see on the CT scans than on the plain film is small bullae. These are manifested as well-circumscribed, clear black areas, often marginated by vessels curving around their periphery, standing out clearly against the normal gray background (Fig. 9-50), the "black cherry" appearance. In addition, the visual impact of bullous emphysema is usually much more dramatic on CT scans than

Table 9-3 Plain films versus CT in diagnosis of COPD

| | Observer 1 | | Observer 2 | | Observer 3 | |
	Plain film	CT	Plain film	CT	Plain film	CT
Sensitivity	88%	60%	86%	56%	91%	80%
Specificity	77%	68%	67%	63%	68%	51%
Accuracy	83%	63%	78%	61%	82%	72%

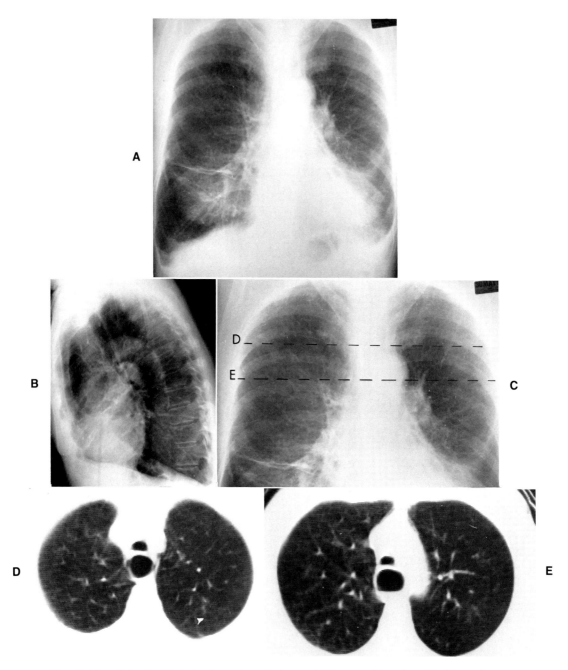

Fig. 9-46 **A** to **C,** PA, lateral, and spot views of 62-year-old male with 60-pack-year smoking history. This was read by all three observers as grade 3 (severe) mixed emphysema and chronic bronchitis. **D** and **E,** CT scans of the same patient (10 mm sections, window width 1200) made within 7 days of the plain film. Read by two observers as normal and by one as 1+ emphysema. The levels of the cuts are indicated on the PA film by dotted lines. This patient had end-stage oxygen-dependent COPD.

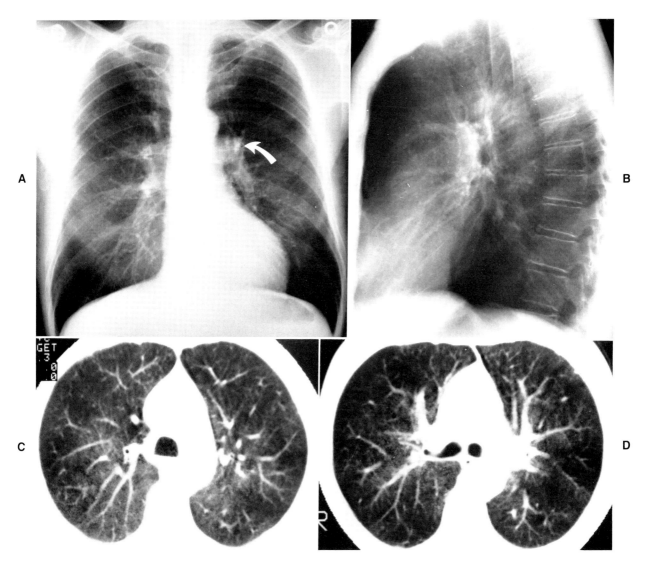

Fig. 9-47 **A** and **B,** PA and lateral views of a 49-year-old male with an 80-pack-year smoking history. All three observers diagnosed moderate generalized emphysema and mild chronic bronchitis on the basis of generalized attenuation of sharply defined vessels and loss of background pattern, as well as bronchial wall thickening *(arrow)* and mild to moderate pulmonary arterial hypertension. The cardiac size is atypical for patients with pure emphysema. The lateral view does reveal an enlarged retrosternal space and some loss of diaphragmatic curvature. **C** and **D,** CT scans (10.0 mm sections, window width 1200) of same patient confirm vascular attenuation and minimal increase in branching angles with some loss of side branches but also reveal more clearly than the plain films the bronchial wall thickening and inflammatory interstitial changes. All three observers read mixed emphysema and chronic bronchitis on these scans, but all three also reversed the order of predominance and diagnosed this as predominantly chronic bronchitis.

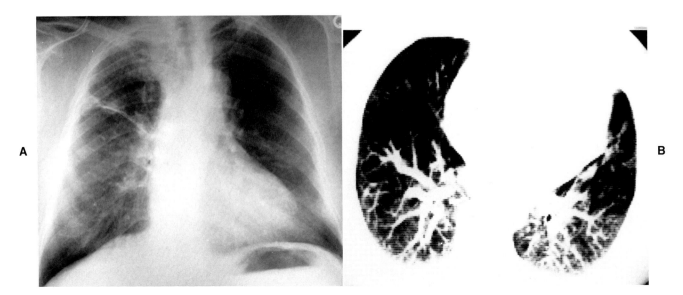

Fig. 9-48 **A,** Radiograph of 60-year-old male with 40-pack-year smoking history. PFTs show FVC of 64% of predicted normal value and FEV_1 of 95%. The plain film was read as showing previous granulomatous disease on the right superimposed on mild chronic bronchitis. No emphysema was diagnosed. **B,** CT scan at a window width of only 500 exaggerates the changes of chronic bronchitis and of the ventral/dorsal gradient.

on plain films. If a bullectomy is planned, a CT scan provides the surgeon with a much better "road map" than conventional films, although not much better than a conventional tomogram. It is particularly important for the surgeon to know that the *nonbullous* portions of the lungs are not affected by emphysema, which would rapidly worsen after bullectomy.[43]

Thick-Section Versus Thin-Section Computed Tomography. Our study used conventional 10 mm thick-section CT scans in patients in whom COPD was *not* being searched for specifically and in whom the optimum window width for displaying the lung parenchyma had not been selected. One might anticipate a somewhat different result if one screened for COPD using optimum window width, with thin section (1.5 mm) cuts and bone algorithm reconstruction. Such a technique demonstrates the texture of the lung parenchyma quite dramatically. Even with this expensive (in terms of dollars and radiation) and time-consuming technique, however, using careful comparisons between the thin-section CT cuts and exactly comparable pathologic sections of the lung, the results for detecting emphysema have not been very good.[44]

One carefully executed study[44] found a correlation coefficient of $r = 0.81$ ($p < 0.001$) between the CT evaluation of emphysema and the pathologic quantification. This appears to be a good correlation but reveals the drawbacks of accepting only correlation coefficients as evidence that the radiologic technique is satisfactory. If instead one examines the data for each patient individually in this study, one finds only 3 of 33 patients in whom the grading of the CT slice and the corresponding pathology slice was the same. In 29 of 31 patients the amount of emphysema was underestimated by the CT scan by a factor of 5. In the 6 patients in whom *no* emphysema was seen on CT, one patient had *severe* and another moderately severe emphysema. Regrettably, this excellent study did not include a comparison of the results of plain film readings in these same patients with the CT scans or pathologic sections. The level of success achieved in diagnosing emphysema with thin-section CT appeared to be little better than we were able to achieve by analyses of the plain chest radiograph, using the vascular criteria we have described.

This thin-section CT study[44] was limited to the diagnosis of emphysema, whereas in our study we were

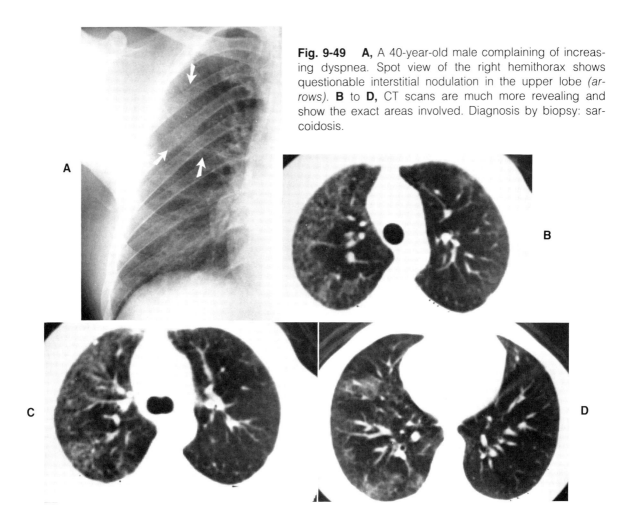

Fig. 9-49 **A,** A 40-year-old male complaining of increasing dyspnea. Spot view of the right hemithorax shows questionable interstitial nodulation in the upper lobe *(arrows).* **B** to **D,** CT scans are much more revealing and show the exact areas involved. Diagnosis by biopsy: sarcoidosis.

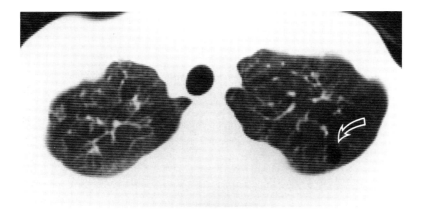

Fig. 9-50 CT scan of patient with moderate emphysema. Attenuation and displacement of vessels, patchy decrease in attenuation, and black cherry appearance *(arrow).*

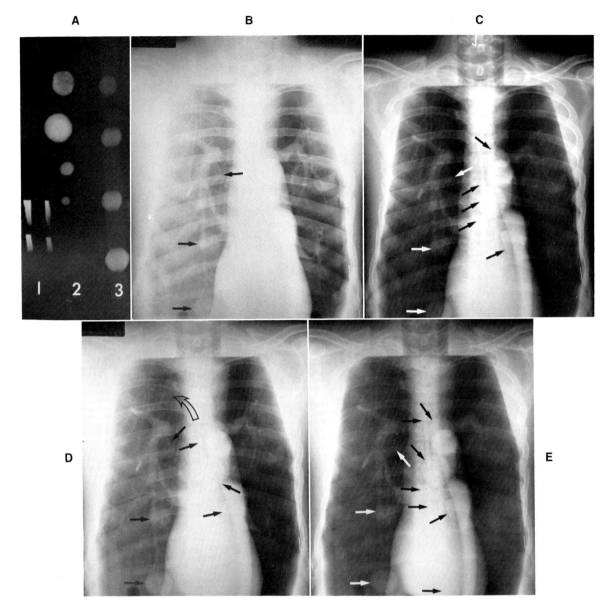

Fig. 9-51   A, Set of imaging tasks. *Vertical row 1:* four bone wedges, 4, 3, 2, and 1 mm thick. *Vertical row 2:* set of four different-sized spheres made of tissue-equivalent plastic containing flecks of bone and calcium. *Vertical row 3:* Four spheres of tissue-equivalent material containing increasing amounts of Hypaque to increase density. All three sets are fastened to a radiolucent backing strip and can be easily inserted into an anthropomorphic phantom containing fixed, inflated, blood-filled lungs and tissue-equivalent heart and mediastinum **(B).** In addition, a "posterior junction line" has been fabricated and 1 cm holes drilled in two vertebral bodies. One has been left empty and the other filled with tissue-equivalent material rendered more opaque by mixing with iodine salts. **B,** Exposure factors, 75 kV and 10 mA. PA film of anthropomorphic phantom with the three sets of imaging tasks in situ. Row 3 overlies the right lung (three nodules faintly visible—black arrows), and rows 1 and 2 overlie the mediastinum. The same screen-film combination and 12:1 grid are used for films **B** to **E.** Right chest wall is thicker than the left, causing the differential density. Vessels of the left lung are ideally displayed. No mediastinal lesions are visible. Three of the four spheres on the right can be seen *(arrows).* Three of 15 lesions are visualized. **C,** Exposure factors, 75 kV (unchanged) and 32 mA.

The difference between the right and left hemithoracic densities is lost. Vessels in the left lung are very poorly seen. Three or four right lung lesions still faintly visible *(white arrows)* and five mediastinal lesions *(black arrows)* seen faintly. Eight of 15 lesions are visualized. **D,** Exposure factors, 120 kV and 3 mA. Density difference between right and left hemithoraces is preserved. Left lung vessels are still poorly seen, but right lung vessels are well seen. Three of four right lung lesions are seen *(arrows),* with questionable visualization of the fourth *(open arrow).* Three mediastinal lesions are seen, but very faintly *(arrows).* Six of 15 lesions visualized. **E,** Exposure factors, 120 kV and 6 mA. Vessels in both lungs are very poorly seen. Three of the four lesions in the right lung can be seen *(white arrows);* the third is very faint. Seven mediastinal lesions are seen *(black arrows).* (Note one lesion at the base, well seen on the film, does not reproduce on this print.) Ten of 15 lesions visualized. For visualizing the lung vessels, in which we are principally interested, to diagnose COPD, the low kilovoltage, low milliampere "window" chest film is clearly the best. In clinical practice, however, this information is invariably sacrificed so that the mediastinum can be seen. The newer techniques of scanning equalization radiography may be the answer to this problem.

considering the early diagnosis of emphysema, chronic bronchitis, and mixed disease. Although we found both thick-section and thin-section CT less valuable than the plain film for the diagnosis of emphysema, this was reversed for the diagnosis of chronic bronchitis and for fine nodular interstitial disease. Early peribronchial inflammatory change, which may be seen only with difficulty on the plain film as faint blurring and thickening of the bronchial walls, in our experience can be very clearly seen on the CT scan, on either 10 mm or 1.5 mm sections (Figs. 9-47 and 9-48).

As a screening procedure for COPD, we do not believe CT has a valuable role to play. For patients with clinical or physiologic deficits (e.g., dyspnea and lowered perfusion capacity) and a negative chest film, however, thin-section CT can reveal the presence of interstitial disease and provide a map of the best areas to biopsy. At present the scan itself, no matter how technically dramatic, still cannot provide a specific diagnosis. One can hope that with further improvements in resolution, such as using fine focal spots and magnification techniques, patterns may be recognized that are so characteristic that a single diagnosis can be offered. Currently the main value of thin-section CT appears to be as a guide for biopsy in patients without COPD. If the scan is completely negative, however, it is not yet clear whether it is justifiable to omit biopsy. Nevertheless, a negative thin-section CT scan in a patient with physiologic abnormalities, particularly reduced diffusion capacity, would suggest that biopsy should be open, not percutaneous.

Improving Effectiveness of Plain Film. When one is attempting to obtain a diagnosis from a thin-section CT, one usually has a priori knowledge that some disease is probably present. One then fine-tunes the technique to the utmost, looking at a range of window widths to "make" the abnormal texture appear. The plain chest radiograph, however, with which CT is so often compared, is usually not tuned at all. If one wanted to abstract the utmost from the plain film, one could do the following:

1. Improve the x-ray beam quality with copper filtration of the tube
2. Use an air-gap technique and 9-foot AFD to remove scatter
3. Employ new generator technology to remove all voltage fluctuations
4. Use a round or square fine focal spot with homogeneous or gaussian distribution of radiation
5. Employ high-resolution film-screen combinations
6. Develop slowly and at lower temperatures
7. Attempt several kilovoltages (as one would try several windows) to show the parenchyma in a patient to maximum advantage (Fig. 9-51)
8. Take inspiration and expiration views to exaggerate air trapping and reveal blebs and bullae
9. Take oblique views to draw the lungs off the spine
10. Return to the dramatic stereoscopic chest radiographs that were common practice 30 to 40 years ago, when the radiologist had more time and could spend almost as long on the plain films as one presently does on a single CT scan

Even with all these radiographic image manipulations, the cost in radiation dose and dollars would still be less than a CT scan.

The plain chest film remains the premier tool for the diagnosis of chest disease and is responsible for approximately 98% of all chest images. Much information can be abstracted from it with the requisite training. Therefore it would be worthwhile for us to institute some of the improvements just suggested. A small gain in our plain film interpretive abilities applied to the millions of chest films taken yearly throughout the world (70 million in the United States alone) would effect a major clinical improvement.

REFERENCES

1. Santolicandro A, Ruschi S, Fornai E, Giuntini C: Imaging of ventilation in chronic obstructive pulmonary disease, *J Thorac Imaging* 1(2):36, 1986.
2. Pratt PC: Role of conventional chest radiography in diagnosis and exclusion of emphysema, *Am J Med* 82:998, 1987.
3. Pratt C: Radiographic appearance of the chest in emphysema, *Invest Radiol* 22:927, 1987.
4. Sutinen S, Christaforidis AJ, Klugh GA, Pratt PC: Roentgenologic criteria for the recognition of non-symptomatic pulmonary emphysema: correlation between roentgenologic findings and pulmonary pathology, *Am Rev Respir Dis* 91:69, 1965.
5. Shanks SC, Kerley P: Emphysema, lung cysts: blebs and bullae, the vanishing lung. In *Chest: a textbook of x-ray diagnosis*, vol. II, Philadelphia, 1962, WB Saunders.
6. Pratt JC, Jutabha O, Klugh GA: Quantitative relationship between structural extent of centrilobular emphysema and postmortem volume and flow characteristics of lungs, *Med Thorac* 22:197, 1965.
7. Milne ENC, Bass H: The roentgenologic diagnosis of early chronic obstructive pulmonary disease, *J Can Assoc Radiol* 20:3, 1969.
8. Milne ENC, Bandler M, Chen Li: The plain film versus CT in the diagnosis of COPD. In *Categorical course on chest radiology*, American Roentgen Ray Society, *AJR*, suppl, 1986, p 143.
9. Burki NK, Krumpelman JL: Correlation of pulmonary function tests with the chest roentgenogram in chronic airways obstruction, *Am Rev Respir Dis* 121:217, 1980.
10. Thurlbeck WM, Simon G: Radiographic appearance of the chest in emphysema, *AJR* 130:429, 1978.
11. Reid L: Chronic obstructive lung diseases. In Fishman AP, editor: *Pulmonary diseases and disorders*, New York, 1980, McGraw-Hill.
12. Simon G: Radiology and emphysema, *Clin Radiol* p 293, 1964.
13. Foster WL, Pratt PC, Roggli VL et al: Centrilobular emphysema: CT-pathologic correlation, *Radiology* 159:27, 1986.
14. Nagai A, West WW, Thurlbeck WM: The National Institutes of

Health intermittent positive-pressure breathing trial: pathologic studies. II. Correlation between morphologic findings, clinical findings and evidence of expiratory air-flow obstruction, *Am Rev Respir Dis* 132:946, 1985.

15. Murray JF. The limitations of pulmonary function testing. In Wilson AF, editor: *Pulmonary function testing: indications and interpretations*, New York, 1985, Grune & Stratton.

16. Ingram RH: Chronic bronchitis, emphysema and airways obstruction.

17. Staub NC: Clinical use of lung water measurements: report of a workshop, *Chest* 90:589, 1986.

18. Sutinen S, Pääkko P, Lohela P, Lahti R: Pattern recognition in radiographs of excised air-inflated human lungs. IV. Emphysema alone and with other common lesions, *Eur J Respir Dis* 62:297, 1981.

19. American Thoracic Society: Statement on definitions and classifications of chronic bronchitis, asthma and pulmonary diseases, *Am Rev Respir Dis* 85:762, 1962.

20. Snider GL, Kleinerman J, Thurlbeck WM, Bengali ZW: The definition of emphysema: report of a National Heart, Lung and Blood Institute, Division of Lung Diseases, workshop, *Am Rev Respir Dis* 132:182-185, 1985.

21. Bates DV, Gordon CA, Paul GI et al: Chronic bronchitis: report on the third and fourth stages of the coordinated study of chronic bronchitis in the Department of Veterans Affairs, Canada Medical Service, *J Can* 22:5, 1966.

22. Fraser RG, Fraser RS, Renner JW et al: The roentgenologic diagnosis of chronic bronchitis: reassessment with emphasis on parahilar bronchi seen end-on, *Radiology* 120:1-9, 1976.

23. Fraser RG, Paré JAP, Paré PD et al: Diseases of the airways. In *Diagnosis of diseases of the chest*, ed 3, vol. III, Philadelphia, 1990, WB Saunders, p 1969.

24. Milne ENC, Bass H: The roentgenological and functional analysis of combined left heart failure and chronic obstructive pulmonary disease, *Invest Radiol* 4:129, 1969.

25. Rao SB, Cohn KE, Eldridge FL, Hancock EW: Left ventricular failure secondary to chronic pulmonary disease, *Am J Med* 45:229, 1968.

26. Burrows B, Fletcher CM, Heard BE et al: The emphysematous and bronchial types of airways obstruction: a clinicopathologic study of patients in London and Chicago, *Lancet* 1:830, 1966.

27. Reid L: Measurement of the bronchial mucous gland layer: a diagnostic yardstick in chronic bronchitis, *Thorax* 15:132, 1960.

28. Simon G: The plain radiograph in relation to lung physiology, *Radiol Clin North Am* 11:3, 1973.

29. Hublitz WF, Shapiro JH: Atypical pulmonary patterns of congestive heart failure in chronic lung disease: the influence of pre-existing disease on the appearance and distribution of pulmonary edema, *Radiology* 93:995, 1969.

30. Milne ENC: Correlation of physiologic findings with chest roentgenology, *Radiol Clin North Am* 11:17, 1973.

31. Nordenström B: Personal communication, 1969.

32. Assman H: *Die Klinische Röntgendiagnostik der Inneren Erkrankungen*, Leipzig, 1929, Verlag Von FCW Vogel.

33. Blair DN, Coppage L, Shaw C: Medical imaging in asthma, *J Thorac Imaging* 1(2):23, 1986.

34. Hungerford GD, Williams HBL, Gandevia B: Bronchial walls in the diagnosis of asthma, *Br J Radiol* 50:783, 1977.

35. Wasson C: *The auxiliary heart*, Springfield, Ill, 1954, Charles C Thomas.

36. Wagner EW, Mitzner W: Interaction of bronchial blood flow, left atrial pressure and lung lymph flow. In Serikov VB, editor: *Book of abstracts of the 31st IUPS Congress*, 1989, Leningrad.

37. Goddard PR, Nicholson EM, Laszlo G, Watt I: Computed tomography in pulmonary emphysema, *Clin Radiol* 33:379, 1982.

38. Carr DH, Pride NB: Computed tomography in pre-operative assessment of bullous emphysema, *Clin Radiol* 35:43, 1984.

39. Bergin CJ, Müller NL, Miller RR: CT in the qualitative assessment of emphysema, *J Thorac Imaging* 1(2):94, 1986.

40. Sider L, Dennis L, Smith LJ, Dunn MM: CT of the lung parenchyma and the pulmonary function test, *Chest* 92:406, 1987.

41. Sanders C, Nath PH, Bailey WC: Detection of emphysema with computed tomography, correlation with pulmonary function tests and chest radiography, *Invest Radiol* 23:262, 1988.

42. Zerhouni EA, Naidich DP, Stitik FP et al: Computed tomography of the pulmonary parenchyma. Part II. Interstitial disease, *J Thorac Imaging* 1(1):54, 1985.

43. Gaensler EA, Jederlinic PJ, FitzGerald MX: Patient work-up for bullectomy, *J Thorac Imaging* 1(2):75, 1986.

44. Miller RA, Müller NL, Vedal S et al: Limitations of computed tomography in the assessment of emphysema, *Am Rev Respir Dis* 139:980, 1989.

10 Intensive Care Unit Radiology

To understand the phenomena one by one as they are written down and explained is not difficult; to think that such understanding can be brought at once into full play in practical work is to underestimate the situation and to fail in the application; a full grasp and working knowledge can be attained only by diligent observation and thought, in which the abnormal is accurately weighed against, and considered with, the normal.[1]

Since we have already discussed in previous chapters how to detect and quantify edema, intravascular and extravascular water, and pulmonary vascular pressure and flow and how to differentiate between edema caused by pressure and that caused by injury, it might seem that there is not enough left to write about to warrant a separate chapter on intensive care unit (ICU) radiology. However, the preceding chapters can be likened to target practice on a shooting range (the general hospital and clinic environment) compared with actually hunting in the forest (the ICU environment). Although learning to hit the target accurately on a shooting range is fundamental, experience in the forest is essential to make a proficient hunter. In the ICU environment, activities can occur with much greater rapidity and complexity than in the general hospital environment. Radiographic images made with portable apparatus and noncooperative patients are inevitably poorer in quality, but the data that must be abstracted from them by the film reader is of even greater value and usually more urgently needed than in the general hospital, clinic, or practice environment. These are the reasons for the inclusion of this chapter on ICU radiology.

It is even more important that the film reader responsible for the ICU have a comprehensive knowledge of cardiac and pulmonary pathophysiology and know precisely what radiologic features must be looked for and evaluated to draw valid physiologic conclusions from the radiograph. We disagree with the frequently expressed view that the principal value of the radiograph in the ICU is to identify such complications as malpositioned intravenous catheters and pacemakers, and we are opposed to the emphasis that some authors place on the "limitations" of the portable ICU chest film.[2] In this chapter we offer a different emphasis: that excellent quantitative data can be obtained from the radiograph and that limitations to the derivation of this objective data from portable films in the ICU are more likely to result from the training of the film reader than from the inadequacy of the film.

In previous chapters we have presented evidence that the data one can derive from chest films are much more objective than is usually recognized. In contrast, at least some of the pressure and flow data derived by *interventional* means may be *less* objective than presently believed. Too much reliance on interventional measurements and the impressiveness of numbers is not new in the world of medicine. In 1928 Sir Thomas Lewis in response to the question, "What is the capacity of the heart for work?" wrote[1]:

Innumerable tests have been and continue to be devised to answer this question; they are based mainly upon pulse and blood pressure readings taken in various circumstances of posture, exercise, etc. One danger of these tests is that, as they are frequently presented by means of formulae, they are apt to create an impression of scientific accuracy that they are far from possessing . . . tending as they often do to become rule of thumb, they likewise become most undesirable.

A similar situation may exist today in many ICUs, with possibly excessive dependency on numbers that can often lead to fallacious deductions, coupled with a deemphasis on the value and objectivity of data revealed by the chest radiograph. In our view the chest radiograph should be viewed not so much as an image but as a complex, integrated physiologic tracing of that patient frozen at a precise instant in time, taken without intervention and with no perturbations of the data introduced by the recording process.

Various reasons offered as "evidence" that sophisticated analysis of ICU films is not possible include (1) that the film reader does not know the patient's exact position (for example, erect, supine, partially erect), (2) that we do not know whether the patient is on mechanical ventilation and, if so, at what pressures, and (3) that the quality of ICU films is often poor because of the need to use relatively low-power portable apparatus, leading to motion blurring and large focal spots, which cause poor spatial resolution.

OBTAINING OPTIMAL QUALITY IMAGES

We would agree completely that not having data about the patient's position and ventilatory status would make it impossible to read the film correctly. Our reaction to this objection is not that we must accept the lack of information and abandon the chest films but that it is *mandatory* for the ICU radiologist to ensure he or she *does* have these data. This is easily achieved by having the radiologic technologist affix to each film an adhesive label that contains all the necessary information[3] (Fig. 10-1). The labels illustrated are only 3 × 1 inches in size, are self-adhesive, and are carried by all technologists. At in-service sessions held every 6 months, a respiratory technologist teaches the radiologic technologists where to find the ventilatory pressure information. The ICU radiologist emphasizes the technologist's role in taking good-quality films and providing the correct data concerning position, technique, and ventilation and how important this is to successful patient treatment. One important element in obtaining good imaging data in the ICU that is often disregarded (possibly because it seems too elementary) is to ensure that the *best* technologists are employed to take these ICU films. If technologists are shown as graphically as possible how important and creative their role is in helping to direct the treatment of these critically ill patients, the quality of the films taken in the

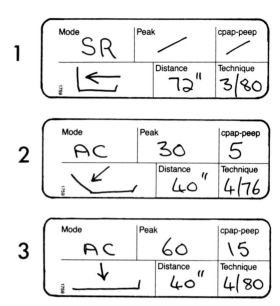

Fig. 10-1 Adhesive labels that are attached to each ICU film. *Mode* indicates type of ventilation. Lower left-hand box is for the technologist to enter a sketch of the patient's position. The arrow indicates the position of the x-ray beam in relation to the patient. Examples *1* to *3* are for the same patient. *1,* The patient is sitting up and breathing spontaneously *(SR).* Tube-to-film distance (TFD), 72 inches; technique, 3 mA at 80 kV. *2,* The mode of ventilation has changed from spontaneous to assist control *(AC)* with peak pressure of 30 cm H_2O and positive end-expiratory pressure (PEEP) of 5 cm H_2O. These are normal physiologic levels indicating that the lung compliance is normal if the lung is expanded to its normal volume. The patient is leaning back, and the x-ray beam is at right angles to the chest (i.e., the beam is no longer horizontal). *3,* Ventilatory pressures have been raised to peak of 60 and PEEP of 15 cm H_2O, indicating a considerable loss of compliance. The radiograph will help to show whether this is caused by changes in the lung, chest wall, abdomen, or all three. The patient is supine and the beam vertical. Technique increased to 80 kV.

ICU setting is typically much better than those usually obtained.

Fig. 10-1 shows that, in addition to knowing the distance of the patient from the film and the degree of erectness, one must know whether the x-ray beam is horizontal, vertical, or somewhere in between. If one does not know this, the ability to diagnose or exclude pneumothoraces and effusions is diminished and the ability to see fluid levels is lost.

With regard to ventilatory pressures, we require that technologists record both peak (or plateau) pressure and positive end-expiratory pressure (PEEP). We virtually never take a chest film on expiration (when PEEP is operating) but always at full inspiration (when peak pressure is operating). As confirmed by published data,[3a,3b] barotrauma is much more likely to result during full inspiration with alveoli dilated by a peak pressure of, for example, 80 cm H_2O than on expiration, with alveoli nondilated and at the much lower level of PEEP (e.g., 10 to 20 cm H_2O). However, since the peak pressure and PEEP are always related, some relationship, although less strong, must also exist between barotrauma and PEEP. Also, if we record the pressure (peak) at which the radiograph is taken, we can compare this with the radiographic lung volume and obtain an instant appreciation of that lung's compliance.

For example, if between films, peak pressure changes from 40 to 80 cm H_2O but *no* change occurs in volume between the film taken at 40 and that taken at 80 cm H_2O, the lung compliance must have diminished greatly by the time the second film was taken (Fig. 10-2). Where there are regional changes in compliance

(very common in patients with adult respiratory distress syndrome [ARDS]), these changes are exaggerated at the point of full lung expansion by peak pressure and are much easier to recognize. At times one whole lung is much more compliant than the other (see Fig. 6-22, *A* to *C*). Under such circumstances, since the gas under pressure travels preferentially to the "good" lung, there is the risk of simultaneous damage to the good lung and inadequate ventilation of the "bad" lung. This highly undesirable situation, when it has been recognized by the film reader and communicated to the clinician, can be greatly improved by using a split endotracheal tube of the Carlens type to ventilate each lung separately at different pressures appropriate to its compliance. Also, the regional distribution of the more compliant portion of the lungs may

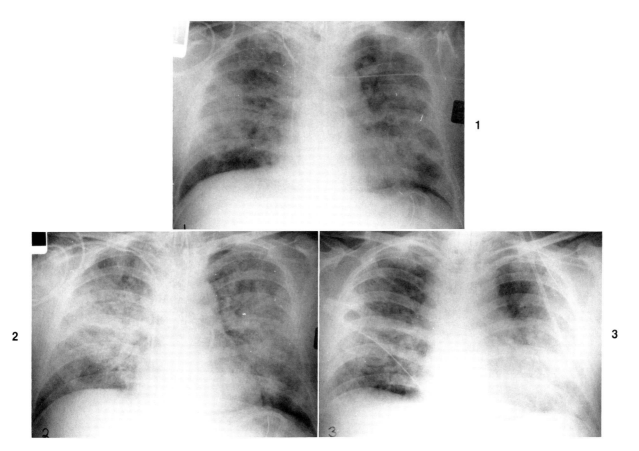

Fig. 10-2 Radiographs of 41-year-old man with head and skeletal injuries and hypotension after motor vehicle accident. **1,** Peak pressure of 40 and PEEP of 10 cm H_2O, indicating a slight loss of compliance. Diagnosis: aspiration pneumonia. The patient is sitting up. **2,** Two days later, very little change in the consolidation and no change in lung volume, but peak pressure now 65 and PEEP 19 cm H_2O, indicating extremely stiff lung. The patient is in the erect position. Diagnosis: adult respiratory distress syndrome (ARDS) secondary to aspiration pneumonia. **3,** Three days after **2.** Peak pressure of 83 and PEEP of 18 cm H_2O, indicating very poor compliance. Diagnosis: severe ARDS initiated by aspiration pneumonia. Note that pure "benign" aspiration pneumonia would have cleared several days before this and would not cause this severe loss of compliance.

be such that repositioning the patient is possible, resulting in perfusion being delivered gravitationally to the "good" lung. This can sometimes improve oxygenation dramatically.[4] We consider later how this knowledge of the lung compliance may also modify the interpretation of wedge pressure data.

A further advantage of instructing radiologic technologists to take the film when the respiratory cycle is at its highest pressure is that they do not have to watch chest wall motion to decide when to "shoot" and virtually never take an "expiratory" film.

"EXPIRATORY" FILMS

Many subtle diagnoses may be missed by radiologists who looked at chest films in which the lung volume is smaller than anticipated for the patient's build and immediately explain the small volume as being caused by expiration or "lack of inspiratory effort." In contrast to the apparently universal belief that expiratory (or at least inadequate inspiratory) films are frequently seen, we believe it is extraordinary how often people breathe in to almost exactly the *same* level (within millimeters) year after year, without being coached on how to take a deep breath.

In a review of 3540 films of 300 faculty and staff members in whom annual chest radiographs were taken over 12 years, we found 120 films (3.4%) that the surveying radiologists agreed could have been called "expiratory." On review, we found that 105 of these smaller lung volumes were caused by intraabdominal changes, including considerable weight gain in 102 patients. Of the remaining 15 patients, 11 had cardiorespiratory problems, including bronchitis with mucous plugging and cardiac decompensation, that decreased their lung volumes. This left only 4 of 3540 films in which no cause for the decreased lung volume could be found, leaving the explanation of "poor inspiratory effort."

One could argue correctly that these data do not apply to ill, uncooperative ICU patients and that films taken in the seated or supine position must show smaller lung volumes because of "poorer inspiration." Radiographic lung volumes in the seated position may be smaller, but the reduction in radiologic lung volume is still not caused by poor inspiratory effort but by changed intraabdominal compliance. If the position of any given patient remains constant (whether erect, seated or supine), the level of the diaphragms should also remain constant on successive films.

Why are patients able to achieve so precisely the same lung volume (diaphragmatic level) every time they inhale? We believe that they normally breathe in to the level of transpulmonary pressure that is comfortable for them. When lung, chest wall, or abdominal abnormalities cause a decrease in compliance (the reciprocal of elasticity), although patients continue to breathe

in to their usual transpulmonary pressure and stop at that "comfortable" point, this point now occurs at a lower lung volume. Therefore the inspiration has been stopped at a lung volume smaller than normal, *not* because the patient made a lesser inspiratory effort (the effort was the same as always), but because of the change in lung compliance. These valuable data concerning compliance are lost to the film reader who constantly attributes low lung volumes to "poor inspiratory effort."

Certain characteristics help to differentiate a true *poor* inspiratory effort with lungs of normal compliance from a *normal* inspiratory effort with lungs of diminished compliance. In a healthy chest, on either mild expiration or "poor inspiration," the blood volume tends to be slightly less than on a full inspiratory film, the vascular pedicle stays unchanged, bronchial wall thickness increases slightly, and the diaphragm is higher than normal in position. However, all these features, apart from the high diaphragms, are difficult to recognize and are much less important than the change in the maximum *width* of the thorax. On a *true* expiratory ("inadequate inspiration") film with a lung of normal compliance, the thoracic diameter is always reduced. On a normal inspiratory effort with a lung of *reduced* compliance, however, although the diaphragm (a very thin muscular sheet) is not strong enough to descend to its usual level because of the lung's increased stiffness, the stronger chest wall muscles *are* still able to expand the thorax to its normal transverse dimension. Therefore, where the lung volumes are small and the diaphragm high because of diminished compliance, the chest's transverse diameter is *not* diminished (Fig. 10-3).

"ENLARGED" HEART

In addition to "the patient has not taken a full breath" phrase, another frequently heard phrase in the ICU is, ". . .well, the heart looks large, but this is an AP film and it is also supine, so I cannot tell you whether the heart is truly enlarged or not." This statement contains at least two assumptions that need examination. The first assumption is that, even if one knows TFD, which one does from the label, one cannot make an appropriate correction for the geometric magnification and state with confidence whether the heart is or is not enlarged. The acceptance by both clinicians and radiologists of the inability to do this seems surprising when you consider that chest films have been read for almost 100 years. Why have radiologists not learned how to do this? The second assumption is that the *supine* position itself affects cardiac size.

Let us examine both these assumptions. We will discuss the effects of geometric magnification and the supine position on cardiothoracic (CT) ratios rather than on cardiac size alone because:

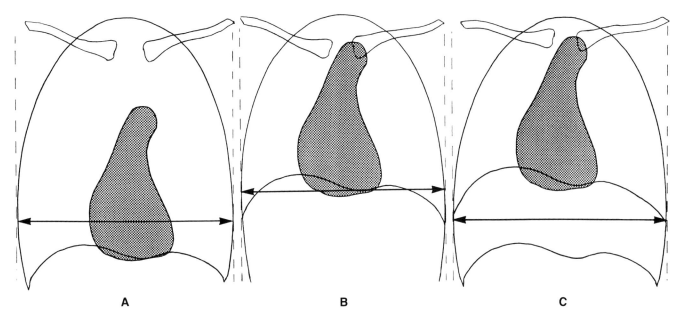

A   **B**   **C**

Fig. 10-3   A, Normal *inspiration.* Note maximum width of thorax *(arrows).* **B,** Normal *ex-piration.* In addition to the elevation of the diaphragm, note that the maximum transverse diameter of the thorax *(arrows)* has decreased. **C,** Normal inspiratory *effort* with a lung of low compliance. Note that the diaphragm is high (as in **B**), but the maximum transverse thoracic diameter *(arrows)* is the same as in a normal inspiratory film (compare with **A**).

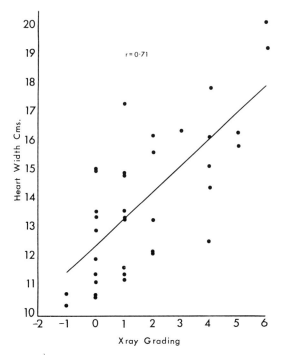

Fig. 10-4   Five radiologists were asked to "grade" cardiac size from −2 (very small) to 6 (grossly enlarged) on 40 films with the thoracic outline blacked out. Correlation coefficient, $r = 0.71$, but note the very wide spread of *true* (measured) sizes corresponding to each estimated grading. For example, at grade 0 (normal) the sizes range from 10.5 to 17.0 cm; therefore, in the absence of "clues" from the patient's chest wall size, film readers are poor at estimating cardiac size.

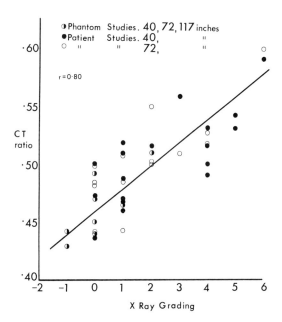

Fig. 10-5   On the same 40 films assessed in Fig. 10-4, the same film readers graded cardiac thoracic (CT) ratio from −2 (extremely reduced) to 0 (normal) to 6 (grossly increased). The correlation coefficient, $r = 0.80$, is improved over Fig. 10-4. More importantly, however, there is much less spread in true (measured) CT ratio at each grading level. For example, the grading of "normal" was associated with a spread of CT ratios from 0.43 to 0.50.

1. Radiologists are somewhat less accurate at assessing cardiac size alone, without reference to the chest's diameter (Fig. 10-4), than they are at assessing CT *ratios* (Fig. 10-5).
2. The different degrees of magnification of the heart versus the thoracic cage can produce unexpected changes in the CT ratio, sometimes even *reducing* it when one would expect the ratio to be increased.

Effects of Radiographic Projection on Cardiac Size

It would seem initially that knowing the TFD, one should be able to calculate magnification and create a nomogram, relating the CT ratio seen on portable 40-inch (or 72-inch) anteroposterior (AP) films to the CT ratio which would have been obtained in the same patient if one had been able to take a 72-inch posteroanterior (PA) film with the patient erect. Unfortunately, several factors make the creation of a satisfactory nomogram impossible.

First, the heart's maximum transverse diameter varies in its distance from the film, depending on the heart's *size*. On an AP film a large heart has its transverse diameter closer to the film than a small heart and actually is magnified *less* than the small heart (Fig. 10-6).

Second, changing from the PA to the AP projection has much more effect on the CT ratio than changing the TFD from 72 to 40 inches (Fig. 10-6). Also, the change that occurs in the CT ratio by altering the TFD from 72 to 40 inches is in opposite directions, depending on whether the projection is PA or AP. That is, changing the TFD from 72 to 40 inches in the *PA* position causes a *reduction* in the CT ratio, whereas changing the TFD from 72 to 40 inches in the *AP* position causes an *increase* in the CT ratio (Fig. 10-7).

Third, changing from the PA to the AP position has a much greater effect on the CT ratio if the heart is small than if it is large (Fig. 10-6).

Fourth, the chest's cross-sectional shape can vary greatly from one individual to another (Figs. 10-8), which directly affects how far the maximum transverse

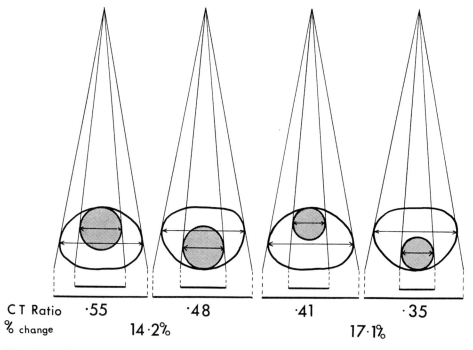

Fig. 10-6 Four diagrams showing (1) a large heart radiographed at 72 inches in anteroposterior (AP) and posteroanterior (PA) projections and (2) a smaller heart also radiographed at 72 inches in AP and PA projections. The transverse diameter (TD) of the large heart on the "normal" projection (72 inches PA) is 16.0 cm and its projected image 20.0 cm, yielding a 25% magnification. The TD of the smaller heart is 12.0 cm and its projected image 16.0 cm, yielding a 33% magnification. Similarly, the larger heart is further from the film in the PA projection than the small heart, and therefore in the AP projection the large heart is magnified slightly more (12.5%) than the small heart (8.3%). The maximum TD of the thorax from the film also varies depending on whether the projection is PA or AP. The change in CT ratio from 72 inches PA to 72 inches AP is 14.2% for the large heart and 17.1% for the small heart.

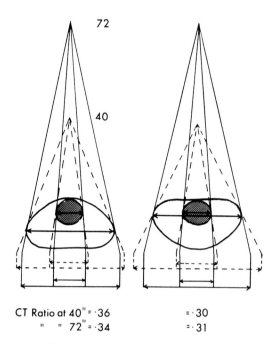

CT Ratio at 40" = ·36   = ·30
 "   " 72" = ·34   = ·31

Fig. 10-7   The first diagram shows the effects of changing TFD from 72 to 40 inches in the PA projection, with the maximum transverse diameter of the thorax in its usual position (see Fig. 10-8, A, B, and C). The CT ratio *reduces* from 0.36 to 0.34. In contrast, if TFD is changed from 72 to 40 inches in the *AP* position, the CT ratio *increases*.

diameter of that chest is from the film. This again affects the relative magnification of the heart versus the thorax and changes the CT ratio (Fig. 10-8).

Using both human patients and anthropomorphic lung phantoms, we found such a wide variation exists in the degree of magnification, even at the same tube-to-patient distance, depending upon the AP diameter of the thorax, the size of the heart, and the location of the maximum diameter of the chest, that it is impossible to predict with any accuracy how much magnification will be present, even when we know the TFD and tube-to-patient distances exactly.[5] We could achieve somewhat greater accuracy by taking lateral films to determine where the heart's maximum transverse diameter lies in relation to the film and the x-ray tube. However, this would be too time-consuming for daily use and still would not tell us where the chest's maximum transverse diameter lies.

We have been able to determine *approximate* correction factors to convert CT ratios measured on portable 40-inch and 72-inch AP films into the "correct" ratios (i.e., those that would have been obtained if the erect patient had a 72-inch PA film taken) (Fig. 10-9). The derived correction factors are, *−12.5%* of the CT ratio for a 40-inch AP film and *−10%* for a 72-inch AP film. For example, if the CT ratio was 0.58 on a 40-inch AP

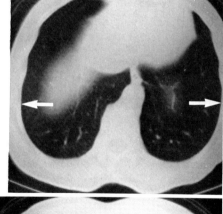

Fig. 10-8   CT scans through the thoraces of three different patients, showing variation in distance of the maximum thoracic diameter (TD) *(arrows),* from the back of the thorax. **A,** Maximum TD dorsally located. **B,** Maximum TD ventrally located. **C,** Maximum TD half-way between ventral and dorsal surfaces.

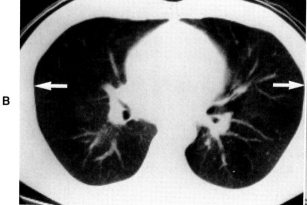

B

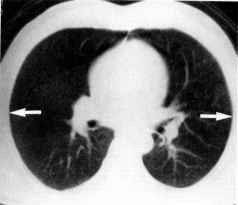

C

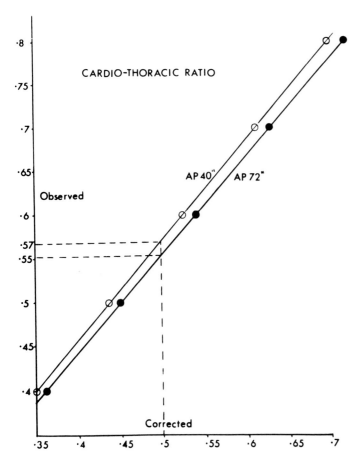

Fig. 10-9 Graph relating observed CT ratio (vertical axis) on an AP film at 40 inches (open circles) and 72 inches (closed circles) to "corrected" CT ratio (that is, as it would be on an erect PA 72-inch film). Note at 40 inches AP a ratio of .57 corrects to a ratio of .5 on a 72-inch PA film, and at 72 inches AP a ratio of .55 corrects to .5 on a 72-inch PA film.

film, it would be corrected to 0.58 (−12.5%) = 0.52 on a 72-inch PA film. The actual mean percentage magnifications found in our research were 13.0% for a 40-inch AP film and 10.5% for the 72-inch AP film. However, amending these figures to 12.5% and 10%, respectively, makes very little difference to the final results while making the mental arithmetic easier, an important point when one reads many portable chest films. Using these factors, corrected CT ratios closely approximate the true CT readings from the 72-inch PA film.

It would be somewhat tedious and time-consuming to have to make a mathematic calculation on each portable film to determine whether the heart is enlarged. However, if we plot the mean enlargement of the CT ratio measured on 40-inch and 72-inch AP films with that measured on 72-inch *PA* films (Fig. 10-9), it becomes clear that a CT ratio of 0.5 on a 72-inch PA film

corresponds to a CT ratio of 0.57 on a 40-inch AP film and 0.55 on a 72-inch AP film. Therefore, if the CT ratio measurement on a portable 40-inch film is 0.57 or less, it will be 0.5 or less (i.e., normal) on a 72-inch PA film. Similarly, a CT ratio of 0.55 or less on a portable 72-inch AP film equals a CT ratio of 0.5 or less (normal) on the 72-inch PA film. *Thus a CT ratio up to 0.57 is normal on a 40-inch portable film, and a CT ratio of 0.55 is normal on a 72-inch portable film.*[5]

These correction factors, although approximate, are clinically valid, rapid, and simple to apply. Applying these average correction factors rarely corrects the magnification of the CT ratio exactly but in our experience rarely causes an enlarged heart to be read as normal.

Since the more powerful portable apparatus now available allows us to shoot all chest films at a 72-inch distance, we had hoped this would remove much of the cardiac magnification problem. However, our experiments with both patients and chest phantoms[5] showed that increasing the distance from 40 to 72 inches on an AP film has only a minor effect on CT ratio (see Fig. 10-6) and that the effect is inconsistent and its magnitude unpredictable. Taking ICU chest films routinely at 72 inches therefore has limited value, particularly since many ICU films must be taken with the patient supine, when it is usually impossible to use a 72-inch TFD. The value of *consistency* for comparison of sequential films in the same patient is greater than the value of taking only some of the films at a 72-inch TFD.

Effects of Patient Position on Cardiac Size

It is widely believed that the heart enlarges when persons assume the supine position because of increased venous return from the lower limbs. The vascular pedicle enlarges and the pulmonary blood volume becomes greater in the supine position,[6] but both these anatomic structures act simply as collecting pools, whereas the heart is a pump and is supposed to deal with an increased preload by pumping out more. Then why *should* the heart enlarge in the supine position?

We have shown that changing from the PA to the AP projection greatly increases the CT ratio, particularly at a 40-inch distance.[5] We wondered if the belief that the heart enlarges in the supine position might be based erroneously on a comparison of 72-inch PA films with 40-inch AP films. Working with Tikhonov at the Leningrad Institute of Radiologic Sciences, we examined 20 normal volunteers and 10 patients with angina and/or questionable cardiac decompensation by taking chest films in the 6-foot lateral and AP *erect* positions and 6-foot lateral and AP *supine* positions.[7] For each position two films were taken, triggered by the electrocardiographic (ECG) tracing in ventricular diastole and ventricular systole. On comparing the erect 6-foot AP and supine 6-foot

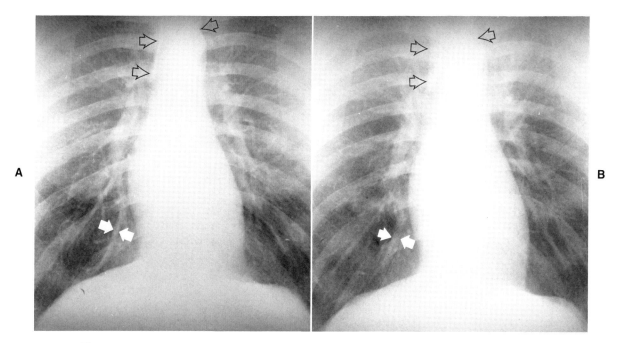

Fig. 10-10   Healthy young volunteer. **A,** Erect 72-inch AP film triggered in systole. Note width of lower lobe vein (white arrows) and vascular pedicle and azygos vein (open arrows). **B,** Supine 72-inch AP film of same volunteer, triggered in systole. Note no change in cardiac size but increase in venous size (white arrows) and in width of the pedicle and azygos vein (open arrows)]

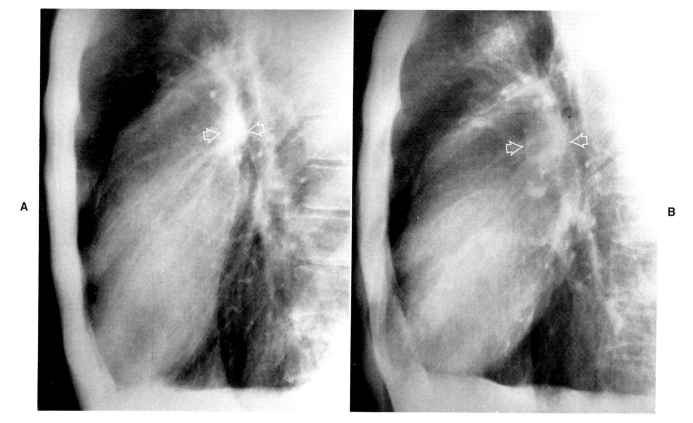

Fig. 10-11   **A,** Same patient in Fig. 10-10. Patient *erect,* 72-inch left lateral film. **B,** Patient *supine,* 72-inch left lateral film. Note increase in AP diameter of the heart and also in the size of the pulmonary vessels *(arrows).* Both films ECG triggered in diastole.

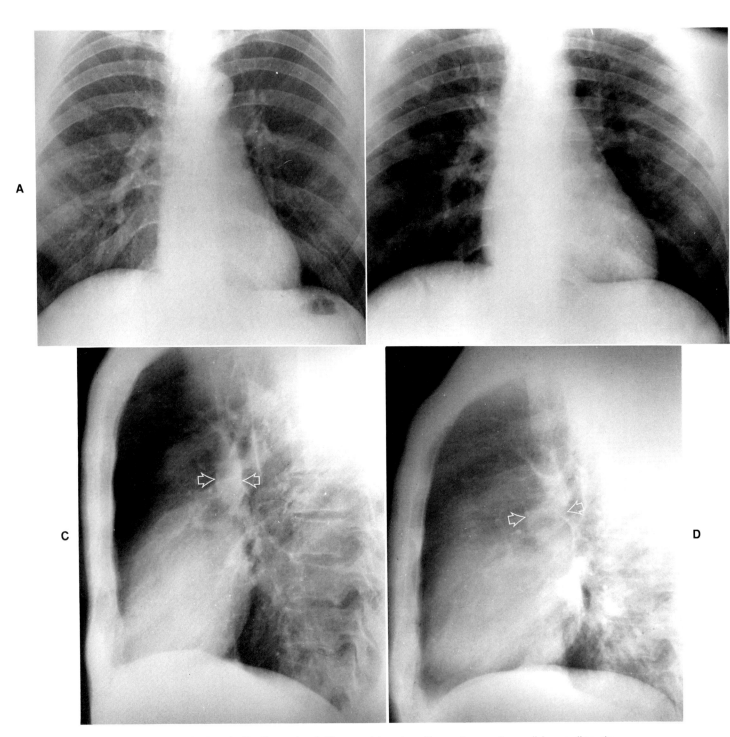

Fig. 10-12 A, Radiograph of 48-year-old male with angina and possible cardiac decompensation, 72-inch AP projection with patient *erect.* **B,** Same patient, 72-inch AP film with patient *supine.* Note increase in the heart's transverse diameter (compare with Fig. 10-10, *A* and *B*). Note also change in flow distribution to a mild degree of inversion. **C,** Same patient, 72-inch left lateral film in *erect* position. **D,** Same patient, 72-inch left lateral film in *supine* position. Note considerable increase in the heart's AP diameter. As with the normal patients (Fig. 10-11), the pulmonary blood volume can be seen to enlarge on the supine film *(arrows).* All films ECG triggered in diastole.

AP films, we found *no* radiologically detectable increase in heart size in the AP supine view of normal heart (Figs. 10-10 and 10-11), but if the heart was unhealthy, the it *does* enlarge (Fig. 10-12, *A* and *B*). Also, the increase in the heart's front-to-back diameter seen in normal subjects on the supine lateral view becomes much greater in abnormal hearts (Fig. 10-12, *C* and *D*). We hypothesize that assuming the supine position could be used as an inexpensive, stress test, but we examined only 30 patients and the hypothesis requires further testing.

Up to the time of performing this study, we had subscribed to the general radiologic view that differences in cardiac volume can be seen in normal erect chest radiographs in the same patient depending on whether the film is exposed while the heart was in ventricular systole or diastole. Much literature states that there *is*

such a difference in cardiac volume, usually quoted as a maximum of 1.5 cm in the normal persons. However, we rarely *see* a difference in cardiac size on successive chest films in the same individual, even though the heart is theoretically alternately larger and smaller. The explanation has been offered that since the heart dwells longer in diastole, the statistical probability of radiographing the heart in diastole rather than in systole is much greater.

When we carefully controlled our triggering of the radiographs so that we knew exactly when the heart was in diastole and in systole, we were initially surprised to find that there was rarely any visually detectable difference in heart size on the frontal film between systole and diastole (Fig. 10-13). To explain this, one must remember that as ventricular volume diminishes

Fig. 10-13   A, Radiograph of 48-year-old male, 72-inch AP supine film triggered in *systole*. Transverse diameter (TD) of heart, 10.3 cm. Note width of right lower lobe artery *(double-ended arrow)* and convexity of main pulmonary artery *(single arrows)*. **B,** Same patient, 72-inch AP supine film triggered in *diastole*. TD of heart, 10.6 cm. Note that width of right lower lobe artery *(double-ended arrow)* is slightly reduced compared with **A,** and that the convexity of the main pulmonary artery *(single arrows)* is also reduced. The difference between the systolic and diastolic phases is very difficult to detect without careful measurements. (Note that **B** is the same as Fig. 10-12, *B*.)

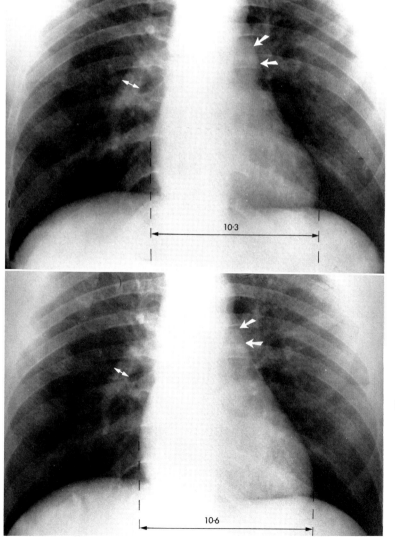

in systole, atrial volume is *increasing* to the same extent. Also, when the ventricular volumes increase in diastole, the atrial volumes are simultaneously diminished by systolic contraction. One therefore would not expect to see much change in cardiac size because of contraction. However, sometimes a change occurs in cardiac diameter on the frontal film, possibly because of rotation during systole or change in left ventricular transverse diameter during isovolumic systole.[8] We also noted a small but constant increase in pulmonary blood volume on the radiograph during each ventricular systolic contraction. This was better seen on the lateral view as an increase in size of the "tache pulmonale" (the right pulmonary artery silhouette seen end-on).

A false radiologic impression that the heart is enlarged can be obtained if for some reason the diaphragms are symmetrically high in position (e.g., because of ascites). Although the heart is not enlarged, when its position is unusually high in the thorax, the eye tends to compare the size of the heart at this level with the transverse diameter of the thorax at the same level, where it is narrower than at the bases, giving the visual "impression" of an increased CT ratio (Fig. 10-14). The heart's transverse diameter should always be compared with the *maximum* transverse diameter of the thorax at whatever level this lies.

Although the previous data may seem somewhat elementary, the film reader must be completely familiar with the effects of position, TFD, and assisted ventilation on lung volumes, cardiac size, and vascular pedicle and azygos vein width. This is particularly true in the ICU, where *all* these factors may be varying simultaneously and normal changes must be distinguished from the effects of the patient's disease process.

Although consistency in positioning the patient (e.g., always erect or always supine, and always with the same TFD) appears to be optimal, sometimes this is impossible to achieve. However, at times the *lack* of consistency can provide additional information. For example, an overpenetrated film with black, unreadable lungs may provide a much better view of mediastinal and retrocardiac pathology (e.g., a paravertebral hematoma extending upward from an injury in the abdomen). Also, an underpenetrated film that shows no mediastinal detail may show the soft tissues much better and exaggerate differences in lung density, perhaps permitting a previously unseen unilateral effusion on a supine film to be detected.

RELIABILITY OF RADIOGRAPHIC DATA

The more the film reader knows about the effects of position, technique, and ventilation on the image, in addition to his or her knowledge of pathophysiology, the "harder" (more objective) the radiologic data will be. An objection frequently raised about the objectivity of data derived from radiologic imaging in the ICU is the nonstandardization of the radiographic technique.[9] However, unlike most other laboratory-derived data, where physicians have no way of knowing how much laboratory error has affected the figures they receive, errors or variations in radiologic technique do not usually *change* the data. The lung volume, vascular pedicle width, soft tissue thickness, and heart size remain the same. Also, perturbations of the imaging technique can usually be easily recognized as such by the reader (e.g., rotation, supine position, underexposure, overexposure) and can then be factored into the radiographic analysis.

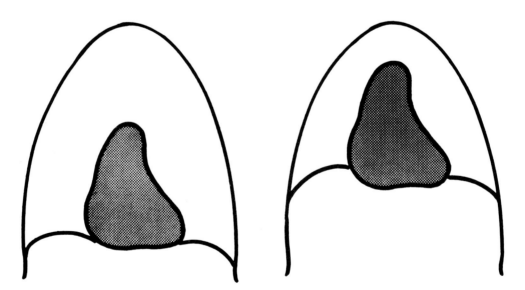

Fig. 10-14   The thoracic dimensions and heart size are identical in both diagrams. The high diaphragm gives the illusion of an increase in cardiac size or CT ratio.

In contrast, with interventionally acquired data, the clinician may be completely unaware that the numbers are wrong because of faulty measurement techniques. For this and other reasons the data may be less "hard" or objective than is generally thought. For example, critical care unit specialists widely recognize that fluid input/output data in the ICU is unreliable. Fortunately, as we have shown in previous chapters, radiologic data concerning intravascular and extravascular volume is reliable and becomes even more so if sequential films are integrated with daily weighing of the patient. Total fluid balance and the ability to recognize what proportions of the fluid are intravascular and extravascular are of considerable diagnostic value in the ICU. From our observations, however, these easily acquired, accurate data about fluid balance, which can be derived nonin-terventionally from changes in the vascular pedicle and soft tissues, are seldom used. This is possibly because the radiologic criteria are not widely known, having been published more in the radiologic literature rather than the intensive care literature.[3,6,10-12]

Our ability to determine left atrial pressure (LAP) also becomes much more objective if we are able to recognize what *type* of edema is present. As stated in other chapters, each type of edema (injury, renal, cardiac) is associated with a different range of LAPs. Before film readers can hope to assess LAP, they first must be able to determine which type of edema is present. Table 10-1 illustrates how the type of edema affects LAP assessment in both pure and complex edemas.

Table 10-1 Radiographic estimation of left atrial pressure (LAP): examples in 5 different patients

Observations	Patient number 1	2	3	4	5
1. Vascular pedicle width	+++	Normal	+++	+	Normal
2. Azygos width	+++	Normal	+++	+	Normal
3. Distribution of flow	Inverted	Normal	Balanced	Balanced	Normal
4. Distribution of edema	Basal	Random	Central	Random	Random
5. Quantity of edema	+++	+++	+++	+++	+++
6. Pulmonary blood volume	+	Normal	++	+	Normal
7. Chronic obstructive pulmonary disease	None	None	None	None	None
8. Peribronchial cuffing	++	None	+	+	++
9. Pleural effusions	+++	None	+	++	+++
10. Septal lines	+	None	None	None	+
11. Air bronchograms	None	Yes ++	None	Yes	++
12. Cardiac size	++	Normal	++	+	Normal
13. Cardiac shape	LV ++	Normal	RV++LV+	R + L normal	Normal

Conclusions	Type of edema				
	Cardiac	Injury	Renal	Injury plus overhydration	Injury plus osmotic
LAP pressure range	10-40	3-10	10-25	10-25	3-10
Assessed pressure for this patient	30 mm Hg	Normal	20 mm Hg	20 mm Hg	Normal

Observations 1 to 13 permit determination of the *type* of edema. Knowing the type of edema, one then knows the associated usual pressure range for that type of edema. The gradation (normal to 4+) of changes allows assessment of LAP. Patients 1, 2, and 3 exhibit uncomplicated cardiac, injury, and renal (overhydration) edema, respectively. In patient 4, to the pattern of injury edema is added peribronchial cuffing and pleural effusions, indicating superimposed hydrostatic edema. Overhydration edema is suggested by the "balanced" flow distribution, widened pedicle, and heart enlarged more to the right than to the left. In patient 5, to the pattern of injury edema is added peribronchial cuffing, septal lines, and pleural effusion, indicating superimposed hydrostatic edema. However, no increase occurs in vascular pedicle width, pulmonary blood volume, or heart size to indicate overhydration and no redistribution of flow or increase in cardiac size to indicate cardiac failure; this suggests that the superimposed edema is probably osmotic in origin. Note that the *quantity* of edema in (5) all five patients is the *same*, but the LAP estimate varies because of the cause of the edema.

LV, Left ventricle; *RV*, right ventricle; *L* and *R*, left and right sides of heart.

RADIOLOGIC VERSUS INTERVENTIONAL DATA

We have already covered in detail the radiologic methodologies for detecting and quantifying edema, deciding whether it is caused by pressure or injury, and quantifying arterial and venous pressures. Now we must examine how these noninterventional assessments may be integrated with interventionally derived data, especially data derived from Swan-Ganz catheterization, and what reliance the referring clinician should put on the radiologic data versus catheter data.

In the box below, we have attempted to provide "reliability indices" for all the physiologic data we are able to abstract noninterventionally from the chest radiograph.

It is just as important for the radiologist to know how much reliance he or she can place on the *interventional* data as it is for the referring clinician to know how "hard" (or otherwise) the radiologic data are. When discrepancies arise, as they frequently do, it is essential to the patient that the clinician and radiologist integrate their information and decide from this integrated data, rather than from the interventional data alone, which data are correct.

In previous chapters we have supplied clinical and experimental evidence concerning the accuracy of noninterventional radiologic determination of pressures, flows, and volumes and accuracy of the differentiation of pressure versus injury edema. We should now consider the reliability of data acquired by interventional monitoring of these same parameters and particularly by the use of the Swan-Ganz catheter.

Data from Swan-Ganz catheterization are widely regarded as being valid and objective. However, many authors have reexamined this reliability in regard to both the methodology of acquiring the data and the conclusions derived from the data and have frequently found both to be "wanting."[13-18a] Sources of errors in collecting Swan-Ganz catheterization data include:

1. Dampened tracings
2. Poor dynamic response
3. Overinflation of the balloon
4. Spontaneous variation in wedge pressure at end expiration
5. Intermediate waveforms
6. Air bubbles, clots, or kinks in the catheter
7. Positioning the catheter in zones 1 or 2
8. Inaccurate calibration of the pressure transducer
9. Using "mean" digital readout instead of the actual tracing
10. Inadequate excursion of the tracing
11. Permanent wedging of the catheter
12. Eccentrically inflated balloon
13. Catheter tip against the wall
14. Unfamiliarity of ICU staff with the technology

In 286 pulmonary wedge pressure (WP) measurements, Morris et al.[17] found 93 with initial technical problems. They calculated the probability of a measurement error equal to or greater than 4 mm Hg as being 33% for these 93 measurements with technical problems and 14% for the entire set of WP measurement attempts. Brandstetter and Gitler[15] note that, despite 2 million catheters having been inserted at a cost of more

---

RELIABILITY INDICES OF RADIOLOGIC EVALUATIONS IN THE ICU

Excellent
Detect pulmonary edema.
Quantify edema.
Differentiate pure pressure and injury edema.
Assess changes in intravascular volume.
Assess pulmonary blood flow (regional).
Detect soft tissue emphysema.
Detect pneumomediastinum.
Assess cardiac volume.
Detect and quantify pulmonary emphysema.
Assess state of hydration.

Very good
Assess change in extravascular volume.
Assess global pulmonary blood flow.
Quantify pulmonary blood volume.
Assess pulmonary artery pressure.
Assess pulmonary venous pressure.
Detect pleural effusions.
Detect pneumothorax.
Quantify pneumothorax.
Diagnose and quantify chronic bronchitis.

Good
Quantify pleural effusions.
Differentiate etiologies of compound edemas.
Assess lung compliance.
Assess cardiac output (except in septic shock).
Detect ascites.
Assess individual cardiac chamber size.
Assess systemic/pulmonary shunt ratios.
Differentiate consolidation from atelectasis.
Differentiate aspiration from infection.

Fair
Differentiate cardiac from renal or overhydration edema.
Assess pulmonary vascular resistance.
Differentiate blood from water in the lung.
Differentiate infection from mucus.
Detect pulmonary interstitial emphysema.
Detect left-sided heart failure in chronic obstructive pulmonary disease.

Poor to useless
Assess cardiac output in septic shock.
Detect and assess size of pericardial effusion.

than $2 billion, amazingly there have been no controlled clinical trials examining the effects that the pulmonary artery catheter has on the patient's status. The technique has not been proven to improve survival rates but has been associated with much morbidity and many deaths,[15] some of which have resulted from the procedure and others from erroneous therapy based on the catheter results.[13,18] Some of these latter deaths might have been prevented if the proper attention had been given to the chest radiograph.[18]

Errors in Interpreting Swan-Ganz Data

In expert hands, if close attention is paid to how the catheter is inserted and to the tip's correct final position, correct calibration, and so on, errors in the actual collection of data diminish. However, even when the data are free from technical error, problems exist with the interpretation of these data.[14]

The Swan-Ganz catheter is generally thought to provide a reliable assessment of left ventricular preload. However, Roper and Sibbald[14] note that assessing left ventricular end-diastolic volume (LVEDV) from the measured WP carries several assumptions: (1) WP must be accurately measured, (2) WP must reflect LAP, (3) LAP must reflect the left ventricular end-diastolic pressure (LVEDP), and (4) LVEDP must relate directly to LVEDV.[14] In clinical practice, errors may be encountered at each step of this progression, thus invalidating the primary inference. WP may not adequately reflect LVEDP, and LVEDP in turn may be unrelated to LVEDV.[18] In addition to the *technical* problems in acquiring data listed earlier, several other problems may make it difficult to *interpret* the data (e.g., to estimate LVEDP from the acquired WP). These problems include:

1. Pulmonary venous obstruction
2. Valvular heart disease
3. Increased pericardial pressure
4. Altered left ventricular compliance

Integrating Swan-Ganz Data and Radiologic Data

Of particular importance to the film reader is the effect of high ventilatory pressure (correlation between WP and LVEDP is lost at high levels of PEEP) and failure to place the catheter tip in zone 3. The usual result of these perturbations is a falsely *high* WP reading. A result of this may be that the film reader's diagnosis of injury lung edema (ARDS) may be ignored because the WP is "too high" to be compatible with this diagnosis, in which LAP should not be elevated. If it is assumed, on the basis of the false WP, that LAP is elevated because of heart failure, overhydration, or renal failure, the patient will usually receive diuresis or dialysis, which can have fatal results[13-18] (Fig. 10-15).

Because of technical faults, it is equally possible for the WP to be falsely low. For example, the radiologist may read the film as showing flow inversion, gravitational distribution of edema, cuffing, and septal lines and conclude that the patient has severe cardiac failure. Reliance on the Swan-Ganz data, indicating a low WP, may lead the clinician to reject this diagnosis and conclude that the patient's edema is caused by *injury*. The patient may therefore be overhydrated, possibly to death. This "drowning in bed" is probably not rare[18] (Fig. 10-16).

These are both instances in which the radiologic data are *hard*; the ability to distinguish between pure injury and pure hydrostatic edema has been proved to be excellent (see box on p. 324), and the radiologic data therefore should not be immediately dismissed. At the very least, when such a discrepancy between the Swan-Ganz data and the radiographic data arises, all the technical factors that might have led to an erroneous Swan-Ganz reading should immediately be checked. This will frequently remove the discrepancy. In particular, a visual (radiographic) determination of the position of the catheter tip should be made. Regrettably, this is done infrequently.

Many authors believe that radiography is unnecessary because the pressure tracing is said to give accurate information about catheter placement. Unfortunately, this is often not true.[16] Over the last 17 years, whenever we have found a Swan-Ganz catheter in a bizarre position, we have made it a practice to phone the ICU immediately. We do not say that the catheter is misplaced but simply ask, "Can you tell us the wedge pressure?" To date we have done this 24 times, and the WP has always been quoted to us confidently, occasionally to two decimal points! These quotes have been given with catheters ranging in position from impaction in the liver to lying free in the pleural space (Fig. 10-17). Despite a universal emphasis on the need to place the catheter tip in zone 3, only one author of the many we have quoted advocates using a lateral radiograph to ensure this.[14] In most publications, radiology is regrettably totally ignored, not simply for catheter positioning but also for all the other valuable physiologic data it can provide.

With current high-power maneuverable portable machines, taking lateral views in the ICU is not particularly difficult. The film quality, except in extremely obese patients, should be more than adequate to indicate where the catheter tip lies. This information is so vital to the patient that any technologic objection that it is too "difficult" to do *cannot* be accepted.

In addition to improving the accuracy of acquiring Swan-Ganz data, the chest radiograph can also assist in solving the problems of data interpretation listed earlier:

1. *Pulmonary venous obstruction.* The radiologic di-

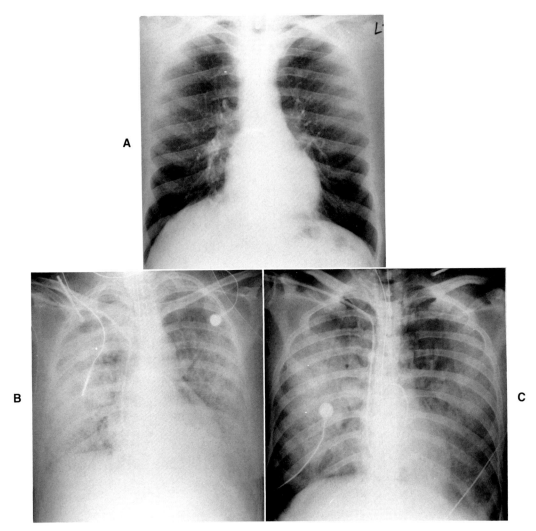

Fig. 10-15 **A,** Film made before development of present illness in 33-year-old male. **B,** Same patient in septic shock showing severe lung edema caused by injury. Peak pressure, 72 cm H$_2$O; PEEP, 18 cm H$_2$O. Wedge pressure (WP) read as 30 mm Hg. The classic radiologic appearance of injury lung edema was ignored, and the patient received *diuresis* on the basis of the Swan-Ganz reading. **C,** Same patient immediately after diuresis. Peak pressure, 100 cm H$_2$O; PEEP, 20 cm H$_2$O. Making allowance for the effects of the very high peak pressure, which caused the lung's periphery to become lucent, edema is not reduced. Note, however, the reduction in vascular pedicle width and cardiac volume (i.e., reduced circulating blood volume). The patient became severely hypotensive but survived after vigorous resuscitation, including fluid replacement.

agnosis of lung edema caused by injury is usually synonymous in the ICU with a diagnosis of ARDS. In the presence of this radiologic diagnosis, which we have shown can be made with a high level of accuracy, the known presence of venospasm or vascular thrombosis in patients with ARDS (see Fig. 3-20) should be taken into consideration in interpreting the Swan-Ganz numbers. Therefore, even though the catheter tip is correctly in zone 3, if venospasm or vascular thrombosis is present, there is no continuous column of blood connecting the catheter tip to the left atrium, and the WP reading will reflect only alveolar pressure.[16]

2. *Valvular heart disease.* This diagnosis can usually be readily made from the chest film. If mitral stenosis is present, the WP clearly will not correctly reflect LVEDP. The radiologic diagnosis of valvular heart disease must therefore be considered in using the WP as a basis for therapy.

3. *Increased pericardial pressure.* This may arise from abrupt cardiac dilatation "stretching" the pericar-

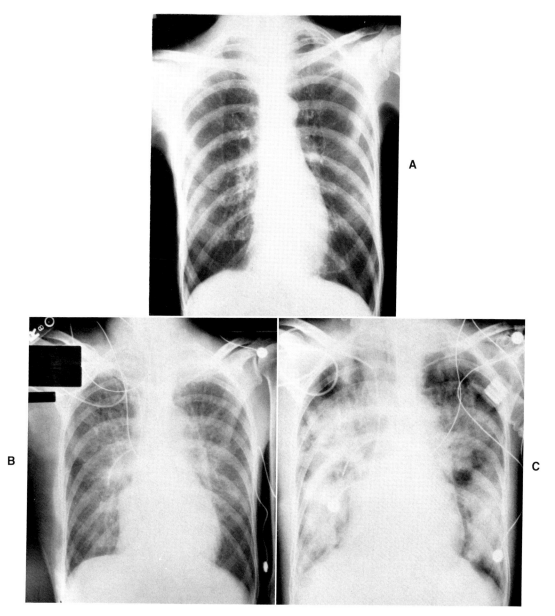

Fig. 10-16   Cachectic 54-year-old woman admitted for ovarian neoplasm. **A,** Admission film showing the very oligemic lungs of dehydration. **B,** The patient began to have episodes of atrial fibrillation, and the film was read as showing "cardiac failure modified by COPD." The reading was ignored because the Swan-Ganz was read as 5.0 mm Hg, and the patient was vigorously hydrated. **C,** As a result of the hydration superimposed on cardiac failure, gross alveolar edema is now present.

dium or from pericardial effusion. Abrupt increases in cardiac volume can be readily detected on sequential films. However, the plain film is poor for confirming or excluding the presence of pericardial effusions, and this should be done immediately by ultrasound.

4. *Altered left ventricular compliance.* A component of ventricular wall compliance depends on the compliance of the surrounding lung, which, as mentioned, is

quite easily determined if the patient is on a ventilator by comparing peak pressure and lung volume taken at full ventilator inflation. Ventricular compliance is also closely related to ventricular filling. Again, a chronologic survey of the patient's previous films can provide evidence about increasing cardiac volume, which must be factored into any deductions about left ventricular compliance.

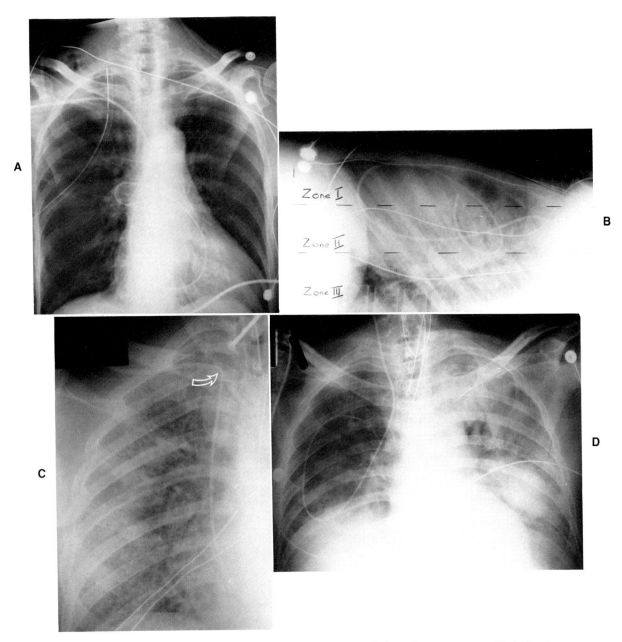

Fig. 10-17 **A,** Swan-Ganz catheter coiled up within right pulmonary artery. **B,** Lateral cross-table view of **A** shows tip of catheter. The usual position of the three flow zones in the supine position is also shown. **C,** At the point of emergence from the introducer *(open arrow)* the Swan-Ganz catheter is severely kinked. This is a typical site for kinking unless the introducer sheath is pushed farther on to turn down into the right brachiocephalic vein. Occasionally, however, this kinks the introducer itself. **D,** Swan-Ganz catheter in the right pleural space (note also feeding tube coiled up in the piriform fossae). When each of these bizarre or kinked catheters was in place, a "wedge pressure" was confidently offered by the referring physician, and the patient's treatment was being based on these figures.

Complex Edema

The approach to diagnosing multifactorial edemas, frequently seen in the ICU, has been fully covered in Chapter 8. Complex edemas most often result in situations in which the interventional data may be *correct* but appear to be discordant with the radiologic findings. For example, a patient with severe ARDS may have been extremely overhydrated with crystalloids, causing a drop in oncotic pressure and resulting in severe edema. The radiologist would read the film at this stage as *hydrostatic* edema, and the concealed ARDS might not be diagnosed. Normally the WP measurement would show some increase, reflecting the increase in LAP usually caused by overhydration, and would therefore not be discrepant with the radiologic diagnosis. However, the presence of severe hypoxemia and diminished pulmonary compliance would *not* be in accord with the radiologic diagnosis of hydrostatic edema. This discrepancy is rarely a problem for the film reader if previous films are available, since a chronologic review of the films shows the initial injury edema and the subsequent changes of superimposed overhydration (Fig. 10-18).

Also, the clinician usually knows from the ventilator data, and presumably from the patient's immediate history, that injury edema was present before the reading of hydrostatic edema. In fact, the superimposition of overhydration edema on injury edema occurs so often in the ICU that it is the *usual* rather than the unusual picture. This "constellation" of discrepancy between the radiologic picture indicating hydrostatic edema and interventional data indicating a very stiff lung with arteriovenous shunting should provide the correct diagnosis of *combined* pressure and injury edema when the two sources of information are integrated (see Figs. 11-20 to 11-22).

Other typical situations in which the radiologic diagnosis may begin to diverge from the diagnosis suggested by the ventilatory data involve pneumonia, either infective or aspiration, and contusion. Aspiration of "benign" material may appear severe radiologically but cause little dysfunction and may clear fairly rapidly. If, however, the aspirated material is septic or of very low pH, ARDS may develop, with little chronologic radiologic alteration. The radiologic diagnosis may continue to be aspiration, although the ventilatory data clearly indicate that ARDS is now present (see Fig. 10-2). It may also be impossible to recognize solely from the radiologic image when a previously uncomplicated infective or aspiration pneumonia begins to develop into ARDS. Similarly, an initially simple lung contusion may become ARDS without significant radiologic

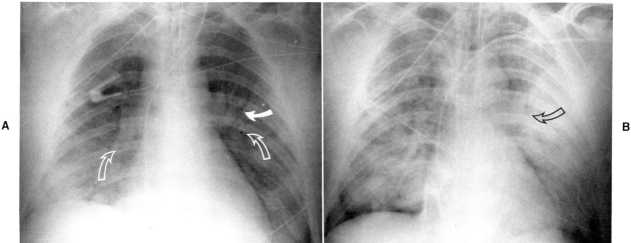

Fig. 10-18 **A,** Radiograph of a 41-year-old man after motor vehicle accident, 40-inch AP projection with the patient seated erect. The gravitational distribution of edema and peribronchial cuffing *(open arrows)* indicate *hydrostatic* edema. Note, however, that injury edema may *also* be present because a faint bronchogram is seen in the left upper lobe *(closed arrow)*. The WP was 18 mm Hg, which would confirm overhydration, but the peak ventilatory pressure was 60 and PEEP 20 cm H_2O, not compatible with pure hydrostatic edema. **B,** Review of previous films taken 3 days earlier in same patient shows nongravitational edema, no cuffing, no effusions, but marked air bronchograms *(open arrows)*, all indicating *injury* edema (wedge pressure, 7.0 mm Hg; peak pressure, 60 cm H_2O; PEEP, 20 cm H_2O).

change. Note that lung contusions should begin to resolve within 3 days,[19] and if they do not do so or begin to increase in extent, ARDS must be suspected.

Oncotic Edema

As we have indicated, the role of oncotic pressure in the production of edema appears to be understated. In ICU patients in particular, decreases in colloid osmotic pressure frequently occur because of increasing capillary permeability, failure of the liver to produce or metabolize albumin, loss of blood or plasma, or reduction in plasma proteins by administration of large amounts of crystalloids.[20] A loss of 1.0 g/dl of plasma protein causes an effective increase in transmural microvascular pressure of approximately 3.5 mm Hg; therefore a reduction in plasma proteins from 7 to 4 g/dl would cause a transmural pressure change equivalent to an increase of 11 mm Hg in LAP, which would not be reflected by any change in the WP.

Colloid oncotic pressure in patients with ARDS has been shown to be closely related to their survival.[21] A good relationship also exists between the amount of injury edema seen on the chest radiograph in ARDS patients and the level of colloid oncotic pressure.[21] In these patients the combination of a reduction in plasma protein and only a small increase in LAP can cause severe edema to develop, with considerable discrepancy between the low WP and the large quantity of edema. The radiograph in such a patient reveals features of both pressure (oncotic) and injury edema.

Severe oncotic edema can also be present in the *absence* of any lung injury, with no evidence of an increased circulating blood volume and with normal or only slightly elevated WPs, if the oncotic pressure is extremely low. In such circumstances the radiologist's diagnosis of "pure" pressure (hydrostatic) edema may not be accepted by the clinician because the Swan-Ganz reading appears to be "too low" to be compatible with such severe edema if it were purely hydrostatic (Fig. 10-19). However, the radiologic data showing gravitational distribution of edema, cuffing, septal lines, effusions, and soft tissue edema are so "hard" that the radiologic diagnosis of hydrostatic edema should not be in question. Instead, the finding of pressure edema as described, in association with a *normal* WP and normal lung compliance, should be accepted as strongly suggesting oncotic edema.

If the low oncotic pressure is caused by fluid replacement while fluid loss *continues* (e.g., severe hemorrhage), the circulating blood volume will be normal or reduced, causing a narrow vascular pedicle; body weight will remain unchanged or reduced; and fluid input will be extremely high but fluid *output* will be the same or possibly greater (Fig. 10-20). (Note that the patient in Fig. 10-20 is the same shown in Fig. 4-18, but the effects are so striking, correlated with the change in oncotic pressure over 24 hours, that we thought it was appropriate to show it again at this point.)

If the oncotic pressure primarily results from renal failure or simple overhydration, the circulating blood volume usually increases, resulting in a wide pedicle, large azygos vein, and 1:1 flow distribution (see Fig. 11-17). The patient's body weight increases; fluid input exceeds output.

Effects of High Ventilatory Pressure

Most aspects of barotrauma have been thoroughly described in the literature[9] and generally are not within the scope of this book. However, two areas are appropriate to consider: quantification of pneumothorax and "tension" pneumothorax.

Quantification of Pneumothorax. When a pneumothorax is detected, the decision whether or not to put in a chest tube is usually based on several criteria. For example, is the patient about to be placed on positive-pressure ventilation? Is the patient about to undergo surgery? Does the patient have some risk (e.g., rib fractures) of developing a pneumothorax on the opposite side? Is the patient manifesting respiratory distress or vagal stimulation from the pneumothorax? In the absence of these special circumstances, however, the decision on inserting a chest tube is frequently based on the size of the pneumothorax, with 25% usually being the key figure. Therefore the film reader should be able to quantify a pneumothorax with a reasonable degree of accuracy.

Rhea et al.[22] have published a nomogram by which the percentage of a pneumothorax can be read from the plain film after making simple measurements and taking their mean value. For a time we carried this nomogram with us and used it whenever we required to quantify a pneumothorax. Frequently, however, we would estimate the pneumothorax first without using the nomogram. On comparing this simplified estimate with the nomogram, we found only small differences between our estimates and the nomogram figures, never large enough to change the therapeutic approach. We therefore stopped using the nomogram and now use only the elementary approach shown in Fig. 10-21.[3,12]

No one has any problems quantifying a pneumothorax as 0% when the lung is fully expanded to the chest wall or 100% when the lung is totally collapsed (Fig. 10-21). We simply interpolate from these end points. If the lung is collapsed to a point halfway between the chest wall and hilum, the pneumothorax is 50%; halfway between this and the chest wall the pneumothorax is 25%; and so on. Since the lung is not a regular cylinder but has an irregularly conical configuration, these arbitrary estimates can only be approximate. However,

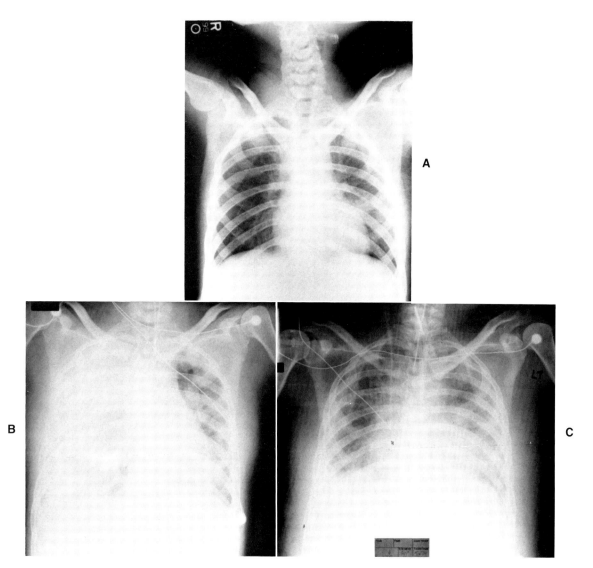

Fig. 10-19 Radiographs of 19-year-old male with Down's syndrome and chronic hepatitis. **A,** AP 40-inch chest film on day of admission. **B,** Severe bilateral edema with large right pleural effusion 24 hours later. Note that the vascular pedicle width and cardiac volume are actually slightly *less* than on admission, indicating a drop in total blood volume, whereas the soft tissues are increased in thickness, indicating increasing *systemic* extravascular water in addition to the pulmonary edema. The edema has all the characteristics of hydrostatic (pressure) edema. The reduction in total blood volume indicates the edema is *not* caused by overhydration/renal failure. The edema distribution is not that of acute cardiac failure. The very abrupt appearance of an effusion, with no *lag* between the appearance of edema and the effusion, also suggests strongly that the effusion is not a result of cardiac failure. The diagnosis of *oncotic* edema was made. (The patient's plasma proteins were subsequently shown to be 2.1 g.) The Swan-Ganz reading, however, was so low (3.0 mm Hg) that the clinician believed this was injury edema from sepsis and hydrated the patient. **C,** After hydration the patient has great increases in soft tissue edema *(arrows)* and circulating blood volume (evidenced by extremely widened vascular pedicle). No decrease in lung compliance. Diagnosis: oncotic edema exaggerated by overhydration.

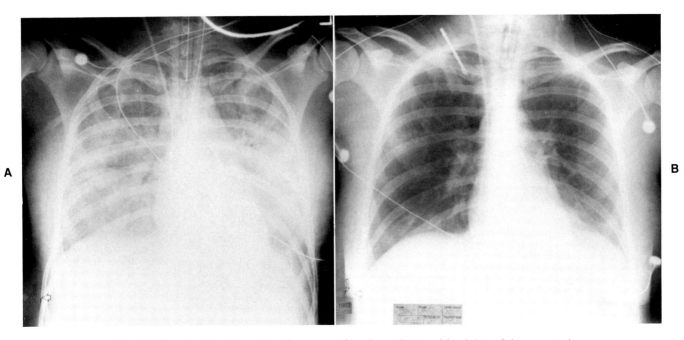

A

B

Fig. 10-20   A, Admission film of a young female patient stabbed 1 to 2 hours previously. She has received several liters of low-molecular-weight fluid, but the circulating blood volume is very low. Note the narrow pedicle and small heart, indicating strongly that the fluid input is not keeping up with fluid loss (i.e., bleeding). The edema is caused by lowered oncotic pressure. It is occurring *much* too rapidly to be injury edema. **B,** The very low hematocrit was recognized on admission, and plasma and packed cells were given, raising the oncotic pressure. The edema in this film only 24 hours later has gone with the elevation of oncotic pressure, but the circulating blood volume remains low (narrow vascular pedicle) and the soft tissues are thin, despite the patient being 9.0 liters "ahead" on fluids. At surgery, 9.0 liters of blood were found in the abdomen from unsuspected liver puncture.

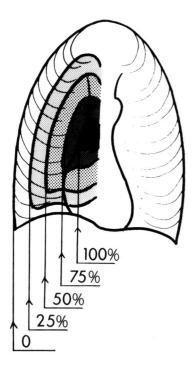

Fig. 10-21   Simplified but clinically valid method of quantifying pneumothorax. Note that this method applies only to a film with the patient *erect*. When the lung edge lies halfway between the chest wall and the hilum, the pneumothorax is assessed as 50%. When it is one-quarter the way from the chest wall to the hilum, the pneumothorax is 25%, and so on. With these "end points" in mind, one can easily extrapolate to degrees of collapse of greater or lesser extent. If the lung collapses irregularly (e.g., if the pneumothorax is larger at the apex than the base), the percentage of pneumothorax can still be assessed by visually averaging the distances at the apex (e.g., 30%) and base (e.g., 5%), yielding a value of approximately 18%. If a much greater length of the lung's upper portion (the 30% area) is stripped away from the chest wall than the lower (5%) area, the estimate is revised upward (e.g., the 25%). If the length of the 30% portion is much smaller than the 5% area, the estimate is revised downward (e.g., to 10%).

they do correlate well with the nomogram technique, the accuracy of which in turn has been proved by summating contiguous serial computed tomographic (CT) slices through the pneumothorax. We therefore now use this simple technique of estimating percentage of pneumothorax in preference to the nomogram.[3,12] Using CT to estimate the volume of a pneumothorax appears to be expensive, time-consuming overkill.

"Tension" Pneumothorax. We believe that this diagnosis is often made incorrectly; that is, when the pleural space is intact, the lung is "held out" to the chest wall by the negative intrapleural pressure, and the chest wall in turn is "held in" slightly by the same negative pressure.[3] Similarly, the diaphragm is held *up* in apposition with the lung by the negative pressure. If this pressure is released or simply made slightly less negative by a pneumothorax, the diaphragm will drop, the chest wall will expand outward, and the mediastinum will shift somewhat away from the pneumothorax as a result of the still intact negative pressure on the contralateral side.

This combination of findings often leads the film reader to make a diagnosis of tension pneumothorax, even though the underlying lung is still partially inflated, indicating that the pressure surrounding it within the pneumothorax must be *negative*.[3] The lung's continued partial expansion is often not taken into account, and on the basis of the depressed diaphragm, widened rib spaces, and displaced mediastinum, a firm (but incorrect) diagnosis of tension pneumothorax is made (Fig. 10-22). The belief that these appearances indicate a tension pneumothorax is so strong that persons inserting the chest tubes often say that they hear air "rushing out," when this is manifestly impossible (unless the patient is simultaneously on positive-pressure ventilation, which, at full inflation, will increase the pressure of the incompressible air in the pneumothorax to the same level as the peak pressure).

A tension pneumothorax usually should not be diagnosed if the underlying lung remains partially expanded. The two exceptions to this are (1) the infrequent patient with valvular obstruction of the bronchus

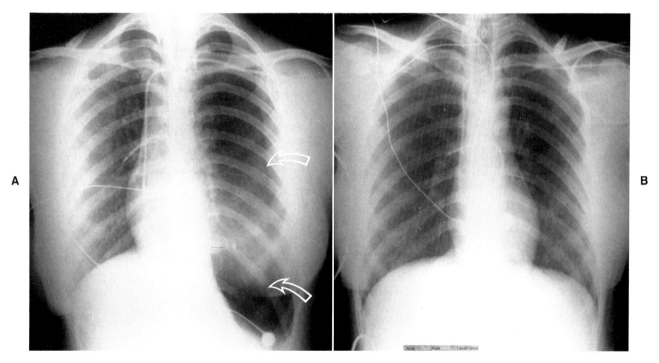

Fig. 10-22 Radiographs of 25-year-old female. **A,** After insertion of a left subclavian line, a large pneumothorax has developed, as shown in this 72-inch AP chest film. The mediastinum is deviated to the right, and the left diaphragm is very low in position. This was diagnosed as a tension pneumothorax, but the underlying lung is still well inflated *(open arrows),* indicating that the pressure in the left pleural space is still negative. In this particular patient the interrib spaces have not increased appreciably; when they do increase, less tendency exists for the diaphragm to descend or the mediastinum to be pulled across by the more negative pressure in the contralateral pleural space. **B,** Follow-up films 36 hours after insertion of a chest tube. Chest tube has been removed, and no pneumothorax is seen.

and (2) the more frequent patient with ARDS whose lung is so airless and dense that it will not collapse even when removed from the thorax.[3] In these patients, tension pneumothorax can be present *without* the lung being fully collapsed.[12] This situation is easy to recognize in patients with ARDS because the partially collapsed lung, which should be of normal radiolucence because blood has been shifted from it to the contralateral lung, is opaque (Fig. 10-23).

Another fallacy is the belief that the inflated cuff around an endotracheal tube prevents aspiration. In fact, an endotracheal tube causes a *predilection* for aspiration because it keeps the vocal cords apart, removing this defense mechanism against aspiration and permitting aspirated material to pass through the cords and impinge on the easily irritated tracheal mucosa. If the patient is not completely unconscious, this will trigger abrupt inspiration, but otherwise the

material can leak slowly past the balloon with every inspiration (Fig. 10-24). As can be seen on rapid cine studies of the bronchi and trachea, at the moment of inspiration the tracheal diameter easily increases to exceed that of the tracheal balloon, and material can readily be aspirated past it into the lungs. The combination of a nasogastric tube keeping the esophagogastric junction open and an endotracheal tube keeping the cords open is a powerful promoter of aspiration. In our experience, when a feeding tube's tip is not in the desired location (the gastric antrum) but in the fundus, close to the esophagogastric junction, the incidence of aspiration is 75% or greater.

APPROACH TO READING INTENSIVE CARE UNIT FILMS

"Looking" is not synonymous with seeing, and seeing in turn is not synonymous with recognizing or perceiving. A regrettable but not immutable fact of life is that

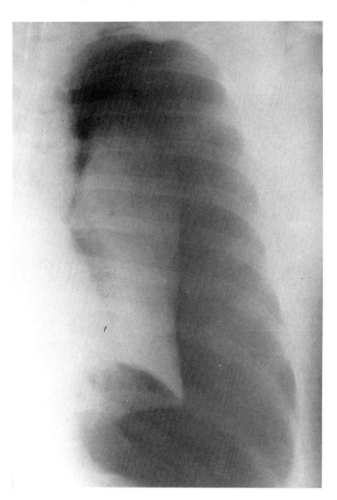

Fig. 10-23 Tension pneumothorax in a patient with ARDS caused by postpneumococcal pneumonia. The underlying lung is so noncompliant that it *cannot* collapse, even if the pressure in the pleural space is positive. The abnormality of this lung is indicated by its great density (compare with the partially collapsed lung in Fig. 10-22, *A*).

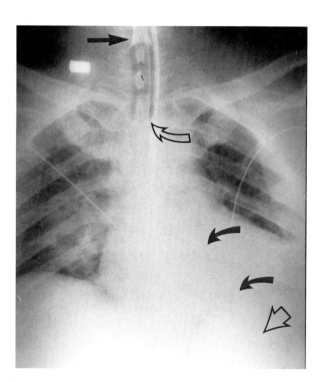

Fig. 10-24 After a bullet wound to the neck, this patient is intubated and has a nasogastric feeding tube inserted. Contrast medium has been injected through the tube into the stomach fundus *(open straight arrow)*. As the film is being taken, some of the contrast medium is refluxing around the nasogastric tube, up the esophagus, and into the trachea, where it can be seen lying on top of the inflated endotracheal tube balloon *(closed straight arrows)*. The contrast medium has also gone past the balloon, outlining its lower aspect *(open curved arrows)* and filling the left lower lobe *(closed curved arrows)*.

when we look at films, we all can *see* much detail, but we may be unable to *recognize* its significance even though we may presently be quite convinced that we *can* recognize the significance.

The previous chapters have been devoted to providing the reader with some pathophysiologic knowledge required (1) to transform the physical act of seeing into the psychophysiologic act of recognition and (2) to further the integration of this recognized visual data with the cerebral store of anatomic/pathologic/physiologic and clinical data to facilitate first perception and second diagnosis. Although one might think a film reader should have a consistent habitual search pattern, designed so that he or she at least does not fail to *look* at all the radiologic features necessary to make diagnoses, this is unfortunately not possible. The human eye-brain combination automatically leaps to focus on whatever instantly appears aberrant, interesting, anomalous, or unusual and often totally "forgets" any imposed search pattern. However, one can use a form of "checklist," programmed so that one asks oneself, "Did I remember to look at the liver, the bones . . . .

In the ICU we find the following simplistic approach helpful in ensuring that we have at least looked at (or "for") all the diagnostic data we require to make a diagnosis or to offer a logically weighted differential diagnosis.

1. Make a global survey of the film from a 6-foot distance.
2. Return to a comfortable viewing distance and make your detailed regional analysis.
3. Make sure you not only look *at* the film but look *through* the film.
4. Before you leave the film, look at "all four corners."
5. "Look back."

Global Survey at 6-foot Distance

Some diagnoses are easier to make at 6 feet than when one is close to the film (e.g., absent pectoralis muscle, mastectomy, McLoud syndrome). Most of these diagnoses are based on a comparison of symmetry. This comparison is greatly facilitated by the 6-foot distance because the *entire* chest image falls on the retina. The areas best compared at this distance are:

1. Lungs. One looks for size, lucency, gradation of density from apex to base, blood volume, and flow distribution in each lung; hilar size and symmetry, looking at each lung first separately and then comparatively; and the lung's overall texture.
2. Heart. The size and shape should be compared with the individual's build and weight.
3. Vascular pedicle width. This should be compared with the individual's physical type, size, and degree of obesity.

4. Diaphragm. The shape and level of each diaphragm should be viewed individually and then compared. It is often accepted that the left diaphragm can occasionally be at the same level or even slightly higher than the right and still be normal.[23] However, we believe subtle but important diagnoses can be missed by too ready an adherence to this belief. We prefer to state that, whenever the left hemidiaphragm is at the same level or higher than the right, the reason *must* be sought. The most common and usually most benign reason for elevation of the left hemidiaphragm is a gas-filled stomach or splenic flexure, which should be immediately obvious. If this is not the case, the differential should include enlarged spleen (increasingly seen, since intravenous drug users and approximately 75% of patients with AIDS have large spleens), subpulmonic effusions, early atelectasis of the left lower lobe, and subdiaphragmatic irritation (e.g., abscesses, splenic hematoma, pancreatitis). Note that spleen size is evaluated much better on the radiograph than by palpation. Even in cachectic patients, the spleen can be felt in only 25% of patients in whom it is manifestly enlarged on the plain radiograph. This has been proven by isotopic "sizing" of the spleen and by CT and ultrasound.[24]

It is often suggested that chest wall pain causes "splinting" of one diaphragm so that it cannot move down and remains high in position relative to the other diaphragm. However, the logic of this seems somewhat faulty. The diaphragm's innervation does not permit one diaphragm to descend less than the other, unless the phrenic nerve is directly involved. Therefore, if pain stops *one* diaphragm from descending, the other diaphragm will also stop descending, and although both diaphragms may be high in position, one will not be abnormally higher than the other.

A common, rather powerful optical illusion can make assessment of the relative levels of the diaphragms erroneous.[3] Fig. 10-25 graphically shows that the film should be positioned not so that the *film* is vertical but so that the patient's *spine* is in its normal vertical position before the diaphragmatic level is assessed.

Survey at Normal Viewing Distance

The hemodynamic features that should be looked for include size of the main pulmonary artery and its central divisions, pulmonary blood volume, blood flow distribution, arterial sinuosity, arterial/venous ratio, sharpness of vessel margins, visibility of small background vessels, cuffing, septal lines, lung lucency, presence and distribution of edema and effusions, width of the vascular pedicle and azygos vein, and thickness of the chest wall's soft tissues. All these features have been fully discussed previously, but we should mention a special role for the vascular pedicle, azygos vein, and right paratracheal stripe in patients with trauma.

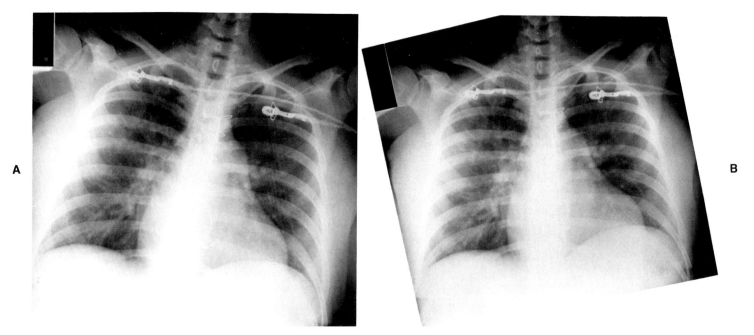

Fig. 10-25 **A,** Diaphragm appears to be approximately equal in height. **B,** Left hemidiaphragm is now clearly much higher than the right. Note that this is the same film shown twice and hung vertically on the viewbox with the film edges vertical.

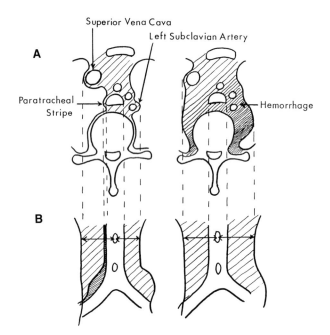

Fig. 10-26 **A,** Normal paratracheal stripe and azygos vein on CT scan and plain film shown diagrammatically. The paratracheal stripe is normally seen because it is outlined from the inside by air within the tracheal lumen and from the outside by air in the lung. In this example the distance from the heart's midline to its right side's border (MR) is greater than distance from the heart's midline to the pedicle's left border (ML), the normal appearance for a supine patient. **B,** When the aorta tears, this usually occurs just distal to the origin of the left subclavian artery. The diagram shows blood flooding the pedicle, causing ML to be larger than MR and the paratracheal stripe and azygos vein to "vanish."

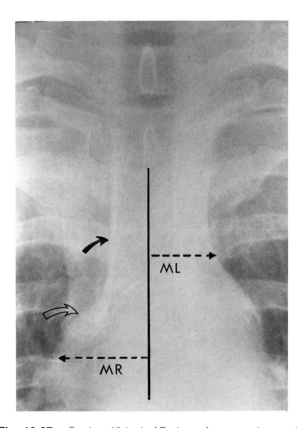

Fig. 10-27 Supine 40-inch AP view of a normal vascular pedicle. MR is greater than ML. The paratracheal stripe *(black arrow)* runs into the azygos vein *(open arrow),* resembling the shaft and head of a golf club.

Normally the trachea's right wall and its thin layer of overlying soft tissues can be seen easily because the trachea on the right is outlined by air on both sides (Fig. 10-26). A *left* paratracheal stripe is not usually seen because the left common carotid and subclavian arteries pass lateral to the trachea and intervene between it and the lung (Fig. 10-26). Followed caudally, the right paratracheal stripe appears to lead into the azygos vein's silhouette, giving an appearance resembling a golf club, with the azygos vein as the head of the club (Fig. 10-27). If any fluid is present (usually blood) within the upper mediastinum, the paratracheal stripe and azygos vein can no longer be seen, a diagnostic sign we have called the "vanishing azygos."[11] The most common cause of this in a hospital population is right-sided hematoma formation from a traumatic right subclavian or sometimes jugular catheter insertion (Fig. 10-28). Under these circumstances the distance from the midline of the vascular pedicle, judged by the spinous processes, and the distance from the heart's midline to its right side's border (MR) become much greater than the distance from the heart's midline to the pedicle's left border (ML)[3,11,12] (Fig. 10-28). Such hematomas are usually benign and resolve within 7 to 14 days; rarely, they become organized and persist as a paratracheal mass.

In contrast, if a tear of the aorta is present, even if this is clinically unsuspected, ML will be wider than MR (an abnormal finding in a supine patient), and the paratracheal stripe and azygos will simultaneously "vanish" (Fig. 10-29). Table 10-2 shows a comparison of the visibility of the vascular pedicle and paratracheal stripe in 108 patients with increased *intra*vascular volume and 54 patients with *extra*vascular fluid in the mediastinum. Of 27 patients with a proven torn aorta, the paratracheal stripe vanished in 26 and was seen but greatly widened in one (Fig. 10-29, *A*). In all 27 patients with aortic tears, ML either exceeded MR (93%) or equaled MR (7%). We have found these vascular pedicle changes to be superior to any other published sign for the diagnosis of an aortic tear.[11] These changes can frequently be present when *no* other radiologic sign of aortic tear is present. In a patient with trauma to the

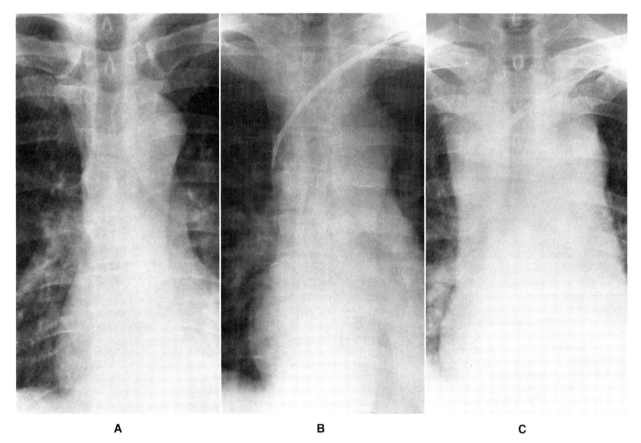

A   **B**   **C**

Fig. 10-28 **A,** Erect 72-inch PA view of normal vascular pedicle. ML is slightly greater than MR (compare with Fig. 10-27). Normal paratracheal stripe. **B,** Left subclavian catheter has been inserted. Its tip appears to overlie the wall of the right brachiocephalic vein. The paratracheal stripe has greatly widened, and the azygos vein is beginning to "vanish." **C,** Hours later the paratracheal stripe and azygos vein have vanished, and MR now exceeds ML. Diagnosis: large right paratracheal hematoma.

A

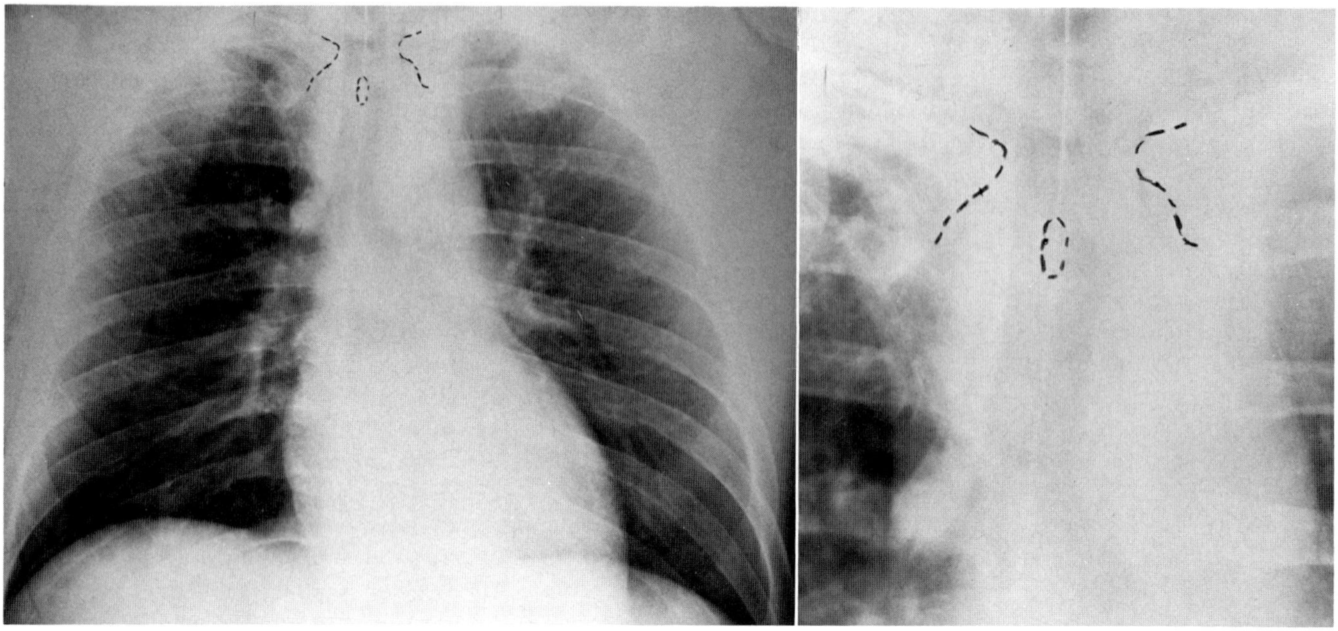

B

Fig. 10-29 **A,** Young male patient immediately following abrupt deceleration injury. Although this is a supine film (with little rotation; see dotted outline of clavicles and spinous process), ML is clearly much greater than MR, the paratracheal stripe is extremely thickened, and the azygos vein's upper border is beginning to be obscured. **B,** Magnified view of **A.** The patient had a normal hematocrit and no clinical suggestion of aortic tear. In view of the radiologic findings, however, an angiogram is mandatory and was performed (against clinical objections) (see Fig. 10-30, *A*).

Table 10-2

Clinical information:	Number	Paratracheal stripe and azygos vein seen	MR > ML	MR = ML	ML > MR
Normals: 2 L IV saline in 20 minutes	3	3 (100%)	3 (100%)	0 (0%)	0 (0%)
Chronic or recurrent cardiac failure	40	31 (77%)	37 (92.5%)	1 (2.5%)	2 (5%)
Renal failure (before dialysis)	30	26 (87%)	18 (60%)	12 (40%)	0 (0%)
Overhydration	30	28 (93%)	28 (93%)	2 (6.6%)	0 (0%)
Polycythemia rubra vera	5	5 (100%)	3 (60%)	2 (40%)	0 (0%)
Total	**108**	**93 (85%)**	**89 (82.4%)**	**17 (15.7%)**	**2 (1.9%)**
Posttraumatic bleeding into pedicle:		**Increased intravascular volume**			
Proven aortic tear	27	1 (3.4%)	0 (0%)	2 (6.8%)	25 (92.6%)
Small vessel bleeding	13	2 (15.4%)	0 (0%)	2 (15.4%)	11 (84.6%)
Subtotal	**40**	**3 (7.5%)**	**0 (0%)**	**4 (10%)**	**36 (90%)**
Iatrogenic infusion into mediastinum	10	0 (0%)	1 (10%)	2 (20%)	7 (70%)
Esophageal tear	3	0 (0%)	1 (33.3%)	2 (66.6%)	0 (0%)
Infection (osteitis)	1	1 (100%)	1 (100%)	—	—
Total	**54**	**4 (7.4%)**	**3 (5.6%)**	**8 (14.8%)**	**43 (79.6%)**

MR, Distance from the heart's midline to its right side's border; *ML*, distance from the heart's midline to the pedicle's left border.

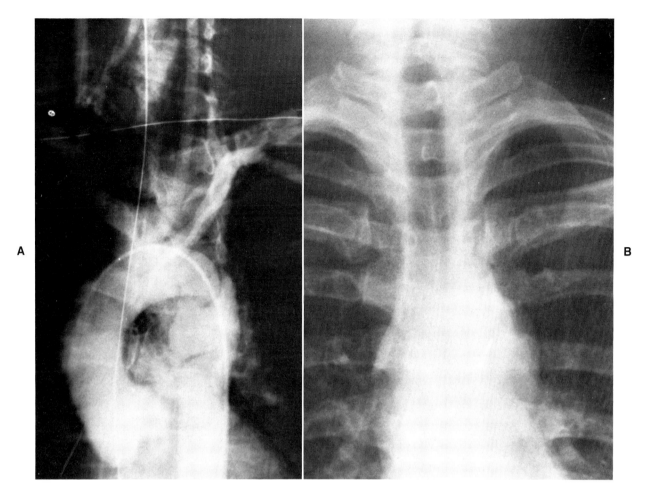

Fig. 10-30 **A,** The angiogram reveals complete transection of the aorta. **B,** One week later, after prosthetic grafting of the damaged aorta, the vascular pedicle returns to normal. Note especially the "reemergence" of the right paratracheal stripe and azygos vein.

thorax, regardless of the presence of any clinical evidence, a vascular pedicle widened to the left (ML greater than MR) with a vanished paratracheal stripe and azygos vein should indicate a *mandatory* angiogram (Fig. 10-30) or at least a CT scan with contrast medium.

These findings are crucial to the management of trauma patients. If the area of the vascular pedicle is not adequately penetrated on the first supine chest film made in the emergency room, the film should *immediately* be repeated with overpenetration to visualize the pedicle's structures. In the past the indications for angiography in patients with suspected aortic tear have been so nonspecific that 65% of angiograms performed for suspected tears were negative. Also, 20% of patients who *did* have an aortic tear did not receive an angiogram and were discharged from hospital without the diagnosis being made.[11,12] Using the paratracheal stripe and vascular pedicle to decide whether to perform angiography, we have reduced the number of negative (unnecessary) examinations and increased the percent-

age of necessary (positive) examinations. To date, from angiograms done for these vascular pedicle indications only, with *all* other signs absent, we have diagnosed six aortic tears that otherwise would have been unsuspected clinically or radiologically.[11]

"Looking Through" the Film

On the chest radiograph, large areas of the lungs and spine are concealed at least partially by the diaphragm and heart and in the upper abdomen by dense abdominal contents. One therefore must make a deliberate effort to "look through" these structures to visualize as much of the lungs and spine as can be seen with the technique employed. In particular, the left paravertebral stripe and left phrenicovertebral angle, seen through the heart, can yield valuable data about paravertebral hematomas. These may result from thoracic spine fractures, postsurgical complications, or retroperitoneal extension from the abdomen, and occasionally are totally unsuspected clinically. In the same area be-

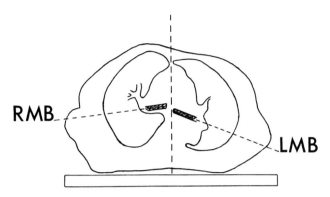

Fig. 10-31 Diagram of a CT scan through the carina. The left main bronchus *(LMB)* slopes downward (mean, 40 degrees) more steeply than the right main bronchus *(RMB)* (mean, 4 degrees), causing a predilection for aspiration and militating against drainage.

hind the heart, left lower lobe atelectasis is frequently revealed.

Left lower lobe atelectasis is an extremely frequent finding after cardiac or abdominal surgery; right lower lobe atelectasis is much rarer. The literature discusses the possible causes for the high incidence of left lower lobe atelectasis; we add two further pertinent observations.

1. It is well known that in the erect position the right main bronchus is more vertical than the left, and therefore aspirated material tends to migrate to the right lung. However, it is much less well known that in the *supine* position the left main bronchus slopes downward (i.e., toward the dorsum of the chest) more steeply than the right, which is frequently horizontal[3, 12] (Fig. 10-31). As a result, aspiration in the supine position tends to favor the left lower lobe. Also, accumulating mucus has more difficulty draining from the left lower lobe against the steeper gradient.

2. In the supine position the posterior half of the diaphragm is pushed cranially by gravitational shift of the intraabdominal contents. On the right side the diaphragm's anterior half can still maintain a good excursion, but on the left side the upward motion of the diaphragm's anterior half is prevented by the heart. As a result, in the supine position the left hemidiaphragm cannot move as well as the right.

The combination of these two factors, poor diaphragmatic motion and steeper left main bronchus, would appear to cause a predilection for mucus accumulation and atelectasis at the left lung base.

"Looking at All Four Corners"

We do not know whether the late Ben Felson originated this phrase, but we certainly learned it from him

and have been grateful many times for its getting us out of trouble or preventing us from getting into trouble. Specifically, before we leave a film, believing that the film has yielded up all the information it contains, we deliberately check or recheck each of the film's "four corners" (the outer quadrants) for the following features.

Right Lower Quadrant. Soft tissues for thickness, texture, air, foreign bodies, or edema. The liver for calculi, drains, stents, calcifications, and air within the liver (e.g., gas in the bile ducts) or above the liver (e.g., colon in suprahepatic position versus pneumoperitoneum). The bones for fracture or metabolic abnormalities and inflammatory or neoplastic change.

Left Lower Quadrant. The stomach bubble for indentations, abnormal rugae, and extraluminal air. The pancreatic tail for calcification and the spleen for its size and the presence of calcifications. The soft tissues and bones as for the right lower quadrant.

Left Upper Quadrant. The humerus, shoulder girdle, acromioclavicular joints, clavicle, companion shadow of the clavicle, and relative density of the tissues on both sides of the neck. Moving toward the right upper quadrant, the trachea, particularly for stenosis and thyroid nodules; vocal cords; piriform fossae; and mandibular arch and teeth if seen on the film.

Right Upper Quadrant. As for the left upper quadrant.

"Looking Back"

In the heat of the battle the ICU film-reading boards, it is easy to compare the film of the day only with films taken during the preceding few days. However, ICU patients, especially long-term patients, can, in addition to their acute disease, change some radiographic features slowly enough so that they can only be recognized by looking at films made early in the course of the patient's disease and reviewing what has occurred since that time. *Gradual* increases in cardiac, vascular pedicle, and soft tissue width and hepatic and splenic enlargements may be dramatically displayed by this comparison with early films. These changes are impossible to detect if comparison is made only with recent films.

It is also film reader's responsibility to know in detail the radiologic history of each patient within the ICU since he or she entered the unit. For example, over a 3 to 4 week period, a patient with septic shock and ARDS may have had several episodes of transitory deterioration which were originally a diagnostic problem but in retrospect were clearly caused by cardiac decompensation, successfully handled by diuretics. When deterioration occurs *again*, the radiologist who knows the patient's history since entering the unit is in a much better position to pinpoint the diagnosis rapidly and to state what treatment has been successful previously.

This is particularly valuable when a patient's long-term care may involve a succession of different physicians. Sometimes only the radiologist knows the patient's entire course since admission and can provide a helpful summary of this to the "new" physician.

The ICU film-reading board can also provide a valuable *demographic* function. For example, a single referring physician may see only one or two patients with nosocomial pulmonary infections a month, but the radiologist sees *all* the patients with infections from every surgical intensive care, cardiac care, medical intensive care, and burn unit physician. The radiologist may therefore be able to recognize a trend toward an epidemic of a particular infection (e.g., *Klebsiella*, *Legionella*) long before any individual referring physician has accumulated enough cases to be aware of the trend.

CREDIBILITY OF RADIOLOGIC DATA IN THE INTENSIVE CARE UNIT

Noninterventionally acquired radiologic data are only of value when they are acted on to the patient's benefit. These data will only be *acted on* if they are believed by the referring clinician, which in turn devolves on:

1. The *clinician's* prior experience with what happens to morbidity and mortality rates in his or her patients when the clinician accepts and acts on the radiologic/physiologic data.
2. The depth of the *radiologist's* physiologic knowledge, which allows him or her to explain in pathophysiologic terms the logic and validity of his or her deductions
3. The clarity and confidence with which the radiologist offers his or her diagnoses

In regard to this last point, a diagnosis weakly phrased, such as "bilateral basal densities are present that may be compatible with edema or pneumonia," is certainly "safer" for the radiologist, since he or she has made no commitment and cannot therefore be called wrong at a later date. However, this type of report (which is, unfortunately, common practice) has much less impact, believability, or value as a guide to therapy than an informed report on the same film, such as:

There are symmetric bilateral basal densities. The differential diagnoses of these should still include pneumonia, but the bronchial cuffing and gravitational distribution provide strong evidence that this is edema. The presence of flow inversion indicates that the cause is left-sided heart failure. The degree of flow inversion and quantity of edema agree with a left atrial pressure in the 25 to 30 mm Hg range. The absence of enlargement of the vascular pedicle, azygos vein, or soft tissues strongly suggests there is no component of right-sided heart failure.

We have already addressed the issue of the accuracy of such radiologic assessments. If the film reader has the requisite knowledge of cardiopulmonary pathophysiology, the physiologic assessments made from the radiograph are usually in the correct range (see the box on p. 324).

Quite often it well not be possible for film reader to be completely positive about the radiologic findings. In these cases, a relative level of certainty or uncertainty should be expressed clearly in the radiologic report. The patient benefits optimally when the referring physician is aware of the strengths and weaknesses of his or her data *and* of the radiologic data and confers freely and frequently with a radiologist who is equally well informed about the strengths and weaknesses of both the interventional and the radiologic data. Frequent integration of the clinical, interventional, and radiologic data and combined analysis of discordance in these data lead to improved patient care.

Much information can be derived from the chest film at minimal cost to the patient in terms of dollars and discomfort, and rapidly changing physiologic and hemodynamic alterations can be monitored well by the radiograph. Therefore one should not hesitate, particularly during rapid deterioration in a patient's status, to take chest films much more frequently than the usually mandated one per day. In many urgent situations a film every 20 to 30 minutes is of such diagnostic value that the cause of the deterioration may be detected and, it is hoped, halted and reversed at a much earlier stage in the course of the disease.

REFERENCES

1. Lewis Sir T: Early signs of cardiac failure of the congestive type, *Br Med J* 36:849, 1930.
2. Savoca CJ, Gamsu G, Rohlfing BM: Chest radiography in intensive care units, *West J Med* 129:469, 1978.
3. Milne ENC: A physiological approach to reading critical care unit films, *J Thorac Imaging* 1(3):60, 1986.
3a. Kolobow T, Moretti MP, Fumagalli R et al: Severe inpairment in lung function induced by high peak airway pressure during mechanical ventilation: an experimental study, *Am Rev Respir Dis* 135:312, 1987.
3b. Dreyfuss D, Soler P, Basset G, Savmon G: High inflation pressure pulmonary edema: respective effects of high airway pressure, high tidal volume, and positive end-expiratory pressure, *Am Rev Respir Dis* 137:1159, 1988.
4. Remolina C, Khan AU, Santiago TJ, Edelman NH: Positional hypoxemia in unilateral lung disease, *N Engl J Med* 304:523, 1981.
5. Milne ENC, Burnett K, Aufrichtig D et al: Assessment of cardiac size on portable chest films, *J Thorac Imaging* 3(2):64, 1988.
6. Milne ENC, Pistolesi M, Miniati M, Giuntini C: The vascular pedicle of the heart and the vena azygos. Part I. The normal subject, *Radiology* 152:1, 1984.
7. Milne ENC, Tikhonov KB: Cardiac dimension and volume—effects of the supine position. In *Proceedings of the Fleischner Society Scientific Meeting*, Scottsdale, Ariz, April 1990.
8. Tikhonov KB: The geometry of the left ventricle in the isovolumic period, *Radiologe* 26:446, 1986.
9. Goodman LR, Putman CE, editors: *Intensive care radiology: imaging of the critically ill*, St Louis, 1978, Mosby–Year Book.

10. Pistolesi M, Milne ENC, Miniati M, Giuntini C: The vascular pedicle of the heart and the vena azygos. Part II. Acquired heart disease, *Radiology* 152:9, 1984.

11. Milne ENC, Imray TB, Pistolesi M et al: The vascular pedicle of the heart and the vena azygos. Part III. In trauma—the "vanishing" azygos, *Radiology* 153:25, 1984.

12. Milne ENC: Chest radiology in the surgical patient, *Surg Clin North Am* 60:1503, 1980.

13. Robin ED: The cult of the Swan-Ganz catheter: perspective, *Ann Intern Med* 103:445, 1985.

14. Roper R, Sibbald WJ: Misled by the wedge? Review, *Chest* 89:427, 1986.

15. Brandstetter RD, Gitler B: Thoughts on the Swan-Ganz catheter, *Chest* 89(1):5, 1986 (editorial).

16. Quinn K, Quebbeman EJ: Pulmonary artery pressure monitoring in the surgical intensive care unit: benefits v. difficulties, *Arch Surg* 116:872, 1981.

17. Morris AH, Chapman RH, Gardner RM: Frequency of wedge pressure errors in the ICU, *Crit Care Med* 13:705, 1985.

18. Eaton RJ, Taxman RM, Avioli LV: Cardiovascular evaluation of patients treated with PEEP, *Arch Intern Med* 143:1958, 1983.

18a. Gates LM, Matthay MA: Central intravascular pressure measurements: when should we believe them? *J Thorac Imaging* 1(3):52, 1986.

19. Milne ENC, Dick A: Circumscribed intrapulmonary hematoma, *Br J Radiol*, October 1961, p 2.

20. Overland ES, Severinghaus JW: Noncardiac pulmonary edema, *Adv Intern Med* 23:307, 1976.

21. Weil MH, Henning RJ, Morissette M, Michaels S: Relationship between colloid osmotic pressure and pulmonary artery wedge pressure in patients with acute cardiorespiratory failure, *Am J Med* 64:643, 1978.

22. Rhea JT, DeLuca SA, Greene RE: Determining the size of pneumothorax in the upright patient, *Radiology* 144:733, 1982.

23. Felson B: *Chest roentgenology*, Philadelphia, 1973, WB Saunders.

24. Pugh P, Milne ENC, Brenner M: Splenic size on routine chest films in AIDS: diagnostic and prognostic significance, *J Thorac Imaging* 3(2):40, 1988.

11 Compendium of Pathophysiologic Patterns

When one attempts to derive physiologic information from the plain chest film, one must look for and quantify at least 15 factors. The number of permutations (constellations) of so many factors is extremely large and many of the variations so subtle that it is virtually impossible to convey the changes in radiologic appearances with verbal descriptions alone. Often, however, a differentiation that would appear to be difficult from pure verbal description is relatively easy to make from a picture or diagram that presents the complete constellation of findings to the eye in one instant.

Since, as we stated in the preface, this book is designed to be "how to do it" as well as "why does it happen," we include the following compendium of pathophysiologic patterns in the form of diagrams. These are meant to assist the film reader in more rapidly establishing his or her own visual store of these patterns and of subtle variations in patterns that are essential to recognize to make physiologic diagnoses. Each compendium diagram relates back to cases and material illustrated throughout the book (see table below).

No complete substitutes exist for experience, but if a pattern has been seen before, it becomes much easier to recognize it when the pattern is seen again. We hope this compendium assists the reader in future pattern recognition.

The radiologic features that must be analyzed and integrated in every patient include:

1. Pulmonary blood volume
2. Pulmonary blood flow distribution
3. Vascular pedicle width
4. Azygos vein size
5. Main pulmonary artery
6. Peripheral divisions
7. Arterial/venous size ratio
8. Aorta
9. Peribronchial cuffing
10. Septal lines
11. Pulmonary edema
12. Distribution of edema
13. Pleural effusions
14. Soft tissue thickness
15. Cardiac size and shape

Compendium figure	Text figures
11-1	4-1 to 4-3, 4-6 to 4-10, 4-16 to 4-18, 4-28, 4-30, 4-31, 4-37 to 4-39, 4-42, 6-1
11-2	3-5, 3-8, 4-17, 4-41, B-C, 5-14, 6-6, 7-17, 8-13
11-3	4-37, 7-7B, 7-36
11-4	1-4, 4-24C, 4-27A, 6-19, 7-3A, 7-28,
11-5	4-36
11-6	1-4, 4-10, 6-3, 6-20, 6-30, 9-3, 9-5, 9-11A
11-7	7-37, 7-39
11-8	6-4B, 7-1A, 7-13, 7-41, 7-43, 9-15A, 9-19A, 9-21A
11-9	7-4, 9-9B-C, 9-21C-D
11-10	2-11B, 2-12, 7-30
11-11	2-13, 2-21, 4-35A, 7-29
11-12	2-24, 2-26, 4-32, 5-9A-C, 8-12A-B, 8-20
11-13	2-16, 4-33, 6-36A, 7-12, 8-1
11-14	4-35B, 6-36, 7-44
11-15	6-4B, 7-1A, 7-7, 7-13, 7-41, 7-43, 8-16, 9-19A, 9-21A
11-16	6-9, 7-1B, 7-11, 7-36
11-17	3-5B, 3-8, 4-17, 4-41B, 5-14, 6-17A, 7-1C
11-18	8-13
11-19	4-41C
11-20	1-5, 2-25, 2-28, 2-29, 3-10 to 3-15, 3-19, 5-21, 10-2(1-3), 10-15
11-21	2-25, 4-9
11-22	2-31, 8-8B, 10-15, 10-18A
11-23	4-28, 4-30, 4-31, 4-42, 10-19C
11-24	8-8
11-25	10-2(1-3)
11-26	5-15

Fig. 11-1

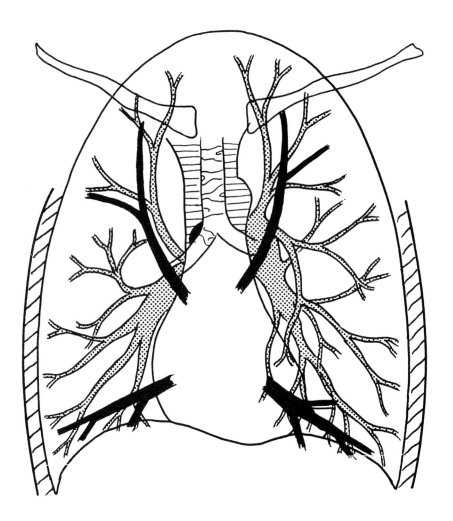

Observations. The vascular pedicle width (VPW), azygos vein, aorta, and pulmonary blood volume (PBV) are all normal. Blood flow distribution, arterial/venous (A/V) ratio, and cardiac size are all normal, and no soft tissue edema or pulmonary edema is present.

Discussion. A completely normal film of this type would rarely be associated with any physiologic abnormality. However, a profound physiologic defect with a virtually normal chest film may be present in patients with (1) the first stage of developing adult respiratory distress syndrome (ARDS), (2) massive pulmonary embolism, or (3) status asthmaticus.

Diagnosis. In the absence of any physiologic or clinical data indicating one of the three diagnoses just listed, the pattern indicates *normal physiology*.

Fig. 11-2

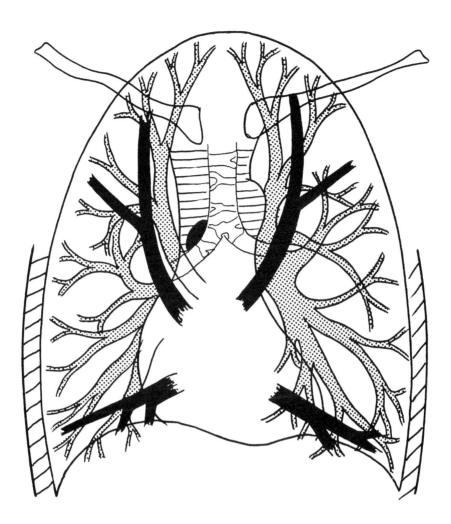

Observations. The VPW, azygos vein, and PBV are very large; flow distribution is "balanced"; the A/V ratio is 1:1; and no edema exists.

Discussion. The wide pedicle and large PBV indicate a marked increase in total blood volume (TBV). The absence of edema tells us that the increase in TBV is not caused by renal failure or overhydration with low-molecular-weight solutes. This leaves only overhydration with oncotically active fluid, such as blood (e.g., iatrogenic, midtrimester of pregnancy).

Diagnosis. *Physiologic or iatrogenic increase in blood volume.*

Fig. 11-3

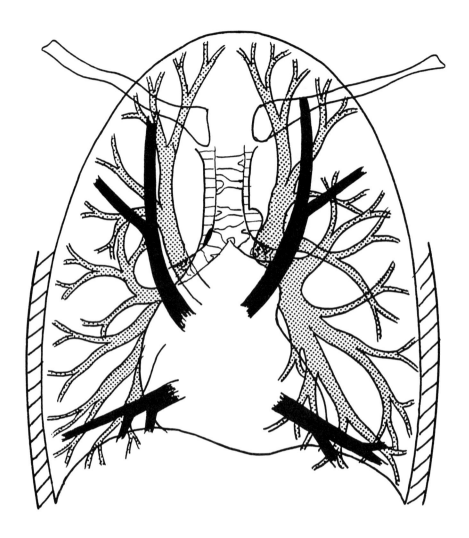

Observations. The PBV and flow distribution are identical with Fig. 11-2. No edema is present, but the VPW, azygos vein, and aorta are very small and the main pulmonary artery (MPA) very large. Since no tortuosity or pruning of peripheral vessels is seen and the A/V ratio is 1:1, no pulmonary arterial hypertension is present and therefore the MPA enlargement must be caused only by high flow. The very small VPW and aorta indicate a small systemic blood volume.

Discussion. The *only* pathophysiology that permits a simultaneous reduction in systemic blood volume and increase in PBV is an intrathoracic left-to-right shunt. There is no differential diagnosis. (Note: if edema had been present, one would have to consider the differential diagnosis of end-stage renal failure with high vasomotor tone.)

Diagnosis. *Intrathoracic left-to-right shunt without pulmonary arterial hypertension.*

Fig. 11-4

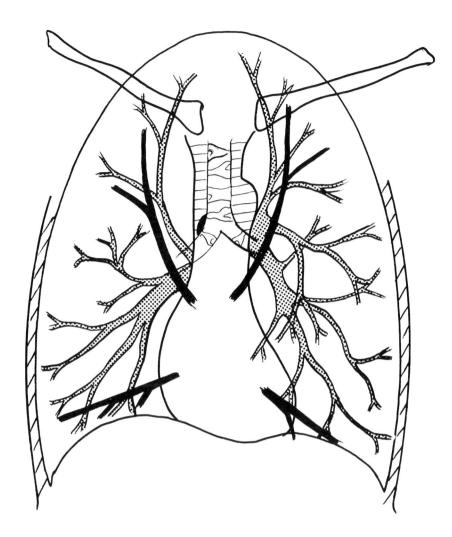

Observations. The VPW and azygos vein are very small, and both the pulmonary arteries and the pulmonary veins are unusually small. The A/V ratio is normal. No edema is present, and the soft tissues appear slightly reduced in thickness.

Discussion. The simultaneous reduction in size of the VPW and the pulmonary blood vessels indicates a reduction in TBV. The dry lungs and the narrow soft tissues suggest a general reduction in extravascular water.

Diagnosis. *Dehydration, either iatrogenic* (e.g. for head trauma) *or secondary to fluid loss* (e.g., hemorrhage, addisonian crisis) (Compare with Fig. 11-5.)

Fig. 11-5

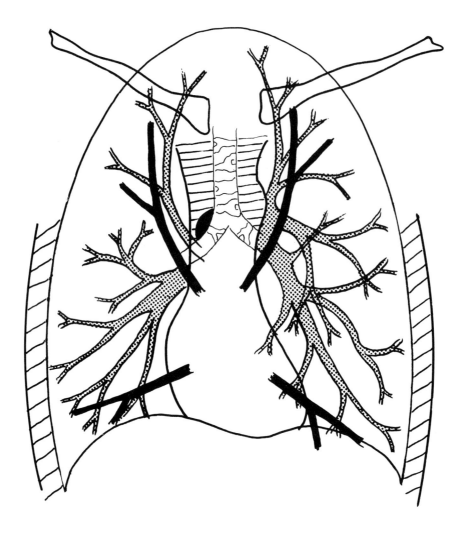

Observations. The PBV is the same as in Fig. 11-4 (i.e., reduced), and no edema is present. However, the VPW and azygos vein are large, indicating increased *systemic* blood volume, and the soft tissues have increased in thickness.

Discussion. Almost the only condition that dissociates systemic blood volume and PBV in this way is pericardial tamponade. Blood has difficulty entering the right atrium and is dammed back, increasing the systemic blood volume and pressure and causing evidence of right-sided heart failure (RHF), while cardiac output decreases, causing diminished PBV.

Diagnosis. *Pericardial tamponade.*

Fig. 11-6

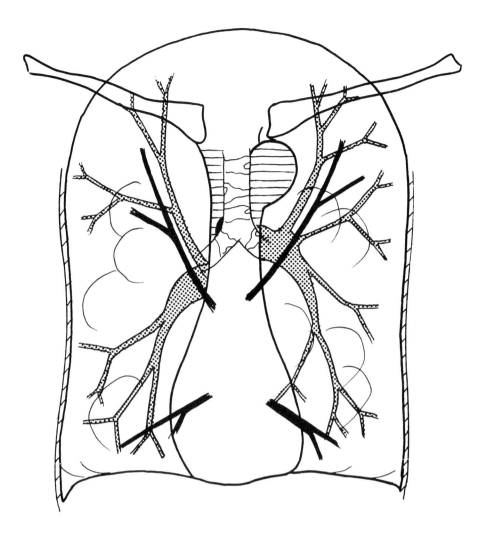

Observations. The lungs are oligemic, but the character of the pulmonary vessels has changed; they have lost their sinuosity, and their branching angles have increased. Many small vessels have disappeared. The VPW and azygos vein are very small, but the aorta is very large. The A/V ratio is 1:1, and the soft tissues are very thin. The vessels have very sharp margins, and no bronchial cuffing is seen. The heart is small and vertical, and no edema is present.

Discussion. Virtually the only pathology that can cause this straightening of pulmonary vessels is emphysema. Status asthmaticus or a Valsalva maneuver results in large, oligemic black lungs, but the vessels never lose all their sinuosity and do not increase their branching angles. The lack of any vascular tortuosity and the 1:1 A/V ratio indicate that no pulmonary arterial hypertension exists.

Diagnosis. Classic picture of *generalized emphysema* ("pink puffer").

Fig. 11-7

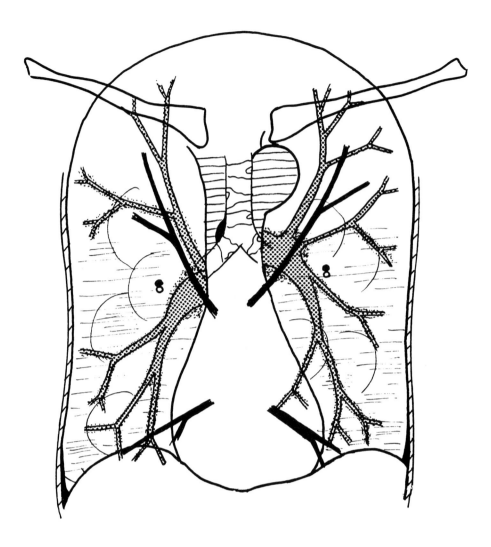

Observations. The picture is almost the same as Fig. 11-6, but the VPW and azygos vein have increased somewhat (although still within normal limits), the heart has increased to normal size, peribronchial cuffs have developed, the vessel margins are faintly blurred, and lamellar effusions are present. Note also that the previously hyperinflated lungs have reduced in volume toward normal.

Discussion. The diagram retains all the features necessary to diagnose emphysema. However, the vessel margins are now blurred and peribronchial cuffing has developed, indicating that hydrostatic edema is superimposed.

Diagnosis. *Left-sided heart failure (LHF) superimposed on emphysema.* This can be a very difficult diagnosis to make unless a film of the patient *without* edema is available for comparison or a film is taken after diuresis. Emphysema vessels should be *unusually* sharply defined, and no suggestion of bronchial wall thickening should exist, unless bronchitis is also present. The presence of such changes should cause a high suspicion of LHF.

Fig. 11-8

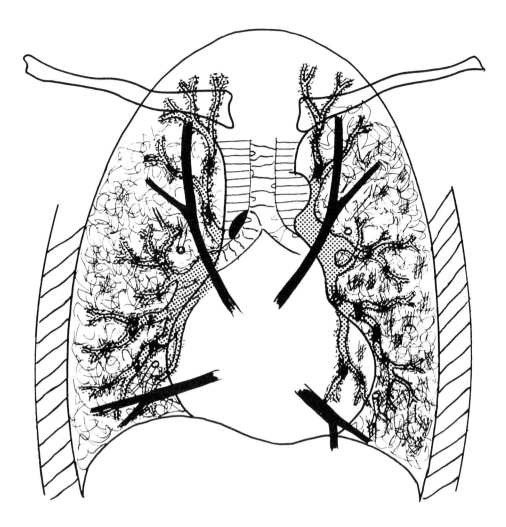

Observations. There is a wide VPW, a large azygos vein, enlarged MPA, and right ventricular enlargement, manifested by outward and *upward* displacement of the cardiac apex. Tortuous pulmonary arteries with apparent "segmentation," marked blurring of vessel margins, thick bronchial walls, and small patches of lobular atelectasis are present. Note slight reduction in venous size relative to arterial size (A/V size greater than 1:1) and the 1:1 flow distribution. The soft tissues are thick.

Discussion. These appearances of apparent "segmentation" of the vessels, with increased tortuosity, and bronchial wall thickening strongly suggest chronic bronchitis. The diagnosis is reinforced by the presence of right ventricular hypertrophy, which frequently occurs in patients with chronic bronchitis secondary to ventilation/perfusion mismatch, leading to hypoxemic arteriolar constriction.

Diagnosis. *Chronic bronchitis with pulmonary arterial hypertension.* Reduced pulmonary vascular bed capacity caused by recurrent infective damage to the lung parenchyma results in a 1:1 flow distribution. The appearances are classic for a "blue bloater" (see Fig. 11-9).

Fig. 11-9

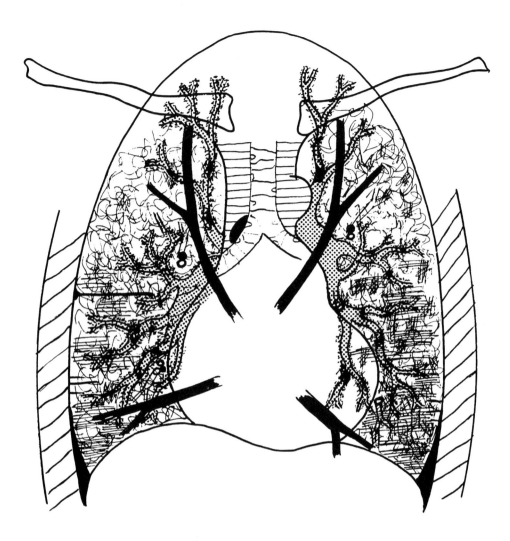

Observations. Subpleural edema abutting the horizontal fissure, peribronchial cuffing, septal lines, small effusions, and increased "veiling" of the lungs with a patchy distribution are superimposed on all the changes illustrated in Fig. 11-8.

Discussion. All the features necessary to make the diagnosis of chronic bronchitis and pulmonary arterial hypertension are present, but now there is additional evidence of superimposed hydrostatic edema. Although this edema may be caused by overhydration or renal failure, one should recognize that LHF occurs very often in patients with chronic obstructive pulmonary disease (COPD).

Diagnosis. *Chronic bronchitis with LHF.* As with emphysema or mixed bronchitis and emphysema, this is a very difficult diagnosis to make, particularly if effusions are absent, as they often are. The patchiness of the edema relates to underlying random damage to the capillary bed, making it even more difficult to differentiate edema from pneumonia. The diagnosis is much easier if previous films are available for comparison, or a test of diuresis may be made, followed by another film. If the diagnosis of LHF superimposed on chronic bronchitis was correct, the improvement will be evident on the postdiuresis film.

Fig. 11-10

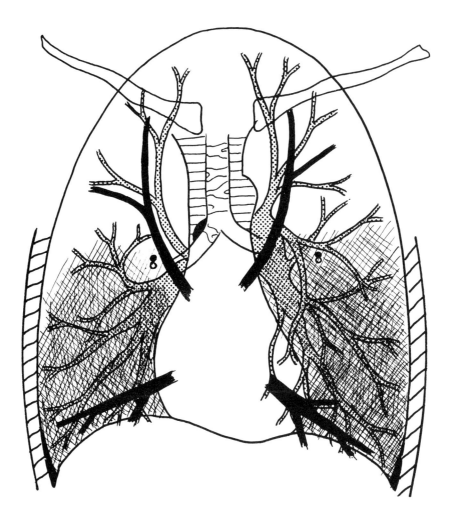

Observations. Normal PBV and flow distribution. The VPW and azygos vein are normal, but peribronchial cuffing is present, with lamellar effusions and gravitationally distributed edema. No soft tissue enlargement is seen.

Discussion. The gravitational distribution of edema, cuffing, and effusions indicate hydrostatic edema (no differential diagnosis). Besides rare conditions such as postglottic obstruction and high-altitude edema, this edema can be caused only by renal failure/overhydration, low oncotic pressure, or cardiac failure. Renal failure/overhydration would usually cause an increase in VPW and PBV and a 1:1 flow distribution, none of which is present. Oncotic edema would apply here but would usually cause soft tissue edema, which is not present. The only remaining diagnosis therefore is cardiac failure. The presence of pulmonary edema indicates that this is *left-sided* heart failure. The absence of soft tissue edema and the normal VPW and azygos vein rule out RHF. We have already deduced that no renal involvement is present (i.e., no evidence of increased TBV). This suggests that the LHF is not chronic. This is supported by the absence of flow inversion.

Diagnosis. *Acute LHF.*

Fig. 11-11

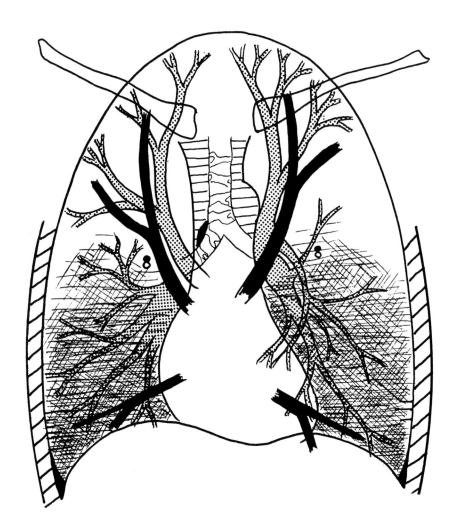

Observations. The appearances are exactly the same as in Fig. 11-10, with the addition of flow inversion.

Discussion. Flow inversion would normally suggest chronic elevation of left atrial pressure, but we have already deduced from the normal VPW and normal soft tissues that this is *not* chronic LHF.

Diagnosis. One of the small percentage of patients with *acute LHF* who do have flow inversion.

Fig. 11-12

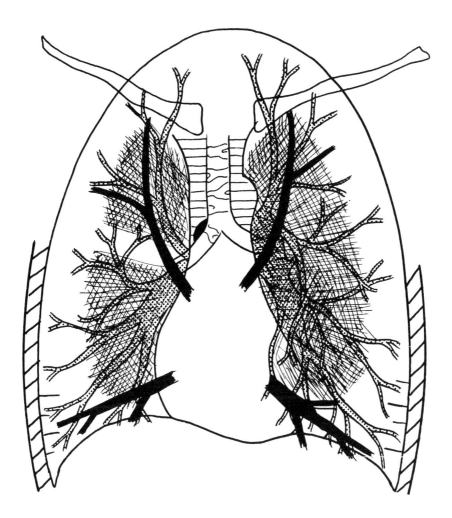

Observations. All the radiologic features are identical with Fig. 11-10, except that effusions and cuffing are not seen, and the edema has a "bat's wing" configuration.

Discussion. Bat's wing edema indicates either acute cardiac decompensation or renal decompensation. The small VPW, azygos vein, PBV, and normal soft tissues all indicate this is not renal failure. Pleural effusions are absent because no edema is contiguous with the visceral pleura and therefore no fluid is present to pass through the pleura into the pleural space. Cuffing can be absent in rapidly developing edema. This edema tends to bypass the interstitial stage and become instantly alveolar.

Diagnosis. *Acute LHF* (severe, abrupt decompensation).

Fig. 11-13

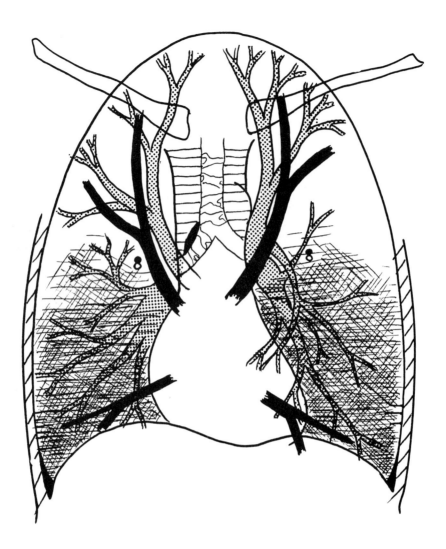

Observations. The VPW and azygos vein are large. Flow inversion is present, with gravitational distribution of edema, bronchial cuffing, septal lines, and lamellar effusions. The A/V ratio remains 1:1 in both upper and lower regions. Soft tissues are normal.

Discussion. Gravitational distribution, cuffing, septal lines, and effusions all indicate hydrostatic edema. The possible causes are renal failure overhydration, oncotic edema, or cardiac failure. If this were only renal failure, there would be a 1:1 flow distribution (not inversion), and in 80% to 90% of patients the edema would be central. If the edema were oncotic, the VPW would not be wide, the soft tissues would not be normal, and no flow inversion would occur. The only remaining diagnosis is cardiac failure. The flow inversion suggests that the failure is *chronic*, which is supported by the wide VPW, indicating renal hypoperfusion. The absence of soft tissue edema militates against any RHF.

Diagnosis. *Chronic LHF.*

Fig. 11-14

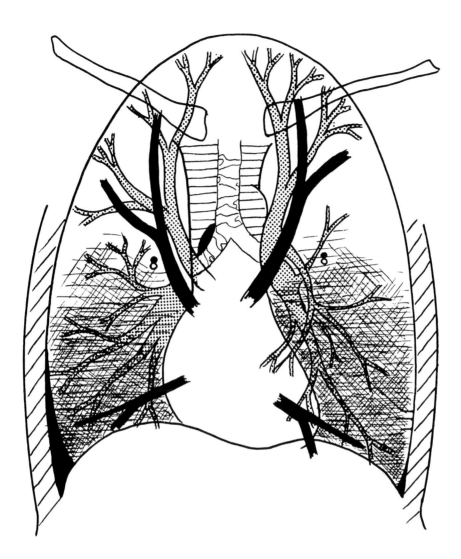

Observations. The appearances are identical to Fig. 11-13 with two additions: (1) the soft tissues have widened and (2) the right pleural effusion has become larger.

Discussion. As discussed for Fig. 11-13, the diagnosis would be chronic LHF, but the added soft tissue thickness strongly suggests that RHF now is also present. This is supported by the larger right pleural effusion, suggesting hepatic engorgement, ascites, and transfer of fluid through the right hemidiaphragm into the right pleural space.

Diagnosis. *Biventricular cardiac failure.* (Note: although biventricular failure occurs often clinically, a clear-cut progression of *radiologic* change from LHF to biventricular failure unfortunately occurs infrequently, and the diagnosis of RHF radiologically remains poor.)

Fig. 11-15

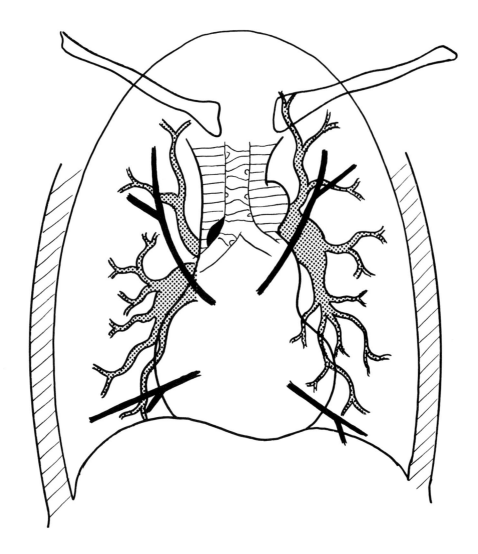

Observations. The VPW and azygos vein are normal, but the MPA is massive; very large central pulmonary arteries are present, and the peripheral divisions are tortuous and "pruned." The A/V ratio is much greater than 1:1, and the upper lobe/lower lobe (UL/LL) flow ratio is 1:1. No edema is present.

Discussion. The large MPA and central divisions, with the addition of the peripheral tortuosity, increase the pulmonary artery pressure to greater than 60 mm Hg (systolic). The presence of precapillary arterial narrowing is confirmed by the small size of the pulmonary veins. The 1:1 flow ratio is caused by loss of pulmonary vascular bed capacity, resulting in complete filling of all the pulmonary vascular bed. Note that a 1:1 flow ratio is *usual* in patients with pulmonary arterial hypertension and can be easily distinguished from the 1:1 distribution of a high-flow state by the small size of the pulmonary veins (i.e., by the large A/V ratio).

Diagnosis. *Pulmonary arterial hypertension.* The *severity* of the hypertension can be judged by the relative sizes of the MPA and the central divisions, the size discrepancy between the central and peripheral divisions, the degree of tortuosity and pruning, and the A/V ratio. The degree of the changes shown indicates that the pulmonary arterial hypertension is severe.

Fig. 11-16

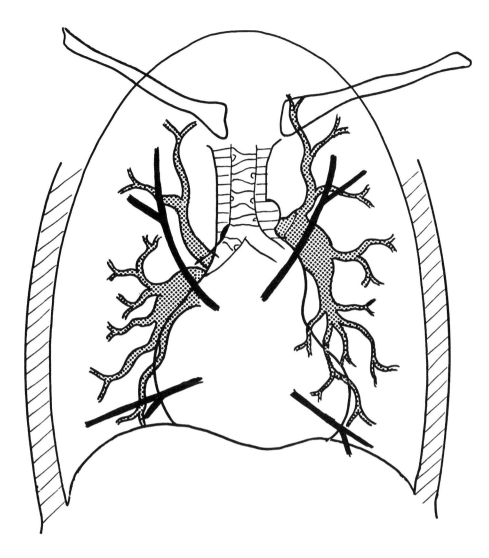

Observations. All the radiologic features are identical to Fig. 11-15, except that the VPW, azygos vein, and aorta are now very small.

Discussion. The small VPW and aorta indicate that systemic blood volume is greatly reduced. This, in conjunction with the large pulmonary arteries and small veins, indicates pulmonary arterial hypertension superimposed on a prior left-to-right shunt.

Diagnosis. *Left-to-right shunt with pulmonary arterial hypertension.* The degree of narrowing of the pulmonary veins would indicate that the shunt is reversing (Eisenmenger syndrome). Occasionally a mixture of chronic bronchitis, emphysema, and cardiac failure (often called "increased markings" emphysema) will mimic these appearances.

Fig. 11-17

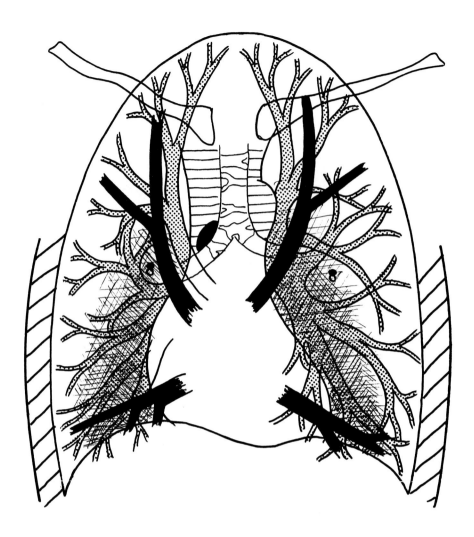

Observations. Very large VPW, azygos vein, and PBV are present. The flow distribution is 1:1 ("balanced") and the A/V ratio 1:1. Cuffing is present, and pulmonary edema has a central distribution. Soft tissues are increased.

Discussion. The cuffing indicates that the edema is hydrostatic. Again, the differential diagnosis is renal failure/overhydration, oncotic edema, or cardiac failure. The very large VPW, azygos vein, and PBV indicate a greatly increased TBV, which would not agree with oncotic edema (the absence of effusions also would not). The appearances would fit biventricular cardiac failure, except for the 1:1 flow distribution and central edema, changes that are much more characteristic of renal failure/overhydration.

Diagnosis. *Renal failure/overhydration.* (Note the similarity of this diagram to Fig. 11-14, biventricular failure.) If the lower vessels are concealed by edema and a clear *central* edema pattern is not present, it is very difficult to differentiate renal failure from cardiac failure. Note, however, that this much edema in a patient with *cardiac* failure implies serious decompensation. The patient is usually in a cardiac care unit, whereas the patient with renal failure has minimal physiologic abnormalities and can easily walk to the radiology department to have erect posteroanterior (PA) films taken. A further distinguishing feature of renal edema occasionally seen is "nodularity" (see Fig. 11-19). Note also that pleural effusions *are* often seen in patients with renal edema despite the predominant central location of edema. Central edema in patients with cardiac failure is more frequently caused by *acute* decompensation, in which case the VPW is usually normal and effusions absent.

Fig. 11-18

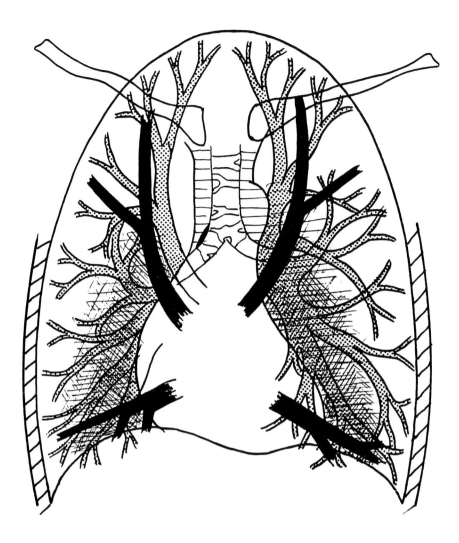

Observations. The appearances are very similar to Fig. 11-17, but the VPW is now slightly narrower than normal and the azygos vein is small. The soft tissues are no longer edematous.

Discussion. Evidence of a large PBV still exists, but the VPW is now small, suggesting a small systemic blood volume. If the systemic blood volume is truly small, a left-to-right shunt would have to be considered. However, edema is present, so this would have to be a left-to-right shunt in a patient with heart failure, which does not usually occur until structural vascular changes have developed. However, this patient shows no evidence of pulmonary arterial hypertension. Also, the edema is central, which would be *very* unusual for a left-to-right shunt with renal failure.

Diagnosis. The appearances agree best with *late-stage renal failure*, in which systemic vasospasm causes the VPW to become smaller while the PBV remains large. Note: this is one of the few instances in which renal failure can be differentiated radiologically from iatrogenic overhydration.

Fig. 11-19

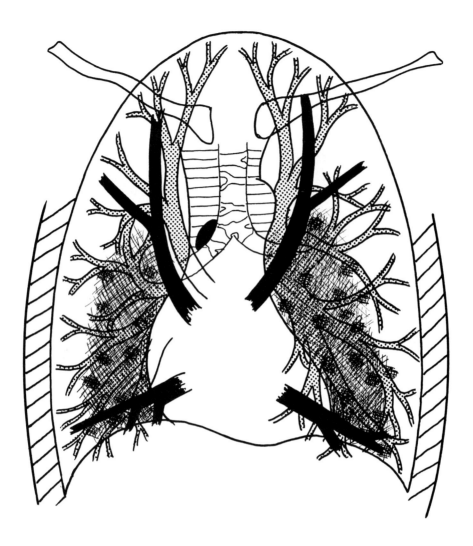

Observations. All features are identical to Fig. 11-17, except the central edema has a "nodular" appearance.

Discussion. The cause for the nodularity, which may be seen in patients with renal edema, is unknown, but it can be so dramatic that it can be readily mistaken for metastases.

Diagnosis. *Renal edema.* Note that nodularity is the second way in which renal edema can sometimes be differentiated from iatrogenic overhydration (see Fig. 11-18). However, if a patient has underlying emphysema or chronic bronchitis, superimposed iatrogenic overhydration can also have a bizarre patchy or nodular appearance.

Fig. 11-20

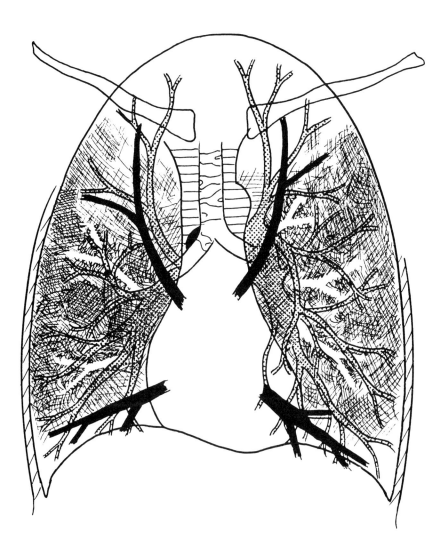

Observations. VPW is normal, as are the azygos vein and aorta. PBV and flow distribution are normal. No cuffing, septal lines, or effusions are present. Edema is present, but with no evidence of a gravitational distribution. Air bronchograms are very evident. The A/V ratio is 1:1, and soft tissues are normal.

Discussion. The absence of gravitational effect on the edema distribution is good evidence that this is not hydrostatic edema. The suspicion that this may therefore be edema caused by lung injury is greatly strengthened by the absence of cuffing, septal lines, and effusions and by the presence of air bronchograms. Hydrostatic edema cannot cause this constellation of findings, and the differential diagnosis therefore does not include renal failure/overhydration, oncotic edema, or cardiac failure. However, several alternative diagnoses could fit this picture, including diffuse severe interstitial symmetric bilateral pneumonia (a form of permeability edema), hypersensitivity pneumonias (sometimes accompanied by septal lines), and diffuse bilateral interstitial hemorrhage.

Diagnosis. *Nonhydrostatic, "injury" lung edema.* Etiology must be determined.

Fig. 11-21

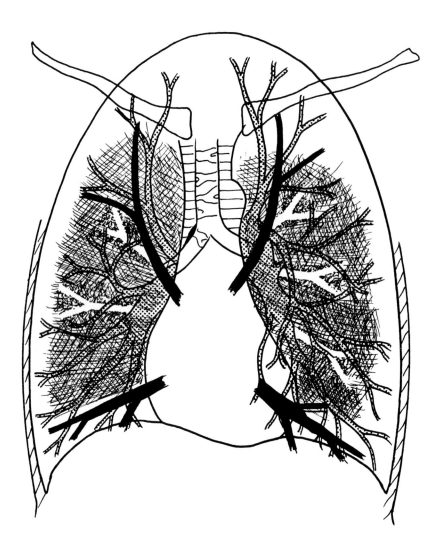

Observations. All features are identical to Fig. 11-20, except the intensity of edema in the peripheral portion of the lung edema appears to have lessened dramatically.

Discussion. This would be an unusual presentation of injury edema *except* when positive-pressure ventilation is applied, which frequently results in increased air content in the periphery of the lungs. The amount of edema is not actually decreased, but the amount of air is increased, giving a spurious visual appearance and suggesting central edema.

Diagnosis. *Injury lung edema subjected to high positive-pressure ventilation.*

Fig. 11-22

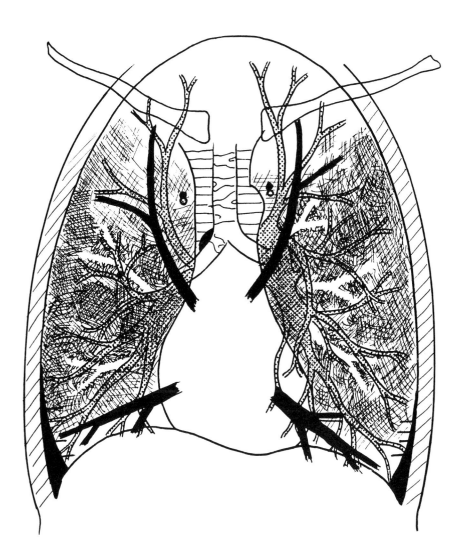

Observations. Most of the features seen in Fig. 11-20 are still present. In addition, cuffs and lamellar effusions are present, and the VPW and azygos vein have increased slightly in size. Soft tissue thickness has also increased.

Discussion. The cuffs, effusions, and occasionally the septal lines indicate that hydrostatic edema *is* present. The normal PBV and VPW indicate that this hydrostatic edema is not caused by simple renal failure/overhydration or chronic LHF. Acute LHF could cause some of these appearances but would rarely show air bronchograms and would not increase soft tissue thickness. Also, the edema distribution would not be so patchy. Oncotic edema would fit many of the appearances but would not be patchy and would not result in air bronchograms.

Diagnosis. *Injury edema with superimposed hydrostatic edema, probably overhydration.* The VPW and PBV remain normal or smaller than normal because of the positive-pressure ventilation. This combination of edemas is the rule rather than the exception in the earlier stages of treatment of patients with ARDS in the intensive care unit (ICU). This would be a difficult diagnosis to make if one had only this single film to read, but it becomes much easier if a previous film is available (see Fig. 11-20). The original radiograph of pure injury edema has clearly become overlaid by some of the features of hydrostatic edema.

Fig. 11-23

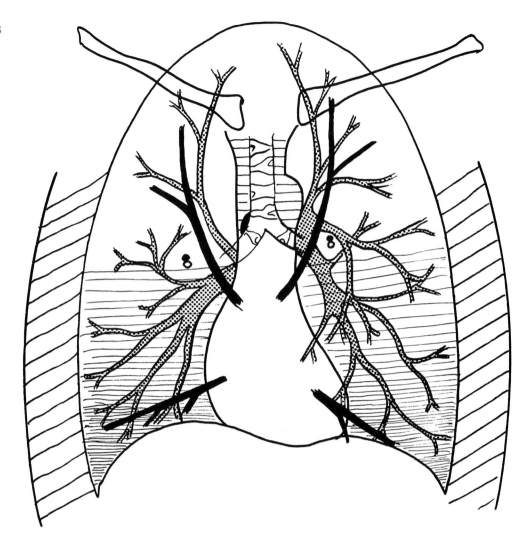

Observations. A slightly narrowed VPW and azygos vein, reduced PBV, normal flow distribution, and normal A/V ratio are present. Cuffing is accompanied by faint gravitational edema, and the soft tissues are *greatly* thickened.

Discussion. The lung changes, if one disregards the thickened soft tissues, are those of very mild hydrostatic edema. Because of the narrow VPW and small PBV, this is not renal failure or overhydration. It could be mild first-episode LHF or mild oncotic edema. However, neither of these could explain the extreme soft tissue edema, which indicates that the patient *is* overhydrated but must be third-spacing all the extra fluid, causing a reduction in the TBV. This explains the narrowed VPW, reduced PBV, and normal pulmonary blood flow distribution. The soft tissue edema is clearly *not* caused by increased generalized capillary permeability because the lungs show only *hydrostatic* edema.

Diagnosis. *Overhydration with soft tissue third-spacing* (e.g., into burned chest wall).

Fig. 11-24

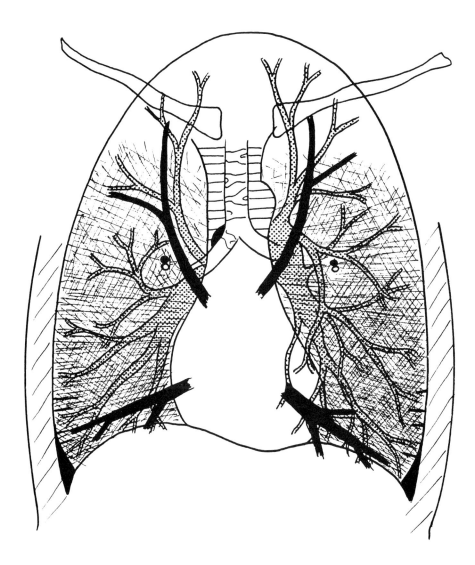

Observations. The appearances are superficially similar to Fig. 11-23 (third-spacing), but the VPW and azygos vein are normal (not reduced), the PBV is normal, effusions are present with cuffing and gravitational distribution of edema, and the soft tissues are thickened but not grossly.

Discussion. The gravitational distribution, cuffing, septal lines, and effusions all confirm that this is *hydrostatic* edema. Renal failure/overhydration are unlikely in this patient because the systemic and pulmonary blood volumes are normal. There is not sufficient soft tissue thickening, to be concerned about third-spacing. First-episode acute LHF would fit most of the appearances but not the soft tissue edema, which is discrepant with the normal VPW and azygos vein. This leaves oncotic edema, which fits all of the observations.

Diagnosis. *Oncotic edema.* Note: a common cause of oncotic edema is hepatic disease, but the normal heart size, lung volumes, thoracic configuration, and diaphragmatic level do not agree with a history of alcoholism or hepatic disease (see Fig. 11-26). The most frequent cause of low oncotic pressure in the ICU is rapid replacement of blood loss with low-molecular-weight fluid while the patient continues to lose blood. The TBV therefore does not increase, but oncotic edema develops.

Fig. 11-25

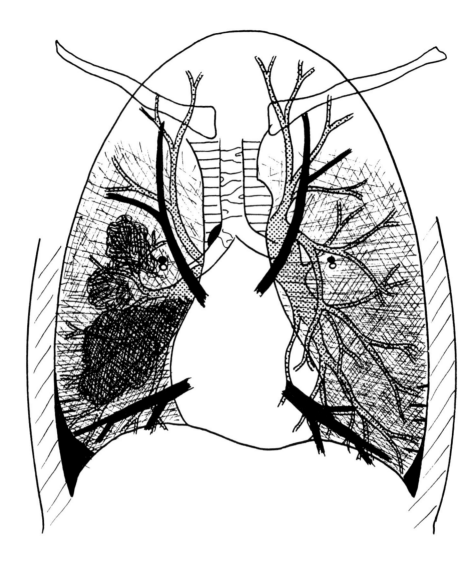

Observations. Every feature is the same as Fig. 11-24, with an added nongravitational density in the right lung.

Discussion. The logic of analysis remains the same as in Fig. 11-24, culminating in a diagnosis of oncotic edema but with some local superimposed pathology. The differential diagnosis of the added pathology includes primarily aspiration, pneumonia, intrapulmonary hemorrhage, and infarction, usually in that order.

Diagnosis. *Oncotic edema with superimposed consolidation.* The differential diagnosis of what type of consolidation is present depends on comparison with previous films and correlation with patient history. (Note: if the patient is endotracheally intubated and has a nasogastric tube in situ, the potential for aspiration is extremely high.) If no consolidation was present the day before, bacterial pneumonia is a much less likely diagnosis, but infarction or hemorrhage remain possibilities. Note that the right pleural effusion has increased in size; this should not occur with intrapulmonary hemorrhage or *benign* aspiration and indicates an irritative process, such as pneumonia or an irritant (because of pH or septic content) aspirate, or an infarct. The speed with which the process has developed helps to separate these possibilities.

Fig. 11-26

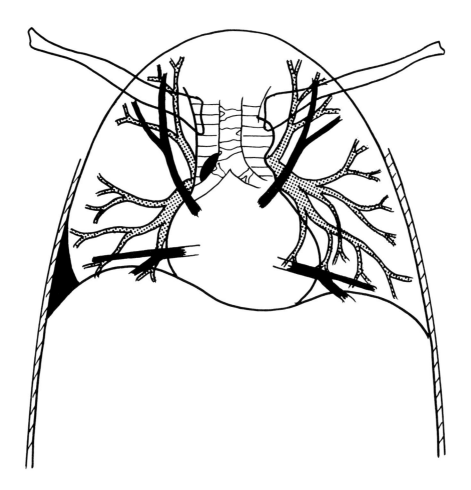

Observations. The normal thoracic "waist" has disappeared, and the chest walls continue to slope outward below the high diaphragm, resulting in a shape resembling the nose cone of a rocket. Despite the very wide thorax, the diaphragm is high. The VPW is normal, but the azygos vein is somewhat large. The PBV and flow distribution are normal, and the A/V ratio is 1:1. There is *no* edema, but a right pleural effusion is present. The soft tissues are very thin (cachectic).

Discussion. The enlarged azygos vein in the face of normal VPW and PBV is discrepant and suggests *intraabdominal* pathology involving the inferior vena cava (IVC) extrinsically or intrinsically and causing increased azygos flow. The presence of a right pleural effusion in the *absence* of edema indicates that the effusion does not have a cardiac, renal, or oncotic etiology and is probably coming through the diaphragm from an ascitic collection. The flaring "nose cone" chest configuration and high diaphragms suggest that abdominal contents are increased, pushing the ribs out. This supports the diagnosis of ascites, and the very thin soft tissues, very discrepant with the large abdomen, suggest the cachexia of liver disease, probably alcoholic.

Diagnosis. *Ascites with possible IVC compression.*

Index